Reducing Dietary Sodium and Improving Human Health

Special Issue Editor
Jacqui Webster

MDPI • Basel • Beijing • Wuhan • Barcelona • Belgrade

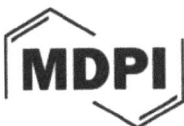

MDPI

Special Issue Editor
Jacqui Webster
The George Institute for Global Health
Australia

Editorial Office
MDPI
St. Alban-Anlage 66
Basel, Switzerland

This edition is a reprint of the Special Issue published online in the open access journal *Nutrients* (ISSN 2072-6643) in 2017–2018 (available at: http://www.mdpi.com/journal/nutrients/special_issues/ nutrients_sodium).

For citation purposes, cite each article independently as indicated on the article page online and as indicated below:

Lastname, F.M.; Lastname, F.M. Article title. *Journal Name* **Year**, *Article number*, page range.

First Editon 2018

ISBN 978-3-03842-925-8 (Pbk)
ISBN 978-3-03842-926-5 (PDF)

Table of Contents

About the Special Issue Editor

Jacqui Webster, Head of Advocacy and Policy Impact, The George Institute for Global Health A/Prof Jacqui Webster (BA Sociology, MA Development, PhD Public Health, RPHNut) is Head of Advocacy and Policy Impact and Director of the World Health Organization Collaborating Centre on Population Salt Reduction at the George Institute for Global Health. She is Associate Professor at the University of New South Wales with an honorary conjoint position at the University of Sydney. Her primary research interests are advocacy, food policy and implementation science and for the last 13 years her main focus has been on increasing the evidence relating to successful implementation of salt reduction interventions. Since 2017, Jacqui has chaired the World Hypertension League's Science of Salt Advisory Group and contributed to regular systematic reviews to update the evidence to support salt reduction interventions. She is currently supported by a four year co-funded Australian National Health and Medical Research Council/National Heart Foundation Career Development Fellowship and receives additional funding from the World Health Organization and the Victorian Health Promotion Foundation. Jacqui has previously worked for a range of NGO, government and international organisations on food policy, including implementing the UK government's salt reduction strategy from 2003–2006. She grew up on a farm in Yorkshire, England and moved to Australia in 2007.

Preface to "Reducing Dietary Sodium and Improving Human Health"

When we launched the special edition on reducing dietary sodium and improving health in January 2017, it was with a view to increasing the knowledge base about how to effectively implement salt reduction interventions. In 2013 The World Health Organization established a global target for all countries to reduce salt by 30% by 2025. The following year, our comprehensive review showed that 75 countries already had a strategy and were implementing one or more interventions to try and reduce population salt intake. However, most of these strategies were in their infancy and only a handful had been underway for long enough to demonstrate a reduction in population salt intake.

The UK government salt reduction strategy is often cited as one of the most successful strategies to date, having reduced population salt intake by 15% between 2003 and 2011, with parallel reductions in blood pressure during the same period. Most salt reduction strategies to date build on the UK model, combining policy programs to engage the food industry to reduce salt in foods and meals, behaviour change programs, labelling and settings based interventions. As these programs mature and additional countries embark upon efforts to reduce salt, it is important that we understand what interventions are likely to be most effective for different groups of the population in different countries and settings including low and middle income countries.

The 29 papers published in the Special Edition provide a wealth of new insights on implementation of salt reduction strategies from all regions of the globe. From the sodium content of street foods in Tajikistan and Kyrgyzstan, to evaluation of mass media campaigns in South Africa, to understanding whether salt reduction was a priority for manufacturers in Australia, the papers covered the broad spectrum of salt reduction interventions, highlighting the many implementation challenges, at the same time as a wealth of lessons on how these might be overcome.

This highly successful special edition of Nutrients has attracted papers on a range of issues relating to effective interventions. One major focus is on establishing salt intake and sources of salt in the diet (7 papers), and related to that establishing or monitoring changes in salt levels in foods (9 papers). 5 studies focus on understanding patterns of knowledge and behaviour. 9 studies evaluate changes over time based on either salt levels in foods or consumer knowledge attitudes and behaviour. Somewhat surprisingly only one study, from our own research project in Fiji, evaluated changes in salt intake over time based on 24 hour urine samples. The lessons from this project will be useful in informing future projects. However, the challenge of accurately measuring salt intake in order to monitor the impact of national strategies and programs and assess progress towards the WHO targets, is one of the areas in urgent need of further research and would be worthy of a future special edition of Nutrients.

This book showcases work from experts and opinion leaders as well as policy makers and program managers from more than 20 countries. I want to take this opportunity to thank all of the contributors and reviewers for the high quality contributions. Finally, this initiative would not have been possible without the dedication, expertise professionalism and technical support of the Nutrients editorial team. It has been an interesting and rewarding learning experience acting as Guest Editor for this Nutrients special edition on salt and health which has made an important contribution to the knowledge on salt reduction.

Jacqui Webster
Special Issue Editor

nutrients

MDPI

Article

The Association of Knowledge and Behaviours Related to Salt with 24-h Urinary Salt Excretion in a Population from North and South India

Claire Johnson [1,2,*], Sailesh Mohan [3], Kris Rogers [1], Roopa Shivashankar [3,4], Sudhir Raj Thout [5], Priti Gupta [3], Feng J. He [6], Graham A. MacGregor [6], Jacqui Webster [1,2], Anand Krishnan [7], Pallab K. Maulik [5,8], K. Srinath Reddy [3], Dorairaj Prabhakaran [3,4] and Bruce Neal [1,2,9,10,11]

[1] The George Institute for Global Health, Box M201 Missenden Rd, Sydney 2006, Australia; krogers@georgeinstitute.org (K.R.); jwebster@georgeinstitute.org.au (J.W.); bneal@georgeinstitute.org.au (B.N.)
[2] School of Public Health, Department of Medicine, The University of Sydney, Sydney 2006, Australia
[3] Public Health Foundation of India, New Delhi 110070, India; smohan@phfi.org (S.M.); roopa@ccdcindia.org (R.S.); priti@ccdcindia.org (P.G.); ksrinath.reddy@phfi.org (K.S.R.); dprabhakaran@ccdcindia.org (D.P.)
[4] Centre for Chronic Disease Control, New Delhi 122002, India
[5] George Institute for Global Health, Hyderabad 500034, India; traj@georgeinstitute.org.in (S.R.T.); pmaulik@georgeinstitute.org.in (P.K.M.)
[6] Wolfson Institute of Preventive Medicine, Barts and The London School of Medicine & Dentistry, Queen Mary University of London, London EC1M 6BQ, UK; f.he@qmul.ac.uk (F.J.H.); g.macgregor@qmul.ac.uk (G.A.M.)
[7] All India Institute of Medical Sciences, New Delhi 110029, India; kanandiyer@yahoo.com
[8] George Institute for Global Health, University of Oxford, Oxford OX1 3PA, UK
[9] Charles Perkins Centre, University of Sydney, Sydney 2050, Australia
[10] School of Public Health, Imperial College, London SW7 2AZ, UK
[11] Royal Prince Alfred Hospital, Sydney 2050, Australia
* Correspondence: cjohnson@georgeinstitute.org.au; Tel.: +61-435131858; Fax: +61-299934502

Received: 19 December 2016; Accepted: 3 February 2017; Published: 15 February 2017

Abstract: Consumer knowledge is understood to play a role in managing risk factors associated with cardiovascular disease and may be influenced by level of education. The association between population knowledge, behaviours and actual salt consumption was explored overall, and for more-educated compared to less-educated individuals. A cross-sectional survey was done in an age-and sex-stratified random sample of 1395 participants from urban and rural areas of North and South India. A single 24-h urine sample, participants' physical measurements and questionnaire data were collected. The mean age of participants was 40 years, 47% were women and mean 24-h urinary salt excretion was 9.27 (8.87–9.69) g/day. Many participants reported favourable knowledge and behaviours to minimise risks related to salt. Several of these behaviours were associated with reduced salt intake—less use of salt while cooking, avoidance of snacks, namkeens, and avoidance of pickles (all $p < 0.003$). Mean salt intake was comparable in more-educated (9.21, 8.55–9.87 g/day) versus less-educated (9.34, 8.57–10.12 g/day) individuals ($p = 0.82$). There was no substantively different pattern of knowledge and behaviours between more-versus less-educated groups and no clear evidence that level of education influenced salt intake. Several consumer behaviours related to use of salt during food preparation and consumption of salty products were related to actual salt consumption and therefore appear to offer an opportunity for intervention. These would be a reasonable focus for a government-led education campaign targeting salt.

Keywords: India; salt; urinary sodium excretion; knowledge; attitude; behaviour

1. Background

Knowledge, attitudes, and behaviours can play an important role in preventing and managing risk factors associated with cardiovascular disease [1]—the leading cause of mortality globally [2,3]. In India, ischaemic heart disease and stroke are leading causes of death and hypertension is a key risk factor [4]. The prevalence of hypertension in India has increased over the past 30 years from less than 5% of adults overall to 34% of urban and 28% of rural adults today. The total numbers with hypertension are expected to almost double from 118 million in 2000 to 214 million by 2025 [5].

Eating too much salt has a clear adverse effect on blood pressure and is likely a leading cause of cardiovascular disease and stroke [6–8]. In 2010, 1.65 million deaths from cardiovascular causes worldwide were attributed to salt consumption of more than 5 g/day [3]. There is strong scientific evidence to show that reducing salt in the diet reduces blood pressure [9–12] and the anticipated magnitude of the vascular risk reduction that could be achieved has been defined previously: a reduction of 3 g/day over 30 years is anticipated to avert nearly 400,000 cases and about 81,000 deaths from myocardial infarction and stroke in India [13]. Additionally, the likely cost-effectiveness of national salt reduction strategies is well documented with data for India suggesting a cost of less than Rs.4400 (US$ 65) per disability-adjusted life year (DALY) averted, and great potential to prevent very large numbers of premature cardiovascular deaths [14]. All Member States of the World Health Organization (WHO), including India, have adopted a 30% reduction in mean population salt consumption by 2025 as part of the "25 by 25" initiative for the control of non-communicable diseases. This is towards the recommendation for a maximum dietary salt intake of 5 g/day for adults [15].

Over the past 20 years, National Nutrition Surveys (NNS) have shown a shift in food consumption patterns in urban and rural areas in India, largely driven by increased per capita income and changes in the food environment, making accessible a wider range of food products including highly processed products, and restaurant and fast foods [16]. Traditionally characterised by high intake of fruit, vegetables and unprocessed coarse cereals and pulses [17], the Indian diet now shows increases in average intake levels of adverse nutrients such as saturated fats, sugars and salt, now above recommended levels [8]. Concurrently, half of the population surveyed in a recent National Family Health Survey (NFHS-3) consumed less than one serving of fruit per week with individuals in the lowest socioeconomic strata consuming very low quantities, in part due to the high cost of fresh fruit and vegetables [18]. In addition, the vegetables that are consumed are often overcooked in Indian meals, leading to vital loss of micronutrients [19].

Observed differences in dietary behaviours are often attributed to socio-demographic factors such as age, sex, education and income [20–23]. Similarly, use of "discretionary" salt at the table or during food preparation is also associated with socio-economic factors, whereby individuals with lower levels of education have higher levels of discretionary salt use [24–26]. Knowledge, self-efficacy, attitudes and beliefs are identified reasons for diet quality variation among the different socio-economic groups [27–29]. Specifically, knowledge about salt has been found to be higher among older people and those with higher levels of education [30].

Health-related behavioural risk factors are widely prevalent in India but there are no related population-wide efforts for prevention targeting salt [31]. Several population surveys assessing dietary salt consumption in India estimate mean intake as >5 g/day [32,33] with results from our cross-sectional study reporting mean 24-h urinary salt excretion as 9.27 (8.87–9.69) g/day [34]. These data make a strong case for the development and implementation of a national salt reduction program; however, the identification of modifiable, mediating factors for salt intake based upon population knowledge, attitudes and behaviours would provide further insight for the development of a salt reduction strategy specific to the Indian context [1,35]. This study aimed to determine the association of knowledge, attitudes and behaviours towards salt with actual salt intake as measured by 24-h urinary sodium excretion, and to assess whether associations differed between more-educated versus less-educated individuals drawn from populations in urban and rural areas in Delhi and Haryana and Andhra Pradesh, India.

2. Methods

Data were collected through a cross-sectional survey in an age-stratified and sex-stratified random sample drawn from urban (slum and non-slum) and rural areas of North and South India. Ethics approval was obtained by the Human Research Ethics Committees of the Centre for Chronic Disease Control in New Delhi (approval number CCDC_IEC_10_2012) and the University of Sydney in Australia (approval number 2012/887), as well as by the Indian Health Ministry's Screening Committee. Written informed consent was obtained from all participants. The survey was conducted between February and June 2014. The methods for participant selection and study conduct have been published elsewhere [34,36].

2.1. Participant Selection and Recruitment

Recruitment of participants was stratified by gender and age as well as area (urban, urban slum and rural). In North India, census enumeration blocks (CEBs) and villages were sampled at random from within the study area. Households were then selected at random and an individual from within each household was selected at random until recruitment numbers in each stratum were fulfilled. In the South, the CEBs and villages were selected to be broadly representative of those in the State using a purposive process. A census list including information about the age and sex of all inhabitants was compiled for each CEB and village and a random sample of the population was invited to participate until recruitment numbers in each stratum were filled.

2.2. Data Collection

Before data collection began, the local administrative body was engaged and permission to conduct the study in each area was obtained. Trained field researchers conducted interviewer-administered questionnaires over two visits within one week. Initially, consenting participants were asked questions relating to demographics, lifestyle behaviours, disease history, medication use, and knowledge, attitudes and behaviours related to salt, followed by a physical examination. Instructions to undertake a single 24-h urine collection were given. Questions about knowledge, attitudes and behaviours were adapted from the World Health Organisation/Pan American Health Organisation (WHO/PAHO) protocol for population level sodium determination [37]. The questionnaire contained 15 questions; 4 specifically on dietary habits and personal consumption; 2 relating to knowledge; and 9 assessing behaviours relevant to lowering salt intake. The participants answered on a range of different scales such as "rarely, sometimes, often", "yes, no" and "too much, just the right amount or too little" (Table S1).

The physical examination comprised measurement of body weight (using calibrated portable Omron weight scale HN-288), and height (using calibrated Seca Brand-214 Portable Stadiometer) to the nearest 0.1 kg and 0.1 cm respectively. Weight and height were used to calculate body mass index (BMI) as weight in kilograms divided by squared height in meters. Dietary salt intake was estimated by 24-h urine collection. Urinary sodium and creatinine were determined using the ion selective electrode method for sodium analysis and the buffered kinetic Jaffe reaction without de-proteinisation for urine creatinine assay. Suspected inaccurate urine collections (i.e., urinary creatinine <4.0 mmol/day for women, or <6.0 mmol/day for men, or a 24-h urine collection of <500 mL for either sex) were excluded from the analyses. For each individual, the 24-h sodium excretion value (g/day) was calculated as the concentration of sodium in the urine (g/L) multiplied by the urinary volume (L/day).

2.3. Statistical Analysis

The baseline characteristics of the sample were summarised as proportions and means (95% confidence interval (CI)) overall and for subgroups defined by level of education, defined as more or less than 10 years of schooling, which was the median point in this population. The associations of knowledge, attitudes and behaviours with 24-h urinary sodium excretion were investigated by making comparisons using linear regression. Estimates were adjusted for age, sex and body mass index, which were included on the basis of their observed association with salt consumption. Subgroup analyses were done for participants with more or less than 10 years of education, which was approximately the median point among the participants surveyed. The *p* values < 0.05 were deemed significant but all findings were interpreted in light of the number of comparisons made and the broader pattern of findings across the data. Statistical analyses were conducted using SAS for Windows (version SAS 9.4).

3. Results

There were 1041 persons selected for the survey in Delhi and Haryana and 712 agreed to participate (68% overall response rate). The corresponding numbers for Andhra Pradesh were 1,291 and 840 (65% overall response rate). For those who agreed to take part, complete data (Knowledge, Attitudes and Behaviours (KAB) questionnaire, physical examination and a 24-h urine sample) were available for 710/712 (99%), 710/712 (99%) and 637/712 (89%) respectively in Delhi and Haryana, and 758/840 (90%), 758/840 (90%) and 758/840 (90%) respectively in Andhra Pradesh. Across both regions, there were a total of 157/1552 (10%) persons who did not return a 24-h urine sample and 438/1395 (31%) persons who returned a sample suspected to be incomplete. Participants who did not provide a complete 24-h urine collection were more likely to be older, female or from a rural site.

Accordingly, the primary analyses included 1395. Forty-seven per cent were female and 42% had more than 10 years of formal schooling. There were anticipated demographic differences between the more- and less-educated groups (Table 1). Overall salt intake was 9.27 (8.87–9.69) g/day and was not different between those with <10 years of education (9.34, 8.57–10.12 g/day) versus >10 years of education (9.21, 8.55–9.87 g/day) (*p* = 0.82).

Table 1. Characteristics of population overall and by level of education (*N* = 1395).

Socio-Demographic Characteristics	All %	% <10 Years' Education	>10 Years' Education	*p*-Value *
Region				
Slum	6.1	7.3	4.6	0.001
Urban	29.2	19.2	40.9	
Rural	64.6	73.6	54.4	
Gender				
Male	53	46.9	60.1	0.014
Female	47	53.1	39.9	
Age Group				
20–39 years	60.4	49.7	72.9	<0.001
40–59 years	27.7	36.1	22.3	
60+ years	9.9	14.2	4.8	
Employment Status				
Employed/Domestic Duties	64.4	65.3	63.3	0.779
Unemployed/Student	35.6	34.7	36.7	
Body Mass Index (kg/m^2)				
BMI < 25	59.7	60.9	58.3	0.653
BMI 25–30	29	29.1	28.9	
BMI 30+	11.3	10	12.9	
Blood Pressure				
SBP ≥ 140 or DBP ≥ 90	23.4	28.5	17.5	0.007
SBP < 140 and DBP < 90	76.6	71.5	82.5	
Tobacco Use				
Never	73.5	68.6	79.2	0.042
Not daily	9.6	10.2	9.0	
Daily	16.9	21.2	11.8	
Stroke				
Yes	0.4	0.5	0.3	0.435
No	99.6	99.5	99.7	

Table 1. *Cont.*

Socio-Demographic Characteristics	All %	<10 Years' Education	>10 Years' Education	*p*-Value *
		%		
Diabetes				
Yes	6.4	8.2	4.2	0.020
No	93.6	91.8	95.8	
Chronic Kidney Disease				
Yes	2.2	1.1	3.5	0.221
No	97.8	98.9	96.5	

* *p*-value for differences in frequencies between the education groups; SBP = systolic blood pressure; DBP = diastolic blood pressure.

3.1. Knowledge, Attitudes and Behaviours (KAB) towards Salt

The majority of participants identified the maximum salt consumption recommendation as <5 g/day (70%) and 90% identified that a diet high in salt can cause serious health problems (Table 2). About half (52%) of the participants reported that lowering salt in their diets was important but 78% of participants reported "always" adding salt to cooking. Of those who reported taking action to lower their salt intake, participants did so by using spices other than salt (98%), avoiding eating out (61%) and avoiding eating processed foods (52%).

Table 2. Association between knowledge, attitudes and behaviours (KAB) and salt excretion (g/day) overall.

KAB Questions	Mean Salt (g/Day) 95% CI		
	Frequency (%)		*p*-Value *
Maximum salt consumption recommendation			
Less than 10 g (2 teaspoons or less)	19.2	9.43 (8.39, 10.47)	0.073
Less than 5 g (1 teaspoon or less)	70.0	8.93 (8.34, 9.51)	
Less than 2 g (1/2 teaspoon or less)	10.8	8.27 (7.49, 9.05)	
Does high salt intake cause health problems?			
Yes	89.6	8.66 (8.19, 9.13)	0.643
No	10.4	8.37 (7.06, 9.67)	
How much salt do you think you consume?			
Too much	8.9	9.79 (8.47, 11.10)	0.122
Just the right amount	73.3	8.67 (8.20, 9.15)	
Too little	17.8	8.18 (7.46, 8.89)	
How important to you is lowering salt in your diet?			
Very important	38.7	8.64 (8.05, 9.24)	0.928
Somewhat important	52.1	8.62 (8.00, 9.24)	
Not at all important	9.2	8.91 (7.62, 10.21)	
How often do you add salt to food at the table?			
Rarely	47.5	8.53 (7.90, 9.16)	0.627
Sometimes	20.3	8.45 (7.68, 9.21)	
Always	32.2	8.86 (8.33, 9.38)	
How often do you add salt to food when cooking?			
Rarely	15.3	7.66 (6.96, 8.35)	0.004
Sometimes	6.8	7.77 (6.55, 9.00)	
Always	77.9	8.93 (8.40, 9.45)	
Take regular action to control your salt intake?			
-check labels for sodium levels?			
Yes	3.3	8.74 (6.87, 10.62)	0.897
No	96.7	8.62 (8.14, 9.10)	
-avoid adding salt at the table?			
Yes	39.9	8.50 (7.74, 9.25)	0.571
No	60.1	8.70 (8.26, 9.15)	

Table 2. *Cont.*

KAB Questions	Mean Salt (g/Day) 95% CI		
	Frequency (%)		*p*-Value *
-buy low-salt alternatives?			
Yes	2.9	9.37 (7.78, 10.97)	0.341
No	97.1	8.60 (8.12, 9.07)	
-avoid adding salt while cooking?			
Yes	3.6	7.10 (6.09, 8.11)	0.003
No	96.4	8.70 (8.22, 9.18)	
-use spices other than salt?			
Yes	98.1	8.67 (8.19, 9.14)	0.282
No	1.9	7.17 (4.49, 9.85)	
-avoid eating out?			
Yes	61.3	8.61 (8.10, 9.12)	0.944
No	38.7	8.64 (7.93, 9.35)	
-avoid eating snacks or namkeens?			
Yes	22.0	7.93 (7.29, 8.57)	0.006
No	78.0	8.84 (8.34, 9.35)	
-avoid eating pickles?			
Yes	18.4	7.47 (6.81, 8.13)	<0.001
No	81.6%	8.89 (8.39, 9.39)	
-avoid processed food?			
Yes	51.8	8.75 (8.06, 9.43)	0.512
No	48.2	8.49 (7.97, 9.02)	

* *p*-value for differences in mean salt intake between the responses to KAB questions.

3.2. Associations of Knowledge, Attitudes and Behaviours with 24-h Urinary Salt Excretion

There were four measures of knowledge and behaviour for which there were significantly higher or lower levels of urinary salt excretion (all $p < 0.002$) (Table 2) aligned with the expected effect. These related to less use of salt while cooking, avoidance of snacks and namkeens—a savoury Indian snack—and avoidance of pickles. There were no instances where a significantly higher level of urinary salt excretion was associated with a knowledge, attitude or behaviour expected to reduce intake or vice versa.

3.3. Associations of Knowledge, Attitudes and Behaviours with Education Level

There were several significant differences in the knowledge and behaviours reported by more- compared to less-educated individuals (all $p < 0.017$) (Table 3) and there were three instances where the levels of urinary salt excretion varied in different ways across responses to the questions for more-versus less-educated individuals (all $p < 0.024$). There was, however, no clearly discernible pattern to the variation across more- versus less-educated individuals in terms of the responses to questions and the recorded levels of salt intake (Table 4).

Table 3. Knowledge, attitudes and behaviours by level of education ($N = 1395$).

KAB Questions	% (*n*)			
	Overall	<10 Years	>10 Years	*p*-Value *
Maximum salt consumption recommendation				
Less than 10 g (2 teaspoons or less)	19.2%	22.5%	14.1%	0.053
Less than 5 g (1 teaspoon or less)	70.0%	64.6%	76.5%	
Less than 2 g (1/2 teaspoon or less)	10.8%	12.9%	9.4%	
Does high salt intake cause health problems?				
Yes	89.6%	86.0%	94.7%	0.011
No	10.4%	14.0%	5.3%	

Table 3. *Cont.*

KAB Questions	% (*n*)			
	Overall	<10 Years	>10 Years	*p*-Value *
How much salt do you think you consume?				
Too much	8.9%	10.8%	7.4%	0.448
Just the right amount	73.3%	70.1%	75.0%	
Too little	17.8%	19.1%	17.6%	
How important to you is lowering salt in your diet?				
Very important	38.7%	45.5%	33.4%	0.058
Somewhat important	52.1%	47.8%	55.7%	
Not at all important	9.2%	6.7%	11.0%	
How often do you add salt to food at the table?				
Rarely	47.5%	49.5%	45.7%	0.680
Sometimes	20.3%	17.4%	20.1%	
Always	32.2%	33.1%	34.2%	
How often do you add salt to food when cooking?				
Rarely	15.3%	18.5%	10.4%	0.072
Sometimes	6.8%	6.8%	6.4%	
Always	77.9%	74.6%	83.2%	
Take regular action to control your salt intake?				
-check labels for sodium levels?				
Yes	3.3%	3.9%	3.4%	0.754
No	96.7%	96.1%	96.6%	
-avoid adding salt at the table?				
Yes	39.9%	37.5%	41.8%	0.326
No	60.1%	62.5%	58.2%	
- buy low-salt alternatives?				
Yes	2.9%	4.5%	1.6%	0.006
No	97.1%	95.5%	98.4%	
-avoid adding salt while cooking?				
Yes	3.6%	2.1%	4.8%	0.009
No	96.4%	97.9%	95.2%	
-use spices other than salt?				
Yes	98.1%	99.5%	96.5%	<0.001
No	1.9%	0.5%	3.5%	
-avoid eating out?				
Yes	61.3%	62.5%	56.0%	0.112
No	38.7%	37.5%	44.0%	
-avoid eating snacks or namkeens?				
Yes	22.0%	15.5%	26.2%	0.017
No	78.0%	84.5%	73.8%	
-avoid eating pickles?				
Yes	18.4%	9.6%	26.1%	<0.001
No	81.6%	90.4%	73.9%	
-avoid processed food?				
Yes	51.8%	49.2%	54.8%	0.212
No	48.2%	50.8%	45.2%	

* *p*-value for differences frequencies of responses between the educations groups.

Table 4. Association between KAB and salt excretion (g/day) by level of education.

KAB Questions	Mean Salt Excretion (g/Day) 95% CI		
	<10 Years	>10 Years	*p*-Value *
Maximum salt consumption recommendation			
Less than 10 g (2 teaspoons or less)	10.79 (9.26, 12.31)	9.63 (7.83, 11.42)	0.542
Less than 5 g (1 teaspoon or less)	9.72 (8.52, 10.92)	9.85 (8.96, 10.75)	
Less than 2 g (1/2 teaspoon or less)	9.21 (7.91, 10.52)	8.15 (6.83, 9.46)	

Table 4. *Cont.*

KAB Questions	Mean Salt Excretion (g/Day) 95% CI		
	<10 Years	>10 Years	*p*-Value *
Does high salt intake cause health problems?			
Yes	9.30 (8.38, 10.23)	9.29 (8.38, 10.19)	0.082
No	10.20 (8.38, 12.01)	7.84 (5.96, 9.72)	
How much salt do you think you consume?			
Too much	11.54 (9.77, 13.30)	9.98 (8.41, 11.55)	0.082
Just the right amount	9.19 (8.27, 10.10)	9.70 (8.66, 10.73)	
Too little	9.73 (8.92, 10.54)	7.19 (6.34, 8.05)	
How important to you is lowering in your diet?			
Very important	9.93 (8.92, 10.94)	8.81 (7.79, 9.84)	0.319
Somewhat important	9.37 (8.16, 10.58)	9.50 (8.21, 10.78)	
Not at all important	9.32 (7.74, 10.90)	9.59 (7.01, 12.16)	
How often do you add salt to food at the table?			
Rarely	9.76 (8.92, 10.59)	8.94 (7.89, 9.98)	0.184
Sometimes	8.66 (7.18, 10.15)	10.54 (8.09, 13)	
Always	9.63 (8.79, 10.46)	8.85 (8.01, 9.69)	
How often do you add salt to food when cooking?			
Rarely	10.22 (9.14, 11.31)	8.23 (7.21, 9.25)	0.073
Sometimes	9.22 (6.75, 11.69)	8.10 (6.86, 9.34)	
Always	9.49 (8.57, 10.41)	9.60 (8.65, 10.55)	
Take regular action to control your salt intake?			
-check labels for sodium levels?			
Yes	7.90 (5.70, 10.10)	10.56 (9.01, 12.11)	0.017
No	9.56 (8.73, 10.39)	9.15 (8.27, 10.04)	
-avoid adding salt at the table?			
Yes	9.61 (8.65, 10.57)	8.77 (7.57, 9.96)	0.292
No	9.40 (8.49, 10.30)	9.45 (8.32, 10.59)	
-buy low-salt alternatives?			
Yes	9.35 (7.51, 11.20)	10.84 (8.60, 13.09)	0.282
No	9.50 (8.66, 10.33)	9.11 (8.21, 10.01)	
-avoid adding salt while cooking?			
Yes	8.60 (6.93, 10.27)	8.26 (6.69, 9.82)	0.943
No	9.53 (8.69, 10.36)	9.28 (8.41, 10.14)	
-use spices other than salt?			
Yes	9.51 (8.69, 10.33)	9.22 (8.37, 10.07)	0.208
No	7.09 (5.01, 9.18)	9.03 (6.20, 11.85)	
-avoid eating out?			
Yes	9.79 (8.92, 10.66)	8.57 (7.95, 9.18)	0.024
No	8.89 (7.63, 10.15)	9.89 (8.54, 11.24)	
-avoid eating snacks or namkeens?			
Yes	9.43 (8.34, 10.53)	8.51 (7.62, 9.40)	0.322
No	9.55 (8.69, 10.41)	9.50 (8.46, 10.53)	
-avoid eating pickles?			
Yes	9.10 (8.01, 10.18)	8.33 (7.47, 9.19)	0.416
No	9.56 (8.69, 10.44)	9.54 (8.52, 10.57)	
-avoid processed food?			
Yes	9.11 (8.15, 10.08)	9.96 (8.83, 11.09)	<0.001
No	9.83 (9.02, 10.64)	8.21 (7.45, 8.96)	

* *p*-value for differences in mean salt intake between the education groups.

4. Discussion

There was strong evidence of an association between participant knowledge and behaviours related to salt and actual salt consumption levels as determined from assays of 24-h urine collections. This suggests that modifying population levels of these indicators of knowledge and behaviour might be an effective way of reducing population mean salt intake in India. Further, the substantial gap between the large proportion of people believing themselves to be consuming "just the right amount" of salt, and the very small proportion actually achieving the 5 g/day target, highlights the opportunity for interventions that can translate that intent into reality.

The education level of individuals may influence their acquisition of knowledge about healthy dietary practices [28,38,39] and has been associated with behaviours related to diet [29,40,41]. In this study, groups defined by different levels of education did show somewhat different results both in terms of responses to questions and corresponding levels of salt excretion, but there was no clear pattern identified whereby it was possible to ascertain particular strategies that should be targeted towards more- versus less-educated individuals. So, while any Indian intervention program targeting salt will need delivering in formats suited to individuals with a broad range of educational levels of achievement, it is not possible to specify particular messages or approaches more likely to result in a reduction in salt intake according to level of education.

Dietary patterns vary considerably around India but high levels of salt deriving from salt added during food preparation and as seasoning at the table [42] are common across many communities. In urban areas, populations are making progressively greater use of chain restaurant and fast food outlets, which often add significant quantities of salt during food preparation, whilst in rural areas salt is used in pickled fruit and vegetables dishes which are consumed in large amounts [42]. While the rapid epidemiological and nutrition transition India is undergoing [3,14] means that dietary patterns are going to evolve across the country, dietary habits will remain diverse and education programs will need to be adaptable to quite different settings.

The fairly high levels of knowledge, and the many people reporting actions to reduce salt intake are comparable to that reported in many other countries [24,30,43–45]. In many cases, those jurisdictions also show persisting high levels of average population salt consumption. The key difference of our findings for India compared to other countries like Australia [43] is that favourable knowledge levels and behaviours were actually associated with lower salt intake in India. This could be a chance finding or the consequence of better statistical power, but it may also be that the large proportion of dietary salt added during cooking and at the table in India makes it possible for the Indian population to control their salt intake in a way that Australians cannot. In Australia, most salt consumed is from pre-prepared packaged and restaurant foods [30]. So, while knowledgeable and motivated Indian consumers can simply leave discretionary salt out while cooking or seasoning at the table, it is much harder for Australians who would need to identify the salt content of different foods and meals and then try to find alternative lower-salt options.

This finding has important implications for any intervention to reduce salt in India. The efficacy of behavioural interventions delivered to populations has been studied mostly in high-income countries where programs typically include a combination of media and counselling activities [31]. A systematic review of such programs identified improvements in various risk factors in 22 studies, although in another 14 studies there were no benefits achieved [46]. A meta-analysis of 17 randomized controlled trials including intensive dietary behavioural interventions showed more convincing effects on dietary fat intake, serum cholesterol, urinary sodium and blood pressure [47]. On balance, the data suggest potential benefits for population-based interventions targeting salt intake [31], but data from developing country settings are few. One study undertaken in an urban community in Pakistan evaluated the effects of a household-based intervention delivered by a social worker focussing on fat and salt in a lower-middle class community. After two years, there was a reported 48% lower fat intake and 41% lower salt intake in intervention households as compared to control households [48].

There has been no dedicated population-based study of salt reduction in India, although one intervention study addressing behavioural risks for cardiovascular disease did report more consumption of fruit and vegetables and reduced intake of salt at four-year follow-up [49]. In another study done amongst at-risk Indian women, significant increases in knowledge and behaviours regarding diet-related risk factors for hypertension were observed after a community-wide education intervention that used posters, handouts, public lectures and focus groups [31]. The effectiveness of these types of programs is likely due to the fairly high intensity of engagement with community members, including one-on-one interactions and small group activities in each case.

A scale-up of this type of approach would not be feasible for salt reduction in India [50] and the observed benefits cannot reasonably be generalised to population-wide settings where average exposure of individuals to the program would be much less. It is clear from experiences in Finland and the UK that population-wide salt reduction can be achieved, and community-wide education was almost certainly a key component of the success in both countries, but a novel form of intervention program tailored to India will be required [7,51].

Key strengths of this analysis are the large size of the populations included and the recruitment of individuals from regions in North and South India that span slum, urban and rural populations. This allows some capacity to generalise the findings to diverse population groups in India beyond those studied. Good participant response rates were achieved and we used weighting to control for differences in age, sex and place of residence of those sampled compared with the respective populations of the regions. However, weighting may not have fully adjusted for systematic difference in those who did and did not agree to take part. The survey also benefitted from the use of the accepted best method of quantification of dietary sodium intake based upon 24-h urine collection and the use of standardised questions about knowledge, attitudes and behaviours related to salt which are widely considered valid [43]. Multiple 24-h urine samples are required to get an accurate estimate of an individual's usual salt intake but the associated high participant burden [52] precluded that option and we used single measurements on large numbers instead. For the estimation of average salt intake levels, this is an effective method of investigation although the between-individual variability within the population will have been over-estimated and the strengths of the associations of salt intake with the various exposures studied will probably have been under-estimated.

These data support the inclusion of population-wide education as part of a multifaceted salt reduction program for India that would likely both prevent large numbers of cases of hypertension as well as strokes and heart attacks [53,54]. Furthermore, there is a strong expectation that an intervention program could be achieved at low total cost and in a highly cost-effective way [14], making a significant contribution to the country's efforts to deliver upon its commitment to the "25 by 25" goal of reducing chronic disease burden in the country by one quarter by 2025. The Food Safety and Standards Authority of India (FSSAI) has developed guidelines to decrease availability of foods high in fat, sugar and salt (HFSS) in and around schools through developing school canteen policies, regulating advertisements of HFSS foods to school children, including restricting celebrity endorsements and improving packaged food labelling [54]. These actions illustrate the willingness and capacity of the Government of India to act and, whilst specific to school settings, provide an example of what can be achieved with strong political leadership.

Supplementary Materials: The following are available online at http://www.mdpi.com/2072-6643/9/2/144/s1.

Acknowledgments: This work was supported by a funding award made by the Global Alliance for Chronic Disease through the National Health and Medical Research Council (NHMRC) of Australia (APP1040179). C.J. is supported by a National Health and Medical Research Council postgraduate scholarship (APP1074678). J.W. is supported by a National Health and Medical Research Council/National Heart Foundation Career Development Fellowship (APP1082924). B.N. is supported by a National Health and Medical Research Council of Australia Principal Research Fellowship (APP1106947). He also holds an NHMRC Program Grant (APP1052555). P.K.M. is an Intermediate Career Fellow of the WT/DBT India Alliance. R.S. is supported by a Wellcome Trust Capacity Strengthening Strategic Award Extension phase to the Public Health Foundation of India and a consortium of UK universities (WT084754/Z/08/A).

Author Contributions: C.J. wrote the first draft of this paper, which B.N. edited for important content. K.R. did the statistical analyses. All authors reviewed and provided comments upon subsequent iterations.

Conflicts of Interest: The authors declare no conflict of interest.

References

1. Sarmugam, R.; Worsley, A.; Wang, W. An examination of the mediating role of salt knowledge and beliefs on the relationship between socio-demographic factors and discretionary salt use: A cross-sectional study. *Int. J. Behav. Nutr. Phys. Act.* **2013**, *10*, 25–33. [CrossRef] [PubMed]

2. Lewis, S.; Rodbard, H.; Fox, K.; Grandy, S. Self-reported prevalence and awareness of metabolic syndrome: Findings from SHIELD. *Int. J. Clin. Pract.* **2008**, *62*, 1168–1176. [CrossRef] [PubMed]
3. Lim, S.; Vos, T.; Flaxman, A.; Danaei, G.; Shibuya, K.; Adair-Rohani, H.; AlMazroa, M.; Amann, M.; Anderson, H.; Andrews, K. A comparative risk assessment of burden of disease and injury attributable to 67 risk factors and risk factor clusters in 21 regions, 1990–2010: A systematic analysis for the Global Burden of Disease Study 2010. *Lancet* **2013**, *380*, 2224–2260. [CrossRef]
4. Gupta, R. Trends in hypertension epidemiology in India. *J. Hum. Hypertens.* **2004**, *18*, 73–78. [CrossRef] [PubMed]
5. Prabhakaran, D.; Jeemon, P.; Roy, A. Cardiovascular Diseases in India Current Epidemiology and Future Directions. *Circulation* **2016**, *133*, 1605–1620. [CrossRef] [PubMed]
6. Brown, I.; Tzoulaki, I.; Candeias, V.; Elliott, P. Salt intakes around the world: Implications for public health. *Int. J. Epidemiol.* **2009**, *38*, 791–813. [CrossRef] [PubMed]
7. Cappuccio, F.; Capewell, S.; Lincoln, P.; McPherson, K. Policy options to reduce population salt intake. *BMJ* **2011**, *343*. [CrossRef] [PubMed]
8. World Health Organization (WHO). *Global Action Plan for the Prevention and Control of Noncommunicable Diseases 2013–2020*; WHO: Geneva, Switzerland, 2013.
9. Campbell, N.; Neal, B.; MacGregor, G. Interested in developing a national programme to reduce dietary salt & quest. *J. Hum. Hypertens.* **2011**, *25*, 705–710. [PubMed]
10. World Health Organization (WHO). *Reducing Salt Intake in Populations: Report of a WHO Forum and Technical Meeting, 5–7 October 2006, Paris, France*; WHO: Geneva, Switzerland, 2007.
11. World Health Organization (WHO). *WHO Global Strategy on Diet, Physical Activity and Health: The Americas Regional Consultation Meeting Report*; WHO: Geneva, Switzerland, 2003.
12. Yang, Q.; Liu, T.; Kuklina, E.V.; Flanders, W.D.; Hong, Y.; Gillespie, C.; Chang, M.H.; Gwinn, M.; Dowling, N.; Khoury, M.J. Sodium and potassium intake and mortality among US adults: Prospective data from the Third National Health and Nutrition Examination Survey. *Arch. Intern. Med.* **2011**, *171*, 1183–1191. [CrossRef] [PubMed]
13. Basu, S.; Stuckler, D.; Vellakkal, S.; Ebrahim, S. Dietary salt reduction and cardiovascular disease rates in India: A mathematical model. *PLoS ONE* **2012**, *7*, e44037. [CrossRef] [PubMed]
14. Patel, V.; Chatterji, S.; Chisholm, D.; Ebrahim, S.; Gopalakrishna, G.; Mathers, C.; Mohan, V.; Prabhakaran, D.; Ravindran, R.D.; Reddy, K.S. Chronic diseases and injuries in India. *Lancet* **2011**, *377*, 413–428. [CrossRef]
15. Draft Comprehensive Global Monitoring Framework and Targets for the Prevention and Control of Noncommunicable Diseases. Available online: http://apps.who.int/gb/ebwha/pdf_files/WHA66/A66_8-en.pdf (accessed on 14 February 2017).
16. Food and Agriculture Organization of the United Nations (FAO). *The Double Burden of Malnutrition: Case Studies from Six Developing Countries*; FAO: Roma, Italy, 2006.
17. Misra, A.; Singhal, N.; Sivakumar, B.; Bhagat, N.; Jaiswal, A.; Khurana, L. Nutrition transition in India: Secular trends in dietary intake and their relationship to diet-related non-communicable diseases. *J. Diabetes* **2011**, *3*, 278–292. [CrossRef] [PubMed]
18. Central Statistics Office Ministry of Statistics and Programme Implementation Government of India. *SARRC Development Goals—India Country Report*; Central Statistics Office Ministry of Statistics and Programme Implementation Government of India: New Delhi, India, 2013.
19. Indian Council of Medical Research. *Nutrient Requirements and Recommended Dietary Allowances for Indians*; A Report of the Expert Group of the Indian Council of Medical Research; Indian Council of Medical Research: New Delhi, India, 2009.
20. Groth, M.V.; Fagt, S.; Brøndsted, L. Social determinants of dietary habits in Denmark. *Eur. J. Clin. Nutr.* **2001**, *55*, 959–966. [CrossRef] [PubMed]
21. Hjartaker, A.; Lund, E. Relationship between dietary habits, age, lifestyle, and socio-economic status among adult Norwegian women. The Norwegian Women and Cancer Study. *Eur. J. Clin. Nutr.* **1998**, *52*, 565–572. [CrossRef] [PubMed]
22. Kant, A.K.; Graubard, B.I. Secular trends in the association of socio-economic position with self-reported dietary attributes and biomarkers in the US population: National Health and Nutrition Examination Survey (NHANES) 1971–1975 to NHANES 1999–2002. *Public Health Nutr.* **2007**, *10*, 158–167. [CrossRef] [PubMed]

23. Mullie, P.; Clarys, P.; Hulens, M.; Vansant, G. Dietary patterns and socioeconomic position. *Eur. J. Clin. Nutr.* **2010**, *64*, 231–238. [CrossRef] [PubMed]

24. Grimes, C.A.; Riddell, L.J.; Nowson, C.A. Consumer knowledge and attitudes to salt intake and labelled salt information. *Appetite* **2009**, *53*, 189–194. [CrossRef] [PubMed]

25. Grimes, C.A.; Riddell, L.J.; Nowson, C.A. The use of table and cooking salt in a sample of Australian adults. *Asia Pac. J. Clin. Nutr.* **2010**, *19*, 256–260. [PubMed]

26. Henderson, L.; Gregory, J.; Swan, G. *The National Diet & Nutrition Survey: Adults Aged 19 to 64 Years*; HM Stationery Office: London, UK, 2003.

27. Leganger, A.; Kraft, P. Control constructs: Do they mediate the relation between educational attainment and health behaviour? *J. Health Psychol.* **2003**, *8*, 361–372. [CrossRef] [PubMed]

28. Parmenter, K.; Waller, J.; Wardle, J. Demographic variation in nutrition knowledge in England. *Health Educ. Res.* **2000**, *15*, 163–174. [CrossRef] [PubMed]

29. Wardle, J.; Steptoe, A. Socioeconomic differences in attitudes and beliefs about healthy lifestyles. *J. Epidemiol. Commun. Health* **2003**, *57*, 440–443. [CrossRef]

30. Webster, J.L.; Li, N.; Dunford, E.K.; Nowson, C.A.; Neal, B.C. Consumer awareness and self-reported behaviours related to salt consumption in Australia. *Asia Pac. J. Clin. Nutr.* **2010**, *19*, 550–554. [PubMed]

31. Pandey, R.M.; Agrawal, A.; Misra, A.; Vikram, N.K.; Misra, P.; Dey, S.; Rao, S.; Devi, K.V.; Menon, V.U.; Revathi, R. Population-based intervention for cardiovascular diseases related knowledge and behaviours in Asian Indian women. *Indian Heart J.* **2013**, *65*, 40–47. [CrossRef] [PubMed]

32. Mittal, R.; Dasgupta, J.; Mukherjee, A.; Saxena, B. *Salt Consumption Pattern in India: An ICMR Task Force Study*; Indian Council of Medical Research: New Delhi, India, 1996.

33. Intersalt Cooperative Research Group. Intersalt: An international study of electrolyte excretion and blood pressure. Results for 24 h urinary sodium and potassium excretion. Intersalt Cooperative Research Group. *BMJ* **1988**, *297*, 319–328.

34. Johnson, C.; Mohan, S.; Rogers, K.; Shivashankar, R.; Thout, S.R.; Gupta, P.; He, F.J.; MacGregor, G.A.; Webster, J.; Krishnan, A. Mean Dietary Salt Intake in Urban and Rural Areas in India: A Population Survey of 1395 Persons. *J. Am. Heart Assoc.* **2017**, *6*, e004547. [CrossRef] [PubMed]

35. Talib, R.; Ali, O.; Arshad, F.; Kadir, K.A. The effectiveness of group dietary counselling among non insulin dependent diabetes mellitus (NIDDM) patients in resettlement scheme areas in Malaysia. *Asia Pac. J. Clin. Nutri.* **1997**, *6*, 84–87.

36. Johnson, C.; Mohan, S.; Praveen, D.; Woodward, M.; Maulik, P.; Shivashankar, R.; Amarchand, R.; Webster, J.; Dunford, E.; Thout, S. Protocol for developing the evidence base for a national salt reduction programme for India. *BMJ Open* **2014**, *4*, e006629. [CrossRef] [PubMed]

37. World Health Organization. *World Health Organization and Pan American Health Organization Regional Expert Group for Cardiovascular Disease Prevention through Population-Wide Dietary Salt Reduction Sub-Group for Research and Surveillance*; Protocol for Population Level Sodium Determination in 24-h Urine Samples; World Health Organization: Geneva, Switzerland, 2010.

38. Turrell, G.; Kavanagh, A. Socio-economic pathways to diet: Modelling the association between socio-economic position and food purchasing behaviour. *Public Health Nutr.* **2006**, *9*, 375–383. [CrossRef] [PubMed]

39. Macario, E.; Emmons, K.M.; Sorensen, G.; Hunt, M.K.; Rudd, R.E. Factors influencing nutrition education for patients with low literacy skills. *J. Am. Diet. Assoc.* **1998**, *98*, 559–564. [CrossRef]

40. Wardle, J.; Parmenter, K.; Waller, J. Nutrition knowledge and food intake. *Appetite* **2000**, *34*, 269–275. [CrossRef] [PubMed]

41. Busselman, K.M.; Holcomb, C.A. Reading skill and comprehension of the dietary guidelines by WIC participants. *J. Am. Diet. Assoc.* **1994**, *94*, 622–625. [CrossRef]

42. Ravi, S.; Bermudez, O.I.; Harivanzan, V.; Kenneth Chui, K.H.; Vasudevan, P.; Must, A.; Thanikachalam, S.; Thanikachalam, M. Sodium Intake, Blood Pressure, and Dietary Sources of Sodium in an Adult South Indian Population. *Ann. Glob. Health* **2016**, *82*, 234–242. [CrossRef] [PubMed]

43. Land, M.A.; Webster, J.; Christoforou, A.; Johnson, C.; Trevena, H.; Hodgins, F.; Chalmers, J.; Woodward, M.; Barzi, F.; Smith, W. The association of knowledge, attitudes and behaviours related to salt with 24-h urinary sodium excretion. *Int. J. Behav. Nutr. Phys. Act.* **2014**, *11*, 1. [CrossRef] [PubMed]

44. Webster, J.; Su'a, S.A.F.; Ieremia, M.; Bompoint, S.; Johnson, C.; Faeamani, G.; Vaiaso, M.; Snowdon, W.; Land, M.A.; Trieu, K. Salt Intakes, Knowledge, and Behavior in Samoa: Monitoring Salt-Consumption Patterns Through the World Health Organization's Surveillance of Noncommunicable Disease Risk Factors (STEPS). *J. Clin. Hypertens.* **2016**, *18*, 884–891. [CrossRef] [PubMed]

45. Claro, R.M.; Linders, H.; Ricardo, C.Z.; Legetic, B.; Campbell, N.R. Consumer attitudes, knowledge, and behavior related to salt consumption in sentinel countries of the Americas. *Rev. Panam. Salud Pública* **2012**, *32*, 265–273. [CrossRef] [PubMed]

46. Pennant, M.; Davenport, C.; Bayliss, S.; Greenheld, W.; Marshall, T.; Hyde, C. Community programs for the prevention of cardiovascular disease: A systematic review. *Am. J. Epidemiol.* **2010**, *172*, 501–516. [CrossRef] [PubMed]

47. Brunner, E.; White, I.; Thorogood, M.; Bristow, A.; Curle, D.; Marmot, M. Can dietary interventions change diet and cardiovascular risk factors? A meta-analysis of randomized controlled trials. *Am. J. Public Health* **1997**, *87*, 1415–1422. [CrossRef] [PubMed]

48. Aziz, K.; Dennis, B.; Davis, C.; Sun, K.; Burke, G.; Manolio, T.; Faruqui, A.; Chagani, H.; Ashraf, T.; Patel, N. Efficacy of CVD risk factor modification in a lower-middle class community in Pakistan: The Metroville Health Study. *Asia Pac. J. Public Health* **2003**, *15*, 30–36. [CrossRef] [PubMed]

49. Prabhakaran, D.; Jeemon, P.; Goenka, S.; Lakshmy, R.; Thankappan, K.; Ahmed, F.; Joshi, P.P.; Mohan, B.M.; Meera, R.; Das, M.S. Impact of a worksite intervention program on cardiovascular risk factors: A demonstration project in an Indian industrial population. *J. Am. Coll. Cardiol.* **2009**, *53*, 1718–1728. [CrossRef] [PubMed]

50. Cobiac, L.J.; Vos, T.; Veerman, J.L. Cost-effectiveness of interventions to reduce dietary salt intake. *Heart* **2010**, *96*, 1920–1925. [CrossRef] [PubMed]

51. Tuomilehto, J.; Puska, P.; Nissinen, A.; Salonen, J.; Tanskanen, A.; Pietinen, P.; Wolf, E. Community-based prevention of hypertension in North Karelia, Finland. *Ann. Clin Res.* **1983**, *16*, 18–27.

52. Dennis, B.; Stamler, J.; Buzzard, M.; Conway, R.; Elliott, P.; Moag-Stahlberg, A.; Okayama, A.; Okuda, N.; Robertson, C.; Robinson, F. INTERMAP: The dietary data—Process and quality control. *J. Hum. Hypertens.* **2003**, *17*, 609–622. [CrossRef] [PubMed]

53. Ireland, D.M.; Clifton, P.M.; Keogh, J.B. Achieving the salt intake target of 6 g/day in the current food supply in free-living adults using two dietary education strategies. *J. Am. Diet. Assoc.* **2010**, *110*, 763–767. [CrossRef] [PubMed]

54. Food Safety and Standards Authority of India (FSSAI). *Draft Guidelines for Making Available Wholesome, Nutritious, Safe and Hygienic Food to School Children*; FSSAI: New Delhi, India, 2015.

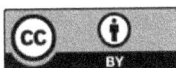

nutrients

MDPI

Article

Effect of 25% Sodium Reduction on Sales of a Top-Selling Bread in Remote Indigenous Australian Community Stores: A Controlled Intervention Trial

Emma McMahon [1,2,*], Jacqui Webster [3] and Julie Brimblecombe [1]

[1] Wellbeing and Preventable Chronic Diseases Division, Menzies School of Health Research, Royal Hospital Campus, 105 Rocklands Dr, Tiwi NT 0810, Australia; Julie.Brimblecombe@menzies.edu.au

[2] Centre for Population Health Research, School of Health Sciences, University of South Australia, City East Campus, North Tce, Adelaide SA 5001, Australia

[3] The George Institute for Global Health, The University of Sydney, Camperdown NSW 2000, Australia; jwebster@georgeinstitute.org.au

* Correspondence: e.j.mcmahon@outlook.com; Tel.: +61-8-8946-4212

Received: 19 December 2016; Accepted: 21 February 2017; Published: 28 February 2017

Abstract: Reducing sodium in the food supply is key to achieving population salt targets, but maintaining sales is important to ensuring commercial viability and maximising clinical impact. We investigated whether 25% sodium reduction in a top-selling bread affected sales in 26 remote Indigenous community stores. After a 23-week baseline period, 11 control stores received the regular-salt bread (400 mg Na/100 g) and 15 intervention stores received the reduced-salt version (300 mg Na/100 g) for 12-weeks. Sales data were collected to examine difference between groups in change from baseline to follow-up (effect size) in sales (primary outcome) or sodium density, analysed using a mixed model. There was no significant effect on market share (-0.31%; 95% CI $-0.68, 0.07$; $p = 0.11$) or weekly dollars (\$58; $-149, 266$; $p = 0.58$). Sodium density of all purchases was not significantly reduced (-8 mg Na/MJ; $-18, 2$; $p = 0.14$), but 25% reduction across all bread could significantly reduce sodium (-12; $-23, -1$; $p = 0.03$). We found 25% salt reduction in a top-selling bread did not affect sales in remote Indigenous community stores. If achieved across all breads, estimated salt intake in remote Indigenous Australian communities would be reduced by approximately 15% of the magnitude needed to achieve population salt targets, which could lead to significant health gains at the population-level.

Keywords: salt; sodium; reformulation; bread; sales; Indigenous Australians; population health

1. Introduction

Excess salt intake is one of the main contributors to the high rates of hypertension, cardiovascular disease, renal disease, and premature mortality experienced by many countries around the world [1]. It is estimated that 2.5 million deaths could be prevented globally each year if population salt intakes were reduced to 5 g/day (2000 mg) [1]. Reformulation to reduce salt added during food processing is a cost-effective and sustainable strategy to reduce population intakes [2].

Australian Indigenous peoples currently experience a highly disproportionate rate of chronic disease and premature mortality, with life expectancy ten years lower than the non-Indigenous Australian population [3,4]. Those living in remote areas of Australia have even higher burden of disease and lower life expectancy than those living in non-remote areas [3,4]. The factors driving these disparities are complex, including cultural and social dispossession; considerable socioeconomic disadvantage; poorer access to health services; and high-risk health behaviours such as smoking, physical inactivity, and poor nutrition [5]. The diet of those living in remote Indigenous communities is characterised by very low intake of fruit, vegetables, and whole grains, and excessive intake of salt, sugar, and nutrient-poor discretionary foods [6–9]. It is likely that even small shifts in dietary intake at the population level could considerably reduce the risk of chronic disease [1,6,10]. We previously modelled dietary change needed to meet dietary guidelines without increasing cost, and found that even with large shifts in modelled dietary intake towards dietary recommendations, estimated sodium intake was still 150% of the upper limit [8], highlighting that changes within food manufacturing are essential to reduce salt intake to a level considered healthy. To address this, the Act on Salt partnership formed in 2014 to investigate opportunities to reduce salt intake in remote Indigenous Australian communities.

Nearly half of all sodium in remote Indigenous communities comes from only three food types [6]. The biggest contributor is discretionary (added) salt (19% of all sodium,), followed by bread (18%, range 13%–25%) and processed meats (9%, range 6%–15%) [6]. We worked with the manufacturer of one of the biggest selling breads in remote Indigenous communities—Bush Oven Outback Bread™ (Bush Oven)—to investigate whether the sodium content could be reduced. Bush Oven bread is primarily distributed to remote Indigenous communities across Australia, and the high fibre white Bush Oven—which currently has 400 mg Na/100 g—represents a considerable proportion of the market share of bread in this population. The manufacturer, Goodman Fielder, developed two levels of reduced salt bread (350 mg sodium/100 g and 300 mg sodium/100 g) without adding or increasing other flavour enhancers or preservatives. After testing that shelf life and microbial quality was retained (internal testing by Goodman Fielder as per standard protocol for recipe formulation), we conducted consumer acceptance testing in one remote Indigenous community. In a triangle test with 62 participants from a remote Indigenous community in Northern Territory, participants were unable to detect a difference between standard bread and reduced salt versions (350 mg or 300 mg/100 g) ($p > 0.05$) [11]. In addition, there were no significant differences in sensory characteristics (appearance, whiteness, flavour, sweetness, saltiness, texture, softness, and overall liking rated a 10-point scale) between standard, 300 mg, or 350 mg sodium breads ($p > 0.05$ using ANOVA) [11].

We calculated that 25% salt-reduction in bread has the capacity to reduce salt intake in remote Indigenous communities by 5%, or an average reduction of 140 mg sodium (0.4 g salt) per day [6]—a reduction that could be clinically significant at the population level [12–14]. However, to maintain commercial viability and to maximise the clinical impact, it is important that consumers continue to purchase the lower salt bread. The aim of this study was to investigate whether 25% salt reduction would affect sales of Bush Oven high fibre white bread (study bread) in remote Indigenous Australian communities. The secondary aim was to examine whether this would significantly reduce the total sodium of purchased food and drinks, and to model impact on total sodium of a 25% sodium reduction across a broader range of breads.

2. Materials and Methods

2.1. Study Design

This study was a non-randomised controlled study examining sales of a reduced salt bread (intervention group) versus the regular salt version (control group) in remote Indigenous Australian community stores. The study included four periods in 2015: baseline (23 weeks, February–July), wash-in (six weeks, July–August), follow-up (12 weeks, August–November), and wash-out (six weeks, November–December). Ethical approval was granted by the Human Research Ethics Committee (HREC) of the Nothern Territory Department of Health and the Menzies School of Health Research (HREC-2014-2311), Central Australian HREC (HREC-14-275), Aboriginal HREC of SA (HREC 04-14-595), Western Australian Aboriginal Health Ethics Committee (HREC-599), and the University of South Australia HREC (04-14-595).

2.2. Participants

Remote Indigenous communities are discrete geographical locations dispersed widely across the remote areas of Australia (mostly Central or Top-End Australia) inhabited predominately by Indigenous Australian peoples [15]. Many communities are serviced by only one or two community stores and are distanced from alternative food sources, meaning that these stores provide the majority of dietary intake [16]. Stores are often owned by the community, and decisions regarding the store are made by a committee of community representatives (store committee). There are several store associations that oversee the management of remote community stores; Outback Stores (OBS) and The Arnhem Land Progress Aboriginal Corporation (ALPA) are two of the largest.

Inclusion criteria were remote Indigenous Australian community stores in the Northern Territory, Western Australia, and South Australia managed by either ALPA or OBS, and where the study bread represented ≥45% of the market share for bread (i.e., ≥45% of total dollars spent on bread was on the study bread, assessed using sales data prior to study commencement). Eligible stores were recruited by representatives of ALPA and OBS (in most cases, the area manager or ALPA/OBS nutritionist) who presented the study to store committees and invited them to participate.

This study was initially designed as a randomised controlled trial; however, changes to the baking location and supply route of the bread during the baseline period (for reasons unrelated to this study) meant that half of the participating stores were unable to receive the reduced salt bread. For this reason, the study was adapted to a non-randomised controlled design, with allocation to intervention or control mostly determined by supply route of study bread for participating stores. Stores were blinded to their allocation, and were asked not to discuss the study with customers.

2.3. Procedures

At baseline, all stores stocked the regular salt study bread (400 mg Na/100 g) as normal. Following this, intervention stores began to receive the 25% reduced salt study bread (300 mg Na/100 g), while control stores continued to receive the regular bread. All stores were asked to order bread as usual throughout the study, but were asked to use a specific order code during the wash-in and follow-up periods when ordering the study bread (with the code differing between control and intervention stores). The reduced salt bread was distributed to the intervention stores for 18 weeks total, the first six weeks of which were designated as a wash-in period to allow for stores to rotate through their existing stock, with the last 12 weeks considered the follow-up period.

The bread packaging was not distinguishable between the regular and reduced salt breads, except for the barcode. The cartons in which the bread was stored prior to delivery were indicated as regular versus reduced salt by a coloured cross marking. The reduced salt study bread was baked, stored, and distributed using the same processes as the regular salt study bread. Bread was distributed from the Independent Grocers warehouse in Darwin with the two types of bread being stored in different locations within the warehouse to prevent the incorrect bread being picked for shipping.

Weekly store sales data on all food and drinks purchased over the study period were collected for the study duration. Data (product codes, description, units sold, and dollar value) were imported into a purpose-built Microsoft Access database (the Remote Indigenous Stores and Takeaways tool) [17]. All food and drink items were linked to nutrient data by assigning a food identification code using the Australian Food and Nutrient database (AUSNUT 2011–2013) [18].

We contacted all stores via telephone fortnightly from the start of washout to the end of the intervention. During these phone calls, store managers were asked if there had been any issues with delivery, any factors that would affect sales of the study bread, and whether there had been any comments from customers about the study bread. Most remote Indigenous community stores operate with a small staff, and in many instances, it was not possible to contact store managers on the first telephone call attempt. Where telephone calls were unsuccessful, there were additional telephone call attempts, and voice messages were left requesting a return call at a convenient time.

2.4. Outcomes and Analyses

Sales-related outcome measures (primary outcomes) were: (1) study bread dollars as a percentage of total dollars spent on food and drink (market share); and (2) average weekly dollars spent on the study bread (weekly dollars). To test if the total sodium of all purchased food and drinks were reduced (secondary outcome), we examined total sodium density per megajoule of energy (sodium density; mg Na/MJ energy).

Analyses were performed using mixed models that included main and interaction terms for period (baseline, wash-in, follow-up, wash-out) and group (control, intervention) and a random intercept for store to account for within-store serial correlation of weekly sales data. *p*-values less than 0.05 were considered statistically significant. The "effect size" was calculated by the difference between the control and intervention group in the change from baseline to follow-up. The main analyses were undertaken using intention-to-treat principle.

We repeated the sodium density analysis to examine the potential change in sodium per megajoule in the following scenarios: (i) if 100% study implementation was achieved (i.e., all bread sold in the follow-up period by intervention stores was reduced salt); (ii) if 25% sodium reduction was also applied to the wholemeal version of the study bread; (iii) if 25% sodium reduction was applied to all breads in the Bush Oven loaf range (high fibre white, wholemeal, and mixed grain); and (iv) if 25% sodium reduction was applied across all breads, regardless of brand.

Comments recorded from phone calls that were related to the quality of the study bread were categorised and reported descriptively. Potential outliers were identified by matching information regarding factors that could affect bread sales (including events in the community, delayed or missed deliveries, or changes to ordering patterns) to anomalies in data.

Sensitivity analyses were performed by repeating the main analyses (i) without outliers and (ii) by dropping individual stores to ensure that results were consistent. All analyses were undertaken using STATA Version 13.1 (StataCorp LLC; College Station, TX, USA).

3. Results

Twenty-nine remote Indigenous community stores (24 OBS and five ALPA-managed) met the inclusion criteria, and were invited to participate. Of these, 26 stores consented to the study (21 OBS and five ALPA). Of the 21 OBS-managed stores that consented to the study, nine could not receive the reduced salt bread due to their supply route and were allocated to the control group; the remaining twelve were allocated to the intervention group. All five ALPA-managed stores could receive the reduced salt bread and were alternately allocated to the intervention or control group. All stores that consented to the study completed the study.

The intervention group had more stores in Top-End NT, while control stores were mostly in central Australia (Table 1). There were no significant differences in total weekly dollars or megajoules of all food and drink purchases (mean difference using mixed model $8962, 95% CI −13,020, 30,943, *p* = 0.42; 8985 MJ, −5949, 23,919, *p* = 0.24). During the baseline period, the study bread contributed a mean 13.9% (range for individual stores 9.2%–17.2%) and 12.8% (range 5.1%–19.2%) of the total sodium in all purchased food and drinks for intervention and control stores, respectively. There were no significant differences between control and intervention groups at baseline in market share (mean difference 0.09%, 95% CI −0.98 to 1.17; *p* = 0.86), weekly study bread dollars ($476, −588 to 1540; *p* = 0.38) or total sodium per megajoule (−7 mg Na, −36 to 21; *p* = 0.63) (Table 2).

Table 1. Baseline characteristics.

Characteristic	Control	Intervention
Store Association (%OBS)	82% ($n = 9/11$)	80% ($n = 12/15$)
Location		
Top-End NT	18% ($n = 2/11$)	73% ($n = 11/15$)
Central NT	55% ($n = 6/11$)	0% ($n = 0/15$)
Central South Australia	9% ($n = 1/11$)	0% ($n = 0/15$)
Western Australia	18% ($n = 2/11$)	27% ($n = 4/15$)
Food and drink purchases		
Dollars ($/week)	28,191 (11,495, 44,887)	37,152 (22,854, 51,450)
Energy (MJ/week)	17,049 (5706, 28,392)	26,034 (16,320, 35,747)

NT = Northern Territory; OBS = Outback Stores; Values are percentages or median (interquartile range).

Table 2. Study outcomes at baseline and follow up.

Outcome	Group	Baseline	Follow-Up	Effect Size
Market share (%)	Control	4.24 (3.43, 5.06)	4.20 (3.48, 4.92)	-0.31 (-0.68, 0.07) $p = 0.11$
	Intervention	4.34 (3.64, 5.04)	3.99 (3.37, 4.60)	
Dollars ($)	Control	1156 (348, 1965)	1106 (376, 1837)	58 (-149, 266) $p = 0.58$
	Intervention	1632 (940, 2325)	1641 (1015, 2266)	
Sodium (mg Na/MJ)	Control	325 (305, 344)	322 (304, 341)	-8 (-18, 2) $p = 0.14$
	Intervention	317 (300, 334)	307 (291, 323)	

Results are margins (95% confidence intervals) from mixed model analysis with group and period as main and interaction terms. Effect size is the difference between control and intervention groups in change from baseline to follow-up periods. Market share (%) is calculated by dollars as a percentage of all food and drink dollars. Dollars ($) indicates average weekly dollars. Sodium (mg Na/MJ) indicates total sodium per megajoule energy of all foods and drinks purchased.

3.1. Main Outcomes

Results of the main analyses are shown in Table 2. We found no significant difference in sales outcomes (percentage market share or weekly average dollars) between control and intervention groups in the change from baseline to follow-up. The effect of all food and drink purchases on sodium density was also not statistically significant. Results across all study periods including wash-in and wash-out are shown in Table S1.

3.2. Simulations and Sensitivity Analyses

We achieved a high level of implementation fidelity; all study bread loaves sold during baseline and by the control stores during the follow-up period were regular salt (100% implementation) and 95% of the total combined study bread loaves sold by the intervention stores during the follow-up period were reduced salt. We simulated change in sodium density if 100% implementation was achieved; however, the effect size was not statistically significant (Table 3). In simulations where 25% sodium reduction was applied to all breads in the Bush Oven loaf range (high fibre white, wholemeal, and mixed grain) or across all breads regardless of brand, the effect size reached statistical significance (Table 3).

Results of sensitivity analyses are shown in Supplement 2. Repeating the main analyses without outliers did not impact the results. Repeating the main analyses with individual stores removed did not impact the results for sales-related outcomes (percentage market share and weekly dollars), however the difference in sodium density reached statistical significance when one of the control stores was dropped (-11 mg/MJ; 95% CI -22 to -1; $p = 0.04$).

Table 3. Simulated effect size for sodium density (mg Na/MJ energy) if sodium reduction were applied to a wider range of breads.

Scenario	Effect Size (95% CI)	*p*
Observed	−8 (−18 to 2)	0.14
100% Implementation	−9 (−19 to 2)	0.11
25% Reduction in wholemeal	−10 (−21 to 0)	0.06
25% Reduction in all Bush Oven loaves	−11 (−21 to 0)	0.05
25% Reduction in all bread	−12 (−23 to −1)	0.03

Effect size is the difference between control and intervention groups from baseline to follow-up periods in change in sodium density (mg Na/100 g) in total food and drink purchases analysed using mixed model analysis with group and period as main and interaction terms.

3.3. Comments about Bread

Of the nine planned calls to each of the store managers, we successfully contacted store managers a median of seven times each, with a median of seven phone calls (range six to eight) in the intervention group and seven (range one to eight) in the control group. Thirteen comments were recorded relating to quality from eight individual stores (Table 4). Of these, one comment from an intervention store was related to improved quality and twelve comments were related to decreased quality (six from intervention; six from control stores). There were an equal proportion of stores in each group that reported comments related to reduced quality of the bread (27%; *n* = 4/15 in intervention and *n* = 3/11 in control groups). Most comments came from store managers, except one comment from customers for each group.

Table 4. Number of stores in each group where customers or store managers made comments related to quality of study bread.

Comment Type	Control (*n* = 11)	Intervention (*n* = 15)
Improved quality	0	1
Tastes better	0	1
Decreased quality	3	4
Tastes worse	2	2
Shelf life/freshness	1	2
Texture	2	1
Size	0	1

Values may not add up to total where a store has made comments across multiple categories.

4. Discussion

We found that 25% salt reduction did not affect sales of one of the top-selling breads in remote Indigenous communities. In addition to no effect on sales, comments from customers did not indicate dissatisfaction with the bread. This is consistent with our consumer acceptance testing, where consumers could not detect the difference between the reduced salt versus regular salt bread [11].

Small incremental sodium reductions (sometimes referred to as step-wise changes) are often preferred by food manufacturers to avoid detection by consumers. Mean sodium levels in bread were decreased by ~40 mg/100 g, or 8.6% over three years in Australia [19], and by 100 mg/100 g or 20% over 10 years in the United Kingdom [20]. However, in a recent meta-analysis, we found that sodium could be reduced by up to 40% in bread (from an average of 692 to 484 mg Na/100 g) in a single step change without affecting consumer acceptance [21]. Quilez and Salas-Salvadó (2015) examined change in sales when salt was reduced in par-baked breads distributed in Spain [22]. In this study, sodium content of nine par-baked breads (delivered to stores frozen and baked on-site to be sold to customers) was reduced by an average of 27.7% from 577 to 417 mg Na/100 g, and potassium citrate was added to partially replace the salt content [22]. Sales in the year following salt reduction (3678 tonnes) were not reduced when compared to the year prior to salt reduction (3577 tonnes). Nor was there an increase in customer complaints. Saavedra-Garcia et al. (2016) also found no reduction in sales when salt was reduced by 20% in a "pan frances" bread sold through a bakery in Peru [23]. Our findings are consistent with these studies, and add to the evidence that considerable sodium reductions in bread can be made in a single step change without affecting commercial viability.

Our study, and the studies by Saavedra-Garcia et al. [23] and Quilez and Salaz-Salvadó [22], did not label the breads as lower salt. Most comments in the present study indicating that the bread was different came from store managers, who were aware of the study, but not of their store's allocation. These comments came in equal proportions from the control group as the intervention group, indicating that store employees perceived a difference because they were expecting the bread to be different or due to attention bias. There is evidence that labelling foods as no/low/reduced salt can influence expectation and taste perception [24,25]. Liem et al. (2012) found that when soups were labelled "now with reduced salt", participants expected to like them less than the same soups without the labelling [25]. They found that this effect persisted after tasting the soups, with participants reporting lower liking of the labelled soups than the same soup without the label [25]. As foods perceived as healthier are often perceived as being less palatable, food manufacturers often prefer to use a "stealth health" approach to salt reduction, without labelling the product as reduced salt or otherwise drawing the sodium reduction to consumers' attention [26,27]. It is likely that adopting this "stealth health" approach was important for maintaining sales.

Reduction to 300 mg Na/100 g would place the Bush Oven high fibre white bread as one of the lowest sodium breads on remote Indigenous community store shelves [6], and the wider Australian market [19,28]. In 2010, the mean sodium content of Australian breads was 435 ± 84 mg Na/100 g in 2010, ranging from 235 to 775 mg Na/100 g [28], while a 2011 estimate indicated a mean sodium content of 415 mg/100 g [19]. By comparison, mean sodium content of breads in the United Kingdom (UK) was 380 ± 70 (range 230–791) mg Na/100 g in 2011 [20]. The UK has achieved this by progressively lowering its target for breads, with the current target of an average of 350 mg/100 g to be achieved by 2017 [29]. The wide range of sodium content in Australian breads, and relatively lower sodium content of breads in the UK, suggest that there is considerable potential for further sodium reductions in bread in Australia.

A secondary aim of this study was to observe the effect on sodium density of all purchased foods and drinks. We projected that reducing sodium in the study bread by 25% would reduce sodium density in purchased foods and drinks by 11 mg Na/MJ. Using an average energy intake of 8.9 MJ/day (based on estimated energy requirements as previously calculated in a similar population [6], and sodium density of purchases of 317 mg Na/MJ (as observed at baseline), this would be equal to a 100 mg/day reduction from 2820 mg/day to 2720 mg/day, or 12% of the reduction needed to reduce sodium to the WHO target. While the values at baseline and follow up in the intervention group correspond with this, the difference from the change in the control group was not statistically significant. It is unlikely that this is due to compensation for the reduced salt bread by increasing the sodium density of other foods purchased, and possibly indicates that we had insufficient power to detect the difference in sodium density.

When we modelled 25% sodium reduction across all breads, significant reductions of -12 (-23 to -1; $p = 0.03$) mg/MJ were estimated, equal to a 3.8% reduction from baseline intake in the intervention group. Using an average energy intake of 8.9 MJ/day, a 12 mg/MJ reduction is equal to approximately 110 mg Na/day, which is 13% of the reduction needed to meet the WHO target. Using an alternative average energy intake of 8.5 MJ/day (as per the remote sample of the Australian Aboriginal and Torres Strait Islander Health Survey 2012–2013) [9], the projected sodium reduction would equal approximately 15% of the reduction needed to meet the WHO target. While a sodium reduction of 3.8% or 110 mg/day may seem small, it has the potential to be clinically significant at the population level [12,13,30]. Cobiac et al. (2010) modelled the health benefits and cost-effectiveness of interventions to reduce sodium intake in the Australian adult population [30]. It was estimated that mandatory reduction of the sodium content of Australian breads (to 450 mg Na/100 g), cereals, and margarines would reduce population sodium intake by 5%, leading to health gains of 110,000 (95% uncertainty index (UI) 53,000 to 180,000) disability-adjusted life years (DALYs) and health care savings of $1.5 (0.7 to 2.8) billion Australian dollars. Even in the voluntary reformulation scenario where sodium intake was reduced by only 0.2%, significant health gains (5300 DALYS, 95% UI 2600 to 9200) and reduction in health care costs (77 (37–140) million AUD) were estimated [30]. Nghiem et al. (2016) modelled salt reduction in bread and found significant health gains of 15,600 quality adjusted life years (95% UI 12,600 to 18,900) and health care savings of $83 million NZD (61 to 110) with only modest reduction in sodium intake of 2.3% or 81.5 mg/day [31]. Salt reduction in bread is a cost-effective intervention that has the potential to reduce sodium intake by small but potentially clinically significant magnitudes in the remote Indigenous Australian population, but more wide-spread reduction across the food supply is needed to meet the WHO target [6].

There are several limitations to this study. It may have been underpowered to detect a difference in the outcomes, particularly sodium density. In sensitivity analysis, there was a significant reduction in sodium density if one control store was dropped. Further, when salt reduction was modelled across all breads, the projected reduction was statistically significant, despite the change in effect size from the original analyses being small. This suggests that the variation in the data may have been larger than the effect size, precluding a significant result. This is less of a concern for the sales-related outcomes; while market share was trending towards a reduction compared to control, average weekly dollars was slightly increased, although neither were statistically significant. Further, sensitivity analyses were consistent in indicating no significant effect on sales; therefore, we are confident in our conclusion that sales were not affected.

A further limitation is that we were unable to randomise the study. Due to this, there was a geographical imbalance between the groups, with more intervention stores located in Top-End Australia, and more control stores located in Central Australia. There is a larger degree of temperature variation in Central Australia compared with the Top-End [32], which may have affected purchasing patterns over the study periods, although this is unlikely to be specifically related to bread purchases. While intervention stores appeared to have higher total food and drink revenue at baseline (indicating they may have been servicing a larger population), this difference was not statistically significant, and the proportion of the study bread sales to total sales (market share) was similar between groups.

Finally, the uniqueness of this population may limit transferability to other settings. Most of the communities in this study had access to only one or two stores from which they could purchase bread; therefore, it would be useful to examine change in sales in an urban setting with easy access to several food vendors and a greater variety of breads from which to choose.

Despite these limitations, our study has several strengths. We tested the bread in a "real-life" setting by replacing the regular product with the lower sodium product on store shelves, rather than conducting testing in a research setting. Our study population included a considerable number of communities spread over a large geographical region with a high proportion of consumers of the study bread. Our main study outcomes were objective, and we collected data on all food and drink sales during the study period, which allowed us to track change in market share of the product and to examine whether sodium reduction was compensated for by increasing sodium density of other purchases. We were also able to determine the impact on sales, an outcome considered of key importance to manufacturers.

5. Conclusions

There is considerable potential for further sodium reduction in breads to reduce population salt intakes in remote Indigenous Australian communities. We found that it was possible to reduce salt by 25% in a top-selling bread without affecting sales in remote Indigenous community stores. This adds to the evidence that considerable sodium reductions can be made in bread without jeopardising commercial viability. Twenty-five percent salt reduction across all breads could reduce estimated salt intake in remote Indigenous Australian communities by approximately 15% of the magnitude needed to achieve the WHO target, which has the potential to lead to health gains at the population-level. More wide-spread reductions across the food supply will help to meet the WHO salt reduction target.

Supplementary Materials: The following are available online at http://www.mdpi.com/2072-6643/9/3/214/s1, Table S1: Outcomes for each of the study periods, Table S2.1: Description of outliers.

Acknowledgments: We are grateful to the Act on Salt research collaborative; Independent Grocers; Goodman Fielder; Arnhem Land Progress Aboriginal Corporation (ALPA); Outback Stores (OBS); and participating communities and store employees. We specifically thank the following people who contributed to study operations: Anthony Gunther, Robyn Liddle, Federica Barzi (statistician), Madelaine Griffith (ALPA), Jen Savenake (OBS), Coral Coyler (Goodman Fielder), Jennie Collis (Independent Grocers) & Shirley Smith (Independent Grocers). E.M. is supported by a NHMRC Program Grant #631947, and the Australian Primary Health Care Research Institute (supported by a grant from the Commonwealth of Australia as represented by the Department of Health). J.B. is supported by a National Heart Foundation (NHF) Future Leader Fellowship (ID: 100085). J.W. is supported by a NHMRC/NHF Career Development Fellowship #172121 and receives additional funds from the NHMRC, the World Health Organization (WHO) and the Victorian Health Promotion Foundation (VicHealth) for work on salt reduction. The funders had no role in study design, data collection and analysis, decision to publish, or preparation of the manuscript. The information and opinions contained in this paper are solely the responsibility of the authors and do not necessarily reflect the views or policy of NHMRC, the Australian Primary Health Care Research Institute, Australian Government Department of Health, NHF, WHO or VicHealth.

Author Contributions: J.B. conceived the study. All authors contributed to study design. E.M. collected and analysed the data. All authors contributed to interpretation of results. E.M. wrote the manuscript. All authors contributed to writing the manuscript and approved the final version.

Conflicts of Interest: We previously conducted a consumer acceptance testing study that was partially funded by Goodman Fielder Limited. Data analysis and interpretation in both the consumer acceptance study and the present study were performed independently from Goodman Fielder.

References

1. Forouzanfar, M.H.; Alexander, L.; Anderson, H.R.; Bachman, V.F.; Biryukov, S.; Brauer, M.; Burnett, R.; Casey, D.; Coates, M.M.; Cohen, A.; et al. Global, regional, and national comparative risk assessment of 79 behavioural, environmental and occupational, and metabolic risks or clusters of risks in 188 countries, 1990–2013: A systematic analysis for the Global Burden of Disease Study 2013. *Lancet* **2015**, *386*, 2287–2323. [CrossRef]

2. Trieu, K.; Neal, B.; Hawkes, C.; Dunford, E.; Campbell, N.; Rodriguez-Fernandez, R.; Legetic, B.; McLaren, L.; Barberio, A.; Webster, J. Salt Reduction Initiatives around the World—A Systematic Review of Progress towards the Global Target. *PLoS ONE* **2015**, *10*, e0130247. [CrossRef] [PubMed]

3. 3302.0.55.003—Life Tables for Aboriginal and Torres Strait Islander Australians, 2010–2012. Available online: http://www.abs.gov.au/ausstats/abs@.nsf/mf/3302.0.55.003 (accessed on 23 February 2017).

4. Australian Burden of Disease Study: Impact and Causes of Illness and Death in Aboriginal and Torres Strait Islander People 2011. Available online: http://www.aihw.gov.au/publication-detail/?id=60129557110 (accessed on 23 February 2017).

5. Australian Institute of Health And Welfare. Australia's Health 2016. Available online: http://www.aihw.gov.au/publication-detail/?id=60129555544 (accessed on 23 February 2017).

6. McMahon, E.; Webster, J.; O'Dea, K.; Brimblecombe, J. Dietary sodium and iodine in remote Indigenous Australian communities: Will salt-reduction strategies increase risk of iodine deficiency? A cross-sectional analysis and simulation study. *BMC Public Health* **2015**, *15*, 1318. [CrossRef] [PubMed]

7. Brimblecombe, J.; Ferguson, M.; Chatfield, M.D.; Liberato, S.C.; Gunther, A.; Ball, K.; Moodie, M.; Miles, E.; Magnus, A.; Mhurchu, C.N.; et al. Effect of a price discount and consumer education strategy on food and beverage purchases in remote Indigenous Australia: A stepped-wedge randomised controlled trial. *Lancet Public Health* **2017**, *2*, e82–e95. [CrossRef]

8. Brimblecombe, J.; Ferguson, M.; Liberato, S.C.; O'Dea, K.; Riley, M. Optimisation modelling to assess cost of dietary improvement in remote Aboriginal Australia. *PLoS ONE* **2013**, *8*, e83587. [CrossRef] [PubMed]

9. 4364.0.55.007—Australian Health Survey: Nutrition First Results—Foods and Nutrients, 2011–12. Available online: http://www.abs.gov.au/ausstats/abs@.nsf/Lookup/4364.0.55.007main+features12011-12 (accessed on 23 February 2017).

10. National Health & Medical Research Council. Eat for Health Educator Guide—Information for Nutrition Educators. Available online: https://www.eatforhealth.gov.au/sites/default/files/files/the_guidelines/n55b_eat_for_health_educators_guide.pdf (accessed on 23 February 2017).

11. McMahon, E.; Clarke, R.; Jaenke, R.; Brimblecombe, J. Detection of 12.5% and 25% Salt Reduction in Bread in a Remote Indigenous Australian Community. *Nutrients* **2016**, *8*, 169. [CrossRef] [PubMed]

12. Gillespie, D.O.; Allen, K.; Guzman-Castillo, M.; Bandosz, P.; Moreira, P.; McGill, R.; Anwar, E.; Lloyd-Williams, F.; Bromley, H.; Diggle, P.J.; et al. The Health Equity and Effectiveness of Policy Options to Reduce Dietary Salt Intake in England: Policy Forecast. *PLoS ONE* **2015**, *10*, e0127927.

13. Wilson, N.; Nghiem, N.; Eyles, H.; Mhurchu, C.N.; Shields, E.; Cobiac, L.J.; Cleghorn, C.L.; Blakely, T. Modeling health gains and cost savings for ten dietary salt reduction targets. *Nutr. J.* **2016**, *15*, 44. [CrossRef] [PubMed]

14. Cobiac, L.J.; Magnus, A.; Lim, S.; Barendregt, J.J.; Carter, R.; Vos, T. Which interventions offer best value for money in primary prevention of cardiovascular disease? *PLoS ONE* **2012**, *7*, e41842. [CrossRef] [PubMed]

15. Australian Bureau of Statistics. 4710.0—Housing and Infrastructure in Aboriginal and Torres Strait Islander Communities, Australia. 2006. Available online: http://www.abs.gov.au/ausstats/abs@.nsf/mf/4710.0 (accessed on 23 February 2017).

16. Wycherley, T.; Ferguson, M.; O'Dea, K.; McMahon, E.; Liberato, S.; Brimblecombe, J. Store turnover as a predictor of food and beverage provider turnover and associated dietary intake estimates in very remote Indigenous communities. *Aust. N. Z. J. Public Health* **2016**, *40*, 569–571. [CrossRef] [PubMed]

17. Brimblecombe, J.; Liddle, R.; O'Dea, K. Use of point-of-sale data to assess food and nutrient quality in remote stores. *Public Health Nutr.* **2013**, *16*, 1159–1167. [CrossRef] [PubMed]

18. Food Standards Australia New Zealand. AUSNUT 2011–2013—Australian Food Composition Database. Available online: http://www.foodstandards.gov.au/science/monitoringnutrients/ausnut/pages/default.aspx (accessed on 23 February 2017).

19. Trevena, H.; Neal, B.; Dunford, E.; Wu, J.H.Y. An Evaluation of the Effects of the Australian Food and Health Dialogue Targets on the Sodium Content of Bread, Breakfast Cereals and Processed Meats. *Nutrients* **2014**, *6*, 3802–3817. [CrossRef] [PubMed]

20. Brinsden, H.C.; He, F.J.; Jenner, K.H.; Macgregor, G.A. Surveys of the salt content in UK bread: Progress made and further reductions possible. *BMJ Open* **2013**, *3*. [CrossRef] [PubMed]

21. Jaenke, R.; Barzi, F.; McMahon, E.; Webster, J.; Brimblecombe, J. Consumer Acceptance of Reformulated Food Products: A Systematic Review and Meta-analysis of Salt-reduced Foods. *Crit. Rev. Food Sci. Nutr.* **2016**. [CrossRef] [PubMed]

22. Quilez, J.; Salas-Salvadó, J. The feasibility and acceptability of reducing salt in partially baked bread: A Spanish case study. *Public Health Nutr.* **2016**, *19*, 983–987. [CrossRef] [PubMed]

23. Saavedra-Garcia, L.; Sosa-Zevallos, V.; Diez-Canseco, F.; Miranda, J.J.; Bernabe-Ortiz, A. Reducing salt in bread: A quasi-experimental feasibility study in a bakery in Lima, Peru. *Public Health Nutr.* **2016**, *19*, 976–982. [CrossRef] [PubMed]

24. Raghunathan, R.; Naylor, R.W.; Hoyer, W.D. The unhealthy = Tasty intuition and its effects on taste inferences, enjoyment, and choice of food products. *J. Mark.* **2006**, *70*, 170–184. [CrossRef]

25. Liem, D.G.; Miremadi, F.; Zandstra, E.H.; Keast, R.S.J. Health labelling can influence taste perception and use of table salt for reduced-sodium products. *Public Health Nutr.* **2012**, *15*, 2340–2347. [CrossRef] [PubMed]

26. Antman, E.M.; Appel, L.J.; Balentine, D.; Johnson, R.K.; Steffen, L.M.; Miller, E.A.; Pappas, A.; Stitzel, K.F.; Vafiadis, D.K.; Whitsel, L. Stakeholder discussion to reduce population-wide sodium intake and decrease sodium in the food supply a conference report from the American Heart Association Sodium Conference 2013 Planning Group. *Circulation* **2014**, *129*, e660–e679. [CrossRef] [PubMed]

27. Mintel Group Limited. Low/No/Reduced Sodium NPD Claims Decline Despite Salt Concerns. Available online: http://www.mintel.com/press-centre/social-and-lifestyle/lownoreduced-sodium-npd-claims-decline-despite-salt-concerns (accessed on 12 October 2016).

28. Dunford, E.K.; Eyles, H.; Mhurchu, C.N.; Webster, J.L.; Neal, B.C. Changes in the sodium content of bread in Australia and New Zealand between 2007 and 2010: Implications for policy. *Med. J. Aust.* **2011**, *195*, 346–349. [CrossRef] [PubMed]

29. Food Standards Agency. Salt Reduction Targets for 2017. Available online: https://www.food.gov.uk/northern-ireland/nutritionni/salt-ni/salt_targets (accessed on 14 October 2016).

30. Cobiac, L.J.; Vos, T.; Veerman, J.L. Cost-effectiveness of interventions to reduce dietary salt intake. *Heart* **2010**, *96*, 1920–1925. [CrossRef] [PubMed]

31. Nghiem, N.; Blakely, T.; Cobiac, L.J.; Cleghorn, C.L.; Wilson, N. The health gains and cost savings of dietary salt reduction interventions, with equity and age distributional aspects. *BMC Public Health* **2016**, *16*, 423. [CrossRef] [PubMed]

32. Bureau of Meteorology. Maps of Average Conditions. Available online: http://www.bom.gov.au/jsp/ncc/climate_averages/temperature/index.jsp (accessed on 10 November 2016).

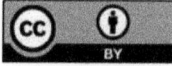

nutrients

MDPI

Article

The Sodium Content of Processed Foods in South Africa during the Introduction of Mandatory Sodium Limits

Sanne A. E. Peters [1,*], Elizabeth Dunford [2,3], Lisa J. Ware [4], Teresa Harris [5], Adele Walker [5], Mariaan Wicks [6], Tertia van Zyl [6], Bianca Swanepoel [6], Karen E. Charlton [7], Mark Woodward [1,3,8], Jacqui Webster [3] and Bruce Neal [3,9,10,11]

1   The George Institute for Global Health, University of Oxford, Oxford OX1 3QX, UK;
    markw@georgeinstitute.org.au
2   Carolina Population Center, University of North Carolina, Chapel Hill, NC 27516, USA;
    edunford@georgeinstitute.org.au
3   The George Institute for Global Health, University of Sydney, Sydney, NSW 2050, Australia;
    jwebster@georgeinstitute.org.au (J.W.); bneal@georgeinstitute.org.au (B.N.)
4   Hypertension in Africa Research Team, North West University, Potchefstroom 2520, South Africa;
    lisa.ware@nwu.ac.za
5   Discovery Vitality, Sandton 2146, South Africa; terryh@discovery.co.za (T.H.);
    adelewa@discovery.co.za (A.W.)
6   Center of Excellence for Nutrition, North West University, Potchefstroom 2520, South Africa;
    13009494@nwu.ac.za (M.W.); tertia.vanzyl@nwu.ac.za (T.v.Z.); biancaswanepoel.nwu@gmail.com (B.S.)
7   School of Medicine, University of Wollongong, Wollongong, NSW 2522, Australia; karenc@uow.edu.au
8   Department of Epidemiology, Johns Hopkins University, Baltimore, MD 21218, USA
9   The Charles Perkins Centre, University of Sydney, Sydney, NSW 2006, Australia
10 Royal Prince Alfred Hospital, Sydney, NSW 2050, Australia
11 Imperial College London, London SW7 2AZ, UK
*   Correspondence: sanne.peters@georgeinstitute.ox.ac.uk; Tel.: +44-1865-617-200; Fax: +44-1865-617-202

Received: 9 March 2017; Accepted: 17 April 2017; Published: 20 April 2017

Abstract: Background: In June 2016, the Republic of South Africa introduced legislation for mandatory limits for the upper sodium content permitted in a wide range of processed foods. We assessed the sodium levels of packaged foods in South Africa during the one-year period leading up to the mandatory implementation date of the legislation. Methods: Data on the nutritional composition of packaged foods was obtained from nutrition information panels on food labels through both in-store surveys and crowdsourcing by users of the HealthyFood Switch mobile phone app between June 2015 and August 2016. Summary sodium levels were calculated for 15 food categories, including the 13 categories covered by the sodium legislation. The percentage of foods that met the government's 2016 sodium limits was also calculated. Results: 11,065 processed food items were included in the analyses; 1851 of these were subject to the sodium legislation. Overall, 67% of targeted foods had a sodium level at or below the legislated limit. Categories with the lowest percentage of foods that met legislated limits were bread (27%), potato crisps (41%), salt and vinegar flavoured snacks (42%), and raw processed sausages (45%). About half (49%) of targeted foods not meeting the legislated limits were less than 25% above the maximum sodium level. Conclusion: Sodium levels in two-thirds of foods covered by the South African sodium legislation were at or below the permitted upper levels at the mandatory implementation date of the legislation and many more were close to the limit. The South African food industry has an excellent opportunity to rapidly meet the legislated requirements.

Keywords: salt intake; sodium legislation; South Africa; packaged food; nutritional composition

1. Introduction

Excess dietary salt intake is associated with elevated blood pressure, a major risk factor for cardiovascular diseases [1,2]. In 2010, an estimated 1.65 million cardiovascular deaths worldwide—or 1 out of every 10 cardiovascular deaths—were attributed to salt consumption above the World Health Organization (WHO) recommended intake of 5 g per day [3,4]. Salt reduction has been described by the WHO as one of the best investments to improve public health and an efficient and cost-effective way to decrease the burden of elevated blood pressure and cardiovascular diseases [5].

In 2013, WHO Member States adopted the global target of a 30% reduction of mean population intake of salt by 2025, as part of a broader set of strategies to reduce premature mortality from non-communicable diseases by 25% in 2025 [6]. A growing number of countries are developing and implementing strategies to reduce salt intake, including, but not limited to, food supply reformulations, front of package labelling, taxation, consumer education, and interventions in public institutions [7,8]. For many countries, these strategies are voluntary or restricted to a limited number of food products [9].

The Republic of South Africa was the first country globally to develop comprehensive, mandatory legislation to reduce sodium levels across a wide range of processed food categories, which involved the co-operation of many food industry members from various sectors [10,11]. It is estimated that about half of daily salt intake in South Africa derives from processed foods, with bread being the greatest contributor to non-discretionary salt intake [12,13]. The South African sodium legislation was passed by the Department of Health in 2013 and set restrictions regarding the maximum levels of sodium allowed in several commonly consumed foods which, in addition to bread, include breakfast cereals, margarines, meat products, snack foods, and soup mixes [10]. A few products that are high in sodium, such as biltong ("jerky") and soy sauce, were exempted due to their relatively low contribution to sodium in the South African diet. The legislation aims to reduce the amount of sodium in specific foods in two waves; the first came into force in June 2016 and the second, with lower sodium targets, will come into effect in June 2019. If successful, this new strategy to reduce sodium in the food supply is expected to save thousands of lives annually and to yield substantial cost savings to the South African health service [14,15].

To measure progress in reducing the sodium levels of foods, identify challenges, and track changes over time, an assessment of the current sodium levels of processed foods in South Africa is needed. In the present study, we used data from nutrition information panels on food labels to evaluate the sodium levels of packaged foods in South Africa during the one-year period leading up to the implementation date for the legislation.

2. Methods

2.1. Data Sources

A database with information on the nutritional composition of packaged foods available for consumer purchase in South Africa was established through in-store surveys and crowdsourcing of food labels by users of the HealthyFood Switch mobile phone app [16]. Store surveys were done through collaboration with Discovery, South Africa's largest private health insurance company. Part of Discovery's health promotion programme is Vitality, which partners with selected South African retailers to offer the HealthyFood benefit [17]. Researchers visited major South African retail stores in Johannesburg, including Woolworths, Pick n Pay, Spar, and Shoprite Checkers, and took photos of all packaged food and beverage items using The George Institute's Data Collector smartphone application and the HealthyFood Switch smartphone application [18]. These applications enable the user to scan the barcode of a packaged food item, and then take multiple photographs of the item to capture the product name, nutritional information, and ingredient list. These data are then used to populate a database from which the HealthyFood Switch smartphone app draws information. Consumers can use this app to scan the barcodes of packaged foods using their smartphone camera, which will then display on-screen, easy-to-interpret nutritional information along with suggestions for similar, but healthier, alternative products. When a product is not present in the database, the user is asked to send photographs of the nutrition information panel (NIP), the list of ingredients, and the front of the package via the crowdsourcing function integrated in the HealthyFood Switch app. Crowdsourcing occurred at a national level, not only in Johannesburg.

2.2. Data Entry

Product images, whether collected by in-store surveys or crowdsourcing, are sent to a central electronic holding area where a group of trained researchers then enter the nutrient data into the HealthyFood Switch database. Data entry and quality checking protocols have been described previously [16]. The current database holds records on ~15,000 food products entered between June 2015 and August 2016. Information on energy, total fat, saturated fat, total carbohydrate, sugars, fibre, protein, and sodium levels of foods are virtually complete as they are required to be declared on all food labels in South Africa. For the present study, only food products with nutritional information, including sodium, presented per 100 g (or per 100 mL) on the package NIP were included. Of these, ~85% of packages had nutritional information per 100 g of product "as sold", the remaining 15% also, or exclusively, reported nutritional information per 100 g of the product, "as prepared". Foods without a NIP or with multiple NIPs (e.g., variety packs) were excluded. In case of exact duplicates, the most recently entered product was used. The data were cross-sectional and reformulations of foods could not be evaluated.

2.3. Definition of Food Categories

Classification of products followed the food categorisation system of the Global Food Monitoring Group; a standardized system set up to systematically and transparently assess the nutrient composition of processed foods around the world [19]. This hierarchical system classifies foods into groups (e.g., bread), categories (e.g., flat bread), and subcategories (e.g., pita bread), thereby allowing for international comparisons of foods at the group level, while leaving flexibility at the category and subcategory level. The South African HealthyFood Switch database categorisation system contains 15 food groups, 57 food categories, and up to three additional levels of increasingly more specific subcategories. For example, pork sausages are classified in the food group 'meat and meat products', food category 'processed meat', level 1 subcategory 'sausages and hotdogs', level 2 subcategory 'sausages', and level 3 subcategory 'pork sausages'. Foods targeted by the South African sodium legislation were identified by mapping the applicable food subcategories to the categories set out in the legislation. A list of the targeted foods and sodium allowances is provided in Table 1.

Table 1. Maximum total sodium levels allowed in certain foodstuffs in South Africa as at June 2016 and June 2019.

Foodstuff Category	Maximum Total Sodium per 100 g per June 2016, Mg	Maximum Total Sodium per 100 g per June 2019, Mg
Bread	400	380
Breakfast cereals and porridges	500	400
Fat and butter spreads	550	450
Savoury snacks, not salt and vinegar flavoured	800	700
Potato crisps	650	550
Savoury snacks, salt and vinegar flavoured	1000	850
Processed meat, uncured	850	650
Processed meat, cured	950	850
Processed meat sausages, raw	800	600
Soup powder, dry	5500	3500
Gravy powders and savoury sauces, dry	3500	1500
Savoury powders with instant noodles, dry	1500	800
Stock cubes, powders, granules, emulsions, pastes, or jellies	18,000	13,000

2.4. Statistical Analyses

Summary statistics of the sodium levels per 100 g were obtained for each food category, and separately for each food group targeted by the sodium legislation. Medians are reported in the text as these are least affected by extreme large or small values and may give more robust 'typical' values. The percentage of targeted foods that met the legislated limits and the amount and percentage by which sodium limits were exceeded were also calculated. For some food groups and categories, only a subset of all foods within that category are targeted by the sodium legislation, that is, the sodium legislation targets a subset of meats and only dry (i.e., powdered) mixes for soups, sauces, stocks, and gravy. For these food categories, we also obtained the summary sodium levels for the individual subcategories. All analyses were carried out in R version 3.3.0 (R Foundation for Statistical Computing, Vienna, Austria).

3. Results

After removing duplicates and products with ineligible or insufficient information on nutritional composition on the NIPs, 11,065 foods were included in the analyses. Of these, 20% were beverages, 16% were processed fruits and vegetable products, 10% were sauces and spreads, 9% were dairy products, 8% were cereal and cereal products, 8% were bread and bakery products, 6% were confectionery, 5% were convenience foods, 5% were meat or meat products, 3% were fish and fish products, and 3% were snack foods.

3.1. Median Sodium Level

There was substantial variation in the sodium level of processed foods within and between food categories (Table A1). The food groups with the highest median sodium level were snack foods (746 mg/100 g), followed by meat and meat products (734 mg/100 g), and sauces and spreads (673 mg/100 g). Cereal and cereal products (70 mg/100 g), fruit and vegetable products (22 mg/100 g), confectionery (66 mg/100 g), and dairy (50 mg/100 g) had relatively lower median sodium levels. Within food groups, food categories with the highest median sodium levels were soups (2017 mg/100 g), sauces (999 mg/100 g), meal kits (939 mg/100 g), cheeses (554 mg/100 g), breads (476 mg/100 g), and noodles (470 mg/100 g). Food categories with the lowest sodium levels included several cereal products (e.g., pasta, maize, rice, couscous; all <10 mg/100 g) and dairy products, excluding cheeses (all <100 mg/100 g).

3.2. Sodium Levels of Foods Targeted by the Sodium Legislation

The median sodium level of foods targeted by the sodium legislation ranged from 171 mg/100 g for breakfast cereals and porridges to 4782 mg/100 g for dry soup powders (Table 2). Other targeted food groups with very high median sodium levels (i.e., >1000 mg/100 g) were stock (3075 mg/100 g), gravy powders and savoury sauces (3029 mg/100 g), instant savoury powders with noodles (1123 mg/100 g), and salt and vinegar flavoured snacks (1094 mg/100 g). Overall, 67% of all targeted foods had a sodium level below the legislated maximum (Figure 1). Categories with less than 50% of all products achieving the legislated maximum sodium level were bread (27%), potato crisps (41%), salt and vinegar flavoured snacks (42%), and raw processed sausages (45%) (Figure 1). Over 90% of breakfast cereals and porridges and uncured processed meats had sodium levels below the legislated maximum allowed.

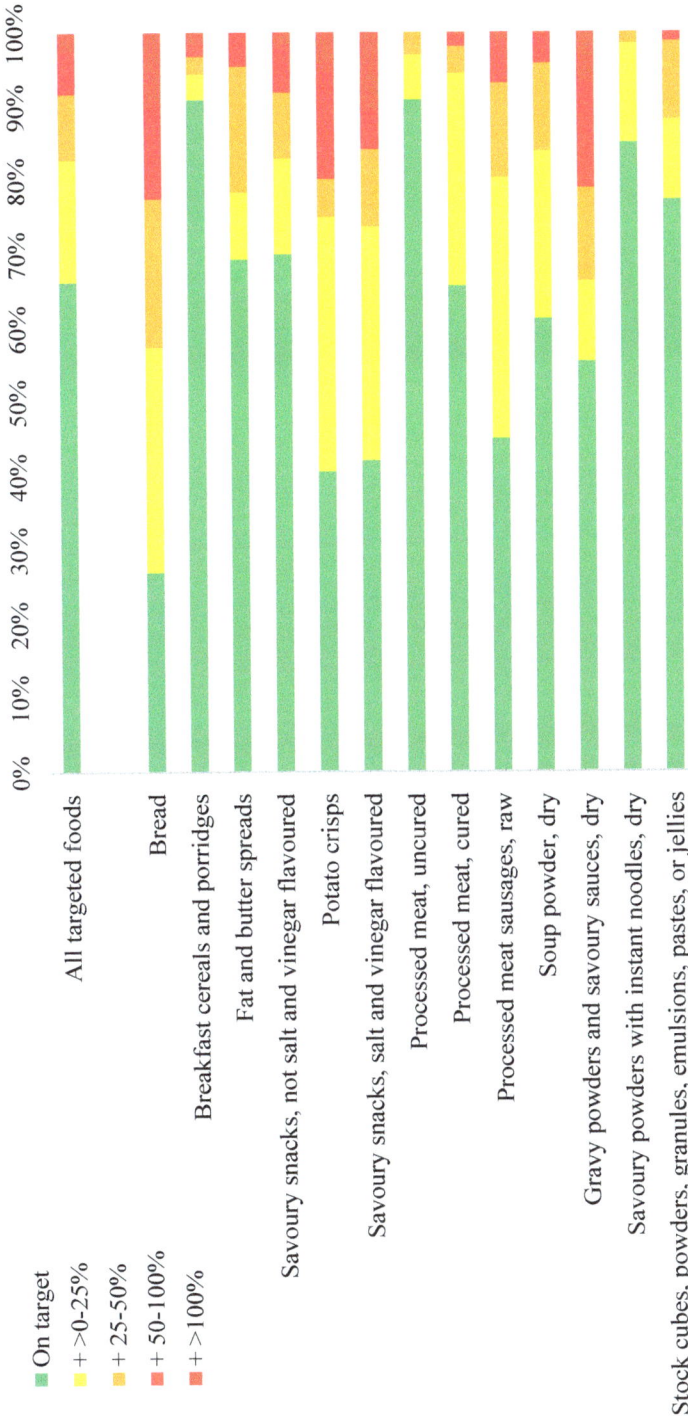

Figure 1. Foods targeted by the sodium legislation according to 2016 sodium limits. Region shaded in green is for foods with sodium levels at or below the sodium limit. The regions shaded in yellow, orange, red, and dark red are for foods with sodium levels 0%–25%, 25%–50%, 50%–100%, or more than 100% above the sodium limit. The maximum total sodium levels allowed in food categories covered by the sodium legislation are given in Table 1. Current sodium levels for targeted foods are provided in Table 2.

Table 2. Sodium levels of soups, stocks, gravies and sauces (*n* = 962), in mg per 100 g.

Foodstuff Category	No. of Products	Minimum	25%	Median	Mean	75%	Maximum
Bread	174	39	388	476	542	593	2470
Breakfast cereals and porridges	376	0	46	171	262	346	4180
Fat and butter spreads	88	0	339	400	428	625	826
Savoury snacks, not salt and vinegar flavoured	417	0	42	480	519	857	2296
Potato crisps	96	175	554	702	721	802	1670
Savoury snacks, salt and vinegar flavoured	19	510	807	1094	1173	1258	2851
Processed meat, uncured	33	44	500	638	618	784	1065
Processed meat, cured	108	0	656	864	836	998	1667
Processed meat sausages, raw	102	426	708	826	851	914	2213
Soup powder, dry	168	123	2842	4782	4505	6366	9180
Gravy powders and savoury sauces, dry	119	186	500	3029	3197	4997	10,960
Savoury powders with instant noodles, dry	67	1	313	1123	887	1314	1876
Stock cubes, powders, granules, emulsions, pastes, or jellies	84	217	1252	3075	9122	17,270	27,010

3.3. Sodium Reductions Needed to Meet the Sodium Target

Of targeted foods exceeding the legislated limits, sodium levels would need to be reduced by a quarter or less for 49% of these foods, by 25%–50% for 26% of foods, by 50%–100% for 17% of foods, and by more than 100% for 7% of foods (Figure 1 and Table A2). In absolute terms, the median reductions in sodium levels required to meet the limits were 110 mg/100 g for breads, 136 mg/100 g for potato crisps, 236 mg/100 g for salt and vinegar flavoured snacks, and 108 mg/100 g for raw processed sausages. Almost 50% of all gravy powders and savoury sauces exceeding the sodium limit, did so by 50% of the limit or more, equating to a median excess sodium level of 1700 mg/100 g.

3.4. Sodium Levels within Categories Partially Targeted by the Sodium Legislation

The sodium legislation only targets a subset of meats and only dry (i.e., powdered) mixes for soups, sauces, stocks, and gravy. The median sodium levels of meat products targeted by the legislation was 638 mg/100 g for uncured processed meats, 864 mg/100 g for cured processed meats, and 826 mg/100 g for raw processed sausages. Sodium levels were higher in meats not targeted by the legislation; bacon, salami, and biltong, had a median sodium level of 1070 mg/100 g, 1674 mg/100 g, and 2079 mg/100 g, respectively (Figure 2 and Table A3). Canned and chilled soups, also not targeted by the legislation, had median sodium levels of 373 mg/100 g, and 303 mg/100 g, respectively. Stocks and gravy sold as liquid contained a median of 4000 mg and 429 mg of sodium per 100 g, respectively. Sauces not covered by the legislation that were high in sodium were curry pastes (2400 mg/100 g), Asian sauces (2499 mg/100 g), mustard (1760 mg/100 g), and table sauces (988 mg/100 g) (Table 3).

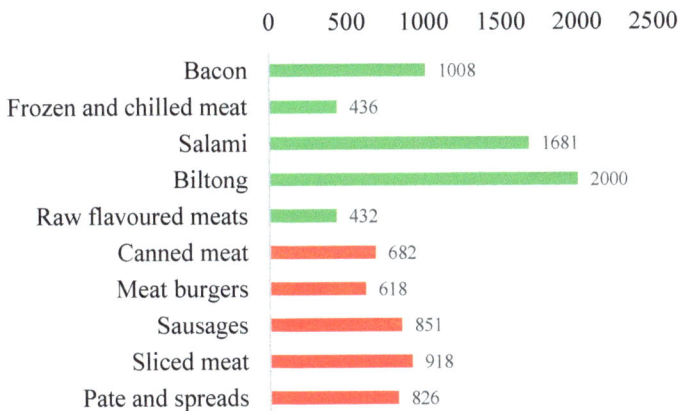

Figure 2. Mean sodium levels of processed meat subcategories in mg per 100 g. Green bars represent meat categories not targeted by the sodium legislation. Red bars represent meat categories targeted by the sodium legislation.

Table 3. Sodium levels of processed foods in South Africa targeted by the sodium legislation (n = 1851), in mg per 100 g.

Food Subcategory	Targeted by Sodium Legislation	No. of Products	Minimum	25%	Median	Mean	75%	Maximum
Soups								
Dry soup mixes	Yes	164	123	2997	4850	4604	6400	9180
Diet soup mixes	Yes	4	312	345	356	442	454	746
Canned soup	No	55	170	260	373	352	418	574
Chilled soup	No	51	1	262	303	328	398	874
Stocks and gravy								
Gravy powders	Yes	30	320	1042	3804	3677	5034	10,960
Stock powders	Yes	36	578	14,780	20,180	18,230	22,810	27,010
Stock liquids	No	21	458	828	4000	4614	8200	9200
Gravy liquids	No	5	429	429	429	447	464	484
Sauces								
Powdered meal-based sauces	Yes	89	186	473	2524	3036	4979	10,600
Marinades	Yes	48	217	1091	1353	2292	1646	11,250
Ambient meal-based sauces	No	66	128	422	563	1423	958	8700
Curry pastes	No	37	47	1217	2400	2597	4000	5770
Liquid meal-based sauces	No	61	0	425	538	1043	806	8100
Asian Sauces	No	49	2	991	2499	3229	5752	9640
Meat accompaniment	No	15	0	12	69	298	353	1770
Mustard	No	23	423	1230	1760	1959	2300	5500
Pasta sauces	No	81	57	438	556	651	710	2050
Table sauces	No	108	0	574	988	1136	1355	5152
Other sauces	No	19	314	474	703	716	899	1634

4. Discussion

South Africa is the first country to adopt mandatory legislation for the reduction of sodium levels across a wide range of processed foods. Findings from this study indicate that two-thirds of targeted food items already met the maximum sodium limits during early stages of policy implementation. However, there was variation in the percentage of foods on target across legislated categories; while over 90% of breakfast cereals and uncured processed meats met the sodium targets, just over 40% of all crisps, salt and vinegar flavoured snacks, and raw processed sausages, and fewer than 30% of breads contained less sodium than the current maximum sodium limit.

Reduction of sodium intake is a global health priority. In 2014, 75 countries representing all WHO regions had national sodium reduction strategies, include food reformulation (81% of countries), front of package labelling (41%), consumer education (95%), and initiatives in public institutions [7,8]. Targets for food reformulation are often voluntary and, in most countries, are only for bread, which is often a large contributor to dietary sodium from processed foods [7]. South Africa, and now also Argentina, are currently the only two countries with mandatory sodium limits for a range of food products across several different food industries. Several other countries have been successful in developing partnerships with the food industry to negotiate voluntary sodium reduction targets for processed foods [9,20]. In the UK, these voluntary sodium reduction targets have led to an estimated 7% decrease in the sodium levels in processed foods and there has been an 8 to 10% decrease in mean population salt consumption between 2006 and 2011 [21,22]. More challenging voluntary sodium targets were set for 2017 in order to achieve further reductions [23,24]. It will be important for the South African government to ensure that the regulated sodium limits are updated regularly to reflect the levels in the current food supply and global best practice. It will also be important to periodically check that the scope of the regulation is adequately capturing all products important to dietary salt consumption in the country.

The ultimate impact of the sodium legislation will be measured by its effect on reducing the burden of cardiovascular disease and associated health care expenditures. A modelling study that informed the development of the sodium legislation in South Africa estimated that a reduction of daily sodium intake of 0.85 g per person per day could avert 7400 cardiovascular deaths; 6400 of which would be due to reducing the sodium levels of bread alone [14]. The additional 4300 non-fatal strokes that could be prevented are projected to save the strained South African health care system 40 million USD a year. An extended cost effectiveness analysis supported these findings and reported that the South African population salt reduction programme could also avert poverty and reduce household out of pocket expenditures, particularly for the middle class, at minimal cost [15]. The impact of the sodium legislation on the burden of cardiovascular disease in South Africa will only become apparent some years after it is implemented. To attribute change in the burden of cardiovascular disease to the sodium legislation, assessment of each step between policy implementation and the anticipated health outcomes is needed, including evaluation of its impact on changes in the sodium levels of foods, population salt intake, and blood pressure levels [25–27]. The HealthyFood Switch technologies used in this study provide an objective, practical, transferable, and scalable approach to assess the nutritional composition of packaged foods, to assess whether targeted food products comply with the legislation, and to facilitate global benchmarking.

This study has some limitations. First, the HealthyFood Switch database mainly comprises foods available from large retailers that predominantly serve the middle to higher socioeconomic urban population. While additional food items were added through crowdsourcing, our data are not necessarily representative of all packaged foods in South Africa. Second, we evaluated the sodium levels of foods available in-store and did not examine actual food purchases or consumption, nor market share of brands. However, there are data from the UK indicating that crude mean sodium levels of product ranges are broadly comparable to the weighted mean sodium levels of products actually sold [28]. Third, since nutritional data were collected between the notification and early implementation period of the sodium legislation, we were unable to determine whether food manufacturers had already commenced reformulating, withdrawing, or replacing high-sodium products before the legislation came into effect. Fourth, sodium levels collected were derived from NIPs of packaged foods, which, although mostly deemed to be accurate [29], are not necessarily derived from chemical analyses. Fifth, in some cases, the availability of 'as prepared' nutrition values alone (<15% of products) limited the capacity for robust comparison because mean sodium levels can be influenced by the recommended method of preparation for which there no agreed standards.

In conclusion, sodium levels of two-thirds of foods covered by the sodium legislation in South Africa already met the sodium target during early stages of policy implementation. Further, only moderate reductions in sodium content will be required to bring many of the currently products in line with the regulation. This represents an excellent opportunity for the South African food industry to make rapid improvements to the national food supply. The high sodium levels of nearly three-quarters of breads, the main contributor to non-discretionary sodium intake in South Africa, will require particular attention and should be an early focus of activity. Continued monitoring of sodium levels in foods is required to support industry action and ensure compliance with the legislation is achieved. Monitoring data will also enable modelled evaluation of the impact of the sodium legislation on dietary sodium intake and its downstream effects on population blood pressure levels and cardiovascular diseases.

Author Contributions: S.A.E.P., E.D., L.J.W., J.W. and B.N. were involved in the concept and design of the study. S.A.E.P. conducted the statistical analyses and prepared the first draft of the manuscript. All authors were involved in the acquisition and/or interpretation of the data, made critical revisions to the manuscript for important intellectual content, and provided final approval of the version to be published. S.A.E.P. and B.N. are responsible for the integrity of the work as a whole.

Conflicts of Interest: The authors declare no conflict of interest.

Appendix A

Table A1. Sodium levels of packaged foods by food category in South Africa (n = 11,065), in mg per 100 g.

Food Group/Category	No. of Products	Minimum	25%	Median	Mean	75%	Maximum
Beverages	2163	0	0	0	31	11	1260
Fruit and vegetable juices	426	0	3	6	18	13	1205
Soft drinks	257	0	2	7	14	13	200
Cordials	113	0	18	56	92	106	667
Coffee and tea	428	0	0	0	73	20	784
Electrolyte drinks	38	0	31	42	192	183	1260
Alcoholic beverages	671	0	0	0	0	0	9
Waters	144	0	0	2	8	9	100
Energy drinks	53	0	7	35	33	56	83
Beverage mixes	18	0	17	205	211	336	667
Bread and bakery products	847	0	250	400	440	582	2827
Bread	174	39	388	476	542	593	2470
Biscuits	526	0	222	378	431	614	2827
Cakes, muffins & pastry	147	20	242	341	353	436	1270
Cereal and cereal products	939	0	6	70	239	296	4180
Cereal bars	78	0	64	168	178	253	850
Noodles	78	0	201	470	737	1314	1876
Breakfast cereals	376	0	46	171	262	346	4180
Pasta	153	0	2	4	78	20	1440
Maize (corn)	41	0	3	5	27	16	193
Rice	64	0	3	8	139	178	1440
Couscous	18	0	3	10	284	532	1262
Unprocessed cereals	131	0	3	9	206	65	3710
Confectionery	645	0	22	66	85	108	1380
Chocolate and sweets	541	0	35	74	95	114	1380
Jelly	49	0	15	26	31	27	93
Chewing gum	44	0	0	1	41	13	616
Cough drops/throat lozengers	11	0	0	0	5	1	49
Convenience foods	586	1	309	442	1624	1887	9180
Pizza	33	377	435	478	477	513	598
Soup	270	1	355	2017	2930	5410	9180
Ready meals	156	12	290	382	422	488	2280
Pre-prepared salads and sandwiches	82	7	240	303	325	454	818

Table A1. *Cont.*

Food Group/Category	No. of Products	Minimum	25%	Median	Mean	75%	Maximum
Meal kits	43	103	554	939	1198	1678	4700
Others	2	329	358	386	386	415	444
Dairy	986	0	39	50	209	270	1820
Cheese	240	0	377	554	654	808	1820
Yoghurt products	339	0	36	43	47	50	514
Milk	253	0	38	48	73	55	822
Cream	30	0	29	36	37	44	142
Desserts	69	0	61	99	154	266	601
Ice cream and edible ices	55	0	18	50	49	78	179
Edible oils and oil emulsions	237	0	0	2	169	390	1706
Butter and margarine	88	0	339	400	428	625	826
Cooking oils	118	0	0	0	2	1	37
All egg products	46	0	126	126	113	131	196
Fish and fish products	284	0	236	328	384	449	4430
Canned fish and seafood	144	0	248	321	387	400	4430
Chilled fish	25	0	162	470	640	876	1620
Frozen fish	94	38	186	284	297	413	670
Other fish products	21	223	359	449	456	502	773
Foods for specific dietary use	320	0	15	102	177	260	2050
Baby foods	203	0	6	27	75	150	306
Meal replacements	117	0	167	347	354	460	2050
Fruit and vegetable products	1815	0	3	22	509	249	38,800
Vegetables	895	0	7	108	288	360	3860
Fruit	466	0	2	8	68	36	3927
Jam and spreads	86	0	6	10	19	24	151
Nuts and seeds	166	0	6	22	123	146	1117
Herbs and spices	202	0	0	0	3028	2444	38,800
Meat and meat products	545	0	464	734	850	1020	4136
Processed meat and derivatives	486	0	477	732	808	1010	3036
Meat alternatives	59	1	359	748	1204	1578	4136
Snack foods	367	0	562	746	785	1020	2851
Sauces and spreads	1059	0	391	673	1981	1634	27,010
Sauces	704	0	482	999	2700	2818	27,010
Mayonnaise/dressings	183	0	311	542	581	805	4500
Spreads	172	0	160	386	531	607	5380

Table A2. Sodium levels of foods covered by the sodium regulation containing higher levels of sodium than the maximum allowed.

	On Target, %	Excess Sodium Level, %				Excess Sodium Level, mg/100 g			
		0%–25%	25%–50%	50%–100%	>100%	25%	Median	Mean	75%
Bread	27	30	20	12	10	68	110	229	225
Breakfast cereals and porridges	91	3	2	2	1	96	148	606	382
Fat and butter spreads	69	9	17	5	0	112	150	161	210
Savoury snacks, not salt and vinegar flavoured	70	13	9	6	2	98	240	289	400
Potato crisps	41	34	5	15	5	71	136	248	377
Savoury snacks, salt and vinegar flavoured	42	32	11	5	11	160	236	487	585
Processed meat, uncured	91	6	3	0	0	24	37	87	126
Processed meat, cured	66	29	4	2	0	48	70	149	201
Processed meat sausages, raw	45	35	13	6	1	75	108	192	276
Soup powder, dry	61	23	12	4	0	553	1184	1385	2192
Gravy powders and savoury sauces, dry	55	11	13	14	7	926	1700	2018	2902
Savoury powders with instant noodles, dry	85	13	1	0	0	26	65	128	181
Stock cubes, powders, granules, emulsions, pastes, or jellies	77	11	11	1	0	3587	4631	5384	8037
Total	67	16	9	6	2	86	211	684	516

Table A3. Sodium levels of packaged meats in South Africa (*n* = 440), in mg per 100 g.

Meat Type	Targeted by Sodium Legislation	No. of Products	Minimum	25%	Median	Mean	75%	Maximum
Bacon	No	22	552	784	1070	1008	1156	1540
Frozen and chilled meat	No	103	39	336	461	436	548	1080
Salami	No	26	1164	1505	1674	1681	1884	2462
Biltong	No	37	975	1763	2079	2000	2231	3036
Raw flavoured meats	No	16	4	315	428	432	497	1080
Canned meat	Yes	25	0	560	657	682	866	974
Meat burgers	Yes	33	44	500	638	618	784	1065
Sausages	Yes	102	426	708	826	851	914	2213
Sliced meat	Yes	70	387	758	942	918	1020	1667
Pate and spreads	Yes	6	550	816	860	826	865	1020

References

1. He, F.J.; Li, J.; Macgregor, G.A. Effect of longer-Term modest salt reduction on blood pressure. *Cochrane Database Syst. Rev.* **2013**, *3*, CD004937.
2. GBD 2015 Risk Factors Collaborators. Global, regional, and national comparative risk assessment of 79 behavioural, environmental and occupational, and metabolic risks or clusters of risks, 1990–2015: A systematic analysis for the Global Burden of Disease Study 2015. *Lancet* **2016**, *388*, 1659–1724.
3. Mozaffarian, D.; Fahimi, S.; Singh, G.M.; Micha, R.; Khatibzadeh, S.; Engell, R.E.; Lim, S.; Danaei, G.; Ezzati, M.; Powles, J. Global sodium consumption and death from cardiovascular causes. *N. Engl. J. Med.* **2014**, *371*, 624–634. [CrossRef] [PubMed]
4. World Health Organization (WHO). *Guideline: Sodium Intake for Adults and Children*; WHO: Geneva, Switzerland, 2012.
5. World Health Organization (WHO). *Global Status Report on Noncommunicable Diseases 2010*; WHO: Geneva, Switzerland, 2010.
6. Sixty-Sixth World Health Assembly. Follow-Up to the Political Declaration of the High-Level Meeting of the General Assembly on the Prevention and Control of Non-Communicable Diseases. 2013. Available online: http://apps.who.int/gb/ebwha/pdf_files/WHA66/A66_R10-en.pdf (accessed on 12 October 2016).
7. Trieu, K.; Neal, B.; Hawkes, C.; Dunford, E.; Campbell, N.; Rodriguez-Fernandez, R.; Legetic, B.; McLaren, L.; Barberio, A.; Webster, J. Salt reduction initiatives around the world—A systematic review of progress towards the global target. *PLoS ONE* **2015**, *10*, e0130247. [CrossRef] [PubMed]
8. Webster, J.L.; Dunford, E.K.; Hawkes, C.; Neal, B.C. Salt reduction initiatives around the world. *J. Hypertens.* **2011**, *29*, 1043–1050. [CrossRef] [PubMed]
9. Webster, J.; Trieu, K.; Dunford, E.; Hawkes, C. Target salt 2025: A global overview of national prog to encourage the food industry to reduce salt in foods. *Nutrients* **2014**, *6*, 3274–3287. [CrossRef] [PubMed]
10. Department of Health. Regulations Relating to the Reduction of Sodium in Certain Foodstuffs and Related Matters (Proclamation No. R. 214, 2013). Available online: http://www.heartfoundation.co.za/sites/default/files/articles/South%20Africa%20salt%20legislation.pdf (accessed on 12 October 2016).
11. Hofman, K.J.; Lee, R. Intersectorial Case Study: Successful Sodium Regulation in South Africa. 2013. Available online: http://apps.who.int/iris/handle/10665/205179 (accessed on 4 April 2017).
12. Charlton, K.; Webster, J.; Kowal, P. To legislate or not to legislate? A comparison of the UK and South African approaches to the development and implementation of salt reduction prog. *Nutrients* **2014**, *6*, 3672–3695. [CrossRef] [PubMed]
13. Charlton, K.E.; Steyn, K.; Levitt, N.S.; Zulu, J.V.; Jonathan, D.; Veldman, F.J.; Nel, J.H. Diet and blood pressure in South Africa: Intake of foods containing sodium, potassium, calcium, and magnesium in three ethnic groups. *Nutrition* **2005**, *21*, 39–50. [CrossRef] [PubMed]
14. Bertram, M.Y.; Steyn, K.; Wentzel-Viljoen, E.; Tollman, S.; Hofman, K.J. Reducing the sodium content of high-Salt foods: Effect on cardiovascular disease in South Africa. *S. Afr. Med. J.* **2012**, *102*, 743–745. [CrossRef] [PubMed]
15. Watkins, D.A.; Olson, Z.D.; Verguet, S.; Nugent, R.A.; Jamison, D.T. Cardiovascular disease and impoverishment averted due to a salt reduction policy in South Africa: An extended cost-Effectiveness analysis. *Health Policy Plan.* **2016**, *31*, 75–82. [CrossRef] [PubMed]
16. Dunford, E.; Trevena, H.; Goodsell, C.; Ng, KH.; Webster, J.; Millis, A.; Goldstein, S.; Hugueniot, O.; Neal, B. FoodSwitch: A mobile phone app to enable consumers to make healthier food choices and crowdsourcing of national food composition data. *JMIR Mhealth Uhealth* **2014**, *2*, e37. [CrossRef] [PubMed]
17. HealthyFood Switch. 2016. Available online: https://www.discovery.co.za/portal/individual/vitality-news-healthyfood-Switch (accessed on 2 November 2016).
18. The George Institute Data Collector App. 2016. Available online: https://itunes.apple.com/us/app/data-collector/id545847554?mt=8 (accessed on 31 October 2016).
19. Dunford, E.; Webster, J.; Metzler, A.B.; Czernichow, S.; Ni Mhurchu, C.; Wolmarans, P.; Snowdon, W.; L'Abbe, M.; Li, N.; Maulik, P.K.; et al. International collaborative project to compare and monitor the nutritional composition of processed foods. *Eur. J. Prev. Cardiol.* **2012**, *19*, 1326–1332. [CrossRef] [PubMed]

20. Trevena, H.; Neal, B.; Dunford, E.; Wu, J.H. An evaluation of the effects of the Australian Food and Health Dialogue targets on the sodium content of bread, breakfast cereals and processed meats. *Nutrients* **2014**, *6*, 3802–3817. [CrossRef] [PubMed]

21. Eyles, H.; Webster, J.; Jebb, S.; Capelin, C.; Neal, B.; Ni, M.C. Impact of the UK voluntary sodium reduction targets on the sodium content of processed foods from 2006 to 2011: Analysis of household consumer panel data. *Prev. Med.* **2013**, *57*, 555–560. [CrossRef] [PubMed]

22. Sadler, K.; Nicholson, S.; Steer, T.; Gill, V.; Bates, B.; Tipping, S.; Cox, L.; Lennox, A.; Prentice, A. *Diet and Nutrition Survey-Assessment of Dietary Sodium in Adults (Aged 19 io 64 Years) in England, 2011*; Public Health England: Endland, UK, 2012.

23. Department of Health. F9. Salt Reduction 2017. Available online: https://responsibilitydeal.dh.gov.uk/pledges/pledge/?pl=49 (accessed on 12 October 2016).

24. Food Standards Agency. Salt Reduction Targets for 2017. Available online: https://www.food.gov.uk/northern-ireland/nutritionni/salt-ni/salt_targets (accessed on 12 October 2016).

25. Christoforou, A.; Trieu, K.; Land, M.A.; Bolam, B.; Webster, J. State-level and community-level salt reduction initiatives: A systematic review of global programmes and their impact. *J. Epidemiol. Community Health* **2016**, *70*, 1140–1150. [CrossRef] [PubMed]

26. Charlton, K.; Ware, L.J.; Menyanu, E.; Biritwum, R.B.; Naidoo, N.; Pieterse, C.; Madurai, S.; Baumgartner, J.; Asare, G.A.; Thiele, E.; et al. Leveraging ongoing research to evaluate the health impacts of South Africa's salt reduction strategy: A prospective nested cohort within the WHO-SAGE multicountry, longitudinal study. *BMJ Open* **2016**, *6*, e013316. [CrossRef] [PubMed]

27. Swanepoel, B.; Schutte, A.E.; Cockeran, M.; Steyn, K.; Wentzel-Viljoen, E. Sodium and potassium intake in South Africa: An evaluation of 24-Hour urine collections in a white, black, and Indian population. *J. Am. Soc. Hypertens. JASH* **2016**, *10*, 829–837. [CrossRef] [PubMed]

28. Eyles, H.; Neal, B.; Jiang, Y.; Ni, M.C. Estimating population food and nutrient exposure: A comparison of store survey data with household panel food purchases. *Br. J. Nutr.* **2016**, *115*, 1835–1842. [CrossRef] [PubMed]

29. Fabiansson, S.U. Precision in nutritional information declarations on food labels in Australia. *Asia Pac. J. Clin. Nutr.* **2006**, *15*, 451–458. [PubMed]

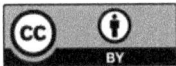

Article

Sodium and Potassium Intake in Healthy Adults in Thessaloniki Greater Metropolitan Area—The Salt Intake in Northern Greece (SING) Study

Eleni Vasara [1], Georgios Marakis [2], Joao Breda [3], Petros Skepastianos [4], Maria Hassapidou [5], Anthony Kafatos [6], Nikolaos Rodopaios [6], Alexandra A. Koulouri [6] and Francesco P. Cappuccio [7,8,*]

[1] Laboratory of Animal Physiology, Department of Zoology, School of Biology, Aristotle University of Thessaloniki, Thessaloniki 54124, Greece; evasara@bio.auth.gr

[2] Nutrition Policy and Research Directorate, Hellenic Food Authority, 124 Kifisias Av. & 2 Iatridou Str., Athens 11526, Greece; gmarakis@efet.gr

[3] Division of Noncommunicable Diseases and Promoting Health through the Life-Course, WHO Regional Office for Europe, Copenhagen DK-2100, Denmark; rodriguesdasilvabred@who.int

[4] Department of Medical Laboratory Studies, Alexander Technological and Educational Institute of Thessaloniki, Sindos, Thessaloniki 57400, Greece; pskep@otenet.gr

[5] Department of Nutrition and Dietetics, Alexander Technological and Educational Institute of Thessaloniki, Sindos, Thessaloniki 57400, Greece; mnhas@gmail.com

[6] Department of Social Medicine, Preventive Medicine and Nutrition Clinic, Medical School, University of Crete, Heraklion 71003, Crete, Greece; kafatos@med.uoc.gr (A.K.); nikow1966@yahoo.gr (N.R.); alexkoulou@yahoo.com (A.A.K.)

[7] Division of Health Sciences (Mental Health & Wellbeing), Warwick Medical School, University of Warwick, Coventry CV4 7AL, UK

[8] University Hospitals Coventry & Warwickshire NHS Trust, Coventry, CV2 2DX, UK

* Correspondence: f.p.cappuccio@warwick.ac.uk

Received: 13 March 2017; Accepted: 20 April 2017; Published: 22 April 2017

Abstract: A reduction in population sodium (as salt) consumption is a global health priority, as well as one of the most cost-effective strategies to reduce the burden of cardiovascular disease. High potassium intake is also recommended to reduce cardiovascular disease. To establish effective policies for setting targets and monitoring effectiveness within each country, the current level of consumption should be known. Greece lacks data on actual sodium and potassium intake. The aim of the present study was therefore to assess dietary salt (using sodium as biomarker) and potassium intakes in a sample of healthy adults in northern Greece, and to determine whether adherence to a Mediterranean diet is related to different sodium intakes or sodium-to-potassium ratio. A cross-sectional survey was carried out in the Thessaloniki greater metropolitan area (northern Greece) (n = 252, aged 18–75 years, 45.2% males). Participants' dietary sodium and potassium intakes were determined by 24-hour urinary sodium and potassium excretions. In addition, we estimated their adherence to Mediterranean diet by the use of an 11-item MedDietScore (range 0–55). The mean sodium excretion was 175 (SD 72) mmol/day, equivalent to 4220 (1745) mg of sodium or 10.7 (4.4) g of salt per day, and the potassium excretion was 65 (25) mmol/day, equivalent to 3303 (1247) mg per day. Men had higher sodium and potassium excretions compared to women. Only 5.6% of the sample had salt intake <5 g/day, which is the target intake recommended by the World Health Organization. Mean sodium-to-potassium excretion ratio was 2.82 (1.07). There was no significant difference in salt or potassium intake or their ratio across MedDietScore quartiles. No significant relationships were found between salt intake and adherence to a Mediterranean diet, suggesting that the perception of the health benefits of the Mediterranean diet does not hold when referring to salt consumption. These results suggest the need for a larger, nation-wide survey on salt intake in Greece and underline the importance of continuation of salt reduction initiatives in Greece.

Nutrients **2017**, *9*, 417

Keywords: salt; sodium; potassium; intake; MedDietScore; Greece

---

1. Introduction

Non-communicable diseases are the leading causes of death in Greece and worldwide. High blood pressure and unhealthy diet are among the risk factors that account for most of the disease burden in Greece [1]. Specifically, according to the most recent nation-wide health and diet survey in Greece, four out of ten adults have raised blood pressure [2] (p. 55). There is compelling evidence from experimental, epidemiological, migration and intervention studies as well as meta-analyses that high salt intake is associated with raised blood pressure and adverse cardiovascular health (i.e., coronary heart disease and stroke) (e.g., [3–6]), despite the publication of a small number of controversial scientific papers using flawed methodologies [7,8]. In addition, high salt intake is related to adverse health effects independent of its effects on blood pressure [9].

The World Health Organization currently recommends that adults should consume no more than 5 g of salt daily [10]. Even though sodium intake varies in populations around the world, in the vast majority of populations, salt intake is high and it exceeds both physiologic requirements and recommendations [11,12]. Greece seems to lack data on actual salt intake [13]. Salt reduction strategies in the European Union, including Greece, encompass monitoring and evaluation actions as one of their important pillars. Hence, comprehensive, current data on salt intake in Greece are urgently needed, using at least one accurately collected 24-hour urine sample for assessing sodium excretion, which is regarded as the gold standard method to assess salt consumption, at least for a population average [14,15].

In contrast to sodium, evidence from epidemiologic studies and randomized trials point to the beneficial effects of dietary potassium on blood pressure and cardiovascular health [16–18]. This effect is more pronounced in those with high sodium intake [19]. It has been suggested that individuals with diets that are low in potassium are particularly vulnerable to the hypertensive effects of high sodium intake [20,21]. Hence, the ratio of sodium-to-potassium may be more reliable than either nutrient alone in predicting the risk of cardiovascular disease [22,23]. In addition to sodium, potassium can also be determined accurately in 24-hour urine collections, hence avoiding the need to rely on reported dietary intake data and national up-to-date food composition tables.

The primary objective of the present study was to estimate the average population sodium and potassium intakes in northern Greece. The study also aimed to investigate whether adherence to a Mediterranean diet is related to different salt intakes or the sodium-to-potassium ratio.

2. Methods

2.1. Participants and Recruitment

Two hundred and seventy-four men and women (aged 18–75 years) participated in the Salt Intake in Northern Greece (SING) study. The investigation took place in northern Greece, mostly in the Thessaloniki greater metropolitan area (the second largest city in Greece). Recruitment was done at various sites and venues including churches and workplaces, based on an opportunistic sampling [15]. This approach has been recently shown to be suitable and free from significant bias when assessing population group average salt consumption [15]. Efforts were taken to avoid recruiting individuals who were particularly worried about their salt intake or their blood pressure and who might, as a consequence, have altered their diet. In order to attain that, adults were initially invited to participate in a nutrition survey, without specifying which nutrients would be investigated or how their intake would be assessed. Once people expressed interest for participating in a nutrition survey, a quick screening took place in order to exclude those who met the exclusion criteria. Pregnant and lactating women were excluded from the study. Other exclusions were those with a medical diagnosis of hypertension (whether on an anti-hypertensive treatment or not), diabetes mellitus as well as those with heart, liver, renal, gastrointestinal or neoplastic diseases.

Eligible volunteers were then told how the study would be conducted and what would be required during their participation. Detailed written and verbal instructions were given to eligible volunteers, before receiving their informed consent to participate. It was carefully explained to participants how to collect their urine for 24 h, emphasizing the importance of providing a complete collection. In an effort to minimise conscious or unconscious modification of their diet or dietary practices (e.g., avoiding adding salt on the plate or avoiding high salt foods), participants were told that the aim of the 24-hour urine collection was to investigate the dietary intake of some nutrients, without specifying that the nutrients of this investigation were sodium and potassium. Participants were also requested not to change their diet before or during the day of the urine collection (e.g., skip a major meal that they normally have or follow a special diet that day).

Sample recruitment and urine collection were confined to one calendar year, commencing in February 2015 and completed in March 2016. No urinary samples were collected during festive seasons. No financial incentive was offered to participants. In order to motivate individuals to participate in this study, it was specified that participants would be notified of their own results as well as the general outcomes of the study. The study was approved by the Ethics Committee of the Alexander Technological and Educational Institute of Thessaloniki, and participants provided written informed consent to take part.

2.2. Data Collection

Height and weight were measured in subjects wearing light clothing, without shoes, using standardized equipment. Body weight was recorded using a Tanita BWB-800S digital scale (Tanita Europe BV, Amsterdam, The Netherlands) to the nearest 0.1 Kg and body height was measured using a stable stadiometer to the nearest 0.1 cm. Body mass index was calculated as weight (Kg)/height (m^2). Waist circumference (in cm) was measured around the midpoint between the costal margin and the iliac crest during expiration. Blood pressure was measured in triplicate, after a 10 min rest, using fully automatic Omron blood pressure monitor (Omron RX Classic II, Kyoto, Japan). The first reading was discarded and the mean of the second and third readings was calculated.

A single 24-hour urine collection was obtained from the participants. The first void upon waking on the day of collection was discarded. Participants then collected all voided urine up to, and including, the first void the following morning in multiple 500 mL screw-cup bottles. The exact times at the beginning and the end of urine collection were noted by the participants. The urine volume of the 24-hour collection was measured in the lab and a 10 mL aliquot was stored at −20 °C until analysis. Urinary sodium and potassium excretions were determined by ion-selective electrode potentiometry (ATVIA 1800 Siemens, ISE buffer Siemens AG, Munich, Germany) and by taking into account the exact 24-hour adjusted urinary volume. The sodium to potassium ratio in the 24-hour urine samples was also calculated.

Urine collections were rejected if the participant admitted that a sample was missed from the collection or if the timing of the collection fell outside the range of 23–25 h. Urine collections were suspected to be inaccurate if urinary volumes were <500 mL. Para-aminobenzoic acid (PABA) marker was not used in this study. Despite its limitation, 24-hour urinary creatinine was used as a means to exclude urine collections judged to be incomplete. Creatinine was measured using the Jaffe method (ATVIA 1800 Siemens AG, Munich, Germany) [24]. If urinary creatinine (UCr) was less than 2 standard deviations from the mean, subjects were excluded from the statistical analysis.

For each individual, the 24-hour sodium or potassium excretion value (mEq/day or mmol/day) was calculated as the concentration of sodium or potassium in the urine (mmol/L) multiplied by the urinary volume (L/day). In order to convert urinary output to dietary intake, the urinary excretion of sodium or potassium values (mEq/day) were first converted to mg/day. Then, sodium values were multiplied by 1.05 (since urine output reflects approximately 95% of intake), while potassium values were multiplied by 1.3 [25]. The conversion from dietary sodium (Na) intake to salt (NaCl) intake was made by multiplying the sodium value by 2.542 (NaCl (g) = Na (g) × 2.542).

2.3. Adherence to Mediterranean Diet

The MedDietScore (MDS) was calculated for each participant to evaluate their adherence to the Mediterranean dietary pattern. The MedDietScore has previously been validated [26] and includes 11 main components. Specifically, it takes into account the frequency of consumption of nine food groups (i.e., servings/week for non-refined cereals, fruits, vegetables, potatoes, legumes, fish, red meat, poultry and full fat dairy products) as well as the frequency of consumption for olive oil (times/week) and alcohol (mL/day). Based on the recommended intake, monotonic ratings (with the exception of alcohol intake) were used in order to score the frequency of consumption of these foods. Individual ratings from 0 to 5 or the reverse were assigned for each of the above food groups/items, according to their position in the Mediterranean diet pyramid. The score ranges from 0 to 55, with higher values indicating greater adherence to the Mediterranean diet.

2.4. Statistical Analysis

In general, to detect approximately 1 g reduction in salt intake over time using 24-hour urinary sodium excretion, with an estimated standard deviation of 75 mmol/day ($\alpha = 0.05$, power = 0.80), a minimum sample of 120 individuals per stratum is recommended [27]. Hence, a minimum sample of 240 men and women participants was expected. Baseline sample characteristics (i.e., age, weight, height, Body Mass Index (BMI), waist circumference, blood pressure and MedDietScore) as well as salt intake, sodium and potassium excretion and intake values and their ratios are presented as mean (standard deviation). Age distribution, level of education and self-assessment of personal diet quality are presented as percentages.

Differences between groups were assessed using independent sample *t*-tests. Differences in sodium intake, potassium intake and sodium-to-potassium ratio across MedDietScore quartiles were assessed by one-way ANOVA. Pearson chi-square test was used to test the association between categorical variables. For all comparisons, significance level was at 5%. Statistical analysis was performed with SPSS statistical software package version 20, IBM (SPSS Inc., Chicago, IL, USA).

3. Results

3.1. Characteristics of Participants

After the initial screening, 274 volunteers gave written consent and provided a 24-hour urine collection. Eight participants were excluded because they admitted that one or more voids were lost or because their urine collection fell outside the range of 23–25 h. Six more were excluded on the grounds of their urinary volume being less than 500 mL per day, despite admitting that no urine was lost. Another six subjects were excluded because their 24-hour urinary creatinine excretion was more than two standard deviations from the mean. One individual was excluded because of low 24-hour urinary creatinine excretion and low urinary volume in spite of high weight, indicating possible under-collection, and finally one was excluded because of low 24-hour urinary creatinine excretion, but very high volume (>two standard deviations) suggesting possible over-dilution. Therefore, 22 participants in total were excluded from the analyses. The final sample comprised of 252 participants (92% of the initial sample) between 18 and 75 years old, of whom 45.2% were men and 54.8% were women.

The characteristics of the participants are shown in Table 1. There was no statistically significant difference in the mean age ($p = 0.701$), mean BMI ($p = 0.234$) and mean urine volume ($p = 0.754$) between male and female participants. Men had higher urinary creatinine excretion compared to women ($p < 0.0001$).

Table 1. Demographic data of the participants (*n* = 252).

	Total (*n* = 252)	Men (*n* = 114)	Women (*n* = 138)
Mean Age (years)	46.6 (16.6)	47.0 (16.2)	46.2 (17.0)
% in the range 18–34	26.8	27.4	27.0
% in the range 35–49	25.6	24.8	25.6
% in the range 50–64	35.6	36.3	35.0
% in the range 65–75	12.0	11.5	12.4
Height (cm)	169.3 (9.5)	176.8 (6.6)	163.1 (6.6) ****
Weight (kg)	77.0 (15.7)	85.2 (14.6)	70.3 (13.1) ****
BMI (kg/m^2)	26.8 (4.7)	27.2 (4.1)	26.5 (5.1)
Waist circumference (cm)	87.6 (14.7)	94.8 (13.1)	81.6 (13.1) ****
Level of education (%)			
Non university graduates	60.3	51.8	67.4
University graduates	39.7	48.2	32.6 *
Self-assessment of personal diet quality (%)			
Good	61.3	62.0	60.7
Moderate	37.1	34.5	39.3
Bad	1.6	3.5	0
Systolic BP (mmHg)	126.5 (16.4)	129.9 (16.8)	123.7 (15.5) **
Diastolic BP (mmHg)	79.8 (11.9)	82.5 (12.5)	77.6 (10.9) ***
MedDietScore	30.5 (5.1)	31.8 (5.4)	29.4 (4.6) ****

BMI, Body Mass Index; BP, blood pressure. Results are presented as means (SD) or %. * $p < 0.05$; ** $p \leq 0.01$; *** $p \leq 0.001$; **** $p \leq 0.0001$ vs. men.

3.2. Sodium and Potassium Intakes

There was a considerable variation in sodium and potassium excretion. Average sodium and potassium excretions were higher in men than in women (Table 2). In men, daily sodium intake ranged from 797 mg to 11,213 mg, while in women dietary sodium ranged from 845 mg to 8489 mg. As far as potassium is concerned, its daily intake ranged from 1221 mg to 9001 mg in men and from 830 mg to 8044 mg in women. Men had significantly higher potassium intake compared to women ($p = 0.001$). The mean salt intake in the SING study was 10.7 (4.4) g/day (Table 2). Men had significantly higher salt intake (11.9 (4.7) g/day) compared to women (9.7 (3.9) g/day) ($p < 0.0001$).

Table 2. Mean sodium and potassium excretion, intakes and their ratio in men and women.

	Total (*n* = 252)	Men (*n* = 114)	Women (*n* = 138)
Urinary excretions			
Volume (mL/24 h)	1800 (807)	1782 (858)	1814 (767)
Creatinine (g/24 h)	1.36 (0.51)	1.66 (0.53)	1.11 (0.33) ****
Sodium (mmol/24 h)	174.7 (72.2)	194.3 (76.8)	158.5 (64.1) ****
Potassium (mmol/24 h)	65.1 (24.6)	70.8 (26.0)	60.5 (22.4) ***
Sodium-to-potassium ratio (mmol/mmol)	2.82 (1.07)	2.87 (1.02)	2.77 (1.12)
Dietary estimates			
Sodium intake † (mg/24 h)	4220 (1745)	4694 (1855)	3828 (1548) ****
Potassium intake † (mg/24 h)	3303 (1247)	3589 (1321)	3067 (1134) ***
Na/K intake ratio (mg/mg)	1.34 (0.51)	1.37 (0.48)	1.32 (0.53)
Salt intake (g/day)	10.7 (4.4)	11.9 (4.7)	9.7 (3.9) ****

Results are presented as means (SD). *** $p \leq 0.001$; **** $p \leq 0.0001$ vs. men. † Intake values were calculated by multiplying urinary excretion values by 1.05 for Na and by 1.3 for K (see Methods).

With regard to the frequency distribution of salt data, only 5.6% of the sample (1.98% men and 3.57% women) had salt intake <5 g per day, which is the target intake recommended by the World Health Organization (WHO) guidelines (Figure 1). Moreover, since the dispersion in our sample (based on person-days of exposure) was substantially greater than the dispersion in a corresponding sample of usual intakes of individuals (due to the subtraction of intra-individual variance), the proportion of "persons" with an intake <5 g per day would be substantially less. In contrast, 50.4% of the study sample had a daily salt intake that exceeded 10 g per day. In a small percentage of participants (3.97%), salt intake exceeded 20 g per day. As far as potassium is concerned, 33.4% of participants had intakes equal or higher than the WHO recommendation of 3510 mg/day.

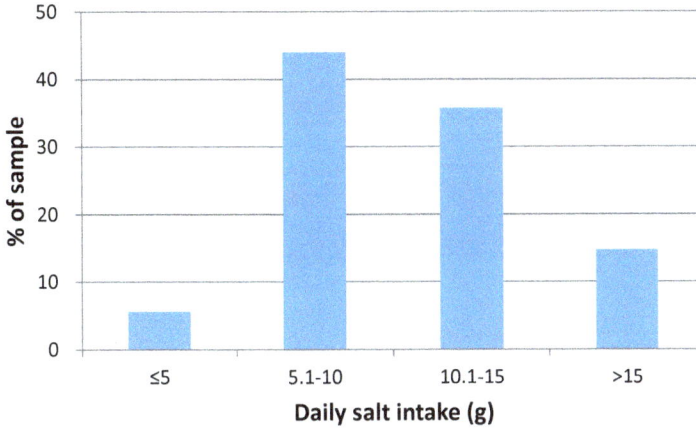

Figure 1. Distribution of single 24-hour salt intake estimates (see text for conversion of urinary excretions to estimates intakes).

3.3. Sodium-to-Potassium Ratio

The urinary sodium-to-potassium ratio was 2.82 (1.07) (Table 2). The dietary sodium-to-potassium intake ratio in the whole group was 1.34 (0.51). In the lowest salt intake quartile, the ratio was 0.98 (0.36), which rose to 1.70 (0.49) in the highest salt intake quartile, a statistically significant difference ($p < 0.0001$) (Figure 2). There was no statistically significant difference in dietary sodium-to-potassium ratio between genders ($p = 0.478$).

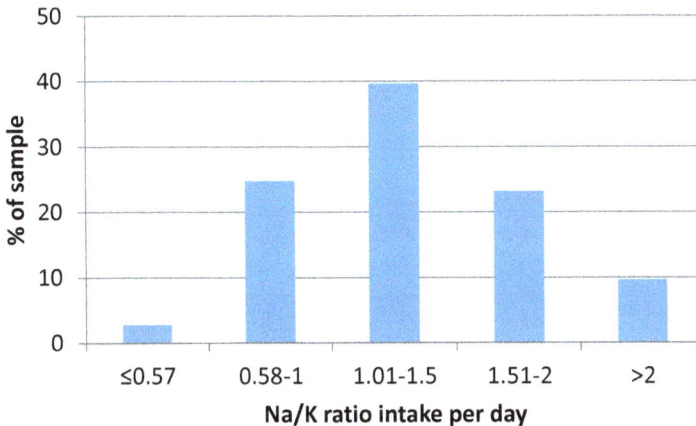

Figure 2. Distribution of dietary sodium-to-potassium ratios (mg/mg) in the sample of 24-hour intake estimates (see text for conversion of urinary excretions to estimates intakes).

For only 2.8% of the sample of 24-hour measurements (1.2% men and 1.6% women) was the dietary sodium-to-potassium intake ratio (mg/mg) less than 0.57 (Figure 2). This chosen cut-off value results from the WHO guidelines on sodium and potassium for adults (i.e., 2000 mg Na/3510 mg K = 0.57).

Finally, we did not detect seasonal variations in estimates of sodium and potassium excretion and dietary consumption between Spring-Summer and Autumn-Winter.

3.4. Salt Intake and Adherence to the Mediterranean Diet

The mean MedDietScore of the sample was 30.5 (5.1), ranging from 14 to 45, with women having a statistically significant lower score compared to men ($p < 0.0001$) (Table 1). There was no statistically significant difference of the MedDietScore between the lowest (29.5 (5.1)) and highest (30.9 (5.1)) quartiles of salt intake ($p = 0.124$). Sodium intake, potassium intake and the sodium-to-potassium ratio by MedDietScore quartiles are shown in Table 3. There were no significant differences in sodium or potassium intake or their ratio across MedDietScore quartiles.

Table 3. Sodium intake, potassium intake and sodium-to-potassium ratio in single 24-hour collections for individuals by MedDietScore quartiles.

MedDietScore Quartiles	Sodium Intake (mg Per Day)	Potassium Intake (mg Per Day)	Sodium-to-Potassium Intake Ratio
1 ($\leq$28)	4079 (1893) 3661–4498	3241 (1268) 2961–3522	1.32 (0.48) 1.21–1.42
2 (>28, $\leq$31)	4361 (1746) 3931–4790	3303 (1369) 2964–3642	1.42 (0.61) 1.27–1.57
3 (>31, $\leq$34)	3972 (1565) 3532–4413	3215 (1275) 2856–3573	1.29 (0.44) 1.17–1.41
4 (>34)	4424 (1636) 3954–4894	3465 (995) 3180–3751	1.33 (0.51) 1.19–1.48
p by ANOVA	0.453	0.735	0.532

Results are presented as means (SD) and 95% confidence intervals (CI).

4. Discussion

This is the first study in northern Greece that estimates salt intake in a group of free-living healthy adults using 24-hour urinary excretion, which is the preferred method of obtaining data on salt intake in population surveys [12]. Furthermore, rigid controls were applied to exclude participants who were suspected of providing a problematic urine collection. While recruitment was done on an opportunistic basis, a recent study carried out in Australia has shown that group estimates of salt intake from such samples are not significantly different from those obtained from "random" samples [15]. If applicable to Greece, this would suggest that the average estimate of salt consumption is unlikely to be biased. In Greece, there are no nationally-specific guidelines or targets regarding sodium and potassium intakes other than those issued by WHO. Salt intake was, on average, double the current WHO recommendations. Less than 5% of the sample will have had usual intakes below the 5 g per day recommended limit, while one third met the current WHO recommendations of 3510 mg per day for potassium [28]. High salt intake was anticipated in this sample, since salt consumption in neighbouring countries with similar dietary habits is also high. For example, in Turkey, the average salt intake is about 15 g per day [29], while in Italy it is approximately 9 g per day [25].

The greater sodium and potassium intakes seen in men compared to women are in line with other studies [11,15,25,30] and may not only reflect differences in food choices but most probably differences in total food consumption, since men have greater energy requirements than women. The higher the body mass index, the greater the salt intake usually is. The mean body mass index of the participants in this study was in the "overweight" range, which is comparable to the mean body mass index of the Greek adult population as a whole, as reported in the first national health and diet survey [2].

It has been suggested that potassium intake should be at a level which will keep the urinary sodium-to-potassium ratio close to 1.0 (mmol/mmol) [31] or the dietary ratio close to 0.57 (mg/mg) to improve blood pressure. However, 97.2% of the sample had a dietary sodium-to-potassium intake ratio (mg/mg) above 0.57. If one considers the sodium-to-potassium excretion ratio, only two participants appeared to meet WHO recommendations (mg/mg). Whether using excretion or intake values, sodium-to-potassium ratio was high. These values are associated with poor cardiovascular outcomes [22,32]. Considering the differences in the ratio values obtained using sodium and potassium excretion from that using sodium and potassium intake, an agreement should be reached on which ratio to use for monitoring population progress [33].

Detailed information on food consumption was not collected and, as a result, the contribution of different dietary sources was not investigated. On average, men met WHO recommendations for potassium intake while women did not. Potassium is particularly abundant in fruits and vegetables, which are also part of the Mediterranean diet model. The mean MedDietScore was 30.5, which is comparable to the scores published for Greek populations in other studies. In the ATTICA study, the mean score was 25.5 (2.9) for men and 27.2 (3.2) for women [26], while in the more recent MEDIS study, participants from the Mani region in Greece (a rural region which keeps old traditions) had a mean MedDietScore of 32 (4.0) [34]. However, in our study, those who appear to adhere better to a Mediterranean diet did not have different salt intake or sodium-to-potassium ratio compared to those who adhere less to a Mediterranean diet. The addition of salt to salads and cooked vegetables as well as the high salt content of some traditional Greek foods, such as cheeses, pies and spreads [35], might account for this lack of association. Therefore, while sustained efforts to promote the traditional Mediterranean model of diet in Greece are important and necessary, these should also be accompanied with specific actions to reduce salt.

Limitations of the Study

Two aspects of the study need further discussion. First, the use of an opportunistic sampling frame may introduce a bias in the overall estimate of salt consumption, affecting the validity of the survey. 24-hour urine collections often are a burden to participants of large population-based dietary surveys so that, despite great efforts and resources, response rates are often low [15,30,36,37]. A recent study has compared the results of an opportunistically recruited volunteer population sample where a random sampling had yielded a 16% response rate [15]. The average estimates of salt intake were comparable, suggesting that such an approach may provide a reasonable estimate of population salt intake. In our study, every possible step was taken to minimize the chance of recruiting individuals who were particularly interested in their salt intake or their blood pressure, and who might unconsciously have modified their consumption of salt during the time of the survey. Still, the possibility of selection bias cannot be excluded, since those who participated expressed interest in taking part in a nutrition-related survey and as a consequence may generally be more cautious about their diet. Similar concerns, however, could be raised for nutrition surveys which do not provide financial or other non-nutrition-related incentives. In addition, although a 24-hour period is necessary to capture the marked diurnal variation in sodium and water excretion, there is day-to-day variation in salt consumption (due to daily variations in salt intake as well as a possible infradian rhythmical variability) [38–40]. The high intra-individual variability, compared to the between-subjects variability, limits the ability to characterize individuals' sodium excretion (i.e., salt intake). However, it does not much limit the ability to identify the average salt intake of groups (like Greek men and women, collectively) to support the valid evaluation of population intervention programmes over time. Finally, the survey was stopped in the months of July and August, to minimize the potential confounding effect of high temperature and excessive sweating. We feel that the estimates obtained in our study, whilst limited, provide enough evidence to support a national programme of population reduction in salt intake.

The second limitation regards the study's representativeness of the whole Greek population. The survey was performed in the urban and suburban areas of Thessaloniki, the largest city in northern Greece. Clearly, it is difficult to infer to the rest of the country. Greece has a widely spread territory, not only spanning from north to south but also with sharp contrasts between mountainous and sea areas and the myriad of islands. Their populations, whilst sharing some national traditions also reflected in common eating habits, do have distinctive local differences that might affect the amount of salt they usually consume. While limited information on dietary habits was obtained to estimate the MedDietScore, detailed long-term data on food consumption, through the use of a food diary or dietary recalls, were not obtained and, as a result, the main contributors to salt intake could not be assessed. Furthermore, university-educated participants were slightly overrepresented compared to the frequency of them in the national census of similar age. As salt consumption was lower in them, the group estimates obtained in our study may be a conservative estimate of an even higher intake in the general population.

5. Conclusions

Measurements of 24-hour urinary sodium and potassium excretion were carried out for the first time in a sample of healthy free-living adults in northern Greece. These measurements revealed that, in this population, salt consumption is high and above the WHO upper limit, whilst potassium consumption is still sub-optimal. No significant relationships were found between salt intake and adherence to a Mediterranean diet, suggesting that the perception of the health benefits of a Mediterranean diet does not hold when referring to salt consumption. These results should provide an impetus for public health authorities in Greece to continue their efforts towards meeting the WHO target of a 30% reduction in salt intake by 2025. In the absence of a more comprehensive national survey of habitual salt intake in Greece, our data provides a useful baseline against which to monitor the impact of future salt reduction initiatives.

Acknowledgments: The WHO Office for Europe provided some financial support for the publication of this study. The present analysis was carried out under the terms of reference of the WHO Collaborating Centre for Nutrition at the University of Warwick.

Author Contributions: E.V. coordinated the study and carried out the fieldwork and all the statistical analyses. G.M. developed the idea and drafted the manuscript. F.P.C. advised on the methodology, carried out data cleaning and contributed to discussions in the analysis and discussion of results. P.S. carried out all urine analyses. A.A.K. and N.R. helped with the fieldwork. All authors contributed to the final version of the manuscript. The authors alone are responsible for the content and views expressed in this publication and they do not necessarily represent the decisions, policy or views of the Hellenic Food Authority or of the World Health Organization.

Conflicts of Interest: G.M. is a scientific officer of the Hellenic Food Authority. J.B. is a staff member of WHO. F.P.C. in an unpaid member of CASH, WASH, the UK Health Forum, the UK Public Health NACD; technical advisor to NICE, the WHO, Vice-President and Trustee of the British and Irish Hypertension Society.

References

1. Global Burden of Diseases, Injuries, and Risk Factors Study (GBD). Available online: http://www.healthdata.org/greece (accessed on 5 March 2017).
2. Hellenic Health Foundation. HYDRIA Project. Conclusions, Remarks and Recommendations for Policy Measures. Available online: http://www.hhf-greece.gr/images/book-hydria-120516print.pdf (accessed on 11 November 2016).
3. Cook, N.R.; Cutler, J.A.; Obarzanek, E.; Buring, J.E.; Rexrode, K.M.; Kumanyika, S.K.; Appel, L.J.; Whelton, P.K. Long term effects of dietary sodium reduction on cardiovascular disease outcomes: Observational follow-up of the Trials of Hypertension Prevention (TOHP). *BMJ* **2007**, *334*, 885–888. [CrossRef] [PubMed]
4. Strazzullo, P.; D'Elia, L.; Kandala, N.B.; Cappuccio, F.P. Salt intake, stroke, and cardiovascular disease: Meta-analysis of prospective studies. *BMJ* **2009**, *339*, b4567. [CrossRef] [PubMed]
5. Aburto, N.J.; Ziolkovska, A.; Hooper, L.; Elliott, P.; Cappuccio, F.P.; Meerpohl, J.J. Effect of lower sodium intake on health: Systematic review and meta-analysis. *BMJ* **2013**, *346*, f1326. [CrossRef] [PubMed]
6. He, F.J.; Li, J.; MacGregor, G.A. Effect of longer term modest salt reduction on blood pressure: Cochrane systematic review and meta-analysis of randomised trials. *BMJ* **2013**, *346*, f1325. [CrossRef] [PubMed]
7. Mente, A.; O'Donnell, M.; Rangarajan, S.; Dagenais, G.; Lear, S.; McQueen, M.; Diaz, R.; Avezum, A.; Lopez-Jaramillo, P.; Lanas, F.; et al. For the PURE, EPIDREAM and ONTARGET/TRANSCEND Investigators. Associations of urinary sodium excretion with cardiovascular events in individuals with and without hypertension: A pooled analysis of data from four studies. *Lancet* **2016**, *388*, 465–475. [CrossRef]

8. Cappuccio, F.P.; Campbell, N.R.C. Population dietary salt reduction and the risk of cardiovascular disease: A commentary on recent evidence. *J. Clin. Hypertens.* **2017**, *19*, 4–5. [CrossRef] [PubMed]
9. Cappuccio, F.P. Cardiovascular and other effects of salt consumption. *Kidney Int. Suppl.* **2013**, *3*, 312–315. [CrossRef] [PubMed]
10. World Health Organization. *Guideline. Sodium Intake for Adults and Children*; World Health Organization (WHO): Geneva, Switzerland, 2012.
11. Brown, I.J.; Tzoulaki, I.; Candeias, V.; Elliott, P. Salt intakes around the world: Implications for public health. *Int. J. Epidemiol.* **2009**, *38*, 791–813. [CrossRef] [PubMed]
12. Cappuccio, F.P.; Capewell, S. Facts, Issues, and Controversies in Salt Reduction for the Prevention of Cardiovascular Disease. *Funct. Food Rev.* **2015**, *7*, 41–61.
13. WHO Regional Office for Europe. *Mapping Salt Reduction Initiatives in the WHO European Region*; WHO Regional Office for Europe: Copenhagen, Denmark, 2013.
14. Intersalt cooperative research group. Intersalt: An international study of electrolyte excretion and blood pressure. Results for 24 hour urinary sodium and potassium excretion. *BMJ* **1988**, *297*, 319–328.
15. Land, M.A.; Webster, J.; Christoforou, A.; Praveen, D.; Jeffery, P.; Chalmers, J.; Smith, W.; Woodward, M.; Barzi, F.; Nowson, C.; et al. Salt intake assessed by 24 h urinary sodium excretion in a random and opportunistic sample in Australia. *BMJ Open* **2014**, *4*, e003720. [CrossRef] [PubMed]
16. Aburto, N.J.; Hanson, S.; Gutierrez, H.; Hooper, L.; Elliott, P.; Cappuccio, F.P. Effect of increased potassium intake on cardiovascular risk factors and disease: Systematic review and meta-analyses. *BMJ* **2013**, *346*, f1378. [CrossRef] [PubMed]
17. Binia, A.; Jaeger, J.; Hu, Y.; Singh, A.; Zimmermann, D. Daily potassium intake and sodium-to-potassium ratio in the reduction of blood pressure: A meta-analysis of randomized controlled trials. *J. Hypertens.* **2015**, *33*, 1509–1520. [CrossRef] [PubMed]
18. Ekmekcioglu, C.; Elmadfa, I.; Meyer, A.L.; Moeslinger, T. The role of dietary potassium in hypertension and diabetes. *J. Physiol. Biochem.* **2016**, *72*, 93–106. [CrossRef] [PubMed]
19. D'Elia, L.; Barba, G.; Cappuccio, F.P.; Strazzullo, P. Potassium Intake, Stroke, and Cardiovascular Disease. A meta-analysis of Prospective Studies. *J. Am. Coll. Cardiol.* **2011**, *57*, 1210–1219. [CrossRef] [PubMed]
20. Young, D.B.; Lin, H.; McCabe, R.D. Potassium's cardiovascular protective mechanisms. *Am. J. Physiol.* **1995**, *268 (4 Pt 2)*, R825–R837. [PubMed]
21. Morris, R.C., Jr.; Schmidlin, O.; Frassetto, L.A.; Sebastian, A. Relationship and interaction between sodium and potassium. *J. Am. Coll. Nutr.* **2006**, *25*, 262S–270S. [CrossRef] [PubMed]
22. Cook, N.R.; Obarzanek, E.; Cutler, J.A. Joint effects of sodium and potassium intake on subsequent cardiovascular disease: The Trials of Hypertension Prevention follow-up study. *Arch. Int. Med.* **2009**, *169*, 32–40. [CrossRef] [PubMed]
23. Weaver, C.M. Potassium and Health. *Adv. Nutr.* **2013**, *4*, 368S–377S. [CrossRef] [PubMed]
24. Jaffe, M. Uber den Niederschlag welchen Pikrinsaure in normalen Harn erzeug und uber eine neue Raction des Creatinins. *Z. Physiol. Chem.* **1986**, *10*, 391–400.
25. Cappuccio, F.P.; Ji, C.; Donfrancesco, C.; Palmieri, L.; Ippolito, R.; Vanuzzo, D.; Giampaoli, S.; Strazzullo, P. Geographic and socioeconomic variation of sodium and potassium intake in Italy: Results from the MINISAL-GIRCSI programme. *BMJ Open* **2015**, *5*, e007467. [CrossRef] [PubMed]
26. Panagiotakos, D.B.; Pitsavos, C.; Arvaniti, F.; Stefanadis, C. Adherence to the Mediterranean food pattern predicts the prevalence of hypertension, hypercholesterolemia, diabetes and obesity, among healthy adults; the accuracy of the MedDietScore. *Prev. Med.* **2007**, *44*, 335–340. [CrossRef] [PubMed]
27. Pan American Health Organization—World Health Organization. *Salt-Smart Americas: A Guide for Country-Level Action*; Pan American Health Organization: Washington, DC, USA, 2013; pp. 1–159.
28. World Health Organization. *Guideline. Potassium Intake for Adults and Children*; World Health Organization: Geneva, Switzerland, 2012; pp. 1–42.
29. Sahan, C.; Sozmen, K.; Unal, B.; O'Flaherty, M.; Critchley, J. Potential benefits of healthy food and lifestyle policies for reducing coronary heart disease mortality in Turkish adults by 2025: A modelling study. *BMJ Open* **2016**, *6*, e011217. [CrossRef] [PubMed]
30. Ribič, C.H.; Zakotnik, J.M.; Vertnik, L.; Vegnuti, M.; Cappuccio, F.P. Salt intake of the Slovene population assessed by 24 h urinary sodium excretion. *Public Health Nutr.* **2010**, *13*, 1803–1809. [CrossRef] [PubMed]

31. World Health Organization (WHO). *Diet, Nutrition and the Prevention of Chronic Disease*; Report of a Joint WHO/FAO Expert Consultation; World Health Organization (WHO): Geneva, Switzerland, 2003.
32. Yang, Q.; Liu, T.; Kuklina, E.V.; Flanders, W.D.; Hong, Y.; Gillespie, C.; Chang, M.H.; Gwinn, M.; Dowling, N.; Khoury, M.J.; et al. Sodium and potassium intake and mortality among US adults: Prospective data from the Third National Health and Nutrition Examination Survey. *Arch. Int. Med.* **2011**, *171*, 1183–1191. [CrossRef] [PubMed]
33. Yi, S.S.; Curtis, C.J.; Angell, S.Y.; Anderson, C.A.; Jung, M.; Kansagra, S.M. Highlighting the ratio of sodium to potassium in population-level dietary assessments: Cross-sectional data from New York City, USA. *Public Health Nutr.* **2014**, *17*, 2484–2488. [CrossRef] [PubMed]
34. Mariolis, A.; Foscolou, A.; Tyrovolas, S.; Piscopo, S.; Valacchi, G.; Tsakountakis, N.; Zeimbekis, A.; Bountziouka, V.; Gotsis, E.; Metallinos, G.; et al. MEDIS study group. Successful Aging among Elders Living in the Mani Continental Region vs. Insular Areas of the Mediterranean: The MEDIS Study. *Aging Dis.* **2016**, *7*, 285–294. [PubMed]
35. Girvalaki, C.; Vardavas, C.I.; Tsimpinos, G.; Dimitreli, G.; Hassapidou, M.N.; Kafatos, A. Nutritional and chemical quality of traditional spreads and pies of Mediterranean diet of Greece. *J. Food Nutr. Disor.* **2013**, *2*, 1.
36. Birukov, A.; Rakova, N.; Lerchl, K.; Engberink, R.H.; Johannes, B.; Wabel, P.; Moissl, U.; Rauh, M.; Luft, F.C.; Titze, J. Ultra-long-term human salt balance studies reveal interrelations between sodium, potassium, and chloride intake and excretion. *Am. J. Clin. Nutr.* **2016**, *104*, 49–57. [CrossRef] [PubMed]
37. Chappuis, A.; Bochud, M.; Glatz, N.; Vuistiner, P.; Paccaud, F.; Burnier, M. Swiss Survey on Salt Intake: Main Results. 2011. Available online: http://my.unil.ch/serval/document/BIB_16AEF897B618.pdf (accessed on 8 March 2017).
38. Ortega, R.M.; Lopez-Sobaler, A.M.; Ballesteros, J.M.; Pérez-Farinós, N.; Rodríguez-Rodríguez, E.; Aparicio, A.; Perea, J.M.; Andrés, P. Estimation of salt intake by 24 h urinary sodium excretion in a representative sample of Spanish adults. *Br. J. Nutr.* **2011**, *105*, 787–794. [CrossRef] [PubMed]
39. Liu, K.; Cooper, R.; McKeever, J.; McKeever, P.; Byington, R.; Soltero, I.; Stamler, R.; Gosch, F.; Stevens, E.; Stamler, J. Assessment of the association between habitual salt intake and high blood pressure: Methodological problems. *Am. J. Epidemiol.* **1979**, *110*, 219–226. [CrossRef] [PubMed]
40. Lerchl, K.; Rakova, N.; Dahlmann, A.; Rauh, M.; Goller, U.; Basner, M.; Dinges, D.F.; Beck, L.; Agureev, A.; Larina, I.; et al. Agreement between 24-hour salt ingestion and sodium excretion in a controlled environment. *Hypertension* **2015**, *66*, 850–857. [CrossRef] [PubMed]

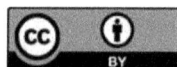

nutrients

MDPI

Article

Changes in the Sodium Content of Australian Processed Foods between 1980 and 2013 Using Analytical Data

Felicity Zganiacz [1], Ron B. H. Wills [2], Soumi Paul Mukhopadhyay [3], Jayashree Arcot [4,*] and Heather Greenfield [4]

[1] Formerly an Honours student within the Food Science and Technology Group, School of Chemical Engineering, UNSW, Sydney, NSW 2052, Australia; felicity.zganiacz@live.com
[2] Department of Food Technology, Faculty of Science and Information Technology, University of Newcastle, Ourimbah, NSW 2258, Australia; ron.wills@newcastle.edu.au
[3] School of Agricultural and Wine Sciences, Charles Sturt University, Wagga Wagga, NSW 2678, Australia; Smukhopadhyay@csu.edu.au
[4] Food Science and Technology Group, School of Chemical Engineering, UNSW, Sydney, NSW 2052, Australia; h.greenfield@unsw.edu.au
* Correspondence: j.arcot@unsw.edu.au; Tel.: +61-2-9385-5360

Received: 14 March 2017; Accepted: 12 May 2017; Published: 15 May 2017

Abstract: The objective of this study was to obtain analytical data on the sodium content of a range of processed foods and compare the levels obtained with their label claims and with published data of the same or equivalent processed foods in the 1980s and 1990s to investigate the extent of any change in sodium content in relation to reformulation targets. The sodium contents of 130 Australian processed foods were obtained by inductively coupled plasma optical emission spectrometry (ICP-OES) analysis and compared with previously published data. The sodium content between 1980 and 2013 across all products and by each product category were compared. There was a significant overall sodium reduction of 23%, 181 mg/100 g (p <0.001, 95% CI (Confidence Interval), 90 to 272 mg/100 g), in Australian processed foods since 1980, with a 12% (83 mg/100 g) reduction over the last 18 years. The sodium content of convenience foods (p < 0.001, 95% CI, 94 to 291 mg/100 g) and snack foods (p = 0.017, 95% CI, 44 to 398 mg/100 g) had declined significantly since 1980. Meanwhile, the sodium contents of processed meats (p = 0.655, 95% CI, −121 to 190) and bread and other bakery products (p = 0.115, 95% CI, −22 to 192) had decreased, though not significantly. Conversely, the sodium content of cheese (p = 0.781, 95% CI, −484 to 369 mg/100 g) had increased but also not significantly. Of the 130 products analysed, 62% met Australian reformulation targets. Sodium contents of the processed foods and the overall changes in comparison with previous data indicate a decrease over the 33 years period and suggest that the Australian recommended reformulation targets have been effective. Further sodium reduction of processed foods is still required and continuous monitoring of the reduction of sodium levels in processed foods is needed.

Keywords: sodium; processed foods; cardiovascular disease; food reformulation; food label accuracy

1. Introduction

The high amount of dietary salt, 9–12 g/day [1], consumed by populations in most countries in the world has been a health issue for decades. This is due to its well-established association with hypertension, which is a major determinant of cardiovascular diseases [2]. In response to the urgency of a reduction in dietary sodium, the World Health Organization (WHO) initiated a global movement. In 2013, all Member States agreed to the target of a 30% reduction in salt intake with the aim of reaching <5 g of salt per day by 2025 [3].

In Australia, the national government and other health authorities have developed and implemented strategies with the aim to reduce the amount of dietary salt. It has been estimated that processed foods contribute to 80% of dietary sodium in Australia [4] and reduction of sodium use in the food industry has been identified as the main approach for addressing this issue. The National Heart Foundation's Tick Program that was implemented over 20 years ago has been successful over the years [5]. Many food companies have taken on the challenge of reducing the salt content of their products in order to meet the "Tick" criteria, which is dependent on the product category [5]. The Australian Division of World Action on Salt and Health (AWASH) and the Australian government's Food and Health Dialogue (FHD) have both published sodium reduction targets. These organizations have been involved in acquiring major food companies to commit to reducing the amount of sodium used in their products until reformulation targets are met [6,7]. The sodium targets (as shown in Table 1) are 400 mg/100 g across bread products, 15% reduction for breakfast cereals exceeding 400 mg/100 g, 1090 mg/100 g for cured meats, 830 mg/100 g for luncheon meats, 10% reduction for wet savoury pies exceeding 400 mg/100 g and dry savoury pies exceeding 500 mg/100 g, 550–800 mg/100 g for potato chips, 950–1250 mg/100 g for extruded snack products, 850–1100 mg/100 g for salt and vinegar snack products, 850 mg/100 g for plain crackers, 1000 mg/100 g for flavoured crackers, 710 mg/100 g for cheddar cheese, and 1270 mg/100 g for other chilled processed cheese [7].

To ensure that the progress towards the sodium reduction targets is made, regular monitoring is essential. There has been a lack of analytical monitoring of sodium changes in processed foods throughout the years. Maples et al. [8] and Wills and Duvernet [9] conducted studies on the sodium content of Australian processed foods in 1980 and 1995, respectively. Both of these studies were conducted prior to the introduction of mandatory nutrition information panel labelling being published in the Commonwealth of Australia Gazette, No. P 30, Wednesday 20 December 2000, as part of Australia New Zealand Food Authority Amendment No. 53 to the Food Standards Code and came into effect from 20 December 2002 [10]. Wills and Duvernet [9] published a comparison of the analytical data from the two studies that presented approximately 10% sodium reduction over the 15 years interval. However, Wills and Duvernet [9] analysed composite samples comprised of all brands of similar food types rather than each product individually, rendering comparison difficult.

Thus, the main purpose of this follow-up study was to determine by chemical analysis the current sodium levels in the same or equivalent processed foods previously analysed. With the introduction of mandatory nutrition information panels [10], it was also considered appropriate to compare the analytical data obtained in the 2013 study with the sodium value declared on the food label.

2. Materials and Methods

The sodium content of 130 different processed foods available in the Australian supermarkets was determined in 2013. The food products were predominately selected based on the availability of those previously analysed by Maples et al. [8] and Wills and Duvernet [9]. The brand and product name of all processed foods were obtained and a market survey was conducted to determine the availability of the products. Products that were no longer obtainable were substituted with an equivalent product. An alternative product by the same manufacturer was selected if available, otherwise the most equivalent product was chosen. The majority of the products were branded products produced by various different manufacturers but some supermarket branded products were also included in the analysis. Two purchases were made of each food product from two different supermarkets in Sydney, ensuring that they were stamped with different batch numbers. The food products were analysed individually, but the results were separated into seven categories: processed meat products, convenience foods (pizza, meat pie, and sausage roll), cheese, bakery products, breakfast cereals, muesli, and snack foods.

Prior to analysis, equal quantities of the two samples purchased for each product were blended to obtain a composite sample with a mass of 100g or more. Sub-samples (0.5 g) of each composite sample were covered with 5 mL of 70% nitric acid and left overnight. They were then heated to 80 °C until the sample became clear in colour (1–3 h) and then cooled prior to adding 2 mL of 30% hydrogen peroxide. The samples were allowed to stand until effervescence ceased before heating for 30 min at 110 °C. They were then made to volume (30 mL) using MilliQ water and left overnight before transferring to 10 mL tubes for analysis by inductively coupled plasma-optical emission spectroscopy (ICP-OES) [11]. Three different blank solutions were also prepared to assist in the calibration of the ICP-OES instrument by negating the effects of background. This method of analysis was used to be consistent with the 1980 and 1995 studies [8,9]. To ensure that the food products were representative of the food as consumed, heating or cooking required by some products was conducted according to the manufacturer's instructions before homogenization. The Standard Reference Material (SRM) 1548a Typical Diet developed by the National Institute of Standards and Technology (NIST) was used to validate the analytical method used for the determination of the sodium content of the food products [12].

Analysis of Variance (ANOVA) and *t*-tests were used for data collected in 2013 as they followed normal distribution for individual category of food products. Hence, mean and range values along with the median values are being reported. For 2013 overall data (Table 1), there were small and varying sample sizes for individual product categories (e.g., 3 salami products; 10 samples each in the pizza, breakfast cereals or sliced white bread categories), normality tests have little power to reject the null hypothesis (that "sample distribution is normal"). Therefore, only results with small sample sizes passed the normality test [13] and have undergone parametric analysis in this instance.

For samples collected from 1980, 1995, and 2013 which were 96, 63, and 116 respectively (Table 2), which represent a large enough sample size (>30 or 40), the normality assumption was not followed [14]. According to the central limit theorem, in large sample sets (>30 or 40), the sampling distribution tends to be normal regardless of the shape of the data [15,16] and means of random samples from any distribution (in this case for Table 2, where mean values from different product categories have been provided) would themselves have a normal distribution [17]. Hence, for all these above reasons, parametric tests have been used in this research.

Independent sample *t*-tests were used to compare the differences in sodium content between 1980 and 2013 overall and by each product category. This data was analysed using the Minitab 17 Statistical Software [18]. The 1995 data could not be included in the statistical analysis as composite samples had been analysed. The 2013 flatbreads and natural muesli data were also excluded from the statistical analyses to ensure products from both data sets included in the analysis were comparable.

3. Results

The sodium contents of the Australian processed foods analysed in 2013 indicate that 62% of the products were compliant when compared to the set targets (Table 1). Overall, the sodium content of the processed foods studied decreased by 23%, 181 mg/100 g ($p < 0.001$, 95% CI, 90 to 272 mg/100 g), since 1980 with most of the reduction (12%, 83 mg/100 g) occurring between 1995 and 2013 (Table 2). Figure 1 indicates an increased density of products appearing toward the lower end of the sodium content scale in 2013 compared to previous years. Table 2 shows the changes in sodium content amongst the different food groups varied considerably with sodium levels of convenience foods (pizza, meat pie, and sausage roll) and cheese increasing by 4% and 50%, respectively.

Table 1. Sodium content of Australian processed foods in 2013.

	Sodium Content (mg/100 g)				
	No. of Products	Mean	Range	Target	% of Products Meeting the Target
Processed meats					
Salami	3	1297	1181–1435	1400 [†]	67%
Ham	4	1131	864–1520	1090 [‡]	50%
Corned beef, canned	1	813			
Luncheon meat, canned	1	793			
Luncheon knobs	5	943	788–1218	830 [‡]	38%
Liverwurst	1	859			
Frankfurts	5	1056	862–1299	1150 [†]	80%
Convenience foods					
Pizza	10	557	412–834		
Frozen/refrigerated	6	540	416–692	390 [†]	0%
Take-away	4	582	412–834	530 [†]	25%
Meat pie	6	395	354–444	400 [‡]	50%
Sausage roll	1	698		450 [†]	0%
Cheese					
Natural cheddar cheese	2	680	670–689	710 [‡]	100%
Other natural cheese	7	597	276–1075		
Processed cheese	2	1535	1242–1828	1270 [‡]	89%
Breads and other bakery products					
Crackers	5	743	572–1024		
Crispbread	3	339	227–513	850 [‡]	88%
Sweet biscuit, plain	4	447	285–523	270 [†]	0%
Sweet biscuit, cream	2	338	291–384	170 [†]	0%
Bread, multigrain, sliced	7	403	358–474		
Bread, white, sliced	10	390	346–511		
Bread, wholemeal, sliced	9	393	321–519		
Fruit bread, sliced	1	220		400 [‡]	65%
Flatbread, white	7	472	151–902		
Flatbread, wholemeal	6	497	163–882		
Cheesecake	2	219	214–223	240 [†]	100%
Breakfast cereals					
	10	401	288–563	400 [‡]	60%
Muesli					
Natural	1	8			
				400 [‡]	100%
Toasted	1	24			
Snack foods					
Potato chips	8	720	483–996	800 [‡]	75%
Salt and vinegar	2	874	751–996	1100 [‡]	100%
Potato straws	1	764		800 [‡]	100%
Extruded products	5	964	674–1169	1250 [‡]	100%
				Overall	62% (80/130)

[†] The Australian Division of World Action on Salt and Health target [19]; [‡] The Food and Health Dialogue target [7].

Table 2. Changes in sodium content of Australian processed foods between 1980 and 2013.

| | | | | Sodium Content Change (mg/100 g) | | | |
| | 2013 | 1995 [9] | 1980 [8] | 1995–2013 | | 1980–2013 | |
				mg	%	mg	%
Processed meats							
No. of products	20	15	24				
Mean sodium content (mg/100 g)	1043	1120	1078	−77	−7%	−35	−3%
Convenience foods (pizza, meat pie, and sausage roll)							
No. of products	17	8	16				
Mean sodium content (mg/100 g)	508	490	700	+18	+4%	−92	−27%
Cheese							
No. of products	11	11	8				
Mean sodium content (mg/100 g)	782	520	725	+262	+50%	+57	+8%
Breads and other bakery products							
No. of products	43	17	23				
Mean sodium content (mg/100 g)	421	550	506	−129	−23%	−85	−17%
Breakfast cereals							
No. of products	10	7	10				
Mean sodium content (mg/100 g)	400	684	806	−284	−42%	−406	−50%
Muesli (toasted)							
No. of products	1	1	2				
Mean sodium content (mg/100 g)	24	250	317	−226	−90%	−293	−92%
Snack foods							
No. of products	14	4	13				
Mean sodium content (mg/100 g)	810	830	1032	−20	−2%	−222	−21%
Overall							
No. of products	116	63	96				
Mean sodium content (mg/100 g)	617	700	798	−83	−12%	−181	−23%

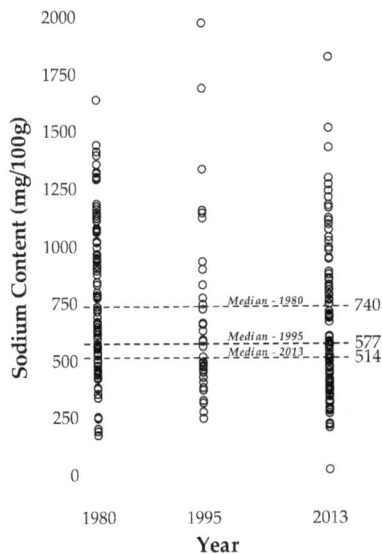

Figure 1. Comparison of the sodium contents of Australian processed foods between 1980 and 2013 where a circle represents each product.

3.1. Sodium Content of Processed Foods in 2013

In 2013, the average sodium content of Australian processed foods was 617 mg/100 g (Table 2). The most significant overall sodium reductions were in the convenience foods (pizza, meat pie, and sausage roll), 27% ($p < 0.001$, 95% CI, 94 to 291 mg/100 g) and breakfast cereals, 50% ($p = 0.001$, 95% CI, 218 to 593 mg/100 g) categories. The muesli category showed a 92% reduction, however it could not be tested for significance due to the low sample size. Conversely, only a slight decrease in the processed meats category, 3% ($p = 0.655$, 95% CI, −121 to 190) was seen, and this was not significant. The results also revealed an 8% ($p = 0.781$, 95% CI, −484 to 369 mg/100 g) sodium increase in the cheese category and this was also not significant. Furthermore, products in the sub-categories within the seven categories presented greater variations in sodium content (Table 1). Among the processed meats, sodium values ranged from 793 mg/100 g in canned luncheon meat up to 1297 mg/100 g in salami. Within the convenience foods group, sausage rolls (698 mg/100 g) contained the highest sodium level and meat pies (395 mg/100 g) contained the lowest. The sodium content of cheese varied greatly, ranging between 267 and 1828 mg/100g overall with processed cheeses—which are typically produced by blending one or more natural cheeses of different ages, emulsifying salts, water, other dairy, and non-dairy ingredients [20]—containing the most sodium. Of the bakery products, crackers had the highest average sodium content of 743 mg/100 g, with the other biscuit subcategories having an average between 338 and 447 mg/100 g. Despite being characterised as "sweet", it is interesting to see that sweet biscuits have high sodium contents. The average sodium level in multigrain (403 mg/100 g), white (390 mg/100 g), and wholemeal (393 mg/100 g) bread was shown to be quite similar. However, the fruit bread analysed was considerably lower with a sodium content of 220 mg/100 g. In comparison to the other types of bread, white (472 mg/100 g) and wholemeal flatbreads (497 mg/100 g) contained the most sodium on average. The cheesecake subcategory had a mean sodium content that is one of the lowest in the bakery products group at 219 mg/100 g. The mean sodium content of breakfast cereals was 401 mg/100 g, which can be considered to be high when evaluated against muesli (16 mg/100 g). In the snack foods category, extruded snack foods had the highest average sodium content, 964 mg/100 g, compared to potato chips (720 mg/100 g) and potato straws (764 mg/100 g).

3.2. Changes in Mean Sodium Content between 1980 and 2013

The changes in the mean sodium content of processed foods between 1980 and 2013 are shown in Table 2. The average sodium content of processed meats in 2013 was lower than the values published in 1980 and 1995 by 3% ($p = 0.655$, 95% CI, −121 to 190) and 7%, respectively, though this was not statistically significant. For convenience foods (pizza, meat pies, and sausage rolls), when compared with the 1980 average sodium content, a 27% ($p < 0.001$, 95% CI, 94 to 291 mg/100 g) reduction is indicated, though there appeared to be a 4% sodium increase between 1995 (by data inspection only) and 2013. The mean sodium content of cheeses is shown to have increased by about 8% ($p = 0.781$, 95% CI, −484 to 369 mg/100 g) since 1980, apparently doubling since 1995, although this was not statistically significant. Continual reduction of sodium used in bakery products was evident, with an overall but not significant reduction of approximately 17% ($p = 0.115$, 95% CI, −22 to 192). Conversely, the sodium content of breakfast cereals had declined significantly by 50% ($p = 0.001$, 95% CI, 218 to 593 mg/100 g). The greatest reduction has occurred within the muesli category, with a 92% decrease. Although the muesli category consisted of a low sample size, the products analysed in 1980 were the same brands re-analysed in 1995 and 2013. Since 1980, the sodium content of snack foods had decreased by 21% ($p = 0.017$, 95% CI, 44 to 398 mg/100 g) though only a 2% reduction may have occurred since 1995 (using data inspection only). Overall, the mean sodium content of processed foods continued to decline over the years (Table 2).

3.3. Proportion of Processed Foods that Met Established Sodium Targets in 2013

The proportion of all Australian processed foods analysed in 2013 that met sodium targets established by the FHD and AWASH was 62% (Table 1). All of the products categorised under natural cheddar cheese, cheesecake, muesli, potato chips (salt and vinegar), potato straws, and extruded products complied in 2013 with the reformulation targets. However, none of the pizza (frozen/refrigerated), sausage roll, or sweet biscuit products met the set targets. The majority of the other categories had ≥50% of products meeting the reformulation targets.

3.4. Comparison of Analytical Sodium Content Data with Label Claims in 2013

The majority of the discrepancies between the actual analytical and label-declared sodium contents of processed foods were within the suggested acceptable range of ±20% [21], with 14% of products being outside the acceptable range (Table 3). The extent of the sodium content variation of both muesli products analysed when compared to the label-declared sodium values were unacceptable, with a 26% under-declaration for the toasted muesli and a 65% over-declaration for the natural muesli. When comparing the analysed and declared sodium content values of convenience foods, 24% of products were shown to have unacceptable label discrepancies. These products were from the pizza sub-category and the differences ranged from 25% less sodium to 26–43% more sodium than the label-declared amount. The breads and other bakery products category had 14% of products testing at unacceptable levels. The greatest discrepancies between analytical data and label claim were most prevalent in the flatbreads sub-category, which were shown to contain 28–47% less sodium than the value declared. The biscuits sub-category had the least amount of variation, ranging between 4% less than the amount declared to 8% more. All breakfast cereals were within ±20% of the sodium content declared on the label. The majority of products contained 1–18% less sodium than the content declared on the label, with a few products containing 2–10% more sodium than declared.

Table 3. Food label discrepancies between the analytical and label-declared sodium contents of processed foods analysed in 2013.

Food Category	Unacceptable ^
Processed meats	10% (*n* = 2/10)
Convenience foods	24% (*n* = 4/17)
Cheese	9% (*n* = 1/11)
Breads and other bakery products	14% (*n* = 8/56)
Breakfast cereals	0% (*n* = 0/10)
Muesli	100% (*n* = 2/2)
Snack foods	7% (*n* = 1/14)
Overall	14% (*n* = 18/130)

^ Unacceptable when exceeding the suggested acceptable discrepancy range of ±20% [21].

4. Discussion

The findings from this study indicate that Australian food companies are making efforts to progressively reduce the amount of sodium added to their processed food products. It is reassuring to observe that the sodium content of processed foods has continued to decline (12%) since the 1995 study. The overall reductions of 12% between 1995 and 2013, and 23% between 1980 and 2013 ($p < 0.001$, 95% CI, 90 to 272 mg/100 g) are positive results. The proportion of products meeting the reformulation targets set is also promising as 80 out of 130 products analysed were within the AWASH and FHD recommendations. Despite this positive result, it is apparent that further improvements are still required. This is achievable if greater emphasis were given to the importance of sodium reduction within the food industry. To maintain momentum, there must be continual monitoring of the progress towards sodium reduction targets using proper methods of reporting as this ensures that companies are fulfilling their pledges [22,23].

Sodium plays various important roles in many food products such as flavour, texture enhancement, and shelf life. This can make sodium reduction difficult when ensuring the acceptability is not affected. For thousands of years, sodium has been used in processed meats to assist in preservation by lowering the water activity and acts as a binding agent [24]. Similarly, salt is used in the production of cheese due to its ability to aid in moisture and microbial control in addition to being an emulsifier [20]. Given that the average sodium content of processed meats only decreased slightly and that there was a considerable increase of sodium in cheese suggests that limitations to the extent of sodium reduction may be responsible. The minimal reduction of sodium in meat products is quite concerning, considering this food group has been assessed as accounting for 21% of Australian's salt intake [25]. However, the overall reduction is still reassuring seeing as Wills and Duvernet [9] previously reported a 30% increase in the sodium content of salami which was likely due to an industry response to the Garibaldi salami food poisoning incident in 1994. The most substantial reductions that have occurred since 1995 are in the bakery products (23%), breakfast cereals (42%), and muesli (90%) categories. This is a good outcome given that cereals and cereal products (grains, bread, pasta, biscuits, etc.) account for 32% of Australian's salt intake and cereal based products and dishes (biscuits, muffins, pizza, etc.) accounted for 17% according to assessments by Webster et al. [25].

It is evident that there are issues and challenges that restrict the extent of sodium reduction achievable for different food groups. Consumer acceptance of sodium reduced products is important, especially when flavour is the major determining factor of food acceptance and consumption [26]. Studies have shown that sodium levels can be reduced by 30% to 50% without influencing the taste and consumer acceptability, where gradual reduction overtime is the key to minimising the noticeability of the change [27–30]. Excessive sodium reduction however, can lead to its replacement at the table where up to 20% can be added [26,31]. This is where consumer education and awareness can be extremely beneficial, where guidance is provided to assist consumers to change their habitual discretionary salt use. Following a national campaign in England, a study revealed that the number of consumers that added salt at the table had decreased by greater than 25% after five years [32]. Where sodium is important for its functional attributes, reduction may result in the requirement of additives to assist in achieving the same favourable characteristics of the product, which can be undesirable [33].

In light of the fact that the nutrition information displayed on the packaging of food products are typically generated theoretically using nutrition databases rather than from actual analysis, discrepancies between the values declared and the analysed contents were assessed. The sodium content of the foods analysed were predominantly within ±20%, which has been suggested to be an acceptable discrepancy range [21]. However, 14% of products were not within this acceptable limit. The issue may be simply due to the use of theoretical nutrition information on the labels. Manufacturers continuously reformulate products [34], therefore it is possible that with changes in the formulation of products, the nutrition labels have not been updated accordingly. Nutrition labels were introduced to assist consumers with their food choices by allowing them to know what they are consuming. It is important that industry declares nutrient content accurately to ensure that consumers can trust the nutrient values declared on labels [35].

5. Conclusions

In conclusion, the analytical data from this study indicates a declining trend in the sodium levels of Australian processed foods. The continual reduction of sodium used during the manufacturing of food products is highlighted, though further reduction is still necessary. Whilst the reduction of salt can reduce the sodium content of a product, it is important to also consider other components in processed foods that contribute to the overall sodium content. Technical limitations may be considered a challenge, however research into new technologies and solutions to the complications that may be faced can assist in developing innovations. The variations between the sodium content of products within categories such as processed meats (793–1297 mg/100 g) and cheese (267–1828 mg/100 g) suggest that reformulation to reduce the sodium content is possible. Gradual reduction of the sodium

Nutrients **2017**, *9*, 501

levels by the food industry will assist in adapting the preference of consumers [29]. The engagement of more food companies in the FHD and AWASH reformulation programs is essential for more consistent reductions. Ongoing salt reduction programs have been most effective in other countries such as the United Kingdom, the United States, Canada, and Finland where the government has been involved [36–38]. Regulation where non-compliance results in some form of penalty is believed to be a strong driver for industry reformulation by public health experts [22,39]. The implementation of mandatory reformulation targets to the entire food industry with the support of the Australian government would be highly beneficial. This would help support continual improvements and ensure that Australia is contributing to the global 30% reduction target set by the WHO. It is also imperative that nutrition information panels are updated when formulation changes are implemented so that consumers are provided with the correct information. However, given that the Australian regulations allow for the nutrition information panels to be theoretically calculated, the use of the sodium content on labels may not be entirely reliable. To track the progress of the food industry accurately and to better monitor the sodium reduction of processed foods, analytical data should be obtained on a regular basis. Conducting future studies to obtain analytical data on the sodium content of the same or similar processed foods included in this study will allow for continuous monitoring of the changes in sodium content in relation to reformulation targets and food labelling. Alternatively, focusing on processed food categories that contribute the most to daily salt consumption—such as bread, bread rolls, processed meat, and cereal products [40]—could allow for more frequent random analysis and comparisons against nutritional information panels to be feasible.

Author Contributions: Felicity Zganiacz did the collection, analyses of the samples, and writing the first draft of the manuscript; Ron B.H. Wills provided advice on the sample collection and types of samples previously analysed; Soumi Paul Mukhopadhyay provided advice and assisted with the statistical analysis; Jayashree Arcot and Heather Greenfield were the main supervisors who advised on sampling and analysis, the management of the project, and writing the manuscript.

Conflicts of Interest: The authors declare no conflict of interest.

References

1. He, F.J.; MacGregor, G.A. A comprehensive review on salt and health and current experience of worldwide salt reduction programmes. *J. Hum. Hypertens.* **2009**, *23*, 363–384. [CrossRef] [PubMed]

2. Morgan, T.; Brunner, H. Hypertension | Etiology. In *Encyclopedia of Human Nutrition, Four-Volume Set*; Allen, L., Prentice, A., Caballero, B., Eds.; Elsevier Science: Cambridge, MA, USA, 2005; ISBN: 9780123750839.

3. The World Health Organization (WHO). Global Strategy on Diet, Physical Activity and Health: Population Sodium Reduction Strategies. Available online: http://www.who.int/dietphysicalactivity/reducingsalt/en/ (accessed on 7 March 2014).

4. Appel, L.J.; Anderson, C.A.M. Compelling evidence for public health action to reduce salt intake. *N. Engl. J. Med.* **2010**, *362*, 650–652. [CrossRef] [PubMed]

5. Williams, P.; McMahon, A.; Boustead, R. A case study of sodium reduction in breakfast cereals and the impact of the pick the tick food information program in Australia. *Health Pr. Int.* **2003**, *18*, 51–56. [CrossRef]

6. The Australian Division of World Action on Salt and Health (AWASH). Our Aims. Available online: http://www.awash.org.au/about-us/our-aims/ (accessed on 7 March 2014).

7. The Food and Health Dialogue (FHD). Summary of Food Categories Engaged under the Food and Health Dialogue to Date. Available online: http://www.health.gov.au/internet/main/publishing.nsf/Content/fhd (accessed on 14th May 2017).

8. Maples, J.; Wills, R.B.H.; Greenfield, H. Sodium and potassium levels in Australian processed foods. *Med. J. Aust.* **1982**, *2*, 20–22. [PubMed]

9. Wills, R.B.H.; Duvernet, L. Update on sodium levels in Australian processed foods. *Food Aust.* **1996**, *48*, 568–569.

10. Food Standards Australian New Zealand (FSANZ). FLMS Overview Fact Sheet. Available online: http://www.foodstandards.gov.au/publications/pages/evaluationreportseries/ foodlabelmonitoringsurvey10/flmsoverviewfactshee3077.aspx (accessed on 14 April 2017).

11. Mark Wainwright Analytical Centre: 2013. DE-23: Microwave Digestion-Closed System without HF, and Final Medium HNO3 and/or HCl. ICP-AES, Certified Method of the Australasian Soil and Plant Analysis. Available online: http://www.aspac-australasia.com/certified-labs/laboratory/30#&ui-state=dialog (accessed on 15 May 2017).

12. The National Institute of Standards and Technology (NIST). Certificate of Analysis: Standard Reference Material 1548a-Typical Diet. Department of Commerce, Ed.; National Institute of Standards and Technology (NIST): United States of America, 2009. Available online: https://www-s.nist.gov/srmors/certificates/1548A.pdf (accessed on 14 May 2017).

13. Oztuna, D.; Elhan, A.; Tuccar, E. Investigation of four different normality tests in terms of type 1 error rate and power under different distributions. *Turk. J. Med. Sci.* **2006**, *36*, 171–176.

14. Pallant, J. *SPSS Survival Manual: A Step by Step Guide to Data Analysis Using SPSS for Windows*; Version 15; Open University Press: Milton Keynes, UK, 2007; pp. 179–200. ISBN: 0335242391.

15. Field, A.P. *Discovering Statistics Using SPSS*, 3rd ed.; Sage Publications, Inc.: London, UK, 2009; ISBN: 978-1-4462-4917-8.

16. Elliott, A.C.; Woodward, W.A. *Statistical Analysis Quick Reference Guidebook with SPSS Examples*, 1st ed.; Sage Publications, Inc.: London, UK, 2007; ISBN: 1-4129-2560-6.

17. Altman, D.G.; Bland, J.M. Detecting skewness from summary information. *Brit. Med. J.* **1996**, *313*, 1200. [CrossRef] [PubMed]

18. Minitab, Inc. *Minitab 17 Statistical Software*; Minitab, Inc.: State College, PA, USA, 2010.

19. The George Institute for Global Health (GIGH). *Interim Australian Targets for Sodium Levels in 85 Food Categories-'Challenging Yet Feasible'*; The George Institute for Global Health: Newtown, Australia, 2011. Available online: https://issuu.com/emmastirling/docs/interim_salt_targets_for_australia (accessed on 14 May 2017).

20. Johnson, M.E.; Kapoor, R.; McMahon, D.J.; McCoy, D.R.; Narasimmon, R.G. Reduction of sodium and fat levels in natural and processed cheeses: Scientific and Technological Aspects. *Compr. Rev. Food Sci. Food* **2009**, *8*, 252–268. [CrossRef]

21. Fabiansson, S. Precision in nutritional information declarations on food labels. *Asia Pac. J. Clin. Nutr.* **2006**, *15*, 451–458. [PubMed]

22. Webster, J.; Trieu, K.; Dunford, E.; Hawkes, C. Target salt 2025: A global overview of national programs to encourage the food industry to reduce salt in foods. *Nutrients* **2014**, *6*, 3274–3287. [CrossRef] [PubMed]

23. Gillespie, C.; Maalouf, J.; Yuan, K.; Cogswell, M.E.; Gunn, J.P.; Levings, J.; Moshfegh, A.; Ahuja, J.K.C.; Merritt, R.; Gillespie, C.; et al. Sodium content in major brands of us packaged foods, 2009. *Am. J. Clin. Nutr.* **2015**, *101*, 344. [CrossRef] [PubMed]

24. Barat, J.M.; Toldra, F. Reducing salt in processed meat products. In *Processed Meats: Improving Safety, Nutrition and Quality*; Kerry, J.P., Kerry, J.F., Eds.; Academic Press: Oxford, UK, 2011; pp. 331–345. ISBN: 978-0-12-384947-2.

25. Webster, J.; Dunford, E.; Huxley, R.; Li, N.; Nowson, C.A.; Neal, B. The development of a national salt reduction strategy for Australia. *Asia Pac. J. Clin. Nutr.* **2009**, *18*, 303–309. [PubMed]

26. Adams, S.O.; Maller, O.; Cardello, A.V. Consumer acceptance of foods lower in sodium. *J. Am. Diet. Assoc* **1995**, *95*, 447–453. [CrossRef]

27. Witschi, J.C.; Ellison, R.C.; Doane, D.D.; Vorkink, G.L.; Slack, W.V.; Stare, F.J. Dietary-sodium reduction among students-feasibility and acceptance. *J. Am. Diet. Assoc.* **1985**, *85*, 816–821. [PubMed]

28. Nolan, A.L. Low sodium foods-where are we headed. *J. Food Eng.* **1983**, *55*, 95–104.

29. Bertino, M.; Beauchamp, G.K.; Engelman, K. Long-term reduction in dietary-sodium alters the taste of salt. *Am. J. Clin. Nutr.* **1982**, *36*, 1134–1144. [PubMed]

30. Hendriksen, M.A.H.; Verkaik-Kloosterman, J.; Noort, M.W.; van Raaij, J.M.A. Nutritional impact of sodium reduction strategies on sodium intake from processed foods. *Eur. J. Clin. Nutr.* **2015**, *69*, 805–810. [CrossRef] [PubMed]

31. Liem, D.G.; Miremadi, F.; Zandstra, E.H.; Keast, R.S. Health labelling can influence taste perception and use of table salt for reduced-sodium products. *Public Health Nutr.* **2012**, *15*, 2340–2347. [CrossRef] [PubMed]

32. Sutherland, J.; Edwards, P.; Shankar, B.; Dangour, A.D. Fewer adults add salt at the table after initiation of a national salt campaign in the UK: A repeated cross-sectional analysis. *Br. J. Nutr.* **2013**, *110*, 552–558. [CrossRef] [PubMed]

33. Dotsch, M.; Busch, J.; Batenburg, M.; Liem, G.; Tareilus, E.; Mueller, R.; Meijer, G. Strategies to reduce sodium consumption: A food industry perspective. *Crit. Rev. Food Sci. Nutr.* **2009**, *49*, 841–851. [CrossRef] [PubMed]
34. Ahuja, J.K.; Pehrsson, P.R.; Haytowitz, D.B.; Wasswa-Kintu, S.; Nickle, M.; Showell, B.; Thomas, R.; Roseland, J.; Williams, J.; Khan, M.; et al. Sodium monitoring in commercially processed and restaurant foods. *Am. J. Clin. Nutr.* **2015**, *101*, 622–631. [CrossRef] [PubMed]
35. Fitzpatrick, L.; Arcand, J.; L'Abbe, M.; Deng, M.; Duhaney, T.; Campbell, N. Accuracy of Canadian food labels for sodium content of food. *Nutrients* **2014**, *6*, 3326–3335. [CrossRef] [PubMed]
36. Pietinen, P.; Valsta, L.M.; Hirvonen, T.; Sinkko, H. Labelling the salt content in foods: A useful tool in reducing sodium intake in Finland. *Public Health Nutr.* **2008**, *11*, 335–340. [CrossRef] [PubMed]
37. Grimes, C.A.; Nowson, C.A.; Lawrence, M. An evaluation of the reported sodium content of Australian food products. *Int. J. Food Sci. Tech.* **2008**, *43*, 2219–2229. [CrossRef]
38. Dunford, E.K.; Eyles, H.; Mhurchu, C.N.; Webster, J.L.; Neal, B.C. Changes in the sodium content of bread in Australia and New Zealand between 2007 and 2010: Implications for policy. *Med. J. Aust.* **2011**, *195*, 346–349. [CrossRef] [PubMed]
39. MacGregor, G.A.; He, F.J.; Pombo-Rodrigues, S. Food and the responsibility deal: How the salt reduction strategy was derailed. *Brit. Med. J.* **2015**, *350*, h1936. [CrossRef] [PubMed]
40. Food Standards Australian New Zealand (FSANZ). How Much Sodium Do Australians Eat? Available online: http://www.foodstandards.gov.au/consumer/nutrition/salthowmuch/Pages/howmuchsaltareweeating/howmuchsaltandsodium4551.aspx (accessed on 11 April 2017).

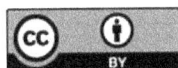

nutrients

MDPI

Article

Know Your Noodles! Assessing Variations in Sodium Content of Instant Noodles across Countries

Clare Farrand [1,*], Karen Charlton [2,3], Michelle Crino [1], Joseph Santos [1], Rodrigo Rodriguez-Fernandez [4], Cliona Ni Mhurchu [5] and Jacqui Webster [1]

[1] The George Institute for Global Health, The University of New South Wales, P.O. Box M20 Missenden Rd, Sydney 2006, Australia; mcrino@georgeinstitute.org.au (M.C.); jsantos@georgeinstitute.org.au (J.S.); jwebster@georgeinstitute.org.au (J.W.)

[2] School of Medicine, Faculty of Science, Medicine and Health, University of Wollongong, Wollongong 2522, Australia; karen_charlton@uow.edu.au

[3] Illawarra Health and Medical Research Institute, Building 32, University of Wollongong Campus, Wollongong 2522, Australia

[4] Non-Communicable Diseases, International SOS, NCD Asia Pacific Alliance, Chiswick Park, 566 Chiswick High Rd, Chiswick, London W4 5YE, UK; rod.rodriguez@ncdapa.org

[5] National Institute for Health Innovation, University of Auckland, Private Bag 92019, Auckland Mail Centre, Auckland 1142, New Zealand; c.nimhurchu@auckland.ac.nz

* Correspondence: cfarrand@georgeinstitute.org.au; Tel.: +61-2-8052-4541

Received: 11 April 2017; Accepted: 8 June 2017; Published: 16 June 2017

Abstract: Reducing salt intake is a cost-effective public health intervention to reduce the global burden of non-communicable disease (NCDs). Ultra-processed foods contribute ~80% of dietary salt in high income countries, and are becoming prominent in low-middle income countries. Instant noodle consumption is particularly high in the Asia Pacific region. The aim of this study was to compare the sodium content of instant noodles sold worldwide to identify potential for reformulation. Analysis was undertaken for 765 instant noodle products from 10 countries using packaged food composition databases of ultra-processed foods compiled by the Global Food Monitoring Group (GFMG) and national shop survey data. Sodium levels were high and variable, within and between countries. Instant noodles in China had the highest mean sodium content (1944 mg/100 g; range: 397–3678/100 g) compared to New Zealand (798 mg/100 g; range: 249–2380 mg/100 g). Average pack size ranged from 57 g (Costa Rica) to 98 g (China). The average packet contributed 35% to 95% of the World Health Organization recommended daily salt intake of <5 g. Forty percent of products met the Pacific Island (PICs) regional sodium targets, 37% met the South Africa 2016 targets, and 72% met the UK 2017 targets. This study emphasises a need for stronger regulation and closer monitoring to drive rigorous reformulation of salt in ultra-processed foods.

Keywords: salt; sodium; salt reduction; ultra-processed food; instant noodles; blood pressure; non-communicable disease (NCDs); burden of disease; nutrition transition; regulation; salt targets

1. Introduction

Cardiovascular disease (CVD) is the number one cause of death worldwide [1], responsible for 17.5 million deaths in 2012. High salt intake raises blood pressure, a major risk factor for CVD. Reducing population salt intake is recognised as a "best buy" for prevention and control of non-communicable diseases (NCDs) by lowering blood pressure and reducing risk of strokes and heart disease [2]. Salt reduction is considered a priority intervention by the World Health Organization (WHO) due to its high feasibility and potential to benefit to the whole population. Many countries are working towards achieving the global target of a 30% relative reduction in mean population salt intake by 2025, towards the WHO recommendation of <5 g/day [3].

Salt is a cheap food ingredient and ubiquitous in the food supply [4]. Salt is added to food products for the purposes of taste and preservation, and to improve technological processes [5]. In most high income countries, the majority of salt in the diet is from ultra-processed foods [6]. Thus, reformulation efforts to reduce the amount of salt added to ultra-processed foods are paramount to reduce population level salt intake. In general, in many low-middle income countries, the major source of salt in the diet is table salt and condiments added during cooking or at the table [6]. However, these countries are increasingly undergoing urbanisation and are experiencing a nutrition transition that is characterised by a marked change in food consumption patterns and a notable shift towards consumption of more ultra-processed foods [7,8].

A key example of this is instant noodles; an ultra-processed ultra-processed food product which is widely available at a low cost [9]. According to the World Instant Noodles Association (WINA), 270 million servings of instant noodles are consumed worldwide each day, with 80% of total consumption in Asian countries [10]. Instant noodles are consumed in more than 80 countries worldwide; China has the highest consumption of instant noodles, followed by Indonesia, Japan, and Vietnam [10].

In many Asian countries, noodles have been a staple food for centuries. Instant noodles are made from wheat flour, starch, water, salt, or kansui (an alkaline mixture of sodium carbonate, potassium carbonate and sodium phosphate), and other ingredients are added to improve the texture and flavour of the noodles [11]. Convenience, prolonged shelf life, taste, and low price make noodles highly popular. They can be eaten as a snack, as a meal or part of a meal, and some people consume them more than once a day.

According to Fu [12], salt is used in the production of instant noodles at concentrations of 1–3% of flour weight, for the purpose of strengthening and tightening the gluten protein of the dough. Salt also serves to reduce cooking time, enhance flavour, provide a softer and more elastic texture, and inhibit enzyme activities and growth of microorganisms [12]. In addition, salt is a major component of the seasoning sachet that is generally included in the packaging of instant noodles and added at the time of consumption.

Despite the widespread consumption of instant noodles in many countries, there has been relatively little assessment of their impact related to total nutritional intake and health. Analysis of dietary data collected in the Korean National Health and Nutrition Examination Survey (KNHANES) III, 2005, identified that consumers of instant noodles, compared to people who did not consume instant noodles, had significantly higher intakes of energy, fat, sodium, thiamine, and riboflavin and lower intakes of protein, calcium, phosphorus, iron, potassium, vitamin A, niacin, and vitamin C [13]. Analysis from KNHANES IV (2007–2009) demonstrated that the consumption of instant noodles two or more times per week was associated with a higher prevalence of metabolic syndrome in women (OR: 1.68; 95% CI: 1.10, 2.55) and that this association was independent of major dietary patterns [14].

Given emerging data of this kind, reformulation of instant noodles is important to reduce their potentially harmful nutritional composition. Programs to engage with the food industry have been undertaken by many countries worldwide, with some countries already, reporting an impact [15]. However, few countries have set targets specifically for instant noodles to date. The United Kingdom (UK) has set an average target of 200 mg of sodium and a maximum of 350 mg of sodium per 100 g of instant noodles "as prepared" (made up according to manufacturer instructions) [16]. South Africa (SA) set legislative targets of 1500 mg of sodium/100 g by 2016 and of 800 mg of sodium per 100 g by 2019 "as sold" [17], similar to the PICs regional target of 1600 mg/100 [18]. "As sold" refers to 100 g of product before it is made up with water, ready to eat.

Through the Global Food Monitoring Group (GFMG) [19], the George Institute for Global Health has been supporting countries to establish comprehensive food composition databases (FCDs) to monitor the nutritional composition of packaged food, which can be used to drive national and international improvements to the food supply, and improve the health of billions of people worldwide.

The aim of this analysis was to assess sodium levels in instant noodles using data from the GFMG national databases as well as from countries that have recently collected sodium data for instant noodles as part of shop surveys. The mean values and ranges of sodium content of instant noodles were compared, both within and between countries, and sodium content was compared against existing sodium targets for instant noodles [16–18]. The purpose of the analysis was to compare the sodium content of instant noodles sold worldwide to monitor sodium levels against existing targets and to identify opportunities to reformulate instant noodles as a means to reduce population level salt consumption.

2. Materials and Methods

Data on instant noodles collected between 2012 and 2016 were extracted from existing packaged food composition databases from countries that are part of the Global Food Monitoring Group (GFMG) [19]. Data on instant noodles were also gathered from countries that have recently been supported by the George Institute to gather shop survey data as part of surveillance activities to monitor sodium contents of the food supply (Table 1). All data were collected systematically by trained research assistants in accordance with the GFMG protocol. Data from the respective databases included brand name, product name, pack size, serving size, sodium mg/100 g "as sold", sodium mg/100 g "as prepared", salt g/100 g "as sold", and salt g/100 g "as prepared".

Table 1. Proportion of instant noodles collected per country and average pack/serving size (g).

Date of Data Collection	Data Source	Country	Total No. of Products Collected	Products with Sodium Data		Products with Sodium Data "as Sold"		Products with Sodium Data "as Prepared"		Average Pack Size (g)	Average Serving Size (g) as Prepared
				n	%	n	%	n	%		
2016	FCD	UK	137	132	96	11	8	121	92	84	282
2015	FCD	New Zealand	85	83	98	42	51	41	49	87	343
2014	FCD	Australia	58	58	100	9	16	49	84	86	308
2015	FCD	China	283	283	100	283	100	0	0	98	-
2012	FCD	India	47	15	32	15	100	0	0	-	-
2013	Shop survey	Samoa	44	43	98	28	65	15	35	69	-
2015	FCD	South Africa	37	37	100	28	76	9	24	72	300
2013	Shop survey	Fiji	28	28	100	23	82	5	18	69	143
2015	Shop survey	Indonesia	28	28	100	28	100	0	0	76	-
2013	FCD	Costa Rica	18	18	100	18	100	0	0	57	-
		Totals	765	725 *	95	485	67	240	33	78	275

- data not available.* Products that listed sodium or salt information, but did not state if as sold or as prepared were excluded from further analysis (*n* = 5).

2.1. Data Categorisation

Instant noodles were defined according to Codex Alimentarius [20], as packaged noodles, with or without additional seasonings provided in separate pouches, ready for consumption after rehydration. Data was categorised into two main groups: "as sold" or "as prepared" according to the listed nutrition information. Products categorised "as sold" listed sodium information based on dry weight including the seasoning. Products that were categorised "as prepared" listed sodium information based on the product as prepared for consumption according to manufacturer instructions, for example, "add x millilitres of water" and included an addition of the seasoning in the sodium value.

2.2. Data Analysis

The total number of instant noodle products and the number of products with sodium or salt information was recorded for each country. Sodium content was calculated from salt where salt information alone was provided on the packaging, using the conversion factor of Na (mg) = salt (mg) (NaCl)/2.5. The mean, median, and ranges of sodium (mg/100 g) were calculated for each category ("as sold" and "as prepared") for each country. Average pack size, "as sold", and average portion size, "as prepared", were derived from available data as given on pack for each country. Mean sodium values of instant noodle products reporting sodium "as sold" were compared against the SA and PICS regional targets, while those reporting sodium "as prepared" were compared against the UK 2017 targets.

The salt targets were converted to sodium for ease of comparison where necessary. The proportion of products known to meet the sodium targets were derived for each country. The contribution of an average packet of instant noodles to the WHO's recommended intake of <2000 mg of sodium (5 g salt) per day was derived using mean sodium values and average pack size for each country.

Sub-analyses comparing sodium content of noodles of countries by income level (based on The World Bank's list of economies [21]) and by whether or not they had specific sodium targets in place for instant noodles were conducted. Median sodium content (mg/100) was compared using the Wilcoxon rank-sum test. The proportion of products meeting the target between groups was compared using the chi-square test. A p-value of < 0.05 was considered significant.

3. Results

Data were collated on 765 instant noodles products from 10 countries. China had the greatest number of noodle products (283 products, 37% total), followed by the UK (137, 18%), New Zealand (85, 11%), and Australia (58, 8%). Indonesia and Costa Rica had the fewest products, 28 and 18 products respectively (Table 1).

3.1. Labelling

Five percent of products did not list sodium or salt content on the nutrition information panel; the majority of these were from India. Sixty-eight percent of instant noodle products in India did not provide sodium content information. Of all the products that did display sodium information, approximately 67% of products listed nutrition information "as sold", while 33% listed nutrition information "as prepared" (Table 1). Most (92%) of the noodle products from the UK listed nutrition information "as prepared", compared to China, Indonesia, India, and Costa Rica, which all listed the nutrition information "as sold". In Australia and New Zealand, 84% and 49%, respectively, of noodle products listed their nutritional content "as prepared".

3.2. Range and Levels of Sodium Per 100 g

There was a wide range in sodium content of instant noodles within and between countries, and the distribution of sodium was not normal, so median sodium values were also reported (Table 2). The highest mean and median sodium content (mg/100 g) of instant noodles "as sold" was found in products in China (mean 1944, median 2062, IQR 757, range 397–3678) followed by Australia, Fiji, Samoa, and Indonesia. The lowest mean sodium content (mg/100 g) was found in products in New Zealand (mean 798, median 508, IQR 429, range 249–2380).

The highest mean sodium content (mg/100 g) of instant noodles "as prepared" was for products in New Zealand (mean 388, median 360, IQR 106, range 222–725), whilst the lowest mean sodium content (mg/100 g) "as prepared" was for products in the UK (mean 220, median 200, IQR 100, range 120–440).

3.3. Percentage of Products which Meet Targets

Forty percent of all products met the PICs targets for instant noodles (1600 mg/100 g "as sold"); 37% met SA 2016 targets (1500 mg/100 g "as sold") and 72% met the UK 2017 maximum target (350 mg of sodium/100 g "as prepared"). Among countries with targets, 26% and 39% of instant noodles in Fiji and Samoa, respectively, met the PICs regional salt targets; 86% of products in SA met the SA salt targets, and 90% of products in the UK met the UK 2017 salt targets.

Sub-analysis comparing countries with sodium targets (either "as sold" or "as prepared") against countries without targets in place showed that countries with targets for instant noodles had a significantly higher proportion of instant noodle products meeting the targets. The proportion of products meeting the PICs, SA, and UK targets in countries with salt targets for instant noodles compared to those without targets were 56% vs. 36% ($p = 0.001$), 47% vs. 34% ($p = 0.031$), and 86% vs. 49% ($p < 0.001$), respectively.

3.4. Average Pack Size

There were large variations in both pack sizes and serving sizes. Average pack size ranged from 57 g in Costa Rica to 98 g in China. Where serving size information was given, average serving size, "as prepared", ranged from 143 g in Fiji to 300 g in South Africa. Six out of 10 countries provided serving size information on the instant noodles packaging (Table 1). Based on an average packet of noodles "as sold", the estimated average contribution of one packet of noodles towards the World Health Organization daily recommended maximum intake of sodium (<2000 mg) ranged from 35% in India and New Zealand (628 mg per pack and 697 mg per pack, respectively) to 95% in China (1905 mg per packet in China) (Figure 1).

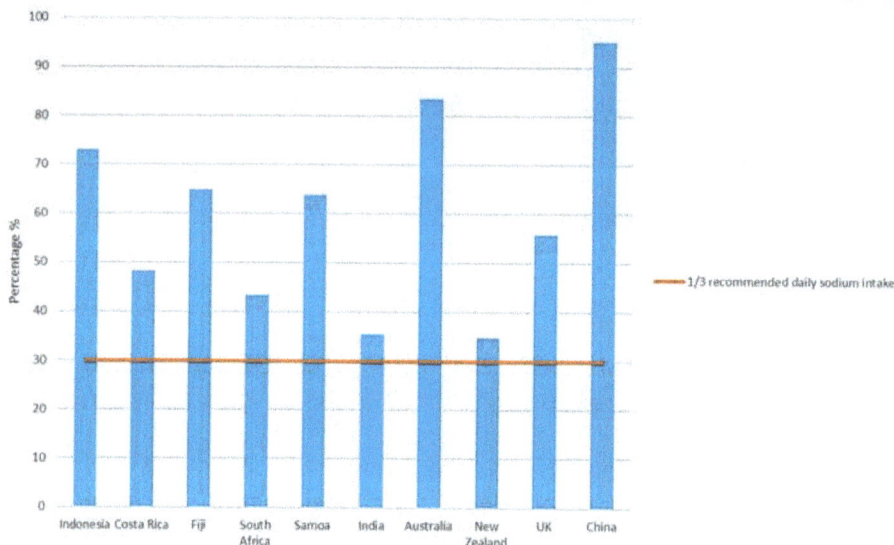

Figure 1. Estimated sodium contribution (%) of an average packet of instant noodles "as sold" with maximum recommended daily sodium intake (2000 mg/day).

3.5. Comparison of Sodium Levels in Instant Noodles between High-Income Countries and Middle-Income Countries

Seven of the 10 countries included in the analysis were classified as middle-income countries (MICs), and 3 classified as high-income countries (HICs); there was no data from low-income countries. Median sodium level of instant noodles "as sold" were significantly higher in MICs (1889 mg/100 g) compared to HICs (605 mg/100 g) ($p < 0.001$). In addition, a significantly higher proportion of products in HICs compared to MICs met the Pacific Island (71% vs. 35%, $p < 0.001$) and South Africa salt targets (71% vs. 32%, $p < 0.001$). There was no significant difference for instant noodles with mean sodium levels "as prepared".

Table 2. Mean, range, median interquartile range, and percentage of products that meet sodium targets.

Country (World Bank Group)	n	Mean Sodium (mg/100 g) as Sold	Range of Sodium (mg/100 g) as Sold	Median Sodium and IQR (mg/100 g) as Sold	Products Known to Meet Pacific Salt Reduction Target (1600 mg/100 g as Sold) n	%	Products Known to Meet South Africa 2016 Target (1500 mg/100 g as Sold) n	%	n	Mean Sodium (mg/100 g) as Prepared	Range (mg/100 g) as Prepared	Median Sodium and IQR (mg/100 g) as Prepared	Products Known to Meet UK 2017 Max Sodium Target (350 mg/100 g as Consumed) n	%
New Zealand (HIC)	42	798	249–2380	508 (429)	35	83	35	83	41	388	222–725	360 (106)	19	46
UK (HIC)	11	1323	488–2650	948 (1620)	6	55	6	55	121	220	120–440	200 (100)	109	90
Australia (HIC)	9	1939	950–3050	2110 (951)	3	33	3	33	49	378	205–635	350 (181)	25	51
China (MIC)	283	1944	397–3678	2062 (757)	74	26	67	24	0	-	-	-	-	-
Samoa (MIC)	28	1854	970–3360	1751 (610)	11	39	6	21	15	334	245–590	280 (75)	12	80
Indonesia (MIC)	28	1916	770–7584	1388 (1025)	15	54	15	54	0	-	-	-	-	-
South Africa (MIC)	28	1206	350–1640	1314 (202)	27	96	24	86	9	331	266–475	290 (90)	5	56
Fiji (MIC)	23	1892	845–3510	1913 (767)	6	26	6	26	5	317	200–443	300 (184)	3	60
Costa Rica (MIC)	18	1703	1148–2278	1766 (242)	4	22	4	22	0	-	-	-	-	-
India (MIC)	15	910	280–1932	590 (1067)	12	80	12	80	0	-	-	-	-	-
HICs sub-total	62	1057	249–3050	605 (1280) *	44	71 *	44	71 *	211	289	120–725	270 (180)	153	73
MICs subtotal	423	1838	280–7584	1889 (926)	149	35	134	32	29	330	200–590	290 (98)	20	69
Totals	485	1738	249–7584	1823 (1029)	193	40	178	37	240	294	120–725	273 (160)	173	72

* Difference between HICs and MICs significant at $p < 0.001$. - data not available.

4. Discussion

This assessment of the sodium content of 765 instant noodles products from 10 countries demonstrated extremely wide variation in sodium content, both between and within countries, according to product ranges and brands. The huge variations in mean sodium content of products in different countries clearly demonstrates significant potential to reduce the sodium content of noodles sold worldwide.

Reasons for the wide range of sodium content of instant noodles between countries cannot be explained solely by taste preferences of consumers, as there were also vast differences in the sodium levels of the instant noodles on the market within each country. For example, the sodium content of instant noodles in Australia ranged from 950 mg/100 g to 3050 mg/100 g ("as sold"), with the highest sodium instant noodle product containing over 3 times more sodium than the lowest sodium instant noodle product. This shows clearly that manufacturers are able to produce instant noodles with far less sodium and that these products are already accepted by consumers. This is evidence that reformulation of instant noodles is feasible, both technologically as well as from a consumer acceptability perspective. Similar results were observed looking at the analyses of median values, which confirms the main findings.

Whilst recognising that the targets only apply to the countries or regions in which they were set, the fact that the sodium content of instant noodles was consistently lower in countries with targets demonstrates the effectiveness of targets as a public policy tool. For example, China, which has the highest number of instant noodle products, does not have targets for sodium levels in foods, and had the lowest proportion of instant noodle products meeting international targets. However, there is scope for greater compliance, as not all products within countries with targets, met the targets, which points toward the need for more concerted efforts to reduce salt by the food industry. This highlights the importance of monitoring frameworks to allow for the transparent and objective evaluation of the food industry towards meeting the targets. In Fiji and Samoa for example, only 39% and 26% of products, respectively, met the PICS regional targets. The targets are part of a voluntary framework in Fiji and are being incorporated into regulations that have yet to be implemented in Samoa. Most Pacific Island countries are also highly dependent on imports, which means they need to work with food importing companies as well as local manufacturers to implement targets and highlights the importance of strong government leadership to support policy implementation. The high level of sodium in instant noodles coupled with their popularity provides a strong case for sodium reduction targets for instant noodles in all countries.

Both voluntary and legislated sodium reduction targets can lead to industry action to reduce sodium; 90% of instant noodle products in the UK met the UK targets (which were voluntary targets to be achieved by 2017), and 86% of products in South Africa met the South African mandatory targets to be achieved by 2016. Public health experts believe that regulation is a much stronger driver for industry reformulation [22], but voluntary programs that are supported by a strong monitoring framework, coupled with strong advocacy efforts, are also making considerable progress [23].

This research also identified that instant noodles in middle-income countries have a significantly higher average sodium content compared to high-income countries. This is of concern, given that nutrition transition is resulting in an increased availability of more ultra-processed foods in these countries [24], and supports the need for robust policies to regulate the food supply to reduce the already overburdened constraints on the healthcare system due to poor diet.

Further to the need for reformulation of instant noodles to contain less sodium, this study highlights the need for clear and consistent nutrition information panels (NIPs) to enable consumers to make healthier food choices. In India, 68% of products did not list sodium data on nutrition information panels, thus failing to meet International Codex Alimentarius requirements [25]. The Food Standards and Safety Authority of India does not currently require reporting of sodium content on food packaging [26]. This lack of nutrition information not only inhibits consumers from making informed choices about food purchases but also prevents any monitoring and evaluation of the food supply.

The fact that some instant noodle manufacturers label sodium information on nutrition information panels "as sold" while others label sodium "as prepared" (as prepared according to manufacturer instructions) within the same country further complicates the picture for both consumers and policy makers. In New Zealand, for example, almost half of the products labelled sodium information "as sold" and half "as prepared". This creates potential confusion for consumers at the point of purchase and makes it difficult to compare nutrition information between brands. Almost a third of all instant noodle products analysed labelled sodium information "as prepared" according to manufacturer instructions. Consumers may not necessarily follow manufacturers' instructions in preparation of the product, which introduces further potential bias in estimates and makes it more difficult for consumers to moderate salt intakes. In countries with interpretive front of pack labelling, for example, the colour coded Front of pack (FOP) nutrition labelling scheme in the UK [27], there is an opportunity for these systems to signpost healthier alternatives and make direct comparisons between products easier for consumers at the point of purchase.

Inconsistent pack sizes provide an additional challenge; the results from this survey showed that pack sizes ranged from 57 g in Costa Rica to 97 g in China and that manufacturers did not always quantify a recommended serve size. A single packet of one brand of instant noodles in China contributes almost the entire (95%) WHO recommended maximum <2000 mg of sodium/day. In Indonesia, Fiji, or Samoa, the average packet of noodles would contribute almost two-thirds of this amount, whereas in India and New Zealand consumers would consume almost one-third.

Ensuring that instant noodles are reformulated to reduce sodium and labelled in a meaningful way is even more important given the fact that they are increasingly being promoted as a vehicle for micronutrient fortification, either added through the flour used to make the product or to the seasoning powders consumed with the noodles [28,29]. This practice may result in contradictory public health outcomes.

There were some limitations to the study. The number of products available in the ultra-processed packaged food composition database may not necessarily reflect the number of products sold in a particular country, but rather those that were captured during shop surveys undertaken within a limited subset of retail outlets, at specific time points. Products were categorised "as sold" or "as prepared" according to the investigators' best interpretation, using mean sodium as a guide. Products that could not be categorised were excluded from further analysis. Products were collected in shop surveys between 2012 and 2016 and may no longer be on sale due to stock changes, and sales data could not be corroborated to assess market share of particular brands. However, the data obtained provides a clear indication of the high levels of sodium in these popular products, which supports the need for reformulation efforts worldwide to reduce sodium in instant noodles to the lowest possible level.

5. Conclusions

The high level of sodium in instant noodles across the world is a major public health concern, given their low cost, convenience, and widespread availability, and the fact that high sodium levels are a key contributor to ill health. There is a need for clear targets coupled with rigorous reformulation efforts to reduce the amount of sodium added to instant noodles. Better regulation of the sodium content of commonly consumed ultra-processed foods is key to reducing population-level salt consumption around the world.

Acknowledgments: This work was supported by a number of organisations listed below as part of the Global Food Monitoring Group (GFMG) and independently by providing data for the survey: Costa Rican Institute of Research and Education on Nutrition and Health (INCIENSA); Discover Vitality, South Africa; The George Institute for Global Health, Australia; The NCD Asia Pacific Alliance, Japan; The Pacific Research Centre for the Prevention of Obesity and Non-communicable Diseases (C-POND), Fiji; The National Institute for Health Innovation, University of Auckland, New Zealand; World Action on Salt and Health, London; Pacific Technical Support Unit, World Health Organization, Fiji; Ministry of Health, Samoa.

Author Contributions: C.F., J.W. and K.C. conceived of the study; M.C. facilitated access to the data; C.F. and J.S. analyzed the data; C.F. drafted the paper. All authors reviewed and provided written comments on subsequent drafts.

Conflicts of Interest: J.W. is Director of the World Health Organization Collaborating Centre on Population Salt Reduction and is supported by a joint National Health and Medical Research Council and National Heart Foundation Career Development Fellowship and receives additional funding from the World Health Organization and Victorian Health Promotion Foundation. All other authors declare no conflict of interest.

References

1. *Global Status Report on Noncommunicable Diseases*; World Health Organization: Geneva, Switzerland, 2014.
2. Wang, G.; Labarthe, D. The cost-effectiveness of interventions designed to reduce sodium intake. *J. Hypertens.* **2011**, *29*, 1693–1699. [CrossRef] [PubMed]
3. *Global Action Plan for the Prevention and Control of Noncommunicable Diseases 2013–2020*; World Health Organization: Geneva, Switzerland, 2013.
4. He, F.J.; MacGregor, G.A. Reducing population salt intake worldwide: From evidence to implementation. *Progr. Cardiovasc. Dis.* **2010**, *52*, 363–382. [CrossRef] [PubMed]
5. Jaenke, R.; Barzi, F.; McMahon, E.; Webster, J.; Brimblecombe, J. Consumer Acceptance of Reformulated Food Products: A Systematic Review and Meta-analysis of Salt-reduced Foods. *Crit. Rev. Food Sci. Nutr.* **2017**, *57*, 3357–3372. [CrossRef] [PubMed]
6. Charlton, K.E.; Langford, K.; Kaldor, J. Innovative and Collaborative Strategies to Reduce Population-Wide Sodium Intake. *Curr. Nutr. Rep.* **2015**, *4*, 279–289. [CrossRef]
7. Popkin, B.M.; Adair, L.S.; Ng, S.W. Global nutrition transition and the pandemic of obesity in developing countries. *Nutr. Rev.* **2012**, *70*, 3–21. [CrossRef] [PubMed]
8. Monteiro, C.A.; Moubarac, J.C.; Cannon, G.; Ng, S.W.; Popkin, B. Ultra-processed products are becoming dominant in the global food system. *Obes. Rev.* **2013**, *14*, 21–28. [CrossRef]
9. Gulia, N.; Dhaka, V.; Khatkar, B.S. Instant Noodles: Processing, Quality, and Nutritional Aspects. *Crit. Rev. Food Sci. Nutr.* **2014**, *54*, 1386–1399. [CrossRef] [PubMed]
10. World Instant Noodles Association. *Global Report*; World Instant Noodles Association: Tokyo, Japan, 2016.
11. Kim, S.G. Instant noodles. In *Pasta and Noodle Technology*; Kruger, J.H., Matsuo, R.B., Dick, J.W., Eds.; American Association of Cereal Chemistry: St. Paul, MN, USA, 1996; pp. 195–225.
12. Fu, B.X. Asian noodles: History, classification, raw materials and processing. *Food Res. Int.* **2008**, *41*, 888–902. [CrossRef]
13. Park, J.; Lee, J.S.; Jang, Y.A.; Chung, H.R.; Kim, J. A comparison of food and nutrient intake between instant noodle consumers and non-instant noodle consumers in Korean adults. *Nutr. Res. Prac.* **2011**, *5*, 443–449. [CrossRef] [PubMed]
14. Shin, H.J.; Cho, E.; Lee, H.J.; Fung, T.T.; Rimm, E.; Rosner, B.; Manson, J.E.; Wheelan, K.; Hu, F.B. Instant noodle intake and dietary patterns are associated with distinct cardiometabolic risk factors in Korea. *J. Nutr.* **2014**, *144*, 1247–1255. [CrossRef] [PubMed]
15. Webster, J.; Trieu, K.; Dunford, E.; Hawkes, C. Target Salt 2025: A Global Overview of National Programs to Encourage the Food Industry to Reduce Salt in Foods. *Nutrients* **2014**, *6*, 3274–3287. [CrossRef] [PubMed]
16. *Public Health Responsibility Deal: UK Salt Reduction Targets for 2017*; UK Department of Health: London, UK, 2014.
17. *Government Gazette: No. R. 214 Foodstuffs, Cosmetics and Disinfectants Act, 1972 (Act 54 of 1972) Regulations Relating to the Reduction of Sodium in Certain Foodstuffs and Related Matters The Heart and Stroke Foundation South Africa*; South Africa Government: Pretoria, South Africa, 2013.
18. *Pacific Salt Reduction Targets: Why Setting Targets for Salt in Food?* Western Pacific Region; World Health Organization: Geneva, Switzerland, 2014.
19. Dunford, E.; Webster, J.; Metzler, A.B.; Czernichow, S.; Ni Mhurchu, C.; Wolmarans, P.; Snowdon, W.; L'Abbe, M.; Li, N.; et al. Maulik PK International collaborative project to compare and monitor the nutritional composition of processed foods. *Eur. J. Prev. Cardiol.* **2012**, *19*, 1326–1332. [CrossRef] [PubMed]
20. *CODEX Alimentarius: Standard for Instant Noodles CODEX STAN 249-2006*; Food and Agriculture Organization of the United Nations and World Health Organization: Rome, Italy, 2016.

21. The World Bank. World Bank List of economies (December 2016). Available online: https://datahelpdesk. worldbank.org/knowledgebase/articles/906519-world-bank-country-and-lending-groups (accessed on 5 June 2017).

22. Moodie, R.; Stuckler, D.; Monteiro, C.; Sheron, N.; Neal, B.; Thamarangsi, T.; Lincoln, P.; Casswell, S. Profits and pandemics: Prevention of harmful effects of tobacco, alcohol, and ultra-processed food and drink industries. *Lancet* **2013**, *381*, 670–679. [CrossRef]

23. Charlton, K.E.; Webster, J.; Kowai, P. To Legislate or Not to Legislate? A Comparison of the UK and South African Approaches to the Development and Implementation of the Salt Reduction Programs Nutrients. *Nutrients* **2014**, *6*, 3672. [CrossRef] [PubMed]

24. Popkin, B.M. The nutrition transition and obesity in the developing world. *J. Nutr.* **2001**, *131*, 871S–873S. [PubMed]

25. *CODEX Alimentarius: Guidelines on Nutrition Labelling*; Food and Agriculture Organization of the United Nations and World Health Organization: Rome, Italy, 2011.

26. *Food Safety and Standards (Packaging and Labelling) Regulations*; Food Safety and Standards Authority of India (FSSAI): New Delhi, India, 2011.

27. Guide to Creating a Front of Pack (FoP) Nutrition Label for Pre-Packed Products Sold Through Retail Outlets. In *Obesity and Healthy Eating Divison*; Department of Health: London, UK, 2013.

28. Kim, S.K. Overview of the Korean noodle industry. *Food Sci. Biotechnol.* **1997**, *6*, 125–130.

29. Spohrer, R.; Larson, M.; Maurin, C.; Laillou, A.; Capanzana, M.; Garrett, G.S. The growing importance of staple foods and condiments used as ingredients in the food industry and implications for large-scale food fortification programs in Southeast Asia. *Food Nutr. Bull.* **2013**, *34*, S50–S61. [CrossRef] [PubMed]

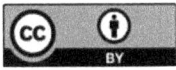

nutrients

Article

Emerging Disparities in Dietary Sodium Intake from Snacking in the US Population

Elizabeth K. Dunford [1,2,*], **Jennifer M. Poti** [2,3] and **Barry M. Popkin** [2,3]

1   Food Policy Division, The George Institute for Global Health, University of New South Wales, Sydney, NSW 2042, Australia
2   Carolina Population Center, The University of North Carolina at Chapel Hill, Chapel Hill, NC 27516, USA; poti@unc.edu (J.M.P.); popkin@unc.edu (B.M.P.)
3   Department of Nutrition, The University of North Carolina at Chapel Hill, Chapel Hill, NC 27516, USA
*   Correspondence: edunford@georgeinstitute.org.au; Tel.: +1-919-903-7863

Received: 17 May 2017; Accepted: 13 June 2017; Published: 17 June 2017

Abstract: Background: The US population consumes dietary sodium well in excess of recommended levels. It is unknown how the contribution of snack foods to sodium intake has changed over time, and whether disparities exist within specific subgroups of the US population. Objective: To examine short and long term trends in the contribution of snack food sources to dietary sodium intake for US adults and children over a 37-year period from 1977 to 2014. Methods: We used data collected from eight nationally representative surveys of food intake in 50,052 US children aged 2–18 years, and 73,179 adults aged 19+ years between 1977 and 2014. Overall, patterns of snack food consumption, trends in sodium intake from snack food sources and trends in food and beverage sources of sodium from snack foods across race-ethnic, age, gender, body mass index, household education and income groups were examined. Results: In all socio-demographic subgroups there was a significant increase in both per capita sodium intake, and the proportion of sodium intake derived from snacks from 1977–1978 to 2011–2014 ($p < 0.01$). Those with the lowest household education, Non-Hispanic Black race-ethnicity, and the lowest income had the largest increase in sodium intake from snacks. While in 1977–1978 Non-Hispanic Blacks had a lower sodium intake from snacks compared to Non-Hispanic Whites ($p < 0.01$), in 2011–2014 they had a significantly higher intake. Conclusions: Important disparities are emerging in dietary sodium intake from snack sources in Non-Hispanic Blacks. Our findings have implications for future policy interventions targeting specific US population subgroups.

Keywords: sodium intake; snacking; race-ethnic disparities

---

1. Introduction

Strong evidence links excessive dietary sodium intake to elevated blood pressure, which is a major risk factor for cardiovascular disease in both children and adults alike [1–4]. Research has also shown that in the US there are large and persistent disparities among race/ethnic subgroups related to hypertension, with the prevalence remaining highest among Non-Hispanic Black adults [5]. Despite the overall improvement of blood pressure control over the past 10 years, Non-Hispanic Blacks and Hispanics continue to have lower control rates than Non-Hispanic Whites [5].

The American Heart Association (AHA), World Health Organization (WHO), and Institute of Medicine all support recommendations to reduce population intake of sodium in the US [4,6,7]. Nonetheless, mean sodium intake in both US adults and children remains too high [8], with approximately two thirds of dietary sodium intake derived from packaged food sources [9,10]. We have shown in a recent publication, that although the sodium content of households' total packaged food purchases decreased significantly between 2000 and 2014, mean sodium intake from packaged food purchases remained far above the AHA recommended intake levels, and the sodium content of processed foods exceeded the 2014 targets established by the National Salt Reduction Initiative [11].

Obesity increases over the past few decades have been attributed to a number of factors, one of which is to an increasing trend of snacking. Coupling this with the fact that the US population is consuming sodium levels in excess of dietary guidelines, it is likely that these increases in snacking behavior are contributing to both excessive dietary sodium intake overall in the US population, as well as within race-ethnic and socio-economic groups, in which health inequality has risen in recent decades [12]. Studies to date have observed inconsistent results in intakes of snacks between different race-ethnic groups and age and weight groups [13], and also demonstrate that a large proportion of snacks still appear to derive from less healthy foods, such as salty snacks, desserts and sweets [14,15]. One study even found that a single snack food item contributed, on average, 14% of a child's daily recommended amount of sodium, with some items providing more than 150% [16] despite data from the most recent National Health and Nutrition Examination Survey (NHANES) indicating that on average, snack food sources contribute 16% of daily sodium intake in children six years and older [17].

To date, there have been no studies examining long term and short term trends in the amount and proportion of daily sodium intake derived from snack food sources, by demographic subgroups. Therefore, we have chosen to examine trends over a period of 37 years, for dietary sodium intake derived from snack food sources in US adults and children by age group, body mass index (BMI), race-ethnicity, household education and income level.

2. Materials and Methods

2.1. Survey Population

Data were obtained from eight nationally representative surveys of food intake in 50,052 US children aged <19 years and 73,179 US adults aged 19+ years. The United States Department of Agriculture (USDA) data come from the 1977–1978 Nationwide Food Consumption Survey (NFCS 1977–1978), the 1989–1991 Continuing Survey of Food Intake by Individuals (CSFII 1989–1991), the 1994–1996 CSFII and the 1997–1998 CSFII (CSFII 1994–1998). From the NHANES, four surveys were used: NHANES 2003–2004, NHANES 2005–2006 (NHANES 03–06), NHANES 2011–2012 and NHANES 2013–2014 (NHANES 11–14). Supplementary Table S1 shows the number of records used in each survey year. The USDA and NHANES surveys are based on a multistage, stratified area probability sample of non-institutionalized US households. Detailed information about each survey and its sampling design has been published previously [18]. By utilizing secondary USDA and NHANES data, we were exempt from institutional review board concerns for this paper.

2.2. Snacking Definition

Each eating occasion was self-defined by the respondent in each survey. Respondents were asked to name the type of each eating occasion, and the main meal planner was asked about intake for any child under the age of 12 [19]. The snack category includes those eating occasions defined by the respondent as "snack" plus the occasions related to snacking, such as food and/or coffee/beverage breaks.

2.3. Dietary Data

All dietary survey data used a comparable food composition table and collection methods developed by the USDA. To examine trends over time from surveys with different collection methods on days 1 and 2, we used only the first day's data (a single, 24-h dietary recall on the basis of interviews) collected from each individual, and used appropriate weights and adjustments for the sample design provided.

2.4. Food Grouping System

To determine those food items contributing to sodium intake from snacking, the food grouping system developed by the University of North Carolina at Chapel Hill (UNC-CH) was used. This food grouping system links all foods from 1977 to 2014. All the foods reported in the USDA surveys were assigned to the 107 UNC-CH food groups. The UNC-CH food grouping system has been described previously [20]. For all participants, the amount of sodium provided by each UNC-CH food group reported consumed as a snack was calculated and then divided by the total sodium from snacking of all individuals. Those food groups contributing the most to sodium intake from snack food sources are reported overall by year and by socio-demographic subgroup.

2.5. Statistical Analysis

Data are presented as means (SE). Snacking trends were studied by dividing the population into age groups (2–5 years old, 6–11 years old, and 12–18 years old for children; 19–29 years old, 30–59 years old and 60+ years old for adults), BMI categories (Underweight, Normal Weight, Overweight and Obese, based on the WHO BMI guidelines), race-ethnic groups (Hispanic, Non-Hispanic White and Non-Hispanic Black), income groups using the Federal Poverty Level (FPL; <185% FPL, 185–350% FPL and >350% FPL) and household education groups (Less than High School, High School Diploma and More than High School). Income definitions used self-reported family income to compute the federal poverty level index. We calculated the mean sodium intake (mg) from snacks per capita per day, and the proportion of dietary sodium intake derived from snack foods overall for adults and children, and separately for each demographic subgroup. Stata version 14.1 was used for all analyses. Survey methods were used within Stata to account for the clustering and weighting that is inherent in the NHANES sampling methodology [21], so as to allow for statistically significant differences between survey cycles to be identified using Student's t-test. A p-value of <0.05 was considered significant.

3. Results

3.1. Overall Trends

For all US adults and children there was a significant increase in per capita sodium intake coming from snacks from 1977–1978 to 2011–2014 ($p < 0.01$) (Table 1). In all age groups the trend was an increase in sodium intake from snacks from 1977–1978 to 2003–2006, followed by a decrease from 2003–2006 to 2011–2014 (significant only in children; $p < 0.01$), except for those in the 60+-year-age group, which was the only group to show an increase in intake from 2003–2006 to 2011–2014 (Table 1). Despite a decrease observed for most age groups in the mean sodium intake derived from snacks from 2003–2006 to 2011–2014, there was little to no change seen in the proportion of the population that consumed snacks from 2003–2006 to 2011–2014.

3.2. Trends by Race-Ethnicity

In all race-ethnic groups for both adults and children, there was an increase in sodium per capita per day from snack food sources between 1977–1978 and 2011–2014 ($p < 0.01$, Table 2), and a decrease from 2003–2006 to 2011–2014, although these decline results were only significant for Non-Hispanic White adults. While in 1977–1978 Non-Hispanic Black adults and children had a significantly lower sodium intake from snacks compared to Non-Hispanic Whites ($p < 0.01$ Figure 1a,b), in 2011–2014 Non-Hispanic Blacks had a significantly higher intake ($p < 0.01$) and had the highest mean sodium intake from snacks out of all race-ethnic groups from 2003 to 2006 onwards. Non-Hispanic Blacks also had the largest increase in mean sodium intake from snacks from 1977 to 2014, with the mean sodium intake more than doubling for Non-Hispanic Black adults and children over the study period.

Table 1. Number of snacks consumed per day, percentage of snackers in the population, and sodium consumed per snacking occasion, by US children and adults from the 1977–1978, 1989–1991, 1994–1998, 2003–2006 and 2011–2014 surveys by age group.

	1977–1978	1989–1991	1994–1998	2003–2006	2011–2014
Age 2–5 years					
Snacks, n/day	1.2 (0.04)[1]	1.4 (0.08)[1]	2.3 (0.05)[1]	3.0 (0.08)	3.0 (0.08)
Per capita mean intake from snacks, mg	157 (7.3)[1]	211 (13.7)[1]	389 (12.2)[2]	444 (18.8)	443 (21.4)
% snackers	63 (1.7)[1]	70 (2.9)[1]	87 (1.2)	96 (0.6)	96 (0.6)
Per capita mean intake from snacks, mg (snackers only)	249 (8.8)[1]	301 (17.1)[1]	445 (11.4)	461 (18.2)	460 (21.8)
Age 6–11 years					
Snacks, n/day	1.0 (0.03)[1]	1.1 (0.07)[1]	1.8 (0.05)[1]	2.7 (0.07)	2.5 (0.06)
Per capita mean intake from snacks, mg	206 (8.9)[1]	281 (28.1)[1]	454 (18.5)	562 (26.6)[1]	468 (18.8)
% snackers	61 (1.3)[1]	64 (2.4)[1]	82 (1.3)[1]	94 (0.9)	94 (0.9)
Per capita mean intake from snacks, mg (snackers only)	336 (12.9)[1]	441 (37.7)	554 (18.5)[2]	598 (29)	498 (20)
Age 12–18 years					
Snacks, n/day	1.0 (0.03)[1]	1.1 (0.05)[1]	1.7 (0.06)	2.3 (0.05)	2.1 (0.06)
Per capita mean intake from snacks, mg	314 (12.3)[1]	367 (35.1)[1]	575 (41)	606 (28.7)[1]	492 (21.2)
% snackers	59 (1.4)[1]	60 (2.2)[1]	77 (1.7)[1]	89 (0.9)	88 (1.1)
Per capita mean intake from snacks, mg (snackers only)	530 (17)	609 (53.2)	748 (40.8)[1]	678 (29.8)	561 (24.8)
Age 2–18 years					
Snacks, n/day	1.1 (0.03)[1]	1.2 (0.05)	1.9 (0.04)	2.6 (0.05)	2.4 (0.05)
Per capita mean intake from snacks, mg	245 (8.4)[1]	295 (18.5)[1]	486 (20.4)	554 (14.5)[1]	472 (13.8)
% snackers	61 (1.3)[1]	64 (1.9)[1]	81 (1.2)[1]	93 (0.5)	92 (0.6)
Per capita mean intake from snacks, mg (snackers only)	405 (11.4)[1]	460 (23.2)	598 (19.5)[1]	599 (14.9)[1]	514 (15.6)
Age 19–29 years					
Snacks, n/day	1.1 (0.03)[1]	1.1 (0.05)[1]	1.6 (0.04)[1]	2.2 (0.07)	2.2 (0.07)
Per capita mean intake from snacks, mg	251 (11.4)[1]	273 (23.5)[1]	473 (25.5)	575 (29.1)[2]	486 (22.3)
% snackers	59 (1.3)[1]	61 (1.8)[1]	72 (1.2)[1]	87 (1.3)	87 (1)
Per capita mean intake from snacks, mg (snackers only)	424 (15.4)[1]	446 (32.7)	653 (35.5)	657 (35.1)	557 (25.6)
Age 30–59 years					
Snacks, n/day	1.2 (0.04)[1]	1.3 (0.06)[1]	1.6 (0.04)[1]	2.4 (0.05)	2.5 (0.05)
Per capita mean intake from snacks, mg	196 (7.3)[1]	238 (10.3)[1]	345 (12.2)[1]	466 (17.8)	440 (15.3)
% snackers	60 (1.3)[1]	64 (1.6)[1]	73 (1)[1]	89 (0.6)	89 (0.8)
Per capita mean intake from snacks, mg (snackers only)	326 (9.3)[1]	373 (13.5)	472 (12.8)	523 (18.4)	494 (15)

Table 1. Cont.

	1977–1978	1989–1991	1994–1998	2003–2006	2011–2014
Age 60+ years					
Snacks, n/day	0.8 (0.02)[1]	1.1 (0.05)[1]	1.3 (0.04)[1]	2.1 (0.05)	2.3 (0.07)
Per capita mean intake from snacks, mg	122 (5.9)[1]	156 (11.3)[1]	226 (9.2)[1]	306 (11.7)	335 (16.4)
% snackers	49 (1.2)[1]	58 (1.9)[1]	68 (1.2)[1]	88 (0.7)	88 (0.9)
Per capita mean intake from snacks, mg (snackers only)	251 (9.7)[1]	270 (15.4)	332 (10.6)	348 (11.9)	381 (17.7)
Age 19+ years					
Snacks, n/day	1.0 (0.03)[1]	1.2 (0.05)[1]	1.5 (0.04)[1]	2.3 (0.04)	2.4 (0.05)
Per capita mean intake from snacks, mg	194 (5.9)[1]	227 (9.3)[1]	347 (10.4)[1]	450 (14.6)	423 (12.1)
% snackers	57 (1.1)[1]	62 (1.4)[1]	72 (0.9)[1]	89 (0.6)	88 (0.6)
Per capita mean intake from snacks, mg (snackers only)	339 (7)[1]	368 (10.9)	482 (11.5)	509 (15.5)	478 (12.7)

[1] Different from 2011–2014, p < 0.01; [2] Different from 2011–2014, p < 0.05. Note: Data from the 1977–1978 Nationwide Food Consumption Survey (NFCS); the 1989–1991 Continuing Survey of Food Intake by Individuals (CSFII), the 1994–1996 CSFII, the 1997–1998 CSFII, NHANES 2003–2004, NHANES 2005–2006, NHANES 2009–2010 and NHANES 2011–2014. Results have been weighted to be nationally representative. Results are presented as mean (SE). NHANES, National Health and Nutrition Examination Survey.

Table 2. Number of snacks consumed per day, percentage of snackers in the population, and sodium consumed per snacking occasion, by US children and adults from the 1977–1978, 1989–1991, 1994–1998, 2003–2006 and 2011–2014 surveys by Federal Poverty Level, race-ethnicity and household education.

	Children					Adults				
	1977–1978	1989–1991	1994–1998	2003–2006	2011–2014	1977–1978	1989–1991	1994–1998	2003–2006	2011–2014
<185% Federal Poverty Level										
Snacks, n/day	0.9 (0.04)[1]	1.2 (0.06)[1]	1.9 (0.05)	2.5 (0.07)	2.3 (0.05)	0.8 (0.03)[1]	1 (0.04)[1]	1.3 (0.04)[1]	2.1 (0.05)	2.2 (0.05)
Per capita mean intake from snacks, mg	198 (11.1)[1]	239 (16.8)[1]	421 (23.2)	547 (24.1)[1]	464 (15.9)	156 (8.2)[1]	185 (11.5)[1]	334 (19.3)[1]	496 (30)	463 (19.9)
% snackers	53 (1.9)[1]	59 (2.1)[1]	79 (1.5)[1]	90 (0.7)	89 (0.7)	49 (1.5)[1]	55 (1.7)[1]	66 (1.2)[1]	87 (0.7)	86 (0.8)
Per capita mean intake from snacks, mg (snackers only)	375 (18)[1]	404 (19.6)[1]	535 (27.2)	608 (24.9)[1]	523 (16.2)	322 (12.7)[1]	333 (14.5)[1]	509 (26.6)	568 (33.6)	539 (22.6)
185–350% Federal Poverty Level										
Snacks, n/day	1.2 (0.03)[1]	1.4 (0.09)[1]	2.2 (0.06)	2.5 (0.09)	2.5 (0.08)	1.1 (0.03)	1.2 (0.07)[1]	1.5 (0.04)[1]	2.2 (0.06)	2.3 (0.06)
Per capita mean intake from snacks, mg	269 (11.2)[1]	327 (30.4)[1]	487 (35)	465 (23.7)	441 (25.7)	205 (6.8)[1]	227 (15.3)[1]	348 (17.6)[2]	419 (19.2)	394 (21.9)
% snackers	65 (1.2)[1]	69 (3.4)[1]	83 (1.4)[1]	90 (1)	88 (1.9)	60 (1.1)[1]	59 (1.8)[1]	72 (1.2)[1]	87 (1.1)	89 (1.2)
Per capita mean intake from snacks, mg (snackers only)	412 (15.5)[1]	475 (35.8)	584 (36.9)	517 (24.1)	500 (25.4)	344 (9.3)[1]	387 (20.5)[1]	486 (21.4)	480 (20.7)	443 (22.1)
>350% Federal Poverty Level										
Snacks, n/day	1.2 (0.04)[1]	1.4 (0.11)[1]	2.2 (0.05)	2.7 (0.07)	2.5 (0.07)	1.2 (0.04)[1]	1.4 (0.05)[1]	1.7 (0.04)[1]	2.4 (0.06)	2.6 (0.06)
Per capita mean intake from snacks, mg	278 (14.6)[1]	297 (26.9)[1]	497 (23.2)	556 (25.7)[1]	427 (25.2)	215 (7.6)[1]	251 (13.7)[1]	354 (13)[2]	435 (18.7)	411 (17.7)
% snackers	69 (1.3)[1]	72 (3)[1]	86 (1.3)[1]	94 (0.9)	94 (0.8)	62 (1.2)[1]	67 (1.7)[1]	76 (1)[1]	90 (0.8)	91 (0.8)
Per capita mean intake from snacks, mg (snackers only)	405 (19.2)[1]	413 (37.6)	574 (24.9)[1]	592 (28.1)[1]	452 (27.2)	345 (9.7)[1]	372 (19.3)[1]	465 (13.7)	481 (19.2)	453 (18.7)

Table 2. *Cont.*

	Children					Adults				
	1977–1978	1989–1991	1994–1998	2003–2006	2011–2014	1977–1978	1989–1991	1994–1998	2003–2006	2011–2014
Less than High School										
Snacks, *n*/day	0.8 (0.04)[1]	1.0 (0.05)[1]	1.5 (0.09)	2.5 (0.1)	2.4 (0.08)	0.8 (0.03)[1]	1.0 (0.04)[1]	1.1 (0.04)[1]	2.0 (0.07)	2.1 (0.07)
Per capita mean intake from snacks, mg	191 (13.6)[1]	284 (29)[1]	408 (28.5)	546 (23.4)[2]	464 (28.6)	142 (7.8)[1]	179 (16.3)[1]	278 (14.1)[1]	436 (28)	409 (21.6)
% snackers	48 (2.2)[1]	56 (3.1)[1]	73 (2.4)[1]	89 (1)	88 (1.2)	47 (1.5)[1]	55 (1.8)[1]	64 (1.4)[1]	84 (0.9)	84 (1.6)
Per capita mean intake from snacks, mg (snackers only)	397 (23.6)	504 (36.9)	556 (37.7)	611 (24.6)[2]	528 (31.7)	303 (13.6)[1]	322 (24.5)[1]	437 (18.6)	517 (32.4)	486 (23.2)
High School Diploma										
Snacks, *n*/day	1.0 (0.03)[1]	1.1 (0.07)[1]	1.7 (0.06)	2.6 (0.08)	2.2 (0.07)	1.0 (0.03)[1]	1.2 (0.07)[1]	1.4 (0.05)[1]	2.2 (0.06)	2.1 (0.07)
Per capita mean intake from snacks, mg	248 (10.5)[1]	267 (27.8)[1]	485 (33.6)	540 (27.7)[1]	434 (20.4)	196 (8.5)[1]	240 (16.5)[1]	347 (17.7)[1]	486 (34.4)	431 (25.5)
% snackers	61 (1.5)[1]	61 (3)[1]	79 (1.9)[1]	90 (1.3)	88 (1.2)	57 (1.2)[1]	61 (2)[1]	70 (1.4)[1]	88 (0.9)	86 (1.4)
Per capita mean intake from snacks, mg (snackers only)	407 (16.3)	439 (36.3)	614 (33.5)[1]	598 (27.1)[1]	492 (21.4)	345 (11.7)[1]	392 (22)[1]	494 (20.9)	549 (36.3)	503 (26.4)
More than High School										
Snacks, *n*/day	1.3 (0.04)[1]	1.2 (0.1)[1]	1.9 (0.05)	2.6 (0.05)	2.4 (0.06)	1.2 (0)[1]	1.3 (0.1)[1]	1.7 (0)[1]	2.2 (0.1)	2.1 (0.1)
Per capita mean intake from snacks, mg	266 (11.3)[1]	314 (24.9)	498 (24.9)	506 (13.3)[1]	448 (15.7)	220.8 (7)[1]	240 (12)[1]	367 (12.8)[1]	439 (13)	424 (13.3)
% snackers	70 (1.7)[1]	68 (2.6)[1]	83 (1.4)[1]	90 (0.6)	89 (1.4)	63.2 (1.3)[1]	65.6 (1.5)[1]	75.8 (1.2)[1]	89.9 (0.7)	90.5 (0.6)
Per capita mean intake from snacks, mg (snackers only)	390 (13.6)[1]	463 (30.8)[1]	594 (23.2)[1]	548 (14.3)[2]	491 (17.1)	349.3 (8.3)[1]	366 (16.3)[1]	484 (14.2)	488 (13.8)	468 (14)
Hispanic										
Snacks, *n*/day	0.9 (0.07)[1]	1.6 (0.18)[1]	2.1 (0.06)	2.6 (0.06)	2.4 (0.05)	0.9 (0.06)[1]	0.9 (0.13)[1]	1.2 (0.05)[1]	2.0 (0.06)[1]	2.3 (0.06)
Per capita mean intake from snacks, mg	187 (18.4)[1]	334 (98.3)[1]	419 (26.5)	534 (27.7)	469 (19.3)	153 (16.4)[1]	222 (63.3)[1]	286 (19.2)[1]	386 (25.1)	403 (12.1)
% snackers	57 (3.1)[1]	75 (6.4)[1]	79 (1.8)	90 (0.9)	88 (1)	52 (2.7)[1]	47 (5.5)[1]	67 (1.9)[1]	83 (1.3)[1]	89 (0.9)
Per capita mean intake from snacks, mg (snackers only)	331 (26.4)[1]	447 (131.2)[1]	529 (29)	590 (28.1)	530 (19.5)	292 (28.2)[1]	472 (122.4)[1]	424 (26.8)	462 (27.6)	455 (15.8)
Non-Hispanic White										
Snacks, *n*/day	1.2 (0.03)[1]	1.3 (0.06)[1]	2.2 (0.04)	2.6 (0.06)	2.5 (0.06)	1.1 (0.03)[1]	1.3 (0.06)[1]	1.6 (0.04)[1]	2.4 (0.06)	2.4 (0.06)
Per capita mean intake from snacks, mg	270 (8.7)[1]	301 (19.8)[1]	487 (24.6)	513 (17.4)[1]	425 (19.5)	202 (6)[1]	239 (10.4)[1]	358 (10.8)[1]	453 (18.1)	419 (15.1)
% snackers	66 (1.2)[1]	68 (2.2)[1]	85 (1.2)	92 (0.8)	92 (0.7)	60 (1.2)[1]	64 (1.7)[1]	74 (1)[1]	90 (0.6)	89 (0.8)
Per capita mean intake from snacks, mg (snackers only)	410 (10.5)[2]	441 (23.7)	572 (23.3)[1]	559 (17.2)[1]	463 (20.6)	335 (6.8)[1]	372 (11.5)[1]	484 (11.7)	505 (18.7)	468 (15.3)
Non-Hispanic Black										
Snacks, *n*/day	0.6 (0.05)[1]	1.1 (0.11)[1]	1.6 (0.06)	2.3 (0.06)	2.1 (0.04)	0.5 (0.04)	1.0 (0.08)[1]	1.1 (0.07)[1]	2.0 (0.04)	2.2 (0.06)
Per capita mean intake from snacks, mg	131 (12.9)[1]	260 (45.1)[1]	411 (26.6)	552 (22.3)	498 (27)	152 (19)[1]	199 (22)[1]	311 (25.2)[1]	541 (30.5)	528 (27.5)
% snackers	39 (2.9)[1]	59 (3.8)[1]	74 (2.2)	88 (1)	86 (0.8)	37 (2.2)[1]	55 (2.8)[1]	61 (2.3)[1]	86 (0.9)	86 (0.7)
Per capita mean intake from snacks, mg (snackers only)	333 (30.7)[1]	441 (66)	556 (30.8)	626 (23.6)	580 (29.5)	415 (44.1)[1]	360 (41.6)[1]	514 (32.4)[2]	633 (31.8)	616 (31.4)

[1] Different from 2011 to 2014, $p < 0.05$; [2] Different from 2011 to 2014, $p < 0.01$; [2] Different from 2011 to 2014, $p < 0.05$. Note: Data come from the 1977–1978 Nationwide Food Consumption Survey (NFCS); the 1989–1991 Continuing Survey of Food Intake by Individuals (CSFII), the 1994–1996 CSFII, the 1997–1998 CSFII; NHANES 2003–2004, NHANES 2005–2006, NHANES 2009–2010 and NHANES 2011–2014. Results have been weighted to be nationally representative. Results are presented as mean (SE).

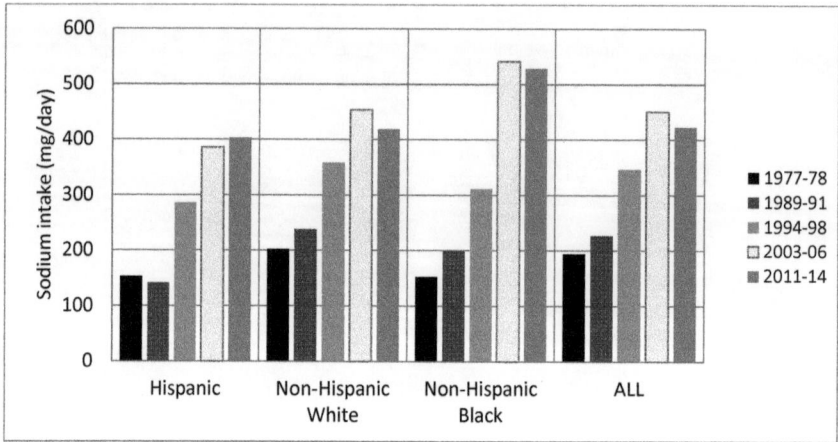

(a)

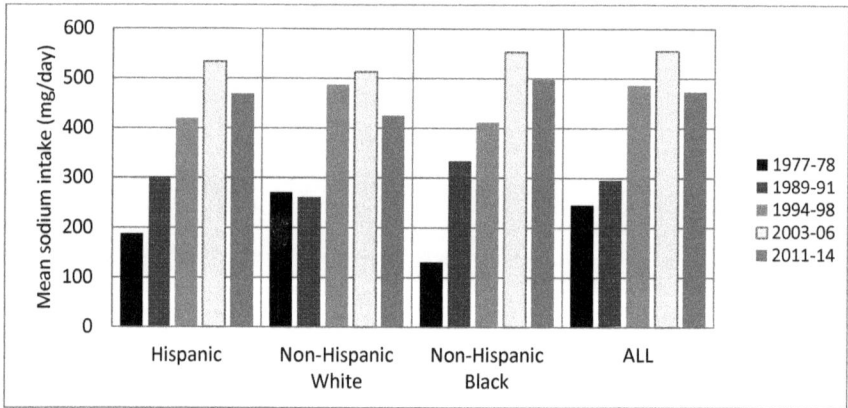

(b)

Figure 1. Sodium intake from snack food sources overall by race-ethnic group in US adults and children (a) Adults; (b) Children.

3.3. Trends by Income Level and Education

All income and education groups showed an increase in sodium intake per capita per day from snacks between 1977–1978 and 2011–2014 (Table 2). The largest increase was seen in the lowest income group (<185% FPL) and the lowest education group (Less than high school). Adults and children in the lowest income group went from the lowest sodium intake from snacks to the highest from 1977 to 2014. Adults in the lowest income group went from a significantly lower intake of sodium from snacks than adults in the highest income group, to a significantly higher intake ($p < 0.01$; Figure 2a). Children in the lowest income group went from a significantly lower intake of sodium from snacks than children in the highest poverty level, to having no difference (Figure 2b). Those in the lowest household education group had the largest increase in sodium intake from salty snacks from 1977 to 2014 (Table 2). No important differences were observed when results were examined by BMI. Results can be seen in Supplementary Table S2.

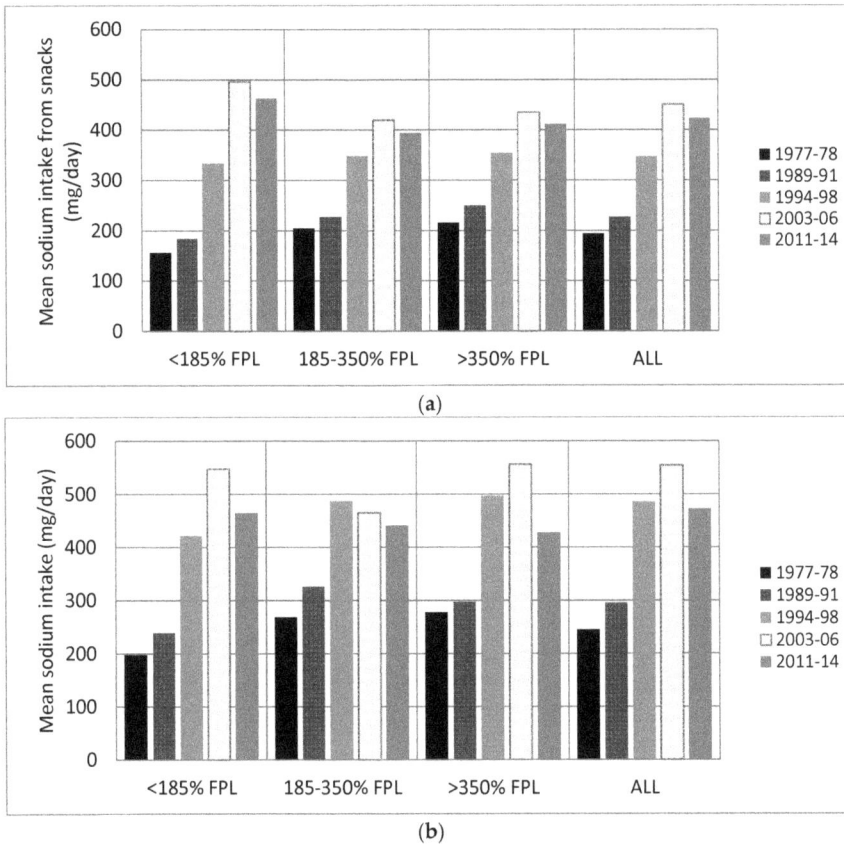

Figure 2. Sodium intake from snack food sources overall by income group in US adults and children (**a**) Adults; (**b**) Children. FPL, Federal Poverty Level.

3.4. Food Sources of Sodium Intake from Snacks

Salty snacks, and desserts and sweets, were the top two food group contributors to sodium intake from snacks in most survey years within most demographic subgroups (Supplementary Tables S3 and S4). Interestingly, either grain-based desserts or salty snacks were the number one contributor to sodium intake from snacks in each survey year in each race-ethnic group. Non-Hispanic Black adults and children had the largest increase in mean sodium intake from salty snacks from 1977 to 2014, compared to Hispanics and Non-Hispanic Whites (Supplementary Figures S1 and S2).

4. Discussion

To the knowledge of the authors, this is the first study to examine both recent and long term trends in sodium intake derived from snack food sources in US adults and children in specific age, race-ethnic, household education and income groups. We found that in all socio-demographic subgroups there was a significant increase in both the per capita sodium intake, and the proportion of sodium intake derived from snacks from 1977–1978 to 2011–2014 ($p < 0.01$); however, in the most recent period following 2003–2006 we found a systematic decline in all socio-demographic subgroups. Most pronounced, were the trends in the Non-Hispanic Black race-ethnic group, that went from the lowest consumption of sodium from snacks to the highest intake of sodium from snacks, which is a marked shift in intake that adds to the evidence base indicating that disparities in sodium intake of this race-ethnic subpopulation are emerging. This was also seen in both adults and children in the lowest household education group of all ages, in sodium intake from snacks over the 37-year period.

A large proportion of sodium intake from snack foods derived from foods generally considered unhealthy, such as desserts/sweets and salty snacks. These two sources alone contributed to more than 25% of sodium from snack foods in both adults and children in 2014. This aligns with both a recent short term study in US children from 2003 to 2010, which showed that although a decrease in total calorie intake from discretionary foods had declined in recent years, that intake was still unacceptably high [13], and a recently published study examining long term trends in energy intake from snack food sources, which showed that grain-based desserts and salty snacks contributed greatly to daily energy intake in US children [22]. In fact, our data showed that for all years examined, either grain-based desserts or salty snacks were the number one source of sodium intake from snacking (Supplementary Table S3). Our findings are also supported by research from other countries which has shown, not only that the foods consumed as snacks are generally from less healthy food groups [23], but that disparities exist between various race-ethnic and education groups [24–27].

This study's results showing that Non-Hispanic Blacks are consuming a higher intake of sodium from snacks than other race-ethnic groups is consistent with recent US research looking at behavioral shifts in food purchases, which found that Non-Hispanic Blacks were the only racial-ethnic group not to follow the overall trend of a decrease in per capita energy intake in the last decade [28] as well as research showing that Non-Hispanic Blacks, overall, have less healthy food purchasing behavior, in comparison to White and Hispanic populations [29]. However, another study examining food purchasing behavior found that Non-Hispanic Blacks actually purchased less sodium from store-bought packaged food sources than other race-ethnic groups, but also purchased much higher levels of salt-laden condiments and salt [30]. This difference might suggest that even though Non-Hispanic Black households may purchase less packaged food sources overall, they may be adding more salt during cooking and at the table [30], or are consuming snack foods from sources other than grocery stores.

Salty snack intake more than doubled from 1977–1978 to 2011–2014 overall in all US adults, and increased by ~75% in children ($p < 0.01$). However, we observed that although Non-Hispanic Blacks had the lowest overall sodium intake from salty snack food sources in 1977–1978, they had the highest sodium intake from salty snacks of all race-ethnic groups in 2011–2014. This is in contrast to prior research which found that the intake of salty snacks over the past 10 years has remained stable in children and adolescents [13], and another study which found that Non-Hispanic Whites had the highest intake of salty snacks [31]. However, prior studies in smaller samples of the US population have supported our results, showing less healthy snacking behaviors in Non-Hispanic Black adolescents [32, 33] than in other groups. This, along with the high intake of sodium from salty snacks and desserts and sweets observed in Non-Hispanic Blacks in this study is concerning, with chronic disease risk factors shown to be considerably higher among Non-Hispanic Blacks compared to Non-Hispanic Whites [34].

Our analysis had some limitations. Collected dietary data has limitations in underreporting, particularly of food and beverages perceived as being less healthy, and these limitations can vary by age, race-ethnicity and body weight status [35–37]. Similar to other studies looking at US trends in dietary intake, different methodologies were used across different survey years. The introduction of the multiple pass method in the 1990s may have resulted in additional snacks identified during that period; however, our finding of a recent decrease in snacking gives us faith that this did not affect our overall findings. Earlier survey years conducted without the multiple pass method may be more prone to issues of recall bias. There is no bridging survey to help understand the impact of this methodological change, meaning that these surveys are the only ones available that use consistent food composition tables developed by the USDA specifically for the food supply at the time of each survey. Dietary intake assessment methods and food composition information have significantly improved over time. Although data presented are based on the first day 24-h recall from all surveys, the recall methodology was modified to include multiple passes through the list of foods and beverages in the CSFII 1994–1998 and to include the USDA's automated collection system in NHANES surveys from 2002 onwards. Validation studies in adults have shown that these newer methods improved completeness of the recall [38]. As such, it is possible that the observed increases in sodium intake from 1977–1978 to 2003–2006 are an artefact of the more complete capture of the data. Each survey was linked to USDA food composition tables, but there may have been changes in nutrient composition based on different assay techniques, for which we cannot account [39,40]. These concerns were addressed by using the food grouping system developed by UNC-CH, which allows foods in each survey year to be linked to one consistent food group to offset changes in food composition table numbering, and to ensure high quality estimates of nutrient values over time [41].

5. Conclusions

Our study found a long term increase in overall sodium intake from snacking, but a declining trend in the last decade, to a lower intake in 2011–2014, and showed important disparities amongst Non-Hispanic Blacks, in particular, and differences between the lower household education and income groups. Importantly, we found that the major foods consumed at these snacking events (desserts and sweets, and salty snacks) are the foods recommended for reduced intake by the US dietary guidelines [42]. These only emphasized, again, the importance of not only focusing on reducing calories, but also improving diet quality. Our findings have major implications for future policy interventions targeting specific demographic subgroups of the US population.

Supplementary Materials: The following are available online at www.mdpi.com/2072-6643/9/6/610/s1, Figure S1: Contribution of salty snacks to sodium intake from snacking by race-ethnic group in US adults; Figure S2: Contribution of salty snacks to sodium intake from snacking by race-ethnic group in US children; Table S1: Socio-demographic characteristics for US adults and children from the 1977–1978 Nationwide Food Consumption Survey (NFCS), the 1989–1991 Continuing Survey of Food Intake by Individuals (CSFII), the 1994–1996 CSFII, the 1997–1998 CSFII, NHANES 2003–2004, NHANES 2005–2006, NHANES 2009–10 and NHANES 2011–2014; Table S2: Number of snacks consumed per day, percentage of snackers in the population and sodium consumed per snacking occasion by US children and adults from the 1977–1978, 1989–1991, 1994–1998, 2003–2006 and 2011–2014 surveys by BMI; Table S3: Top 10 sources of sodium intake from snack foods in US adults overall and by race-ethnic group; Table S4: Top 10 sources of sodium intake from snack foods in US children overall and by race-ethnic group.

Acknowledgments: This work was supported by the Robert Wood Johnson Foundation (grant numbers 67506, 68793, 70017, 71837), NIH (grant numbers R01DK098072; DK56350) and CPC (grant number P2C HD050924). E Dunford is supported by a National Health and Medical Research Council of Australia Early Career Fellowship (APP1088673).

Author Contributions: E.K.D. and B.M.P. conceived and designed the study; E.K.D. performed the analyses; E.K.D. wrote the paper; J.M.P. and B.M.P. provided feedback on the manuscript.

Conflicts of Interest: The authors declare no conflict of interest.

References

1. Aburto, N.J.; Ziolkovska, A.; Hooper, L.; Elliott, P.; Cappuccio, F.P.; Meerpohl, J.J. Effect of lower sodium intake on health: Systematic review and meta-analyses. *BMJ* **2013**, *346*, f1326. [CrossRef] [PubMed]
2. Mozaffarian, D.; Singh, G.M.; Powles, J. Sodium and cardiovascular disease. *N. Engl. J. Med.* **2014**, *371*, 2138–2139. [PubMed]
3. National Heart Lung and Blood Institute. Lifestyle Interventions to Reduce Cardiovascular Risk: Systematic Evidence Review from the Lifestyle Work Group. Available online: https://www.nhlbi.nih.gov/health-pro/guidelines/in-develop/cardiovascular-risk-reduction/lifestyle (accessed on 15 April 2017).
4. Institute of Medicine. Sodium Intake in Populations: Assessment of Evidence. Available online: https://www.nap.edu/catalog/18311/sodium-intake-in-populations-assessment-of-evidence (accessed on 15 April 2017).
5. Centers for Disease Control and Prevention. Prevalence of hypertension and controlled hypertension—United States, 2005–2008. *MMWR* **2011**, *60*, 94–97.

6. Eckel, R.H.; Jakicic, J.M.; Ard, J.D.; de Jesus, J.M.; Houston Miller, N.; Hubbard, V.S.; Lee, I.M.; Lichtenstein, A.H.; Loria, C.M.; Millen, B.E.; et al. 2013 AHA/ACC guideline on lifestyle management to reduce cardiovascular risk: A report of the American College of Cardiology/American Heart Association task force on practice guidelines. *Circulation* **2014**, *129*, S76–S99. [CrossRef] [PubMed]

7. World Health Organization. Guideline: Sodium Intake for Adults and Children. Available online: http://apps.who.int/iris/bitstream/10665/77985/1/9789241504836_eng.pdf (accessed on 15 April 2017).

8. Quader, Z.S.; Zhao, L.; Gillespie, C.; Cogswell, M.E.; Terry, A.L.; Moshfegh, A.; Rhodes, D. Sodium intake among persons aged >/=2 years—United States, 2013–2014. *MMWR* **2017**, *66*. [CrossRef] [PubMed]

9. Drewnowski, A.; Rehm, C.D. Sodium intakes of US children and adults from foods and beverages by location of origin and by specific food source. *Nutrients* **2013**, *5*, 1840–1855. [CrossRef] [PubMed]

10. Mattes, R.D.; Donnelly, D. Relative contributions of dietary sodium sources. *J. Am. Coll. Nutr.* **1991**, *10*, 383–393. [CrossRef] [PubMed]

11. Poti, J.M.; Dunford, E.K.; Popkin, B.M. Sodium reduction in US households' packaged food and beverage purchases from retail food stores, 2000–2014. *JAMA Intern. Med.* **2017**, in press.

12. Deaton, A. On death and money: History, facts, and explanations. *JAMA* **2016**, *315*, 1703–1705. [CrossRef] [PubMed]

13. Bleich, S.N.; Wolfson, J.A. Trends in SSBs and snack consumption among children by age, body weight, and race/ethnicity. *Obesity* **2015**, *23*, 1039–1046. [CrossRef] [PubMed]

14. Piernas, C.; Popkin, B.M. Snacking increased among U.S. adults between 1977 and 2006. *J. Nutr.* **2010**, *140*, 325–332. [CrossRef] [PubMed]

15. Hess, J.M.; Jonnalagadda, S.S.; Slavin, J.L. What is a snack, why do we snack, and how can we choose better snacks? A review of the definitions of snacking, motivations to snack, contributions to dietary intake, and recommendations for improvement. *Adv. Nutr.* **2016**, *7*, 466–475. [CrossRef] [PubMed]

16. Lucan, S.C.; Karpyn, A.; Sherman, S. Storing empty calories and chronic disease risk: Snack-food products, nutritive content, and manufacturers in Philadelphia corner stores. *J. Urban Health* **2010**, *87*, 394–409. [CrossRef] [PubMed]

17. Quader, Z.S.; Gillespie, C.; Sliwa, S.A.; Ahuja, J.K.; Burdg, J.P.; Moshfegh, A.; Pehrsson, P.R.; Gunn, J.P.; Mugavero, K.; Cogswell, M.E. Sodium intake among US school-aged children: National Health and Nutrition Examination Survey, 2011–2012. *J. Acad. Nutr. Diet.* **2017**, *117*, 39–47. [CrossRef] [PubMed]

18. Perloff, B.P.; Rizek, R.L.; Haytowitz, D.B.; Reid, P.R. Dietary intake methodology. II. USDA's Nutrient Data Base for Nationwide Dietary Intake Surveys. *J. Nutr.* **1990**, *120* (Suppl. 11), 1530–1534. [PubMed]

19. National Health and Nutrition Examination Survey. MEC In-Person Dietary Interviewers Procedures Manual. Available online: https://www.cdc.gov/nchs/data/nhanes/nhanes_03_04/dietary_mec.pdf (accessed on 15 April 2017).

20. Slining, M.M.; Mathias, K.C.; Popkin, B.M. Trends in food and beverage sources among US children and adolescents: 1989–2010. *J. Acad. Nutr. Diet.* **2013**, *113*, 1683–1694. [CrossRef] [PubMed]

21. Popkin, B.M.; Haines, P.S.; Siega-Riz, A.M. Dietary patterns and trends in the United States: The UNC-CH approach. *Appetite* **1999**, *32*, 8–14. [CrossRef] [PubMed]

22. Dunford, E.K.; Popkin, B.M. 35 year snacking trends for US children 1977–2012. *Pediatr. Obes.* **2017**, in press.

23. Mercille, G.; Receveur, O.; Macaulay, A.C. Are snacking patterns associated with risk of overweight among Kahnawake schoolchildren? *Public Health Nutr.* **2010**, *13*, 163–171. [CrossRef] [PubMed]

24. Durao, C.; Severo, M.; Oliveira, A.; Moreira, P.; Guerra, A.; Barros, H.; Lopes, C. Association of maternal characteristics and behaviours with 4-year-old children's dietary patterns. *Matern. Child. Nutr.* **2017**, *13*. [CrossRef] [PubMed]

25. Fernandez-Alvira, J.M.; Bornhorst, C.; Bammann, K.; Gwozdz, W.; Krogh, V.; Hebestreit, A.; Barba, G.; Reisch, L.; Eiben, G.; Iglesia, I.; et al. Prospective associations between socio-economic status and dietary patterns in European children: The Identification and Prevention of Dietary- and Lifestyle-induced Health Effects in Children and Infants (IDEFICS) Study. *Br. J. Nutr.* **2015**, *113*, 517–525. [CrossRef] [PubMed]

26. Gates, A.; Skinner, K.; Gates, M. The diets of school-aged Aboriginal youths in Canada: A systematic review of the literature. *J. Hum. Nutr. Diet.* **2015**, *28*, 246–261. [CrossRef] [PubMed]

27. Howe, L.D.; Ellison-Loschmann, L.; Pearce, N.; Douwes, J.; Jeffreys, M.; Firestone, R. Ethnic differences in risk factors for obesity in New Zealand infants. *J. Epidemiol. Community Health* **2015**, *69*, 516–522. [CrossRef] [PubMed]

28. Kant, A.K.; Graubard, B.I. 40-year trends in meal and snack eating behaviors of American adults. *J. Acad. Nutr. Diet.* **2015**, *115*, 50–63. [CrossRef] [PubMed]

29. Stern, D.; Poti, J.M.; Ng, S.W.; Robinson, W.R.; Gordon-Larsen, P.; Popkin, B.M. Where people shop is not associated with the nutrient quality of packaged foods for any racial-ethnic group in the United States. *Am. J. Clin. Nutr.* **2016**, *103*, 1125–1134. [CrossRef] [PubMed]

30. Poti, J.M.; Mendez, M.A.; Ng, S.W.; Popkin, B.M. Highly processed and ready-to-eat packaged food and beverage purchases differ by race/ethnicity among US households. *J. Nutr.* **2016**, *146*, 1722–1730. [CrossRef] [PubMed]

31. Masters, M.A.; Stanek Krogstrand, K.L.; Eskridge, K.M.; Albrecht, J.A. Race/ethnicity and income in relation to the home food environment in US youth aged 6 to 19 years. *J. Acad. Nutr. Diet.* **2014**, *114*, 1533–1543. [CrossRef] [PubMed]

32. Delva, J.; O'Malley, P.M.; Johnston, L.D. Racial/ethnic and socioeconomic status differences in overweight and health-related behaviors among American students: National trends 1986–2003. *J. Adolesc. Health* **2006**, *39*, 536–545. [CrossRef] [PubMed]

33. Ford, M.C.; Gordon, N.P.; Howell, A.; Green, C.E.; Greenspan, L.C.; Chandra, M.; Mellor, R.G.; Lo, J.C. Obesity severity, dietary behaviors, and lifestyle risks vary by race/ethnicity and age in a northern California cohort of children with obesity. *J. Obes.* **2016**, *2016*, 4287976. [CrossRef] [PubMed]

34. Centers for Disease Control and Prevention. Differences in prevalence of obesity among black, white, and Hispanic adults—United States, 2006–2008. *MMWR Wkly.* **2009**, *58*, 740–744.

35. Livingstone, M.B.; Robson, P.J.; Wallace, J.M. Issues in dietary intake assessment of children and adolescents. *Br. J. Nutr.* **2004**, *92* (Suppl. 2), S213–S222. [CrossRef] [PubMed]

36. Schoeller, D.A. Limitations in the assessment of dietary energy intake by self-report. *Metabolism* **1995**, *44*, 18–22. [CrossRef]

37. Heitmann, B.L.; Lissner, L.; Osler, M. Do we eat less fat, or just report so? *Int. J. Obes. Relat. Metab. Disord.* **2000**, *24*, 435–442. [CrossRef] [PubMed]

38. Moshfegh, A.J.; Rhodes, D.G.; Baer, D.J.; Murayi, T.; Clemens, J.C.; Rumpler, W.V.; Paul, D.R.; Sebastian, R.S.; Kuczynski, K.J.; Ingwersen, L.A.; et al. The US Department of Agriculture automated multiple-pass method reduces bias in the collection of energy intakes. *Am. J. Clin. Nutr.* **2008**, *88*, 324–332. [PubMed]

39. US Department of Agriculture. Food and Nutrient Database for Dietary Studies, 2013–14. Available online: https://www.ars.usda.gov/northeast-area/beltsville-md/beltsville-human-nutrition-research-center/food-surveys-research-group/docs/fndds-download-databases/ (accessed on 15 April 2017).

40. US Department of Agriculture. USDA National Nutrient Database for Standard Reference. Available online: https://www.ars.usda.gov/northeast-area/beltsville-md/beltsville-human-nutrition-research-center/nutrient-data-laboratory/docs/usda-national-nutrient-database-for-standard-reference/ (accessed on 15 April 2017).

41. Popkin, B.M.; Haines, P.S.; Reidy, K.C. Food consumption trends of US women: Patterns and determinants between 1977 and 1985. *Am. J. Clin. Nutr.* **1989**, *49*, 1307–1319. [PubMed]

42. US Department of Health and Human Services. Scientific Report of the 2015 Dietary Guidelines Advisory Committee. Available online: https://health.gov/dietaryguidelines/2015-scientific-report/ (accessed on 16 April 2017).

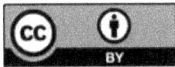

nutrients

MDPI

Review

A Systematic Review of Fatalities Related to Acute Ingestion of Salt. A Need for Warning Labels?

Norm R. C. Campbell [1,*] and Emma J. Train [2]

[1] Department of Medicine, Physiology and Pharmacology and Community Health Sciences, O'Brien Institute for Public Health and Libin Cardiovascular Institute of Alberta, University of Calgary, Calgary, AB T2N 4Z6, Canada
[2] The School of Public Policy, University of Calgary, Calgary, AB T2N 4Z6, Canada; emmajtrain@gmail.com
* Correspondence: ncampbel@ucalgary.ca; Tel.: +403-210-7961; Fax: +403-210-9837

Received: 7 June 2017; Accepted: 20 June 2017; Published: 23 June 2017

Abstract: There are sporadic cases of fatalities from acutely eating salt. Yet, on social media, there are "challenges to" and examples of children and some adults acutely eating salt, and recently a charity advocated eating small amounts of salt to empathize with Syrian refugees. We performed a systematic review of fatalities from ingesting salt to assess if relatively moderate doses of salt could be fatal. In 27 reports, there were 35 fatalities documented (19 in adults and 16 in children). The lethal dose was estimated to be less than 10 g of sodium (<5 teaspoons of salt) in two children, and less than 25 g sodium in four adults (<4 tablespoons of salt). The frequency of fatal ingestion of salt is not able to be discerned from our review. If investigation of the causes of hypernatremia in hospital records indicates salt overdose is relatively common, consideration could be given to placing warning labels on salt containers and shakers. Such warning labels can have the added advantage of reducing dietary salt consumption.

Keywords: salt; sodium; overdose; warning labels; hypertension; hypernatremia

---

1. Introduction

Dietary risks are estimated to be the leading risk for death and disability globally [1]. Among the dietary risks, high intake of dietary sodium is the leading risk, being attributed to over 4 million deaths and 83 million disability-adjusted life years (DALYs) in 2015 [1]. The deaths and disability are considered to be largely related to hypertension and dietary salt intake promoting gastric cancer [1].

Much less attention has been given to the acute toxic effects of dietary salt. Isolated cases of fatalities caused by the acute ingestion of table salt have been reported [2]. These isolated reports were concerning when a Canadian campaign was initiated in August of 2016 to encourage people to eat small quantities of table salt to empathize with the suffering of refugees in Syria [3]. The #Salt4Syria marketing campaign website shows children eating salt out of spoons and pictures of an overflowing spoonful of salt. The campaign encourages children to record and share their salt consumption videos and nominate others to do the same. Further, a brief investigation of social media indicates several children and adults are acutely ingesting salt and challenging others to do so (a google video search of "eat salt challenge" resulted in 313,000 uploaded videos, 20 April 2017). A systematic review of fatalities occurring from acute ingestion of salt was conducted, in part, to assess the potential risk of advocating the acute ingestion of salt. The intent was to assess whether relatively modest ingestion of salt might cause fatalities.

2. Materials and Methods

We systematically searched for all studies that reported fatalities from ingesting salt (sodium chloride). The search strategy included Medline, Embase, Cochrane Register of Control Trials, and the

Cochrane Database of Systematic Reviews using the terms from Table 1 on 23 January 2017 with no time restrictions. NRCC searched all the titles and abstracts identified by the searches, and articles that were identified as potentially eligible were obtained for full review. The articles were reviewed by NRCC. The reference lists of the included studies and reviews were hand-searched for additional studies. Letters to editors and abstracts were included.

Table 1. Literature search terms to identify potential fatalities related to salt ingestion.

1.	((toxic* or intoxic* or overdos*) adj5 salt).mp
2.	((toxic* or intoxic* or overdos*) adj5 Na).mp
3.	((toxic* or intoxic* or overdos*) adj5 sodium).mp
4.	((salt* or Na or sodium) adj5 overdos*).mp
5.	hypernatremia.mp
6.	hypernatremia/
7.	1 or 2 or 3 or 4 or 5 or 6
8.	((dietar* or intake* or food* or consumption or consume* or ingest*) adj5 sodium).mp
9.	((dietar* or intake* or food* or consumption or consume* or ingest*) adj5 salt).mp
10.	((dietar* or intake* or food* or consumption or consume* or ingest*) adj5 Na).mp
11.	8 or 9 or 10
12.	7 and 11
13.	Limit 12 to humans

Articles were included if there was oral ingestion of salt (sodium chloride) that resulted in a fatal outcome. Fatalities related to gastric lavage with salt were included but fatalities related to intravenous and rectal administration of salt and to absorption of salt through the skin (burn treatment) were excluded. There were no exclusion criteria based on language.

Data from manuscripts was extracted by EJT and NRCC, including the first author, year of publication, country where the report originated, location, and the patients' age, gender, weight (kg), category of ingestion (e.g., accidental by patient, intentional by patient (suicide), therapeutic adverse outcome from lavage), estimated dose of salt/sodium ingested, presence of known chronic disease, presence of known prior renal dysfunction, co-ingestion of other toxins, co-ingestion of drugs that impact renal excretion of sodium (e.g., diuretic), mental illness, acute illness, and highest recorded serum sodium level. The fatalities were categorized by age (<5, 5–10, >10 to 18 and >18 years). Where the amount of salt ingested was provided in a range, this was recorded.

Salt and sodium ingestion units were converted to sodium in grams using the conversions: 1 mmol sodium = 1 mEq sodium = 23 mg sodium, and 1 g sodium = 2.54 g salt (NaCl). Where salt ingestion was estimated by table, dessert, or teaspoons, the ingested salt was estimated to be 17.06 g (sodium 6.8 g), 11.4 g (sodium 4.5 g), and 5.7 g (sodium 2.28 g), respectively. Where it was indicated that the spoon was overfilled or "large", 50% more salt was estimated to have been ingested. When estimates were provided both as a weight (e.g., 60 g salt) and a spoon measurement (2 tablespoons), both are indicated as a range. When sodium bicarbonate was co-administered with sodium chloride, the total sodium dose ingested was estimated.

3. Results

The literature search yielded 460 articles (Figure 1) of which 25 articles were selected for full-text review following a review of the title and abstract. Exclusions included 13 articles that did not report fatality from salt ingestion, and one article was a review without original cases reported. Eleven of the included articles reported one or more fatalities from acute ingestion of salt. Review of abstract and titles of the citations in the selected articles obtained in the literature search yielded an additional 24 articles for full text review. Of the 24, 17 contained reports of fatalities from ingesting salt. Thus, 27 manuscripts reporting fatality from ingesting dietary salt were obtained. There were 35 fatalities reported, 19 in adults [2,4–19] and 16 in children [6,20–29]. The fatalities were categorized by age (Tables 2 and 3). There were no fatalities reported in the age category 10–18 years. Nearly all the reported cases had multiple missing values in the data extraction table with, for example, few reporting weights.

Adults (age >18): There were 19 fatalities reported in 16 females and 3 males (average age 40.6, standard deviation (s.d.) 17.9 years, range 19–83) (Table 2). In twelve fatalities, the salt was administered as an emetic, in four the salt was administered as part of an exorcism ritual, in three ingestion was inadvertently mistaking salt for sugar, and in one the reason for ingestion was unknown. The average lower and average higher estimated doses of sodium ingested was 60 and 118 g, respectively. The ingested doses in individuals were estimated to range from 6 g to 400 g. In four fatalities, the estimated sodium dose ingested was under 25 g.

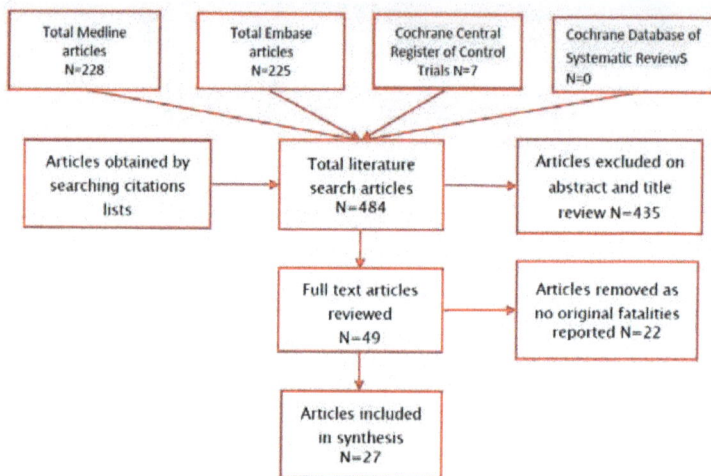

Figure 1. Flow diagram.

In two of the fatalities, sodium bicarbonate was co-ingested with salt (sodium chloride). In the cases where salt was given as an emetic, it was for overdoses with several of the overdoses reported as minor. Although many of the fatalities had histories of prior psychiatric disease, few had chronic medical disease and none were previously known to have renal impairment. The average maximum blood/serum sodium level recorded was 205.51 (s.d. 28.19) mmol/L, with the highest being 255 mmol/L and the lowest 151 mmol/L.

Adolescents (age 10–18 years): There were no reported fatal cases in this age range.

Children (age 5–10 years): There was one reported fatality (female age 5) (Table 3). The dose of sodium ingested was estimated to be a minimum of five teaspoons of table salt given by the parents (approximately 11.4 grams of sodium). The patient had a record of poor growth but was otherwise healthy and had a serum sodium level of 220 mmol/L after ingestion.

Children (age <5 years): There were 15 reported fatalities overall and 13 fatalities that reported some individual details (Table 3). The ages ranged from 1 day to 4 years of age. In eight of the fatalities, salt was mistaken for sugar, with six occurring in a single incident at a hospital. The salt was reported to be administered by parents in many of the remaining fatalities with intent to injure, and as an emetic in four cases. In one fatality, there was a mistake made in the amount of salt added in making a rehydration formula. Most of the doses of sodium ingested were not known, with reported estimates ranging from less than 7 g to 13 g. Similarly, most serum sodium levels were not reported, but reported levels ranged from 178 to 245 mmol/L.

Table 2. Fatal ingestion of salt in adults.

First Author Year of Publication	Age (Years)	Gender	Explanation of Overdose	Estimated Dose Ingested Sodium (g) *	Highest Reported Blood Level of Sodium (mmol/L) **	Co-Ingestion of Other Potential Toxins	Chronic Illness
Engtrom 2008 [4]	83	Female	Mistaken for sugar	13.6–20.4 g	223	None stated	Hypertension, dementia
Raya 1992 [5]	36	Female	Exorcism ritual	273 g	246	Sodium bicarbonate *	None stated
Turk 2005 [6]	34	Female	Health care professional administered emetic	80 g	196	None stated	"Psychomotor retardation"
	69	Male	Health care professional administered emetic	39.4–81.6 g	175	Single table of unprescribed "neuroleptic"	Schizophrenia
Moder 1990 [2]	41	Male	Mistaken for sugar	27.1–34.8 g	209	None stated	Downs Syndrome, lymphoma, hepatitis B, seizures
Johnston 1977 [7]	45	Female	Mistaken for sugar	30.6–40.8 g	190	None stated	Prader-Willi Syndrome, hypertension obesity, impaired glucose tolerance
Bacarreza 2008 [8]	33	Female	Not known	50 g	203	None stated	Alcohol abuse
Ofran 2004 [9]	20	Female	Exorcism ritual	<400 g	255	None stated	Depression
Robertson 1971 [10]	23	Female	Emetic	Not stated	214	Chlordiazepoxide overdose	None stated
Hey 1982 [11]	56	Female	Emetic	27.2–47.2 g	214	"trivial" overdose	Not stated
Hedouin 1999 [12]	19	Female	Exorcism ritual	Not stated	153	None stated	Hydrocephalus, seizures
Bird 1974 [13]	35	Female	Emetic	20.4 g	200	"Overdose"	"Psychiatric patient"
Ward 1963 [14]	74	Male	Emetic	13.6–24.4 g	174	Accidental overdose of imipramine and perphenazine	"Mild depression"
Gresham 1982 [15]	48	Female	Emetic	6.8–10.2 g	166	"Extra dose" of chlorpromazine	Past leucotomy, depression
Laurence 1969 [16]	35	Female	Emetic	69 g	184	Overdose thioridazine	None stated
Goodbody 1975 [17]	35	Female	Emetic and lavage	>17.7 g	226 ***	"Minor" overdose sodium amytal	None stated
	44	Female	Emetic	Not stated	151	Overdose sodium amytal	None stated
Winter 1974 [18]	21	Female	Emetic and lavage	118–236 g	227	Amitriptyline, imipramine, chlorpromazine, diazepam and nitrazepam overdose	Psychiatric disease
Roberts 1974 [19]	26	Female	Emetic	27–60 g	172	Salicylate overdose	Depression

* The sodium in g from the sodium bicarbonate or lavage is included in the estimate of ingested sodium; ** reports did not indicate if blood or serum levels were provided; *** post-mortem value, 210 mmol/L was recorded pre-mortem.

Table 3. Fatal ingestion of salt in children aged 10 years and under.

First Author, Year of Publication	Age (Years) (Months) (Weeks) (Days)	Gender	Explanation of Overdose	Estimated Dose Ingested Sodium (g) *	Highest Reported Serum Level of Sodium (mmol/L) **	Co-Ingestion of Other Potential Toxins	Chronic Illness
Dockery 1992 [21]	5 years	Female	Parental administration	11.4 g	220	None stated	"Poor growth"
Turk 2005 [6]	4 years	Female	Emesis	Not stated	245	None stated	Low body weight
Martos Sanchez 2000 [22]	20 months	Female	Mistaken for sugar	9.12 g	195	None stated	None stated
	7 months	Female	Accidental	5.03 g	178	None stated	None stated
Scott 1947 [23]	2 years	Male	Mistaken for sugar	<7 g	Not stated	None stated	Gastrointestinal strictures
Barer 1973 [24]	3 years	Male	Emetic and lavage	Not stated	188	Aspirin overdose	None stated
Streat 1982 [25]	2 years	Female	Emetic	Not stated	204	Pheniramine overdose	None stated
Finberg 1963 [26]	7 days	Male	Mistaken for sugar	Not stated	Not stated	None stated	Prematurity
	2 months	Female	Mistaken for sugar	Not stated	Not stated	None stated	Congenital neuroblastoma
	3 weeks	Male	Mistaken for sugar	Not stated	Not stated	None stated	None stated
	5 days	Female	Mistaken for sugar	Not stated	Not stated	None stated	None stated
	2 days	Female	Mistaken for sugar	Not stated	Not stated	None stated	None stated
	1 day	Female	Mistaken for sugar	Not stated	244	None stated	None stated
Rogers 1976 [27]	1 year	Female	Parental administration	Not stated	200	None stated	Repeated abscesses
Meadow 1993 [28]***	1.5–9 months	Half were female	Parental administration	Not stated	Not stated	Not stated	Not stated
Smith 1990 [29]	26 months	Not stated	Emetic for minor overdose	6.8–13.6 g	217	None stated	None stated

* The sodium in g from lavage is included in the estimate of ingested sodium where possible; ** reports did not indicate if blood or serum levels were provided; *** two fatalities were reported in a case series but individual data was not provided.

4. Discussion

Relatively modest doses of sodium have been reported to cause fatality. In two children, the lethal dose was estimated to be less than 10 g of sodium (less than five teaspoons of salt) and the lethal dose was estimated to be less than 25 g sodium in four adults (less than four tablespoons of salt). The mechanism of salt ingestion causing death is believed to be related to hypernatremia with the serum sodium levels in reported fatalities ranging from 175 to 255 mmol/L. Ingestion of as little as two tablespoons of salt has been reported to increase serum sodium levels by as much as 30 mmol/L with the potential to cause severe irreversible neurological damage [7,9]. Many of the fatalities were related to the administration of salt therapeutically as an emetic agent, where toxicity may have been, in part, related to co-ingested drugs. Nevertheless, several deaths occurred by accidental ingestion of salt, most where salt was mistaken for sugar without any other co-ingested toxins. While this review found that modest amounts of sodium have been reported to be associated with death, the review design and available information do not allow any estimates of the usual amount of ingested sodium that might be lethal (e.g., lethal dose 50 (LD50); the dose that is lethal in 50% of exposed animals). The media LD50 in rats is 3 g/kg for ingestion over 4 h [30]. Further, the reported deaths and serious illness from using salt as an emetic agent resulted in strong recommendations to no longer use salt for that indication [10]. Historically it has been reported that wealthy Chinese committed suicide by ingesting large amounts of salt [6].

The lower amounts of sodium ingested that were associated with death in this systematic review are only four-fold higher than daily intake levels consumed by the average person in Beijing and less than twice as high as the upper range of daily consumption by individual Chinese [31,32]. Ingestion of sodium in forms that are rapidly consumed and absorbed (e.g., dissolved in water) may acutely overwhelm the ability to excrete sodium resulting in rapidly increasing extracellular (and specifically serum) sodium levels. Humans evolved on much lower amounts of sodium than are currently ingested (0.1 to 1 g sodium/day), and hence we may not have developed the capacity to rapidly excrete large amounts of sodium that are acutely ingested [33,34]. Excretion is by the kidneys, sweating, and gastrointestinal tract [33]. About 90% of ingested sodium is excreted by the kidneys [33]; hence, it is reasonable to hypothesize that individuals with less capacity to excrete sodium (i.e., renal impairment) might be particularly susceptible to toxic effects ingested sodium. In the systematic review, there were no cases where renal impairment was identified before the overdose, although several persons were noted to have a modest elevation in serum creatinine ($\leq$140 µmol/L) during the acute illness following sodium ingestion [2,4,5,9]. A wide variation in ability to excrete sodium has been observed in studies examining genetic variation in the blood pressure increasing effects of dietary sodium [35]. Hence, through genetic variation in renal excretion of sodium, some "salt-sensitive" individuals may be predisposed to, and some "salt-resistant" individuals protected from, the adverse effects of acute sodium ingestion. The sodium content in food is likely to be lower and more slowly absorbed than the ingestion of salt itself or in solutions, hence these findings are not likely to inform the discussion on salt as generally regarded as safe (GRAS) additives which has been ongoing in the United States [36]. Nevertheless, very severe hypernatremia has been reported from drinking food condiments high in sodium (e.g., soya sauce) [37].

There are several weaknesses to this systematic review. For many if not most of the fatalities, the ingested dose of salt could only be estimated based on incomplete information. In particular, the estimated dose of sodium of 6 g causing a fatality in an adult seems implausible. We have also noted that most reports gave incomplete information on the patients, including such important information as weight that could have allowed the doses of salt ingested to be expressed per kg of body weight. The review does not provide useful information on how frequent fatal salt ingestion occurs. Further, the levels of hypernatremia reported are likely underestimates of the true peak blood sodium levels, as in several of the fatalities, blood levels of sodium were not assessed at presentation nor were they closely monitored. Lastly, many of the manuscripts were found by hand-searching reference lists as opposed to the primary literature searches. Factors which may have reduced the sensitivity of the literature searches may include the older age of many publications, the relatively low prominence of several of the journals, and that several of the articles were "letters" to editors rather than full research publications.

If severe hypernatremia is relatively common with doses of salt ingestion as low as reported in this review, it may speak to the need to place warning labels on salt shakers and containers. Several of the reported cases came from a review of single-centre case reviews, suggesting that a systematic examination of patients presenting with hypernatremia may find a higher frequency of fatal sodium overdoses than this systematic review of published literature indicates [6,22,26]. Warning labels could increase the awareness of the acute dangers of salt and reduce the number of people ingesting salt as part of a challenge or ritual and may discourage organizations from using salt ingestion in awareness campaigns. A search on social media finds many recent examples of mostly children and some adults challenging themselves or others to eat amounts of salt that are in the range of the fatalities reported in this systematic review (google search "eat salt challenge", 10 April 2017). An added benefit of warning labels on salt containers relates to evidence that it may reduce salt intake [38–40].

5. Conclusions

This systematic review finds doses of salt that have been reported to cause fatalities are not exceptionally high and accidently replacing sugar with salt can cause fatalities. The prevalence of salt overdose is uncertain, but if it is relatively common as suggested on social media, warning labels on salt and high-salt products (e.g., soya sauce) could be one mechanism considered to reduce the use of salt in rituals and salt challenges.

Acknowledgments: We acknowledge Helen Lee Robertson, MLIS Liaison Librarian, Clinical Medicine at the University of Calgary for providing advice on the literature search strategy and Aaron Lucko conducted the literature search.

Author Contributions: N.R.C.C. reviewed the literature search to select relevant articles, performed data extraction and drafted the manuscript. E.J.T. reviewed the data extraction and revised the manuscript.

Conflicts of Interest: N.R.C.C. is a paid consultant to the Novartis Foundation to support their program to improve hypertension control in low to middle income countries which includes travel support for site visits and a contract to develop a survey. N.R.C.C. has also agree to provide paid consultative advice on accurate blood pressure assessment to Midway Corporation and is an unpaid member of World Action on Salt and Health (WASH); E.J.T. has no funding or conflicts of interest to disclose. E.J.T. is an unpaid volunteer board director of Open Arms Patient Advocacy Society and is a self-employed writer and administrator of the Anthony Train Corp.

References

1. Institute for Health Metrics and Evaluation. *GDB Compare*; Electronic Citation; Institute for Health Metrics and Evaluation: Seattle, WA, USA, 2015.
2. Moder, K.G.; Hurley, D.L. Fatal hypernatremia from exogenous salt intake: Report of a case and review of the literature. *Mayo Clin. Proc.* **1990**, *65*, 1587–1594. [CrossRef]
3. #Salt4Syria. Available online: http://www.salt4syria.com/challenge-accepted/category/take-the-challenge (accessed on 10 April 2017).
4. Engjom, T.; Kildahl-Andersen, O. An 83-year-old woman with coma and severe hypernatremia. *Tidsskr. Nor. Laegeforen.* **2008**, *128*, 316–317. [PubMed]
5. Raya, A.; Giner, P.; Aranegui, P.; Guerrero, F.; Vazquez, G. Fatal acute hypernatremia caused by massive intake of salt. *Arch. Intern. Med.* **1992**, *152*, 640–646. [CrossRef] [PubMed]
6. Turk, E.E.; Schulz, F.; Koops, E.; Gehl, A.; Tsokos, M. Fatal hypernatremia after using salt as an emetic—Report of three autopsy cases. *Leg. Med. (Tokyo)* **2005**, *7*, 47–50. [CrossRef] [PubMed]
7. Johnston, J.G.; Robertson, W.O. Fatal ingestion of table salt by an adult. *West. J. Med.* **1977**, *126*, 141–143. [PubMed]
8. Nunez Bacarreza, J.J.; Remolina Schlig, M.; Zuñiga Rivera, A.; Posadas Callejas, J. Severe hypernatremia due to sodium chloride intake. *Med. Intensiv.* **2008**, *32*, 258–259.

9.   Ofran, Y.; Lavi, D.; Opher, D.; Weiss, T.A.; Elinav, E. Fatal voluntary salt intake resulting in the highest ever documented sodium plasma level in adults (255 mmol L^{-1}): A disorder linked to female gender and psychiatric disorders. *J. Intern. Med.* **2004**, *256*, 525–528. [CrossRef] [PubMed]

10. Robertson, W.O. A further warning on the use of salt as an emetic agent. *J. Pediatr.* **1971**, *79*, 877. [CrossRef]

11. Hey, A.; Hickling, K.G. Accidental salt poisoning. *N. Z. Med. J.* **1982**, *95*, 864. [PubMed]

12. Hedouin, V.; Révuelta, E.; Bécart, A.; Tournel, G.; Deveaux, M.; Gosset, D. A case of fatal salt water intoxication following an exorcism session. *Forensic Sci. Int.* **1999**, *99*, 1–4. [CrossRef]

13. Bird, C.A.; Gardner, A.W.; Roylance, P.J. Letter: Danger of saline emetics in first-aid for poisoning. *Br. Med. J.* **1974**, *4*, 103. [CrossRef] [PubMed]

14. Ward, D.J. Fatal hypernatremia after a saline emetic. *Br. Med. J.* **1963**, *2*, 432. [CrossRef] [PubMed]

15. Gresham, G.A.; Mashru, M.K. Fatal poisoning with sodium chloride. *Forensic Sci. Int.* **1982**, *20*, 87–88. [CrossRef]

16. Laurence, B.H.; Hopkins, B.E. Hypernatraemia following a saline emetic. *Med. J. Aust.* **1969**, *1*, 1301–1303. [PubMed]

17. Goodbody, R.A.; Middleton, J.E.; Gamlen, T.R. Saline emetics and hypernatraemia: Report on 2 fatalities. *Med. Sci. Law* **1975**, *15*, 261–264. [PubMed]

18. Winter, M.; Taylor, D.J. Letter: Danger of saline emetics in first-aid for poisoning. *Br. Med. J.* **1974**, *3*, 802. [CrossRef] [PubMed]

19. Roberts, C.J.; Noakes, M.J. Fatal outcome from administration of a salt emetic. *Postgrad. Med. J.* **1974**, *50*, 513–515. [CrossRef] [PubMed]

20. Kupiec, T.C.; Goldenring, J.M.; Raj, V. A non-fatal case of sodium toxicity. *J. Anal. Toxicol.* **2004**, *28*, 526–528. [CrossRef] [PubMed]

21. Dockery, W.K. Fatal intentional salt poisoning associated with a radiopaque mass. *Pediatrics* **1992**, *89*, 964–965. [PubMed]

22. Martos Sanchez, I.; Ros Pérez, P.; Otheo de Tejada, E.; Vázquez Martínez, J.L.; Pérez-Caballero, C.; Fernández Pineda, L. Fatal hypernatremia due to accidental administration of table salt. *An. Esp. Pediatr.* **2000**, *53*, 495–498. [PubMed]

23. Scott, E.P.; Rotondo, C.C. Salt intoxication; accidental ingestion of a large amount of sodium chloride; report of a case with autopsy of a two year old infant. *Ky. Med. J.* **1947**, *45*, 107–109. [PubMed]

24. Barer, J.; Hill, L.L.; Hill, R.M.; Martinez, W.M. Fatal poisoning from salt used as an emetic. *Am. J. Dis. Child.* **1973**, *125*, 889–890. [CrossRef] [PubMed]

25. Streat, S. Fatal salt poisoning in a child. *N. Z. Med. J.* **1982**, *95*, 285–286. [PubMed]

26. Finberg, L.; Kiley, J.; Luttrell, C.N. Mass accidental salt poisoning in infancy. A study of a hospital disaster. *JAMA* **1963**, *184*, 187–190. [CrossRef] [PubMed]

27. Rogers, D.; Tripp, J.; Bentovim, A.; Robinson, A.; Berry, D.; Goulding, R. Papers and originals: Non-accidental poisoning: An extended syndrome of child abuse. *Br. Med. J.* **1976**, *1*, 793–796. [CrossRef] [PubMed]

28. Meadow, R. Non-accidental salt poisoning. *Arch. Dis. Child.* **1993**, *68*, 448–452. [CrossRef] [PubMed]

29. Smith, E.J.; Palevsky, S. Salt poisoning in a two-year-old child. *Am. J. Emerg. Med.* **1990**, *8*, 571–572. [CrossRef]

30. ScienceLab.com. Material Safety Data Sheet. Sodium Chloride MSDS. Available online: http://www.sciencelab.com/msds.php?msdsId=9927593 (accessed on 11 April 2017).

31. Hipgrave, D.B.; Chang, S.; Li, X.; Wu, Y. Salt and sodium intake in China. *JAMA* **2016**, *315*, 703–705. [CrossRef] [PubMed]

32. Peng, Y.; Li, W.; Wang, Y.; Chen, H.; Bo, J.; Wang, X.; Liu, L. Validation and assessment of three methods to estimate 24-h urinary sodium excretion from spot urine samples in chinese adults. *PLoS ONE* **2016**, *11*, e0149655. [CrossRef] [PubMed]

33. Sterns, R.H. Disorders of plasma sodium—Causes, consequences, and correction. *N. Engl. J. Med.* **2015**, *372*, 55–65. [CrossRef] [PubMed]

34. Campbell, N.R.; Correa-Rotter, R.; Cappuccio, F.P.; Webster, J.; Lackland, D.T.; Neal, B.; MacGregor, G.A. Proposed nomenclature for salt intake and for reductions in dietary salt. *J. Clin. Hypertens. (Greenwich)* **2015**, *17*, 247–251. [CrossRef] [PubMed]

35. Kelly, T.N.; He, J. Genomic epidemiology of blood pressure salt sensitivity. *J. Hypertens.* **2012**, *30*, 861–873. [CrossRef] [PubMed]

36. U.S. Food, Drug Administration. Select Committee on GRAS Substances (SCOGS) Opinion: Sodium Chloride. 2015. Available online: https://www.fda.gov/food/ingredientspackaginglabeling/gras/scogs/ucm260741.htm (accessed on 11 April 2017).
37. Carlberg, D.J.; Borek, H.A.; Syverud, S.A.; Holstege, C.P. Survival of acute hypernatremia due to massive soy sauce ingestion. *J. Emerg. Med.* **2013**, *45*, 228–231. [CrossRef] [PubMed]
38. Karppanen, H.; Mervaala, E. Sodium Intake and Hypertension. *Prog. Cardiovasc. Dis.* **2006**, *49*, 59–75. [CrossRef] [PubMed]
39. Mozaffarian, D.; Afshin, A.; Benowitz, N.L.; Bittner, V.; Daniels, S.R.; Franch, H.A.; Jacobs, D.R., Jr.; Kraus, W.E.; Kris-Etherton, P.M.; Krummel, D.A.; et al. Population approaches to improve diet, physical activity, and smoking habits: A scientific statement from the American heart association. *Circulation* **2012**, *126*, 1514–1563. [CrossRef] [PubMed]
40. Pinjuh Markota, N.; Rumboldt, M.; Rumboldt, Z. Emphasized warning reduces salt intake: A randomized controlled trial. *J. Am. Soc. Hypertens.* **2015**, *9*, 214–220. [CrossRef] [PubMed]

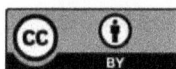

nutrients

MDPI

Review

Time to Consider Use of the Sodium-to-Potassium Ratio for Practical Sodium Reduction and Potassium Increase

Toshiyuki Iwahori [1,2,*], Katsuyuki Miura [1,3] and Hirotsugu Ueshima [1,3]

1   Department of Public Health, Shiga University of Medical Science, Seta Tsukinowa-cho, Otsu, Shiga 520-2192, Japan; miura@belle.shiga-med.ac.jp (K.M.); hueshima@belle.shiga-med.ac.jp (H.U.)
2   Research and Development Department, OMRON HEALTHCARE Co., Ltd., 53 Kunotsubo Terada-cho, Muko, Kyoto 617-0002, Japan
3   Center for Epidemiologic Research in Asia, Shiga University of Medical Science, Seta Tsukinowa-cho, Otsu, Shiga 520-2192, Japan
*   Correspondence: iwahori@belle.shiga-med.ac.jp; Tel.: +81-77-548-2191; Fax: +81-77-543-9732

Received: 12 May 2017; Accepted: 2 July 2017; Published: 5 July 2017

Abstract: Pathogenetic studies have demonstrated that the interdependency of sodium and potassium affects blood pressure. Emerging evidences on the sodium-to-potassium ratio show benefits for a reduction in sodium and an increase in potassium compared to sodium and potassium separately. As presently there is no known review, this article examined the practical use of the sodium-to-potassium ratio in daily practice. Epidemiological studies suggest that the urinary sodium-to-potassium ratio may be a superior metric as compared to separate sodium and potassium values for determining the relation to blood pressure and cardiovascular disease risks. Higher correlations and better agreements are seen for the casual urine sodium-to-potassium ratio than for casual urine sodium or potassium alone when compared with the 24-h urine values. Repeated measurements of the casual urine provide reliable estimates of the 7-day 24-h urine value with less bias for the sodium-to-potassium ratio as compared to the common formulas used for estimating the single 24-h urine from the casual urine for sodium and potassium separately. Self-monitoring devices for the urinary sodium-to-potassium ratio measurement makes it possible to provide prompt onsite feedback. Although these devices have been evaluated with a view to support an individual approach for sodium reduction and potassium increase, there has yet to be an accepted recommended guideline for the sodium-to-potassium ratio. This review concludes with a look at the practical use of the sodium-to-potassium ratio for assistance in practical sodium reduction and potassium increase.

Keywords: sodium-to-potassium ratio; sodium; salt; potassium; dietary intake evaluation; behavior change; self-monitoring; blood pressure; cardiovascular diseases

1. Introduction

Efforts to prevent hypertension and cardiovascular disease (CVD) by dietary improvement have been made for years. In earlier studies, researchers attempted to use dietary intervention as a way of evaluating the effects of a reduced salt intake and an increased fruit and vegetable intakes, while other groups used reduced dietary sodium (Na) combined with the dietary approach to stop hypertension (DASH) diet in order to prevent CVD [1–5]. Since most of these previous interventions showed positive effects and major nutrients affecting blood pressure (BP) became identified in studies [1–8], international recommendations have advised for reducing Na intake and increasing fruit and vegetable intake, i.e., potassium (K) intake [9–12].

For this review, a literature search was performed in PubMed for publications through 12 June 2017 and from our data. Citations were limited to those published in English. The search referenced the sodium-to-potassium (Na/K) ratio and the cardiovascular variables (blood pressure, hypertension, and cardiovascular disease). Of the 426 unduplicated articles, 318 were excluded based on title (or review of abstract if title was unclear) or publication type. An additional 85 articles were excluded after abstract reviews. After the remaining 23 articles were read in full, 6 were excluded. Ten articles were added by searching reference lists of the remaining 17 articles, resulting in a final inclusion of 27 articles.

2. Conventional Dietary Assessment on Sodium and Potassium Separately

Pathogenetic studies have demonstrated that the interdependency of Na and K affects BP [13]. Epidemiological studies have shown that high K mitigates the effect that high Na has on the BP levels, thereby decreasing the risk of CVD [14–17]. The World Health Organization (WHO) has recommended for years that individuals reduce Na intake and increase K intake; recently, WHO has reiterated its guidelines for Na and K [11,12]. Despite rigorous campaigns to reduce Na and increase K intake, a large gap remains between the recommended and actual intakes of both Na and K [18,19]. Thus, the conventional population approaches have not been able to compensate for this gap [20]. Moreover, the awareness of intakes by individuals remain poor, with subjects who reported practicing reduced-salt diets actually showing salt intake levels similar to those who were not practicing a reduced-salt diet [21]. Thus, an individual approach, such as self-monitoring of Na and K intakes, may aid in a timely achievement of the goals set by the World Health Organization (WHO) of intake levels of less than 2 g of Na per day by 2025 [22].

Previous studies have reported that 80–95% of dietary Na is excreted in the urine [23–28]. However, valid estimations of the Na intake can be challenging since random and systematic errors are common [29]. These errors may lead to a paradoxical relationship regarding the Na intake vs. the BP and CVD [30,31]. A prior study reported finding under-collection of the 24-h urine due to limited or no attention to quality control [32]. To reduce both the random error from the high day-to-day variability of Na within an individual and the systematic error due to incomplete urine collection, the use of high quality multiple 24-h urine collection has become the gold standard for estimating the individual daily Na intake [23,24,29,30,33]. Specific approaches that are followed in order to assure the completeness of the 24-h urine collection include asking participants to start and finish the collections in the clinic, and applying rigorous quality control procedures [34,35]. However, collecting repeated high quality 24-h urine is a substantial burden for the study participants. Thus, repeated measurement and high quality measurement for 24-h urine collection in humans are costly, neither easy nor practical to collect.

Single day measurement can be useful for estimating group intake, though it is imprecise to assess as an individual estimate [29,31]. Several suboptimal methods for evaluating Na intake have been suggested, including 24-h urine collected with limited or no attention to quality control, timed overnight urine collection, casual urine collection, 24-h dietary recalls, and the use of food frequency questionnaires. However, the amount of salt used during cooking or added as a table salt is difficult to evaluate when using dietary surveys such as the 24-h dietary recalls and the food frequency questionnaires [36]. One of the major difficulties encountered during public health surveillance studies is the underreporting of the Na intake from the dietary surveys [36]. Although the measurement of casual urine collections is much easier to perform than the other methods, the most commonly used formulas for estimating the 24-h urine Na excretions have a problematic bias [37–39]. Even though these formulas contain less bias for the population mean salt intake level, overestimations in the low salt ranges and underestimations in the high salt ranges are the major factors that can lead to irrelevant conclusions in association studies that examine salt intake and CVD [31,40,41], e.g., findings from PURE (Prospective Urban Rural Epidemiological) study [42,43]. Furthermore, since these formulas depend on other parameters such as body weight and creatinine levels, this makes it uneasy for the patients to undertake self-monitoring [37–39]. Therefore, a more reliable and easier method for assessing the Na levels is required.

Similarly, the amount of K excreted in the 24-h urine is less than that of Na, as relatively more K is excreted in the stool. A previous study reported finding a high correlation between the K intake and the 24-h urinary K excretion [23]. Thus, K excreted in the 24-h urine provides a good estimate of the dietary K intake [23,33,44]. Other reports have also stated that 63–77% of the dietary K is reflected in the urinary K [23,25–27]. The amount of K can also be evaluated by use of 24-h dietary recalls [33,36]. A high correlation is also reported between the actual K intake and the K intake estimated by the 24-h dietary recall [23]. However, obtaining either a 24-h urine collection or a 24-h dietary recall is a major difficulty for public health surveillance studies, as repeated collections are needed in order to reliably estimate the intakes [23,29,44]. Although the measurement of casual urine is much easier than other methods, the formulas for estimating the 24-h urine K excretions are less commonly used compared to those for the evaluation of the 24-h urine Na excretions [37].

3. The Na/K Ratio: A Surrogate Index for Higher Na Intake and Lower K Intake

A high urinary Na/K ratio is an indicator of a higher Na intake and a lower K intake [45–47]. These ratios are easier to measure due to the independence of the urine collection or the creatinine measurements. The present review examines the practical use of the Na/K ratio, which is a surrogate index of the dietary Na reduction and K increase, for supporting dietary change.

3.1. Epidemiological Findings for the Na/K Ratio

Most epidemiological studies have shown that the Na/K ratio in the 24-h urine is cross-sectionally associated with BP [6,8,48–60]. In addition, the Na/K ratio has been reported to be a superior metric vs. either Na or K alone in relation to BP [6–8,55]. Use of the Na/K ratio is resistant to systematic errors related to incomplete urine collection or underreporting of intake from 24-h recalls. These may contribute to diminish the paradoxical results often seen in association studies.

Findings from the large multicenter international cooperative study on salt, other factors, and blood pressure (INTERSALT) population study demonstrated that the change in the urinary Na/K molar ratio from 3.09 to 1.00 delivers 3.36 mmHg of estimated reduction in the population systolic BP (Table 1) [6,7]. The estimated reduction was larger for the Na/K ratio compared to when the Na and K were analyzed separately [6,7]. Reductions of 3–5 mmHg in the population BP has been estimated to lead to reductions of approximately 8–14% in the mortality of stroke, 5–9% in the mortality of coronary heart disease, and 4–7% in the total mortality [61]. Thus, the reduction of the Na/K ratio is indirectly effective for the prevention of CVD. However, the TOHP (Trials of Hypertension Prevention) study reported finding a direct association between the urinary Na/K ratio and the CVD [62–64]. Comparison of the TOHP study data between the lowest (<2) and the highest (≥4) urinary Na/K ratio category determined the hazard ratio (HR) for all-cause mortality was 0.75 (95% confidence interval (CI): 0.47 to 1.20) [63]. There was also a linear relationship observed for the mortality, with an HR of 1.13 per unit increase in the urinary Na/K ratio ($p = 0.035$) [63]. Furthermore, the 10–15 years of post-trial follow-up for the TOHP study showed that a higher Na/K ratio was associated with an increased risk of later CVD, which was greater than that for either Na or K alone [62]. The TOHP follow-up study also found there was a significant trend for the CVD risk regarding the gender-specific quartiles of the Na/K ratio (HR = 1.00, 0.84, 1.18, and 1.50, p-trend = 0.04) [62]. In addition, there was also a statistically significant linear association between the urinary Na/K ratio and the risk of CVD, with an HR of 1.24 per unit (95% CI = 1.05–1.46, $p = 0.012$) [62].

Association studies that utilized the dietary recall and dietary record methods from the national health and nutrition examination survey (NHANES) III and the national integrated project for prospective observation of non-communicable disease and its trends in the aged (NIPPON DATA80) cohort study also reported similar findings on Na/K ratio [65,66]. The report from the NHANES III cohort studies showed that the HR for the highest vs. the lowest quartile of the dietary Na/K ratios were 1.46 (95% CI: 1.27–1.67) for all-cause mortality, 1.46 (95% CI: 1.11–1.92) for cardiovascular diseases, and 2.15 (95% CI: 1.48–3.12) for ischemic heart disease [65]. Similarly, the findings from the

NIPPON DATA80 cohort study showed that the HR for the highest quartile vs. the lowest quartile of the dietary Na/K ratios (mean dietary Na/K molar ratio: 2.72 vs. 1.25) were 1.43 (95% CI: 1.17–1.76) for stroke, 1.39 (95% CI: 1.20–1.61) for cardiovascular diseases, and 1.16 (95% CI: 1.06–1.27) for all-cause mortality [66].

Table 1. Predicted differences in population mean systolic blood pressure with lifestyle variables.

Lifestyle Variable	Present Level	Improved Level	Predicted Difference
Na	170 mmol *	70 mmol	−2.17 mmHg
K	55 mmol *	70 mmol	−0.67 mmHg
Na/K	3.09 *	1.00	−3.36 mmHg
BMI	25.0 *	23.0	−1.55 mmHg
High Alcohol	≥300 mL/week ‡	1–299 mL/week ‡	−2.81 mmHg
Improved levels of both Na/K and BMI	-	-	−4.91 mmHg
Expected difference if heavy drinkers also reduced alcohol	-	-	−5.33 mmHg

* Approximate median level found in INTERSALT. ‡ Reported by 15% of respondents. Na: sodium; K: potassium; Na/K: sodium-to-potassium ratio; BMI: body mass index. INTERSALT: the international cooperative study on salt, other factors, and blood pressure. Tables created based on results from [7].

3.2. Casual Urine Estimates for the 24-h Urine Value for The Na/K Ratio

Higher correlations are seen for the casual Na/K ratio vs. the individual casual Na or K when compared with the 24-h urine values [45]. Furthermore, the population mean of the 1-day 24-h urine Na/K ratio can be estimated from the population mean of the single casual urine Na/K ratio within the diverse worldwide population [45]. High correlation ($r = 0.80$–0.88) and good agreement are seen between the mean value of repeated casual urine Na/K ratio and the 7-day 24-h urine Na/K ratio in Japanese normotensive individuals and Japanese hypertensive individuals (who were primarily taking calcium channel blockers (CCBs), angiotensin 2 receptor blockers (ARBs), or both CCBs and ARBs) (Figures 1 and 2) [67,68]. Evidences showed that the association between casual and 24-h urine Na/K ratio were robust to use of ARB, CCB, and thiazide diuretics [45,68]. The correlation and agreement quality of mean Na/K ratio of 4–7 repeated measurements of casual urine with 7-day 24-*h* urine Na/K ratio were similar to that of 1–2 day 24-h urine Na/K ratio with 7-day 24-*h* urine Na/K ratio [67,68]. There are several benefits for using the casual urine estimate for the 24-*h* urine value used to determine the Na/K ratio. These benefits include the independence of the urine volume, creatinine excretion, and body weight, the fact that repeated random sampling minimizes the systemic error caused by diurnal variation and day-to-day variation in the Na/K ratio [69], that there is less bias observed in the low to high salt range, and that the gold standard set for the casual urine estimate is the 7-day 24-*h* urine when the single day 24-*h* urine value is used for Na and K separately [67,68]. Therefore, the repeated casual urine Na/K ratio measurement may be one of the most reliable individual estimates for assessing intakes involved with Na reductions and K increases in normotensive and hypertensive individuals. Through the use of these estimates, this might make it easier to screen individuals who need to make dietary lifestyle modifications in addition to improving the awareness of an individual's dietary levels. However, the association between the repeated casual urine Na/K ratio and the 24-*h* urine Na/K ratio has yet to be examined in the elderly (ages 70 or older) and in individuals with chronic kidney disease or diabetes, or in subjects being administered several different types of anti-hypertensive medication therapies (loop diuretics, beta-blockers, angiotensin converting enzyme inhibitors, alpha-blockers, central agonists, or combinations of these different drugs). Further validations will need to be performed in all of these areas.

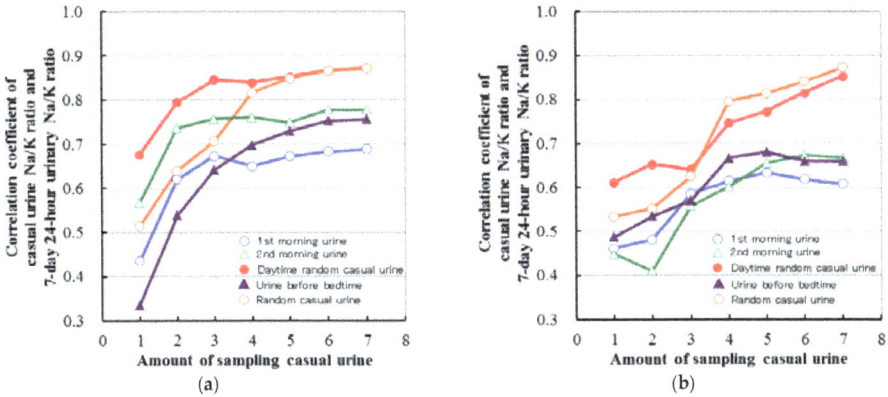

Figure 1. Correlation specification between numbers of repeated casual urine sampling and 7-day 24-h urine of sodium-to-potassium (Na/K) ratio in normotensive and hypertensive individuals (made from data of [67,68]). (**a**) Normotensive individuals; (**b**) Hypertensive individuals.

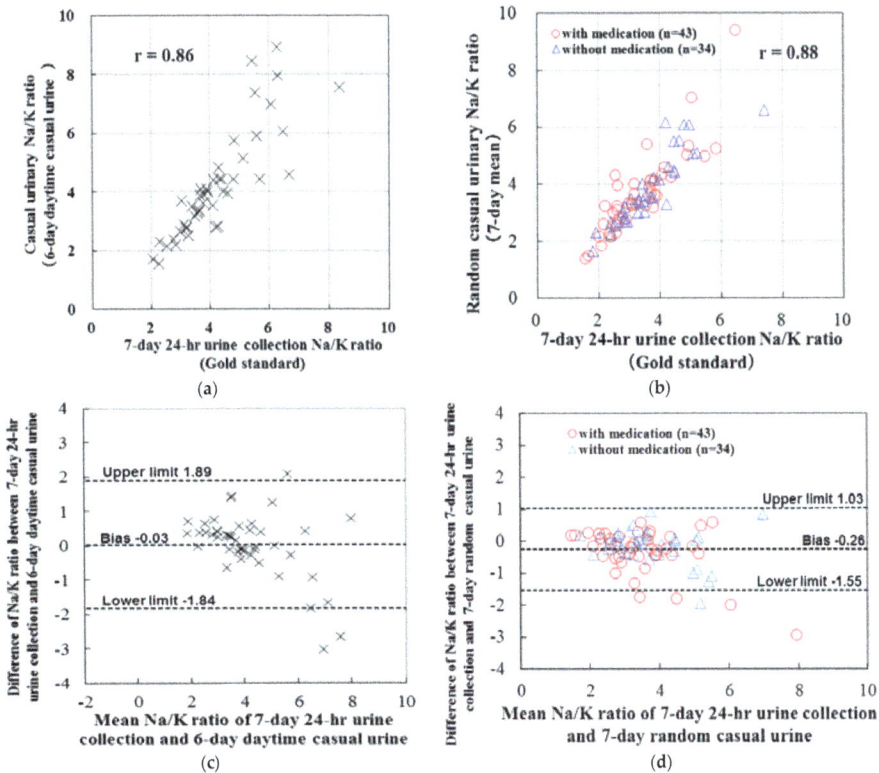

Figure 2. Plots of Na/K ratio of casual urine vs. 24-h urine, and Bland–Altman plots in normotensive and hypertensive individuals (made from data of [67,68]). (**a**) Normotensive individuals (scattered plots, *n* = 45); (**b**) Hypertensive individuals (scattered plots, *n* = 77); (**c**) Normotensive individuals (Bland-Altman plots, *n* = 45); (**d**) Hypertensive individuals (Bland-Altman plots, *n* = 77).

3.3. Target Level of Na/K Ratio

Findings from the INTERSALT study demonstrated that the mean 24-h urine Na/K molar ratio ranged from 0.01 (Yanomamo, Brazil) to 7.58 (Tianjin, China) [6,45]. Mean Na/K ratios in Asian and Western populations were approximately 5 and 3, respectively [6,45]. Considering the ratio calculated by population mean 24-h urine Na/K molar ratio and population mean 24-h urine salt (NaCl) (g/day) may give a rough estimate for predicting NaCl intake from Na/K ratio; population mean 24-h urine Na/K molar ratio was 3.24 and population mean salt intake estimated by 24-h urine was 9.1 (g/day) thus the mean value of the ratio was calculated as 2.8 (ranged from 1.3 to 5.3 among 52 populations (mostly 2 to 4)) in 10,079 individuals among 32 countries in INTERSALT study [45]. Thus, a rough estimate of population mean salt intake (g/day) may be given by approximately 2–4 times of population mean 24-h urinary Na/K molar ratio in the general populations. Furthermore, Yatabe et al. demonstrated that the daily population means of the urinary Na/K ratios traced dietary salt intake within 2–3 days during an experimental feeding study, with 4.2 for the unrestricted diet, 1.1 for the low-salt 3 g/day diet, and 6.6 for the high-salt 20 g/day diet periods [70,71]. Currently, there is no generally accepted recommended guideline for the Na/K ratio. Based on the findings from the INTERSALT study, Stamler et al. recommended that an urinary Na/K molar ratio of 1.0 be used for the target level [7]. Reports from WHO suggested that achieving the guidelines for both the Na and K intakes would yield an Na/K molar ratio of approximately 1.00 [11,12]. Cook et al. also reported that Na/K molar ratios between 1 and 2 exhibited the lowest CVD risk [62]. Therefore, although urinary Na/K molar ratios less than 1 are preferable, ratios less than 2 might be an interim suboptimal goal for most people trying to lower their BP and reduce the CVD risk.

4. Self-Monitoring of the Urinary Na/K Ratio

Reducing the Na/K ratio is essential for preventing hypertension and CVDs prior to clinical onset [6–8,48–60]. Urinary Na/K ratios can be measured by urinary Na and K concentrations, or by performing measurements in a central inspection lab. One of the methods for sampling urine specimens and identifying an individual's Na/K ratio levels is to collect the casual urine specimens using small spout containers, followed by measuring the mean values at the clinician's office. However, due to the time required for the collection, delivery, and measurement, this method may not provide prompt enough feedback for the patients to make further dietary modifications.

Nowadays, urinary Na/K ratio can be measured by a portable self-monitoring device (HEU-001-F, OMRON Healthcare Co., Muko, Japan). This device measures urinary Na/K ratio by the ion electrode method and displays the result within one minute. Since this device provides prompt onsite feedback in personal use, it became evaluated in randomized control trial with a view to support an individual approach for Na reduction and K increase [72]. With regard to the individual approach, it is important that there is a balance between lower effort and financial burden in order to achieve an effective intervention. A recent study that examined this self-monitoring device reported finding a trend for larger reductions in the urinary Na/K ratio in a self-monitoring group under a pure self-management setting. When the baseline urinary Na/K molar ratio level was approximately 3.7, the reductions in the urinary Na/K molar ratio were 0.55 in the intervention group and 0.06 in the control group [72]. However, the intervention effect size was limited due to the lack of an effective education program for reducing the Na/K ratio. Since self-monitoring devices are different from therapeutic devices, these monitoring devices may be powerless unless the subjects also take part in a practical dietary program. Thus, it would be expected that there would be a much larger reduction when these devices are combined with a useful education program. Furthermore, if individuals are able to acquire basic knowledge and skills for Na reduction and K increase, this could be one of the key factors for improving confidence and enhancing motivation for dietary improvements. Therefore, providing feedback to individuals at appropriate times might also help to support the effectiveness of these education programs.

5. Implications for Prevention and Treatment

Na surfeit and K deficit are of worldwide concern for hypertension, cardiovascular diseases, and non-communicable diseases. Measurement of the Na/K ratio is much easier to obtain than trying to perform Na and K measurements separately. Thus, an awareness of dietary levels through the use of this index may lead to improvements in an individual's ratio. The individual estimate of the 24-h urinary Na/K ratio that can be obtained by the repeated casual urine Na/K ratio may be useful in detecting individuals who need an easy dietary lifestyle modification during the prevention stage. For the treatment stage, self-monitoring devices may increase patient awareness of their dietary level and help to maintain appropriate levels since evidences showed that the association between casual and 24-h urine Na/K ratio were robust to class of use of anti-hypertensive medication [45,68]. The urinary Na/K ratio level objectively reflects a patient's recent dietary status [70,71]. Thus, information on the urinary Na/K ratio is essential when trying to determine the types and doses of anti-hypertensive medication therapy. However, dietary K restriction is advised for those with impaired kidney function in advanced stage of chronic kidney disease (CKD). Therefore, it is reasonable to infer that the Na/K ratio may be safe and beneficial index to reduce Na and increase K intake for individuals who has not reached to the advanced stage of CKD.

Use of an individual approach in conjunction with an effective education program for lowering the Na/K ratio and self-monitoring tools for the urinary Na/K ratio may help improve individual's Na and K intake levels and support their attempts at a lifestyle modification. In addition, utilizing a combination of the conventional population approach and the individual approach focused on the Na/K ratio may help to minimize the gap between the actual and ideal ratio levels. Therefore, implementation of the use of the Na/K ratio as a way for practical Na reduction and K increase may be a key factor for reaching the 2025 goal set by WHO of achieving intake levels less than 2 g of Na per day [22].

Acknowledgments: OMRON Healthcare is covering the cost for publishing this study as an open access article.

Author Contributions: T.I. contributed to the drafting of the manuscript. All authors participated in the critical revision of the manuscript. All authors approved the final version of the manuscript for submission.

Conflicts of Interest: Toshiyuki Iwahori is an employee of OMRON Healthcare Co., Ltd. Hirotsugu Ueshima served as a consultant of OMRON Healthcare Co., Ltd. Katsuyuki Miura received a research fund from OMRON Healthcare Co. Ltd.

References

1. Appel, L.J.; Moore, T.J.; Obarzanek, E.; Vollmer, W.M.; Svetkey, L.P.; Sacks, F.M.; Bray, G.A.; Vogt, T.M.; Cutler, J.A.; Windhauser, M.M.; et al. A clinical trial of the effects of dietary patterns on blood pressure. *N. Engl. J. Med.* **1997**, *336*, 1117–1124. [CrossRef] [PubMed]
2. Sacks, F.M.; Svetkey, L.P.; Vollmer, W.M.; Appel, L.J.; Bray, G.A.; Harsha, D.; Obarzanek, E.; Conlin, P.R.; Miller, E.R., 3rd; Simons-Morton, D.G.; et al. Effects on blood pressure of reduced dietary sodium and the Dietary Approaches to Stop Hypertension (DASH) diet. *N. Engl. J. Med.* **2001**, *344*, 3–10. [CrossRef] [PubMed]
3. Pomerleau, J.; Lock, K.; Knai, C.; McKee, M. Interventions designed to increase adult fruit and vegetable intake can be effective: A systematic review of the literature. *J. Nutr.* **2005**, *135*, 2486–2495. [PubMed]
4. Shah, M.; Jeffery, R.W.; Laing, B.; Savre, S.G.; Van Natta, M.; Strickland, D. Hypertension Prevention Trial (HPT): Food pattern changes resulting from intervention on sodium, potassium, and energy intake. Hypertension Prevention Trial Research Group. *J. Am. Diet. Assoc.* **1990**, *90*, 69–76. [PubMed]
5. Jeffery, R.W.; Pirie, P.L.; Elmer, P.J.; Bjornson-Benson, W.M.; Mullenbach, V.A.; Kurth, C.L.; Johnson, S.L. Low-sodium, high-potassium diet: Feasibility and acceptability in a normotensive population. *Am. J. Public Health* **1984**, *74*, 492–494. [CrossRef] [PubMed]
6. Rose, G.; Stamler, J.; Stamler, R.; Elliott, P.; Marmot, M.; Pyorala, K.; Kesteloot, H.; Joossens, J.; Hansson, L.; Mancia, G.; et al. INTERSALT: An international study of electrolyte excretion and blood pressure. Results for 24 h urinary sodium and potassium excretion. *BMJ* **1988**, *297*, 319–328.

7. Stamler, J.; Rose, G.; Stamler, R.; Elliott, P.; Dyer, A.; Marmot, M. INTERSALT study findings. Public health and medical care implications. *Hypertension* **1989**, *14*, 570–577. [CrossRef] [PubMed]

8. Tzoulaki, I.; Patel, C.J.; Okamura, T.; Chan, Q.; Brown, I.J.; Miura, K.; Ueshima, H.; Zhao, L.; Van Horn, L.; Daviglus, M.L.; et al. A nutrient-wide association study on blood pressure. *Circulation* **2012**, *126*, 2456–2464. [CrossRef] [PubMed]

9. World Health Organization. *Diet, Nutrition and the Prevention of Chronic Diseases*; Report of the joint WHO/FAO expert consultation; World Health Organization: Geneva, Switzerland, 2003.

10. U.S. Department of Agriculture and U.S. Department of Health and Human Services. *Dietary Guidelines for Americans*, 7th ed.; U.S. Government Printing Office: Washington, DC, USA, 2010.

11. World Health Organization. *Guideline: Sodium Intake for Adults and Children*; WHO Document Production Services: Geneva, Switzerland, 2012.

12. World Health Organization. *Guideline: Potassium Intake for Adults and Children*; WHO Document Production Services: Geneva, Switzerland, 2012.

13. Adrogué, H.J.; Madias, N.E. Sodium and potassium in the pathogenesis of hypertension. *N. Engl. J. Med.* **2007**, *356*, 1966–1978. [CrossRef] [PubMed]

14. Gay, H.C.; Rao, S.G.; Vaccarino, V.; Ali, M.K. Effects of different dietary interventions on blood pressure: Systematic review and meta-analysis of randomized controlled trials. *Hypertension* **2016**, *67*, 733–739. [CrossRef] [PubMed]

15. He, F.J.; Li, J.; MacGregor, G.A. Effect of longer term modest salt reduction on blood pressure: Cochrane systematic review and meta-analysis of randomized trials. *BMJ* **2013**, *346*, f1325. [CrossRef] [PubMed]

16. Aburto, N.J.; Ziolkovska, A.; Hooper, L.; Elliott, P.; Cappuccio, F.P.; Meerpohl, J.J. Effect of lower sodium intake on health: Systematic review and meta-analyses. *BMJ* **2013**, *346*, f1326. [CrossRef] [PubMed]

17. Aburto, N.J.; Hanson, S.; Gutierrez, H.; Hooper, L.; Elliott, P.; Cappuccio, F.P. Effect of increased potassium on cardiovascular risk factors and disease: Systematic review and meta-analyses. *BMJ* **2013**, *346*, f1378. [CrossRef] [PubMed]

18. Brown, I.J.; Tzoulaki, I.; Candeias, V.; Elliott, P. Salt intakes around the world: Implications for public health. *Int. J. Epidemiol.* **2009**, *38*, 791–813. [CrossRef] [PubMed]

19. Drewnowski, A.; Rehm, C.D.; Maillot, M.; Mendoza, A.; Monsivais, P. The feasibility of meeting the WHO guidelines for sodium and potassium: A cross-national comparison study. *BMJ Open* **2015**, *5*, e006625. [CrossRef] [PubMed]

20. Jacobson, M.F.; Havas, S.; McCarter, R. Changes in sodium levels in processed and restaurant foods, 2005 to 2011. *JAMA Intern. Med.* **2013**, *173*, 1285–1291. [CrossRef] [PubMed]

21. Okuda, N.; Stamler, J.; Brown, I.J.; Ueshima, H.; Miura, K.; Okayama, A.; Saitoh, S.; Nakagawa, H.; Sakata, K.; Yoshita, K.; et al. Individual efforts to reduce salt intake in China, Japan, UK, USA: What did people achieve? The INTERMAP Population Study. *J. Hypertens.* **2014**, *32*, 2385–2392. [CrossRef] [PubMed]

22. World Health Organization. Global Strategy on Diet, Physical Activity and Health. Population Sodium Reduction Strategies. Available online: http://www.who.int/dietphysicalactivity/reducingsalt/en/ (accessed on 7 April 2017).

23. Hunter, D. Biochemical indicators of dietary intake. In *Willet W, Nutritional Epidemiology*, 2nd ed.; Oxford University Press: New York, NY, USA, 1998; pp. 174–243.

24. Pietinen, P.I.; Findley, T.W.; Clausen, J.D.; Finnerty, F.A.; Altschul, A.M. Studies in community nutrition: Estimation of sodium output. *Prev. Med.* **1976**, *5*, 400–407. [CrossRef]

25. Voors, A.W.; Dalferes, E.R., Jr.; Frank, G.C.; Aristimuno, G.G.; Berenson, G.S. Relation between ingested potassium and sodium balance in young Blacks and whites. *Am. J. Clin. Nutr.* **1983**, *37*, 583–594. [PubMed]

26. Clark, A.J.; Mossholder, S. Sodium and potassium intake measurements: Dietary methodology problems. *Am. J. Clin. Nutr.* **1986**, *43*, 470–476. [PubMed]

27. Holbrook, J.T.; Patterson, K.Y.; Bodner, J.E.; Douglas, L.W.; Veillon, C.; Kelsay, J.L.; Mertz, W.; Smith, J.C., Jr. Sodium and potassium intake and balance in adults consuming self-selected diets. *Am. J. Clin. Nutr.* **1984**, *40*, 786–793. [PubMed]

28. Rakova, N.; Jüttner, K.; Dahlmann, A.; Schröder, A.; Linz, P.; Kopp, C.; Rauh, M.; Goller, U.; Beck, L.; Agureev, A.; et al. Long-term space flight simulation reveals infradian rhythmicity in human Na$^+$ balance. *Cell Metab.* **2013**, *17*, 125–131. [CrossRef] [PubMed]

29. Liu, K.; Stamler, J. Assessment of sodium intake in epidemiological studies on blood pressure. *Ann. Clin. Res.* **1984**, *16*, 49–54. [PubMed]

30. Cogswell, M.E.; Mugavero, K.; Bowman, B.A.; Frieden, T.R. Dietary sodium and cardiovascular disease risk—Measurement matters. *N. Engl. J. Med.* **2016**, *375*, 580–586. [CrossRef] [PubMed]

31. Cobb, L.K.; Anderson, C.A.; Elliott, P.; Hu, F.B.; Liu, K.; Neaton, J.D.; Whelton, P.K.; Woodward, M.; Appel, L.J. Methodological issues in cohort studies that relate sodium intake to cardiovascular disease outcomes: A science advisory from the American Heart Association. *Circulation* **2014**, *129*, 1173–1186. [CrossRef] [PubMed]

32. Bingham, S.A.; Cassidy, A.; Cole, T.J.; Welch, A.; Runswick, S.A.; Black, A.E.; Thurnham, D.; Bates, C.; Khaw, K.T.; Key, T.J.; et al. Validation of weighed records and other methods of dietary assessment using the 24 h urine nitrogen technique and other biological markers. *Br. J. Nutr.* **1995**, *73*, 531–550. [CrossRef] [PubMed]

33. Dennis, B.; Stamler, J.; Buzzard, M.; Conway, R.; Elliott, P.; Moag-Stahlberg, A.; Okayama, A.; Okuda, N.; Robertson, C.; Robinson, F.; et al. INTERMAP: The dietary data—Process and quality control. *J. Hum. Hypertens.* **2003**, *17*, 609–622. [CrossRef] [PubMed]

34. The INTERSALT Co-operative Research Group. INTERSALT Study: An international co-operative study on the relation of blood pressure to electrolyte excretion in populations. I: Design and methods. *J. Hypertens.* **1986**, *4*, 781–787.

35. Stamler, J.; Elliott, P.; Dennis, B.; Dyer, A.R.; Kesteloot, H.; Liu, K.; Ueshima, H.; Zhou, B.F. INTERMAP: Background, aims, design, methods, and descriptive statistics (nondietary). *J. Hum. Hypertens.* **2003**, *17*, 591–608. [CrossRef] [PubMed]

36. Buzzard, M. 24-h dietary recall and food record method. In *Willet W, Nutritional Epidemiology*, 2nd ed.; Oxford University Press: New York, NY, USA, 1998; pp. 50–73.

37. Tanaka, T.; Okamura, T.; Miura, K.; Kadowaki, T.; Ueshima, H.; Nakagawa, H.; Hashimoto, T. A simple method to estimate populational 24-h urinary sodium and potassium excretion using a casual urine specimen. *J. Hum. Hypertens.* **2002**, *16*, 97–103. [CrossRef] [PubMed]

38. Kawasaki, T.; Itoh, K.; Uezono, K.; Sasaki, H. A simple method for estimating 24 h urinary sodium and potassium excretion from second morning voiding urine specimen in adults. *Clin. Exp. Pharmacol. Physiol.* **1993**, *20*, 7–14. [CrossRef] [PubMed]

39. Brown, I.J.; Dyer, A.R.; Chan, Q.; Cogswell, M.E.; Ueshima, H.; Stamler, J.; Elliott, P. Estimating 24-h urinary sodium excretion from casual urinary sodium concentrations in Western populations: The INTERSALT study. *Am. J. Epidemiol.* **2013**, *177*, 1180–1192. [CrossRef] [PubMed]

40. Polonia, J.; Lobo, M.F.; Martins, L.; Pinto, F.; Nazare, J. Estimation of populational 24-h urinary sodium and potassium excretion from spot urine samples: Evaluation of four formulas in a large national representative population. *J. Hypertens.* **2017**, *35*, 477–486. [CrossRef] [PubMed]

41. Huang, L.; Crino, M.; Wu, J.H.; Woodward, M.; Barzi, F.; Land, M.A.; McLean, R.; Webster, J.; Enkhtungalag, B.; Neal, B. Mean population salt intake estimated from 24-h urine samples and spot urine samples: A systematic review and meta-analysis. *Int. J. Epidemiol.* **2016**, *45*, 239–250. [CrossRef] [PubMed]

42. Mente, A.; O'Donnell, M.J.; Dagenais, G.; Wielgosz, A.; Lear, S.A.; McQueen, M.J.; Jiang, Y.; Wang, X.Y.; Jian, B.; Calik, K.B.; et al. Validation and comparison of three formulae to estimate sodium and potassium excretion from a single morning fasting urine compared to 24-h measures in 11 countries. *J. Hypertens.* **2014**, *32*, 1005–1014. [CrossRef] [PubMed]

43. O'Donnell, M.; Mente, A.; Rangarajan, S.; McQueen, M.J.; Wang, X.; Liu, L.; Yan, H.; Lee, S.F.; Mony, P.; Devanath, A.; et al. Urinary sodium and potassium excretion.; mortality, and cardiovascular events. *N. Engl. J. Med.* **2014**, *371*, 612–623. [CrossRef] [PubMed]

44. Taylor, E.N.; Stampfer, M.J.; Mount, D.B.; Curhan, G.C. DASH-style diet and 24-hr urine composition. *Clin. J. Am. Soc. Nephrol.* **2010**, *5*, 2315–2322. [CrossRef] [PubMed]

45. Iwahori, T.; Miura, K.; Ueshima, H.; Chan, Q.; Dyer, A.R.; Elliott, P.; Stamler, J. Estimating 24-h urinary sodium/potassium ratio from casual ('spot') urinary sodium/potassium ratio: The INTERSALT study. *Int. J. Epidemiol.* **2016**. [CrossRef] [PubMed]

46. Stamler, J.; Chan, Q. INTERMAP appendix tables. *J. Hum. Hypertens.* **2003**, *17*, 665–758. [CrossRef]

47. Yi, S.S.; Curtis, C.J.; Angell, S.Y.; Anderson, C.A.; Jung, M.; Kansagra, S.M. Highlighting the ratio of sodium to potassium in population-level dietary assessments: Cross-sectional data from New York City, USA. *Public Health Nutr.* **2014**, *17*, 2484–2488. [CrossRef] [PubMed]

48. M'Buyamba-Kabangu, J.R.; Fagard, R.; Lijnen, P.; Mbuy wa Mbuy, R.; Staessen, J.; Amery, A. Blood pressure and urinary cations in urban Bantu of Zaire. *Am. J. Epidemiol.* **1986**, *124*, 957–968. [CrossRef] [PubMed]

49. Kesteloot, H.; Huang, D.X.; Li, Y.L.; Geboers, J.; Joossens, J.V. The relationship between cations and blood pressure in the People's Republic of China. *Hypertension* **1987**, *9*, 654–659. [CrossRef] [PubMed]

50. Dyer, A.R.; Elliott, P.; Shipley, M. Urinary electrolyte excretion in 24 h and blood pressure in the INTERSALT Study. II. Estimates of electrolyte-blood pressure associations corrected for regression dilution bias. *Am. J. Epidemiol.* **1994**, *139*, 940–951. [CrossRef] [PubMed]

51. Elliott, P.; Stamler, J.; Nichols, R.; Dyer, A.R.; Stamler, R.; Kesteloot, H.; Marmot, M. Intersalt revisited: Further analyses of 24 h sodium excretion and blood pressure within and across populations. *BMJ* **1996**, *312*, 1249–1253. [CrossRef] [PubMed]

52. Cook, N.R.; Kumanyika, S.K.; Cutler, J.A. Effect of change in sodium excretion on change in blood pressure corrected for measurement error. The Trials of Hypertension Prevention, Phase I. *Am. J. Epidemiol.* **1998**, *148*, 431–444. [CrossRef] [PubMed]

53. Huggins, C.E.; O'Reilly, S.; Brinkman, M.; Hodge, A.; Giles, G.G.; English, D.R.; Nowson, C.A. Relationship of urinary sodium and sodium-to-potassium ratio to blood pressure in older adults in Australia. *Med. J. Aust.* **2011**, *195*, 128–132. [PubMed]

54. Hedayati, S.S.; Minhajuddin, A.T.; Ijaz, A.; Moe, O.W.; Elsayed, E.F.; Reilly, R.F.; Huang, C.L. Association of urinary sodium/potassium ratio with blood pressure: Sex and racial differences. *Clin. J. Am. Soc. Nephrol.* **2012**, *7*, 315–322. [CrossRef] [PubMed]

55. Perez, V.; Chang, E.T. Sodium-to-potassium ratio and blood pressure, hypertension, and related factors. *Adv. Nutr.* **2014**, *5*, 712–741. [CrossRef] [PubMed]

56. Binia, A.; Jaeger, J.; Hu, Y.; Singh, A.; Zimmermann, D. Daily potassium intake and sodium-to-potassium ratio in the reduction of blood pressure: A meta-analysis of randomized controlled trials. *J. Hypertens.* **2015**, *33*, 1509–1520. [CrossRef] [PubMed]

57. Tabara, Y.; Takahashi, Y.; Kumagai, K.; Setoh, K.; Kawaguchi, T.; Takahashi, M.; Muraoka, Y.; Tsujikawa, A.; Gotoh, N.; Terao, C.; et al. Descriptive epidemiology of spot urine sodium-to-potassium ratio clarified close relationship with blood pressure level: The Nagahama study. *J. Hypertens.* **2015**, *33*, 2407–2413. [CrossRef] [PubMed]

58. Li, N.; Yan, L.L.; Niu, W.; Yao, C.; Feng, X.; Zhang, J.; Shi, J.; Zhang, Y.; Zhang, R.; Hao, Z.; et al. The effects of a community-based sodium reduction program in rural China—A cluster-randomized trial. *PLoS ONE* **2016**, *11*, e0166620. [CrossRef] [PubMed]

59. Ndanuko, R.N.; Tapsell, L.C.; Charlton, K.E.; Neale, E.P.; O'Donnell, K.M.; Batterham, M.J. Relationship between sodium and potassium intake and blood pressure in a sample of overweight adults. *Nutrition* **2017**, *33*, 285–290. [CrossRef] [PubMed]

60. Xu, J.; Chen, X.; Ge, Z.; Liang, H.; Yan, L.; Guo, X.; Zhang, Y.; Wang, L.; Ma, J. Associations of usual 24-h sodium and potassium intakes with blood pressure and risk of hypertension among adults in China's Shandong and Jiangsu provinces. *Kidney Blood Press. Res.* **2017**, *42*, 188–200. [CrossRef] [PubMed]

61. Stamler, R. Implications of the INTERSALT study. *Hypertension* **1991**, *17*, I16–I20. [CrossRef] [PubMed]

62. Cook, N.R.; Obarzanek, E.; Cutler, J.A.; Buring, J.E.; Rexrode, K.M.; Kumanyika, S.K.; Appel, L.J.; Whelton, P.K. Joint effects of sodium and potassium intake on subsequent cardiovascular disease: The Trials of hypertension prevention follow-up study. *Arch. Intern. Med.* **2009**, *169*, 32–40. [CrossRef] [PubMed]

63. Cook, N.R.; Appel, L.J.; Whelton, P.K. Sodium intake and all-cause mortality over 20 years in the trials of hypertension prevention. *J. Am. Coll. Cardiol.* **2016**, *68*, 1609–1617. [CrossRef] [PubMed]

64. Cook, N.R.; Cutler, J.A.; Obarzanek, E.; Buring, J.E.; Rexrode, K.M.; Kumanyika, S.K.; Appel, L.J.; Whelton, P.K. Long term effects of dietary sodium reduction on cardiovascular disease outcomes: Observational follow-up of the trials of hypertension prevention (TOHP). *BMJ* **2007**, *334*, 885–888. [CrossRef] [PubMed]

65. Yang, Q.; Liu, T.; Kuklina, E.V.; Flanders, W.D.; Hong, Y.; Gillespie, C.; Chang, M.H.; Gwinn, M.; Dowling, N.; Khoury, M.J.; et al. Sodium and potassium intake and mortality among US adults: Prospective data from the Third National Health and Nutrition Examination Survey. *Arch. Intern. Med.* **2011**, *171*, 1183–1191. [CrossRef] [PubMed]

66. Okayama, A.; Okuda, N.; Miura, K.; Okamura, T.; Hayakawa, T.; Akasaka, H.; Ohnishi, H.; Saitoh, S.; Arai, Y.; Kiyohara, Y.; et al. Dietary sodium-to-potassium ratio as a risk factor for stroke, cardiovascular disease and all-cause mortality in Japan: The NIPPON DATA80 cohort study. *BMJ Open* **2016**, *6*, e011632. [CrossRef] [PubMed]

67. Iwahori, T.; Ueshima, H.; Miyagawa, N.; Ohgami, N.; Yamashita, H.; Ohkubo, T.; Murakami, Y.; Shiga, T.; Miura, K. Six random samples of casual urine on different days are sufficient to estimate daily sodium/potassium ratio as compared to 7-day 24-h urine collections. *Hypertens. Res.* **2014**, *37*, 765–771. [CrossRef] [PubMed]

68. Iwahori, T.; Ueshima, H.; Torii, S.; Saito, Y.; Fujiyoshi, A.; Ohkubo, T.; Miura, K. Four to seven random casual urine specimens are sufficient to estimate 24-hr urinary sodium/potassium ratio in individuals with high blood pressure. *J. Hum. Hypertens.* **2016**, *30*, 328–334. [CrossRef] [PubMed]

69. Iwahori, T.; Ueshima, H.; Torii, S.; Yoshino, Saito.; Kondo, K.; Tanaka-Mizuno, S.; Arima, H.; Miura, K. Diurnal variation of urinary sodium-to-potassium ratio in free-living Japanese individuals. *Hypertens. Res.* **2017**. [CrossRef] [PubMed]

70. Yatabe, J.; Yatabe, M.S.; Takano, K.; Watanabe, A.; Kurosawa, S.; Yonemoto, M.; Nochi, M.; Ikeda, Y.; Iwahori, T.; Shiga, T.; et al. Newly developed personal device can detect changes and variations of urinary Na/K ratio with standardized low- and high-salt meals in healthy volunteers. *Hypertension* **2014**, *64*, A072.

71. Yatabe, M.S.; Iwahori, T.; Watanabe, A.; Takano, K.; Sanada, H.; Watanabe, T.; Ichihara, A.; Felder, R.A.; Miura, K.; Ueshima, H.; et al. Urinary sodium-to-potassium ratio tracks the changes of salt intake during an experimental feeding study using standardized low-salt and high-salt meals in healthy Japanese volunteers. *Nutrients* **2017**, in press.

72. Iwahori, T.; Ueshima, H.; Ohgami, N.; Yamashita, H.; Miyagawa, N.; Kondo, K.; Torii, S.; Yoshita, K.; Shiga, T.; Ohkubo, T.; et al. Effectiveness of a self-monitoring device for urinary sodium/potassium ratio on dietary improvement in free-living adults: A randomized controlled trial. *J. Epidemiol.* **2017**, in press.

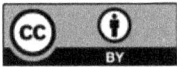

nutrients

MDPI

Article

Taste, Salt Consumption, and Local Explanations around Hypertension in a Rural Population in Northern Peru

M. Amalia Pesantes [1,*], Francisco Diez-Canseco [1], Antonio Bernabé-Ortiz [1,2], Vilarmina Ponce-Lucero [1] and J. Jaime Miranda [1,3]

1   CRONICAS Center of Excellence in Chronic Diseases, Universidad Peruana Cayetano Heredia, Av. Armendáriz 497, Miraflores, Lima 18, Peru; fdiezcanseco@gmail.com (F.D.-C.); antonio.bernabe@upch.pe (A.B.-O.); vponcelucero@gmail.com (V.P.-L.); jaime.miranda@upch.pe (J.J.M.)
2   Faculty of Epidemiology and Population Health, London School of Hygiene and Tropical Medicine, London WC1E 7HT, UK
3   School of Medicine, Universidad Peruana Cayetano Heredia, Lima 18, Peru
*   Correspondence: maria.pesantes.v@upch.pe; Tel.: +511-241-6978

Received: 7 April 2017; Accepted: 28 June 2017; Published: 5 July 2017

Abstract: Interventions to promote behaviors to reduce sodium intake require messages tailored to local understandings of the relationship between what we eat and our health. We studied local explanations about hypertension, the relationship between local diet, salt intake, and health status, and participants' opinions about changing food habits. This study provided inputs for a social marketing campaign in Peru promoting the use of a salt substitute containing less sodium than regular salt. Qualitative methods (focus groups and in-depth interviews) were utilized with local populations, people with hypertension, and health personnel in six rural villages. Participants were 18–65 years old, 41% men. Participants established a direct relationship between emotions and hypertension, regardless of age, gender, and hypertension status. Those without hypertension established a connection between eating too much/eating fried food and health status but not between salt consumption and hypertension. Participants rejected dietary changes. Economic barriers and high appreciation of local culinary traditions were the main reasons for this. It is the conclusion of this paper that introducing and promoting salt substitutes require creative strategies that need to acknowledge local explanatory disease models such as the strong association between emotional wellbeing and hypertension, give a positive spin to changing food habits, and resist the "common sense" strategy of information provision around the causal connection between salt consumption and hypertension.

Keywords: hypertension; low-sodium diet; Peru; health knowledge; attitudes and practices; qualitative methods

1. Introduction

Hypertension is an important public health problem especially in low and middle-income countries [1]. In 2006, approximately 14% of the Peruvian population aged 20 and older had hypertension [2]. There is, however, geographical variation of hypertension rates within the country. For instance, in Tumbes, a region located in Peru's northern coast, one in every four adults aged ≥35 years has hypertension, which is much higher than other regions in the country [3].

There are numerous strategies to prevent and control hypertension. One of the more common approaches focuses on reducing sodium intake [4,5], as recommended by several international bodies [6–8]. In Latin America, such strategies have translated into regulations to change sodium levels in processed foods, such as bread in Argentina, Chile, and Uruguay [9]. A less common initiative has been to alter the amount of daily sodium intake through the promotion of behavioral changes to reduce the amount of salt consumption at the household level [10]. In Peru, our research team is currently implementing an intervention that aims at reducing blood pressure levels through the distribution of a salt substitute containing less sodium than regular salt, in combination with a social marketing campaign weaved around messages that highlight the importance of reducing the amount of salt used at the household level for everyday cooking [11]. Using a random sample of participants from the six villages enrolled in the study, we found that the average potassium intake in the area is 4.4 (±2.1) g per day (equivalent to about 11 g of salt per day) based on a 24-h urine collection.

Sodium in salt does not only preserve food but also enhances the taste of food [12]. A national study in Peru showed that 20% of those interviewed stated that they add extra salt to food on a regular basis [2]. However, very little is known, on a population-wide basis, about the level of salt consumption recommended as per World Health Organization recommendations of 5 g per day [13]. Therefore, changing sodium intake patterns requires carefully designed interventions. One innovative solution for Peru, where over 80% of subjects in coastal cities have lunch and dinner at home [14] and where daily cooking remains a common practice, is to reduce the amount of sodium in the regular salt by replacing a proportion of sodium with another mineral.

Peru has a previous successful experience promoting the consumption of iodized salt, whose price is subsidized by the government to ensure its consumption. This sets a positive precedent for the promotion of salt with lower potassium concentrations once we demonstrate the efficacy of such an approach for reducing high blood pressure at the population level.

To tackle a salt-substitution tactic, the first step was to identify the adequate levels of sodium replacement without compromising preferences on flavor that would limit its uptake. To this end, we conducted experiments with sensory discriminatory tests through gradual reduction on sodium concentration [15]. The sodium was then replaced with potassium, which can reduce mean systolic and diastolic blood pressure levels [16,17] and could contribute to the prevention of hypertension, especially in populations with elevated blood pressure [18,19]. We conducted several tests until we identified the combination of sodium and potassium where people were not able to distinguish a dish prepared with regular salt and one prepared with a sodium-reduced salt [15].

Once the ideal levels of salt substitution were identified, we had to ensure people would uptake and consume the new product on a sustained manner. Two strategies needed to be put in place: a reliable salt distribution system and a social marketing campaign. Social marketing aims to change a behavior, or introduce a new behavior, by getting acquainted with the target audience and their social environment [20]. In this vein, before embarking on developing such a social marketing campaign, the project team needed general information around local explanations about the causes and consequences of hypertension, the impact of local eating habits, including, but not limited to, salt intake, and its relationship with health problems such as hypertension. Furthermore, it was also relevant to learn the local opinions about the introduction of changes to their regular diet. The data we present was collected during the formative phase of our intervention oriented to promote the use of a salt substitute containing less sodium than regular salt in Tumbes, Peru.

2. Materials and Methods

2.1. Study Design

We chose a qualitative approach since our goal was to explore local explanations around specific issues (diet, salt consumption, and hypertension), rather than quantifying or measuring local knowledge on such topics [21].

We used semi-structured interviews and focus groups using a pre-determined set of questions (see Annexes 1, 2, and 3) allowing interviewees to talk about their perceptions around hypertension, diet, salt consumption, and health.

2.2. Study Site

The study was conducted in the Tumbes region, in the north of Peru. Tumbes has an approximate population of 200,000 inhabitants, 90% of which live on urban areas [11]. Recent statistics indicate that 3.5% of the population of Tumbes has no formal education and 14.4% of the population was considered poor and 1.4% extremely poor [22].

We selected six villages for this study and for the salt substitute intervention. They are all located in rural districts and more than 78% of the population earned less than the minimum wage (750 PEN per month ~240 USD per month). The average population in the villages selected was 600 inhabitants: the smallest village had 507 people and the biggest had 788 people [11]. The main economic activity of one of the six villages was fishing and in the other five, people worked in agriculture.

While men are mostly agricultural farmers (of rice and plantains), cattle ranchers, or fishermen, women are usually housewives or—in some few cases—owners of small *bodegas*. Women are responsible for cooking at home on a daily basis.

2.3. Study Participants and Selection Rationale

We aimed to collect information from the local population differentiated by gender and age. We strove to ensure that participants in the focus group were as homogeneous as possible in order to respond to the need to collect common perceptions and opinions about the research topic, and to help promote a comfortable interaction with and among participants [23]. We wanted to know if there were coincidences or differences in their explanations of the stated research topics. Our goal was to conduct four focus groups per village (24 in total), divided along gender and age groups: one focus group of women from 20 to 44, one focus group of women from 45 to 65, one focus group of men from 20 to 44, and one focus group of men aged between 45 to 65 years old (Table A1).

Out of the 24 planned focus groups we were able to conduct 14 since it was difficult for people to take time off from their everyday activities. Half of the focus groups were conducted with men. In the fishermen village (Village 3), male participants of the age group 20–44 failed twice to attend and it was decided to replace that focus group with seven individual interviews with men in that age group. In total, 98 participants participated in focus group discussions.

Besides the focus groups, we conducted interviews with different types of informants: five with health workers from the villages with a primary health care facility (villages: #1, #2, #5, and #6) and twenty with individuals with hypertension.

People with hypertension were a group of special importance because we thought they would be better informed about causes, consequences, and management of hypertension and could share their experiences about the difficulties of incorporating changes in their diets such as salt intake reduction. Fieldworkers had a hard time finding men with hypertension interested in participating in the study and, as a result, all of our interviewees were female. Interviews with health personnel were relevant because they could provide an overview about the local health perceptions and their health and food habits, based on their regular interactions at the health facility.

2.4. Data Collection

2.4.1. Recruitment

Fieldworkers were instructed to go to randomly selected households and ask questions to determine eligibility. If eligible, individuals were invited to participate in the focus group. Fieldworkers faced some difficulties (participants were not at home or declined participation) which affected the randomization process. At the beginning of the focus group session, oral informed consent was obtained. At the end of each session, a short questionnaire containing demographic information (age, sex, and education level) as well as disease status (known hypertension status, years of disease, current treatment if any) was applied.

Individuals with hypertension were recruited from the baseline data, whose hypertension status was known. Fieldworkers were instructed to look for the randomly selected participants' households and ask them some questions to determine eligibility. If eligible, they were invited to participate in the in-depth interview. If the participant agreed to participate, a meeting was scheduled.

2.4.2. Interview and Focus Group Topics

Three different interview guides were developed to collect data about health perceptions, food culture, knowledge of hypertension, and views about salt consumption (whether it is associated with health problems and local perceptions about the amount of salt consumed on a daily basis). There was also a specific question to learn about their expectations around a "new salt" (the salt substitute) which is not part of this analysis. The interview guide for focus groups, individuals with hypertension, and health workers had three common sections: knowledge about hypertension, views about salt consumption, and expectations of a new salt product (Annex 1).

For individuals with hypertension we added questions regarding causes and consequences of hypertension, hypertension management, and experiences with dietary changes for health (Annex 2). For health workers, we added a section about local health needs, local knowledge on hypertension, and their potential role to promote the use of the salt substitute (Annex 3).

2.5. Data Analysis

Interviews and focus groups were transcribed and then analyzed using qualitative analysis software (Atlas-ti 7.1). Researchers created a codebook (list of codes and its definition) (Table A2). These codes were used to analyze the contents of the interviews and focus groups. The transcriptions were read to identify information that was relevant for each topic: (1) causes of hypertension; (2) consequences of hypertension; (3) local eating habits and their impact on health, in general and on the onset of hypertension; (4) opinions about introducing changes in the diet. The sections of the interviews or focus groups that had data related to the research topics were highlighted and received a code. With the help of the software, reports were generated for each code. These reports are a word document with a list of quotes (excerpts) of the interviews and focus groups assigned to each code. The reports were read to identify coincidences, repetitions, similarities, or differences in the data [24].

2.6. Ethics

The study "Launching a Salt Substitute to Reduce Blood Pressure at the Population Level in Peru" was approved by the *Comité Institucional de Ética* (Institutional Review Board) at Universidad Peruana Cayetano Heredia in Lima, Peru on 13 September 2012 (Registration code 58563) and by the Institutional Review Board at Johns Hopkins University in Baltimore, USA on 9 November 2012 (IRB No. 00004391).

3. Results

3.1. Local Diet, Salt Intake, and Hypertension

3.1.1. Local Diet

Both men and women who participated in focus groups stated that women were the ones responsible for preparing the food at home. Most participants said that they usually eat at home and that they only ate outside the home on weekends or for special occasions. Young men stated they usually eat in *"pensiones"* (*pensión* is the local term for having an economic agreement with a person who will prepare homemade food for you on a regular basis) or restaurants near their workplaces.

Both in the interviews and focus groups participants mentioned a wide variety of types of meals consumed regularly. Fish was the most mentioned ingredient, and the most common way of preparing it was stewed (*pescado sudado*). The other ingredients consumed on a regular basis were rice, banana, cassava, and sweet potato. Banana (in its different preparations: boiled, fried, or "majado") was the most consumed carbohydrate. Majado plantain is mashed and then fried with onions and spices. People eat *majado de plátano* both for breakfast and lunch.

Aliño was among the condiments women used the most for cooking. *Aliño* is a combination of onion, garlic, achiote, oregano, salt, and oil that is used as a base for most meals. In addition, there is also a frequent use of processed condiments such as *ajinomoto* (monosodium glutamate) and *sibarita* (spice mix), and natural spices such as cumin and pepper.

"Look, to be honest, I use *aliño* that has onion, garlic, oregano, and a little *achiote*. I grind made it with some oil, a little salt, and I keep it for the week. In my youth, I lived in the countryside (. . .), I do not like food with artificial colors, I do not like that, I use *aliño*." (Woman with hypertension, Village 5)

A few women said they did not use condiments for cooking; these women consider condiments to be harmful to health.

According to the health personnel, the local diet is not balanced, since it is based on big amounts of carbohydrates and little intake of vegetables and fruits. This coincides with the information provided by the local people who mentioned the low consumption of vegetables and fruits. Focus group participants explained that such products are out of reach for people in their villages because they are expensive.

Unlike the general population, people with hypertension did mention that they tried to consume vegetables on a regular basis. People with hypertension specified that they followed a special diet, with low consumption of meat and salt.

3.1.2. Hypertension and Salt

Participants associated certain eating habits with health problems. Hypertension was one of such health problems. Women stated that they have heard that salt and spices are related to the onset of some health problems but did not specify which ones. Male participants mentioned that too many spices could cause hypertension but also stressed that overeating, eating too much food or too much fried food, were the culprits of such disease. Young men mentioned that lack of physical activity coupled with eating too much and eating too much salt could be associated with the development of hypertension.

" . . . factor number one (for getting hypertension) of course are condiments, and salt . . . On the first place is the salt, eating a lot of salt makes you prone to developing high blood pressure, and eating in excess, we eat a lot, and [afterwards] what do we do? (We go) to the hammock. That is the problem, (after eating we go) to the bed, to the floor, to the mat, to rest ..." (Man, 18–44 years group, Village 6)

When asked about the relationship between salt intake and hypertension, only some participants (such as the one in the previous quote) mentioned the excessive intake of salt as a habit associated with the onset of hypertension. Women regardless of their age not only did not understand the process through which salt could cause high blood pressure, but they actually expressed doubts about such a causal relationship. Similarly, male participants explained that they were unclear about the role of salt in relation to illnesses like hypertension.

"It's what is said about common salt (that it can cause hypertension), I mean I don't understand so well how salt influences somebody's blood pressure." (Women, 18–44 years group, Village 5)

"But tell me how can it harm you? . . . I don't see how it (salt intake) could do harm." (Men, 45–65 years group, Village 4)

Overall, we found that the interviewed population was confused by the diversity of information about hypertension and about what are "safe" foods for preventing diseases.

3.2. Knowledge about Hypertension

3.2.1. General Information of the Disease

Men and women did not have a clear understanding about the causes of hypertension. They had many doubts about the role of diet in the onset of disease. However, participants did state that hypertension was a dangerous disease because it could kill you. There were no major differences in the general information managed by men and women regardless of their age.

Unlike the general population, people with hypertension recognized the importance of reducing salt intake to control their blood pressure.

"I eat plain food, I can't eat salty food because they told me to stop taking salt, [I can] not even add spices, pepper, cumin. They told me not to eat any of that at the [health] center," (Woman with hypertension, 66 years old).

Usually it has been the health personnel who have explained to them that high salt intake is associated with their elevated blood pressure.

3.2.2. Causes

According to the general population, the cause of hypertension was related to emotions. Worries, problems, anger, sadness, and strong impressions (getting bad news, for example), were the most frequent explanations for the onset of hypertension. Participants stated that:

"(W)orries can ... (cause high blood pressure), over-thinking, worrying can also bring many other illnesses." (Woman, 45–65 years focus group, Village 5)

"Sometimes (hypertension starts) because of thinking, sometimes because of worries, sometimes because of anger, there are always problems .... (hypertension) comes more from the little outbursts of anger, (or because) you're thinking about something and then the blood pressure starts to rise or go down, it can be both, but that's where this disease comes from. It's not because you eat too much, it's because of anger, because of the worries that overwhelm you." (Men focus group, 45–65 years group, Village 2)

Similarly, those with hypertension also argued that one of the main reasons for having hypertension were worries, stress, and *"la pensadera"*, a local term used that refers to over-thinking about a subject that causes concern:

"It must be that I was thinking about my children. That's why my blood pressure rises...." (Woman with hypertension, 56 years old).

The emotional origin of hypertension seemed to be reinforced by the health personnel, because some of the participants indicated that the doctors had given them that explanation.

"The doctor examines me, takes my blood pressure, and tells me that I have emotional hypertension, that I should control it by taking a lot of liquids ...." (Woman with hypertension, 43 years old).

"Because ... the doctor explained it to me, she said that this (hypertension) sometimes comes from food, too much salt, or maybe you have troubles at home, or maybe you have something (...), I said I did have a lot of problems in my home, maybe that's why it happened, too many worries." (Woman with hypertension, 47 years old).

More than diet, emotional wellbeing was the most common explanation for hypertension in the six villages.

Participants diagnosed with hypertension also acknowledged the role of genetics (e.g., if they had other family members with the disease), being overweight, having a diet based on meat and salt, and having limited physical activity, in the onset and progression of the illness. Some expressed their fear of dying of high blood pressure:

"You know that when you are hypertensive it is like having death between your hands because if I do not take my medication I can die any day." (Woman with hypertension, 58 years old).

3.3. Opinions about the Possibility of Introducing Dietary Changes

Both hypertensive and non-hypertensive participants were asked about their experience and/or their opinion about the possibility of introducing dietary changes to improve their health, such as increasing the intake of fruits and vegetables and reducing the amount of salt they take with their food.

3.4. Salt Intake Reduction

The reduction or elimination of salt from food appears to be a great challenge for those interviewed, both for those diagnosed with hypertension and those who are not:

"I'll never give up salt." (Man, 45–60 group, Village 4).

For some of those interviewed, the idea of stopping their consumption of salt is a saddening one:

"(W)hen you're ... very sick, they take you to the doctor, right? Then they diagnose you with a bunch of illnesses. Then the diet comes. Because all diseases mean diet. Then they tell you to stop taking salt, and that's going to be a problem, you get depressed." (Man, 18–44 group Village 6).

Health personnel state that using a lot of salt on food preparation is part of the local culinary culture and thus very hard to change:

"(T)aking away that [salt] is very difficult, because they are people used to eating everything salty—fish, ceviche, everything. Salt intake is very important here, right?" (Health worker, Village 2).

3.5. Fruits and Vegetables

It was found that not only people with hypertension but many other non-hypertensive participants had received advice from the health personnel to improve their diet (i.e., more fruits and vegetables and less fatty foods). Many of these participants, especially those with hypertension, said that it was hard to follow such advice. The difficulties they expressed were associated with the implications of eating less meat and carbohydrates on their strength and their performance on physical tasks.

"(T)hey told me to eat only carrots ..., only vegetables and nothing else. (They told me) that was my food. (They told me) that I can't eat anything else. But, who is going to live (like that?) ... As I told you, here we work the land, and if you go around with (just) a little bit of carrots ... working hard: how are you going to go [to work] like that?" (Man, 45–60 group, Village 3).

Furthermore, as we have mentioned earlier, the economic cost of introducing fruits in their diets was also identified as a barrier for dietary changes, especially by women. Participants were reticent to the health personnel's suggestion to reduce or stop eating the food they like and enjoy:

"They have already taken away lots of foods from my diet. (It is hard) especially (forme) that I like coffee. They have taken that away from me... the coffee, they have (also) taken away the fish." (Woman, 45–60 group, Village 2).

"(Because I have hypertension) they told me I can't eat chili anymore, but you see I want to eat chili. Even if I die, I want to eat it, it's so good." (Woman with hypertension, 56 years old).

"I was diagnosed (with diabetes), like that, and they said "no sugar for 15 days', and I told the doctor: "I can't take it, I can't take it". They served me my oatmeal without sugar." (Man, 18–44 group Village 3).

Introducing dietary changes such as increasing the amount of fruits and vegetables and reducing salt intake constitutes a challenge both from the perspective of interviewed population as well as the health personnel that advocate for such changes.

4. Discussion

The goal of this study was to learn about local perceptions about hypertension, diet, and salt consumption that could generate insights for later designing a context-relevant social marketing campaign promoting a salt substitution strategy in rural Tumbes in Peru.

4.1. Main Findings

The results present a context with opportunities and challenges for designing a social marketing campaign aimed at introducing a salt substitute with less sodium content.

People in the study have some understanding about the connections between certain food habits and health status. Participants said they have heard that eating too much food (in general) or eating too many fatty foods (specifically) could have a negative impact on health. Young men seemed to have a better grasp of this information. However, there was confusion about the way a high-sodium diet impacts health status, since the connection was not clear for them. A study done in three Latin American countries found that people believed that only those who consumed high quantities of salt were at risk of health problems and that only those with high blood pressure or heart problems had to reduce their salt intake [25]. In our study, people with hypertension did mention the importance of having a low-salt diet to manage their disease, but among the general population very few participants stated that having a diet with high salt content could be harmful.

Similar to other studies [26,27], our study found that local people establish a causal connection between emotional problems and the onset of hypertension. This was common between participants with and without hypertension. Worries, troubles, anger, and bad news were identified by both genders and all age groups as the primary cause of hypertension. It is possible that this association is related to the fact that the word for hypertension in Spanish (*hipertensión*) includes the word tension (*tensión*) which stands for "being tense". A systematic review of qualitative studies around lay perceptions of hypertension (which included 53 studies) found that participants reported stress, food consumption, being overweight, family history, and alcohol as the main causes of hypertension [28]. Participants in the reviewed studies widely and strongly connected stress and worries as a cause, an exacerbating factor, and a consequence of hypertension [28]. We did not find stress being mentioned as a consequence for hypertension, but participants did identify stress as a cause and a worsening factor for hypertension.

Previous experiences of communicational health campaigns suggest that it is important not to assume that because a group is at greater risk of having an illness that they require different communicational strategies [29]. Our results show that there are important similarities in terms of the association between emotions and hypertension among people with and without hypertension. However, besides emotional factors, participants with hypertension in our study mentioned other causes such as salt consumption, genetics, and weight. Weight has been showed to be an important contributing factor of hypertension in the region where this study was conducted [30].

Finally, we found among all participants that introducing changes in their diet was seen as something difficult, saddening, and even negative because agricultural work requires physical strength that is associated with a diet rich in carbohydrates. Decreasing the amount of carbohydrates in the diets appears as unacceptable for participants and increasing their consumption of fruits and vegetables is not affordable. Our results suggest that reducing the amount of salt consumed by this particular population is certainly a challenge but one that does not face economic or idiosyncratic barriers.

4.2. Implications for the Promotion of a Salt Substitute

Social marketing campaigns for reducing sodium intake have been strongly recommended by the World Health Organization [31]. Social marketing aims at changing individual and social behavior through persuasion [32]. Given that the social marketing campaign of our intervention aims at promoting the use of a salt substitute, we cannot overlook the negative attitude towards dietary changes and the value of taste. Thus, the campaign should frame the reduction of salt consumption in a positive way, such as the improvement in health, and avoid talking specifically about hypertension since people do not make this connection. Furthermore, such a marketing campaign ought to stress the good aspects of the substitute that is being promoted, such as the fact that the taste will be the same. This is particularly important given the role of salt and condiments, such as *aliño* or salad dressings, in the local food culture. Learning about the use of salty "seasonings" in food culture has been shown to be relevant for sodium reduction campaigns in other parts of the world, such as in Ghana [33].

In a US setting, the formative study of the campaign "Skip the Salt, Help the Heart" found that it is not uncommon that people associate a low-sodium diet with bland or tasteless foods [34]. The authors state the importance of using messages that highlight an immediate exchange in benefits, such as that "the taste will be good", rather than ones that prescribed the importance of consuming less salt on a regular basis, such as: "you will not develop hypertension". This experience is relevant for our efforts in Peru and shows that despite the geographical differences, there are some relevant lessons when the target population has a high appreciation for salt.

Given that salt is not the only source of sodium, the social marketing campaign could also highlight the importance of learning how to use salty products (such as Monosodium glutamate) moderately as a mechanism for health preservation. One way of helping people to put using less salt into practice could be to introduce a technique for measuring the use of salt during the preparation of meals. Such salt measurements would allow people to identify when they are using too much salt and should consider reducing it. Finally, people should be given alternatives to salt such as other spices available in the local market.

The connection between emotional health and hypertension should not be overlooked. If possible, it could also be part of a social marketing campaign by stating that just as important as it is to take care of their emotional health it is also important to take care of their physical health. The importance of stress and daily worries management could be articulated as relevant elements for good health, while at the same time emphasizing the importance of healthy eating habits.

4.3. Limitations

One major limitation of our study is that all of the hypertensive individuals interviewed were female and we do not know the perspective of men with hypertension in the selected villages. Some studies show that men use health services less than women and have less knowledge of their health status [35–37], however, this cannot be confirmed in our study. Similarly, the study setting and the chosen villages could have flavor preferences and lifestyles that are markedly different from other locations, thus giving a more prominent role to researching local contexts before embarking into behavioral interventions related to the promotion of salt reduction strategies.

Our study was conducted in a rural area where the consumption of processed food with high sodium content such as canned food is rare. Despite this, a lot of sodium seems to be consumed in foods prepared at home such as soup, fried plantains, and *aliño*. In high income settings, most sodium comes from commercial goods and thus if the study was to be replicated in other settings, it should be complemented with questions determining both the total commercial and home cooking sources of sodium in people's diets.

5. Conclusions

This study was nested within the formative phase of an intervention oriented to promote the use of a salt substitute containing less sodium than regular salt. This study clearly showed a number of specific considerations needed to develop a context-relevant social marketing campaign promoting such behavior. First, information about the link between salt intake and hypertension is poor. Yet, proposing a major change in food-related behavior or habit focusing solely on information provision would be inadequate—flavor matters. Second, our findings suggest that a marketing campaign promoting the uptake and acceptance of a salt substitute will not require segmentation of the audience, either by sex or according to hypertensive status. Third, it is relevant to understand local understandings of the disease because despite people with hypertension being more informed about the causes and consequences of hypertension, the primary explanatory model remains the same: emotions are at the root of hypertension. This association is common to findings in other parts of the world, and researchers should make an effort to incorporate it in the strategies for hypertension control.

If the patterns and perceptions around salt intake, wellbeing, and hypertension described in this study are also prevalent in other settings, then these findings can inform similar salt reduction or wellbeing promotion strategies. Most of the paternalistic physician-driven "do not do this" type of messages directly affect the adoption and sustained change towards healthier behaviors, especially if connections between behavior-health-disease are not clear for the target populations, thus limiting the reach and impact of health promotion endeavors. In this sense, conducting preliminary research about the local context and food culture can have a good return for investment in interventions aimed at reducing salt intake, and, importantly, sustaining it over time. As such, either the findings or the approach of this study, or both, can well serve as useful tools in other settings willing to devise similar strategies to stem the tide of hypertension.

Acknowledgments: We are indebted to Miguel Moscoso, Alvaro Taype, and Elizabeth Garby Aliaga Diaz for their support on initial qualitative data analysis. We extend our special gratitude to Gabriela Villarreal for her support with English translations. M.A.P. was supported by a postdoctoral fellowship (2014–2016) from the Peruvian National Council for Science and Technology (Consejo Nacional de Ciencia y Tecnología, CONCYTEC). AB-O is supported by a Research Training Fellowship in Public Health and Tropical Medicine funded by Wellcome Trust (103994/Z/14/Z). This study was conducted as part of a grant from the National Heart, Lung, and Blood Institute (5U01HL114180).

Author Contributions: F.D.-C. participated in the study design and in the making of the data collecting instruments. Data analysis was done by M.A.P. and F.D.-C. The overall project was designed and overseen by A.B.-O., F.D.-C. and J.J.M. The first draft was written by M.A.P. with intellectual contributions from A.B.-O., F.D.-C., V.P.-L. and J.J.M. All the authors participated in the writing and approval of the final version of the manuscript.

Conflicts of Interest: The authors declare that they have no conflict of interest.

Appendix

Table A1. Number and characteristics of focus group participants per village.

Gender/Age Group	Villages	Number of Participants	Focus Groups
Men ≥45 years old	V2	7	2
	V5	6	
Men <45 years old	V1	6	5
	V2	7	
	V4	7	
	V5	7	
	V6	7	
Women ≥45 years old	V2	6	4
	V3	7	
	V4	8	
	V5	6	
Women <45 years old	V2	10	3
	V4	7	
	V5	7	
Average		7	14
Total number of participants		98	

Table A2. Codes used in the qualitative analysis.

CODE	Definition
Perceptions of High Blood pressure	Perceived gravity of having hypertension.
Symptoms of High Blood pressure	Symptoms associated with hypertension.
Causes of High Blood pressure	Ideas about lifestyles or practices deemed to cause hypertension.
Consecuences of High Blood pressure	Ideas about health aspects that are a consequence of hypertension.
Treatment of High Blood pressure	Practices and information around treating high blood pressure.
Food culture at home	Eating practices at home.
Food culture	Descripción de prácticas relacionadas a la preparación y consumo de alimentos en la comunidad
Knowledge healthy food habits	Information about what are healthy foods.
Practices healthy food habits	Habits and attitudes towards the consumption of healthy food practices
Spice use	Regular use of spices in everyday home cooking
Value of salty taste	Value assigned to the use of salty condiments
Typical local meal	Any reference to the preferred local meal (*plato típico*)
Use of salt for food preparation	Any mention to dishes that require a lot of salt and references to the consumption of such dishes
Salt consumption	Perception of the regular use of salt.
Relationship between salt consumption and HBP	Knowledge and ideas regarding the relationship between salt consumption and high blood pressure.
Person responsible of food preparation	*Decision-maker* of the meals at home.

References

1. NCD Risk Factor Collaboration. Worldwide trends in blood pressure from 1975 to 2015: A pooled analysis of 1479 population-based measurement studies with 19.1 million participants. *Lancet* **2017**, *389*, 37–55.
2. Instituto Nacional de Salud. *Encuesta Nacional de Indicadores Nutricionales, Bioquímicos, Socioeconómicos y Culturales Relacionados con las Enfermedades Crónicas Degenerativas*; National Survey of Nutritional, Bioquemical, Socioeconomic and Cultural indicators related to Chronic Degenerative Diseases; Centro Nacional de Alimentación y Nutricion, Instituto Nacional de Salud: Lima, Peru, 2006.
3. Bernabe-Ortiz, A.; Carrillo-Larco, R.M.; Gilman, R.H.; Checkley, W.; Smeeth, L.; Miranda, J.J. Contribution of modifiable risk factors for hypertension and type-2 diabetes in Peruvian resource-limited settings. *J. Epidemiol. Community Health* **2016**, *70*, 49–55. [CrossRef] [PubMed]
4. Liem, D.G.; Miremadi, F.; Keast, R.S. Reducing sodium in foods: The effect on flavor. *Nutrients* **2011**, *3*, 694–711. [CrossRef] [PubMed]
5. Bobowski, N. Shifting human salty taste preference: Potential opportunities and challenges in reducing dietary salt intake of Americans. *Chemosens. Percept.* **2015**, *8*, 112–116. [CrossRef] [PubMed]
6. Beaglehole, R.; Bonita, R.; Horton, R.; Adams, C.; Alleyne, G.; Asaria, P.; Baugh, V.; Bekedam, H.; Billo, N.; Casswell, S.; et al. Priority actions for the non-communicable disease crisis. *Lancet* **2011**, *377*, 1438–1447.
7. Henney, J.E.; Taylor, C.L.; Boon, C.S. (Eds.) *Strategies to Reduce Sodium Intake in the United States*; Committee on Strategies to Reduce Sodium Intake; Institute of Medicine, National Academies Press: Washington, DC, USA, 2010.
8. World Health Organization. *Global Status Report on Noncommunicable Diseases*; World Health Organization: Geneva, Switzerland, 2011.

9.   Ferrante, D.; Apro, N.; Ferreira, V.; Virgolini, M.; Aguilar, V.; Sosa, M.; Perel, P.; Casas, J. Feasibility of salt reduction in processed foods in Argentina. *Rev. Panam. Salud Publica* **2011**, *29*, 69–75. [CrossRef] [PubMed]

10. Brown, I.J.; Tzoulaki, I.; Candeias, V.; Elliott, P. Salt intakes around the world: Implications for public health. *Int. J. Epidemiol.* **2009**, *38*, 791–813. [CrossRef] [PubMed]

11. Bernabe-Ortiz, A.; Diez-Canseco, F.; Gilman, R.H.; Cardenas, M.K.; Sacksteder, K.A.; Miranda, J.J. Launching a salt substitute to reduce blood pressure at the population level: A cluster randomized stepped wedge trial in Peru. *Trials* **2014**, *15*, 93. [CrossRef] [PubMed]

12. Keast, R.S.J.; Breslin, P.A.A. An overview of binary taste-taste interactions. *Food Qual. Prefer.* **2003**, *14*, 111–124. [CrossRef]

13. Saavedra-Garcia, L.; Bernabe-Ortiz, A.; Diez-Canseco, F.; Miranda, J.J. Generating information: What is the average consumption of salt and what are the sources? *Rev. Peru Med. Exp. Salud Publica* **2014**, *31*, 169–180. [PubMed]

14. Ministerio de Salud del Peru. *Sala Situacional Alimentaria Nutricional 2: Consumo Alimentario*; Centro Nacional de Alimentación y Nutrición (CENAN): Lima, Peru, 2012.

15. Saavedra-Garcia, L.; Bernabe-Ortiz, A.; Gilman, R.H.; Diez-Canseco, F.; Cardenas, M.K.; Sacksteder, K.A.; Miranda, J.J. Applying the Triangle Taste Test to Assess Differences between Low Sodium Salts and Common Salt: Evidence from Peru. *PLoS ONE* **2015**, *10*, e0134700. [CrossRef] [PubMed]

16. Whelton, P.K.; He, J.; Cutler, J.A.; Brancati, F.L.; Appel, L.J.; Follmann, D.; Klag, M. Effects of oral potassium on blood pressure. Meta-analysis of randomized controlled clinical trials. *JAMA* **1997**, *277*, 1624–1632. [CrossRef] [PubMed]

17. Whelton, P.K.; Buring, J.; Borhani, N.O.; Cohen, J.D.; Cook, N.; Cutler, J.A.; Kiley, J.E.; Kuller, L.H.; Satterfield, S.; Sacks, F.M.; et al. The effect of potassium supplementation in persons with a high-normal blood pressure. *Ann. Epidemiol.* **1995**, *5*, 85–95. [CrossRef]

18. Geleijnse, J.M.; Kok, F.J.; Grobbee, D.E. Blood pressure response to changes in sodium and potassium intake: A metaregression analysis of randomised trials. *J. Hum. Hypertens.* **2003**, *17*, 471–480. [CrossRef] [PubMed]

19. Dickinson, H.O.; Nicolson, D.J.; Campbell, F.; Beyer, F.R.; Mason, J. Potassium supplementation for the management of primary hypertension in adults. *Cochrane Database Syst. Rev.* **2006**, *19*, CD004641.

20. Roncancio, A.M.; Ward, K.K.; Carmack, C.C.; Munoz, B.T.; Cano, M.A.; Cribbs, F. Using Social Marketing Theory as a Framework for Understanding and Increasing HPV Vaccine Series Completion Among Hispanic Adolescents: A Qualitative Study. *J. Community Health* **2017**, *42*, 169–178. [CrossRef] [PubMed]

21. Green, J.; Thorogood, N. *Qualitative Methods for Health Research*; SAGE: London, UK, 2004.

22. Gobierno Regional de Tumbes. *Programa Regional de Población de Tumbes*; Gobierno Regional de Tumbes: Tumbes, Peru, 2013.

23. Kitzinger, J. The methodology of focus groups: The importance of interaction between research participants. *Sociol. Health Illn.* **1994**, *16*, 103–121. [CrossRef]

24. Creswell, J.W. *Qualitative Inquiry and Research Design*, 3rd ed.; SAGE: Thousand Oaks, CA, USA, 2013.

25. Sanchez, G.; Pena, L.; Varea, S.; Mogrovejo, P.; Goetschel, M.L.; Montero-Campos Mde, L.; Mejía, R.; Blanco-Metzler, A. Knowledge, perceptions, and behavior related to salt consumption, health, and nutritional labeling in Argentina, Costa Rica, and Ecuador. *Rev. Panam. Salud Publica* **2012**, *32*, 259–264. [PubMed]

26. Boutin-Foster, C.; Ogedegbe, G.; Ravenell, J.E.; Robbins, L.; Charlson, M.E. Ascribing meaning to hypertension: A qualitative study among African Americans with uncontrolled hypertension. *Ethn. Dis.* **2007**, *17*, 29–34. [PubMed]

27. Heurtin-Roberts, S.; Reisin, E. The relation of culturally influenced lay models of hypertension to compliance with treatment. *Am. J. Hypertens.* **1992**, *5*, 787–792. [CrossRef] [PubMed]

28. Marshall, I.J.; Wolfe, C.D.; McKevitt, C. Lay perspectives on hypertension and drug adherence: Systematic review of qualitative research. *BMJ* **2012**, *345*, e3953. [CrossRef] [PubMed]

29. Institute of Medicine. *Speaking of Health: Assessing Health Communication Strategies for Diverse Populations*; The National Academies Press: Washington, DC, USA, 2002.

30. Bernabé-Ortiz, A.; Carrillo-Larco, R.M.; Gilman, R.H.; Checkley, W.; Smeeth, L.; Miranda, J.J.; CRONICAS Cohort Study Group. Impact of urbanization and altitude on the incidence of, and risk factors for hypertension. *Heart* **2017**. [CrossRef]

31. Bardfield, L. *Applying a Social Marketing Framework to Salt Reduction*; Family Health International: Washington, DC, USA, 2012.

32. Weinrich, N.K. *Hands-on Social Marketing: A Step-by-Step Guide to Designing Change for Good*; SAGE: Los Angeles, CA, USA, 2011.

33. Kerry, S.M.; Emmett, L.; Micah, F.B.; Martin-Peprah, R.; Antwi, S.; Phillips, R.O.; Plange-Rhule, J.; Eastwood, J.B.; Cappuccio, F.P. Rural and semi-urban differences in salt intake, and its dietary sources, in Ashanti, West Africa. *Ethn. Dis.* **2005**, *15*, 33–39. [PubMed]

34. Health Communication Research Center, Missouri School of Journalism. Skip the Salt, Help the Heart. University of Missouri. Available online: http://hcrc.missouri.edu/case-studies/skip-the-salt-help-the-heart/ (accessed on 16 March 2017).

35. Hamlyn, S. Reducing the incidence of colorectal cancer in African Americans. *Gastroenterol. Nurs.* **2008**, *31*, 39–42. [CrossRef] [PubMed]

36. Teo, C.H.; Ng, C.J.; Booth, A.; White, A. Barriers and facilitators to health screening in men: A systematic review. *Soc. Sci. Med.* **2016**, *165*, 168–176. [CrossRef] [PubMed]

37. Seidler, Z.E.; Dawes, A.J.; Rice, S.M.; Oliffe, J.L.; Dhillon, H.M. The role of masculinity in men's help-seeking for depression: A systematic review. *Clin. Psychol. Rev.* **2016**, *49*, 106–118. [CrossRef] [PubMed]

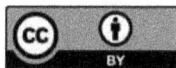

nutrients

MDPI

Article

Sodium Reduction in Processed Foods in Brazil: Analysis of Food Categories and Voluntary Targets from 2011 to 2017

Eduardo A. F. Nilson [1,2,*], Ana M. Spaniol [1], Vivian S. S. Gonçalves [1], Iracema Moura [1], Sara A. Silva [1], Mary L'Abbé [3] and Patricia C. Jaime [4]

1   Ministry of Health of Brazil, Brasilia 70058-900, Brazil; ana.spaniol@saude.gov.br (A.M.S.); vivian.goncalves@saude.gov.br (V.S.S.G.); iracema.moura@saude.gov.br (I.M.); sara.silva@saude.gov.br (S.A.S.)
2   Global Health and Sustainability Program, University of Sao Paulo, Sao Paulo 01255-001, Brazil
3   University of Toronto, Toronto, ON M5S 2E8, Canada; Mary.Labbe@utoronto.ca
4   Department of Nutrition, University of Sao Paulo, Sao Paulo 01255-001, Brazil; constant@usp.br
*   Correspondence: eduardo@saude.gov.br; Tel.: +55-33159022

Received: 15 June 2017; Accepted: 10 July 2017; Published: 12 July 2017

Abstract: Non-communicable diseases, including cardiovascular diseases, are responsible for over 70% of deaths in Brazil. Currently, over 25% of Brazilian adults are diagnosed as hypertensive; overall, current dietary sodium intake in Brazil (4700 mg/person) is over twice the international recommendations, and 70–90% of adolescents and adults consume excessive sodium. National sodium reduction strategies consider the main dietary sources of sodium to be added salt to foods, foods consumed outside of the household, and sodium in processed foods. The national voluntary strategy for sodium reduction in priority food categories has been continuously monitored over a 6-year period (2011–2017) and there was a significant 8–34% reduction in the average sodium content of over half food categories. Different food categories have undergone differing reductions in sodium over time, aiding gradual biannual targets to allow industries to develop new technologies and consumers to adapt to foods with less salt. By 2017, most products of all food categories had met the regional targets proposed by the Pan American Health Organization, showing that voluntary sodium reduction strategies can potentially contribute to food reformulation. Nevertheless, regulatory approaches may still be necessary in the future in order to reach all food producers and to allow stronger enforcement to meet more stringent regional targets.

Keywords: sodium; processed foods; hypertension; cardiovascular disease; food reformulation

1. Introduction

In most countries in the world, there is excessive dietary sodium consumption within the population, which is an important risk factor for the development of hypertension and cardiovascular disease [1]. Accordingly, sodium reduction was prioritized in the United Nations' Global Action Plan for the Prevention and Control of Noncommunicable Diseases (NCD), and the World Health Organization (WHO) has defined a 30% relative reduction in mean population intake of salt/sodium as a global voluntary target for 2025 [2]. The Pan American Health Organization (PAHO) has followed global priorities by urging governments to commit to the global NCD targets and supporting countries of the Americas in reducing dietary sodium to less than 2000 mg per person by 2020 [3].

Diet is an important risk factor for NCDs. Dietary sodium reduction is a modifiable risk factor for hypertension and cardiovascular disease and a highly cost-effective strategy ("best-buy") in non-communicable disease prevention as per the WHO [4]. It has been projected that a 10% worldwide reduction in sodium consumption over 10 years would avert millions of disability-adjusted life years (DALYs) and hundreds of thousands of deaths related to cardiovascular diseases [5]. The epidemiologic and economic burdens of NCDs in Brazil are also substantial. Non-communicable diseases are the main cause of mortality in the country (72.8% of deaths) and cardiovascular diseases have been the leading cause of death since the 1960s, accounting for 20% of total deaths in 2013 [6,7]. The prevalence of diagnosed hypertension in Brazilian adults has increased by over 14%, from 22.5 to 25.7% over a ten-year period (2006 to 2016) according to the 2016 National Telephone Survey (Vigitel) [8]. The overall hospitalization costs due to cardiovascular diseases have increased approximately 40% from 2008 to 2016 (from the equivalent of US$448 million to US$741 million), according to the National Healthcare Expenditure Database (Sistema de Informações Hospitalares do Sistema Único de Saúde/SIH-SUS), which covers more than 70% of all hospital admissions in Brazil.

Over the last decades, food consumption has been changing rapidly in Brazil and processed foods are replacing staple foods in diets [9]. The participation of processed foods in dietary sodium is continuously increasing and excessive sodium consumption has been directly related to the share of processed foods in the diet [10], although salt and salt-based condiments added to foods are the main sodium source in the diet [11].

The need for sodium reduction in processed foods is also supported by recent data on nutritional profiling in Brazil, which evidences the high sodium content of most processed foods [12] and even of foods targeted at children [13]. The average sodium consumption of Brazilians (4700 mg/day) is over twice the World Health Organization maximum recommendation and 70–90% of adolescents and adults consume excessive dietary sodium (over 2000 mg/day) [14]. Nevertheless, in the 2013 National Health Survey, people were asked about their self-perception of salt/sodium consumption, and only 14% of the adults considered their consumption as high and over 80% of the population perceived it as adequate or low [15].

In the last decade, national sodium reduction policies have been implemented by many regions of the world, including multi-component strategies and individual strategies such as mandatory and voluntary food reformulation, taxation of unhealthy foods, school interventions, dietary advice, community-based counseling, and nutritional labeling. Recent evidence suggests that population-wide policies and comprehensive strategies involving food reformulation, food labeling, media campaigns and mandatory reformulation may achieve larger reductions in salt consumption than focused interventions [16,17].

A systematic review of progress in sodium reduction policies in processed foods in 75 countries of all regions in the world showed that voluntary agreements with food industries are more commonly implemented (36 countries), while only nine countries have set mandatory limits for sodium in processed foods [18].

In general, regulatory approaches are able to be enforced more effectively, but it is more difficult for them to be approved and updated regularly. In contrast, voluntary strategies are more easily implemented and adjusted over time, but rely on industry commitment and strong monitoring to achieve changes in the nutritional profile of foods [18,19].

National sodium reduction strategies have been monitored by assessing compliance with sodium reduction targets (voluntary or mandatory) and the changes in sodium levels in foods, mostly using commercial label data.

In the United Kingdom, where a long-term voluntary sodium reduction program coupled with public awareness campaigns has been in place since 2006, a reduction in sodium levels in processed foods has already impacted the overall sodium intake of the population [20]. Voluntary strategies in Australia and New Zealand have also shown a reduction in mean sodium levels in several food categories, both through food label collection [21] and analytical data [22].

In Argentina, mandatory maximum levels for meat and farinaceous products as well as soups and dressings were set in 2013, following previous voluntary agreements. Currently, most of the food groups included in the law already have sodium content within the maximum limits, so further reductions of the existing limits are required, and more food categories should be included in the law [23]. In South Africa, industries are rapidly meeting the mandatory limits for sodium content in processed foods and, one year after the introduction of the national legislation, two-thirds of targeted foods have met the established limits and many others are close to meeting the legislated requirements [24]. The Brazilian Dietary Sodium Reduction Plan takes into account the multiple dietary sources of sodium and the needs of different population groups, and involves consumer education, healthy diet promotion, processed food reformulation, health promotion in school and work settings, food regulation, and healthcare organization [25].

The Dietary Guidelines for the Brazilian Population are the major tool for food and nutrition education and state that salt should only be used in small amounts when cooking and consuming foods and that so called ultra-processed foods, commonly rich in sodium, sugars, and fats, should be avoided [26].

The food reformulation strategies in Brazil have been based on voluntary agreements with the Brazilian Association of Food Industries (ABIA), which accounts for over 70% of the processed food market in the country. Targets were set in order to represent gradual but meaningful reductions in the maximum sodium content of packaged foods through biannual targets for the food categories that most contribute to sodium intake [27], according to national household budget surveys [28]. The Pan American Health Organization has supported sodium reduction policies in the Americas and proposed inaugural regional targets for several food categories in 2014 (breads, cakes, cookies and biscuits, pastas, dairy spreads, breakfast cereals and mayonnaise). These targets were based on the national targets for sodium reduction in the region, either voluntary or regulatory, as in Argentina, Brazil, Canada, Chile and the United States. The maximum values set by the PAHO consist of a general target for each food category. A more stringent target is also proposed, based on the lowest targets in the region, in order to assist countries in starting their national sodium reduction policies and to improve the ongoing policies [29].

Thus the main purpose of this study was to follow-up the changes in sodium content of the main food categories with voluntary sodium reduction targets in Brazil from 2011 to 2017 and to compare the sodium content of food categories in Brazil to the regional targets proposed by the PAHO.

2. Materials and Methods

2.1. Product Selection Criteria

The food categories that were analyzed in this study include breads, cakes and cake mixes, pastas, snacks, mayonnaise, dairy spreads, margarines, salt-based condiments, mozzarella cheese, biscuits, cookies and crackers, and breakfast cereals, which were prioritized for sodium reduction with food industries.

Some food categories were divided into subcategories for specific sodium reduction targets because of technical justifications by food industries when targets were established. Breads include sliced bread and buns, cakes are subdivided into those with or without filling, cake mixes may be aerated or creamy, snacks include extruded corn snacks and potato chips, and condiments include bouillons, paste and rice condiments [30–33]. Prior to data collection, food companies that voluntarily committed to the national sodium reduction targets and their products were listed by the Brazilian Association of Food Industries.

The food subcategories that were included in this study were required to have completed two monitoring cycles, considering the baseline of target setting (in 2011) and data collection rounds every two or three years (2013–2014 and 2017). Food categories that did not complete at least 4 years of target implementation and products belonging to companies that are not members of ABIA were not included in the analysis.

2.2. Data Collection

Data on sodium content were directly obtained from the mandatory food label information of products, mainly from the official company websites. All nutritional information from products that was not available in the websites was collected through the companies' customer services. The products also needed to be available on the market at the time of data collection according to the information provided by ABIA, and in the case of different package sizes for the same product, only one entry was considered. Baseline and follow-up data consisted of records of the manufacturer, brand and commercial product name, as well as the sodium content per sizing and adjusted per 100 g. Data were independently verified for outliers, missing values and data entry accuracy by two study personnel and queries and discrepancies were reviewed from the websites and followed-up directly with the food industries and their association.

2.3. Statistical Analysis

Firstly, data were independently verified for outliers, missing values and data entry accuracy by two study personnel, and queries and discrepancies were reviewed from the websites and directly with the food industries and ABIA when necessary.

The sodium content of all food subcategories in 2017 was directly compared to the PAHO regional targets (lowest and most stringent). Some food subcategories were grouped in order to be compared to the regional food categories (breads, pasta, snacks, mayonnaise, butter/dairy spread, condiments, cookies and sweet biscuits, savory biscuits and crackers, and breakfast cereals) and food categories which did not have corresponding regional targets were compared to the 2016 national targets [29].

For all food categories studied, descriptive statistics were calculated including the total of products for each category, measures of central tendency and dispersion (means and medians, as well as their respective standard deviations and maximum and minimum sodium levels) in 2011, 2013–2014 and 2017. Then, the sodium content of each food category was calculated at the same time points based on variable distribution to verify normality through the Shapiro–Wilk test. After that, we investigated the significance of the differences in sodium content at each data collection point through the Kruskal–Wallis test, a non-parametric test, because the data studied did not meet the normality criteria. For the food categories that presented statistical significance, we conducted the Dunn's test to verify statistical difference in each time period (2011 to 2013–2014, 2013–2014 to 2017 and 2011 to 2017). All analyses considered statistical significance as $p < 0.05$.

Additionally, data were plotted in distribution graphs of sodium values from baseline to the second round of monitoring, displaying the interquartile ranges.

All statistical analyses were conducted using Stata 12 (Stata Corp, College Station, TX, USA).

3. Results

3.1. Proportion of Products Meeting the PAHO Regional Targets

After removing duplicates and products with ineligible or insufficient information on nutritional composition, we analyzed a total of 1067 products at baseline, 1288 products in the first data collection cycle (2013–2014) and 981 products in the second data collection cycle (2017). According to the Brazilian Association of Food Industries, the different number of food products within each time period is due to discontinuity and replacement of products over time.

The sodium content of Brazilian processed foods analyzed in 2017 indicates that in over half of the food subcategories 100% of the products met these targets, and in all except one food subcategory (corn snacks), over 85% of products met the regional targets for 2017.

Considering the more stringent maximum values set by the PAHO for the region, the targets were met by over 70% of the products in half of the food subcategories, and only breakfast cereals had all products meet these maximum values. In addition, nine food subcategories had a less than

50% compliance in their products when compared to the more stringent targets, of which three subcategories had less than 10% of the products meet these targets, as shown in Table 1.

Table 1. Proportion of food categories and subcategories that met the initial and the lower inaugural regional sodium reduction set by the Pan American Health Organization.

Food Categories and Subcategories		Regional Target	% Products That Have Met the Regional Targets (2017)	Lower Target	% Products That Have Met the Lower Regional Targets (2017)
Americas	**Brazil**	mg/100 g	%	mg/100 g	%
Breads	Sliced bread (n = 82)	600	100.0	400	59.8
	Buns (n = 11)		100.0		81.8
Cakes	Aerated cake mixes (n = 135)	400	90.4	205	25.9
	Creamy cake mixes (n = 24)		91.7		45.8
	Cakes without filling (n = 68)		100.0		36.8
	Cakes with filling (n = 48)		100.0		54.2
Shelf-stable pasta and noodles (dry, uncooked)	Instant pasta (n = 87)	1921	98.9	1333	10.3
Snacks	Corn snacks (n = 39)	900	53.8	530	10.2
	Potato chips (n = 29)		100.0		75.9
Mayonnaise	Mayonnaise (n = 28)	1050	85.7	670	17.9
Butter/dairy spread	Dairy spread (n = 45)	800	100.0	500	73.3
	Margarines (n = 46)		95.7		28.3
Cheese *	Mozzarella cheese (n = 28)	559	89.3	512 [b]	50.0
Condiments	Rice condiments (n = 5)	33,100	100.0	9100	0.0
	Bouillon cubes and powders (n = 35) **	1025	97.1	900	11.4
	Paste condiments * (n = 14)	37,901	100.0	33,134	78.6
Cookies and sweet biscuits	Sweet biscuits (n = 52)	485	99.8	265	21.2
	Filled cookies (n = 185)		100.0		86.5
Savory biscuits and crackers	Salted crackers (n = 84)	1340	100.0	700	91.7
Breakfast cereals	Breakfast cereals (n = 15)	630	100.0	500	100.0

* National targets (food categories with no regional targets). ** Adjusted to portion size (5 g) according to Brazilian regulation.

3.2. Analysis of Mean and Median Sodium Content for Each Food Category over Time

The mean and median sodium content of all 20 food subcategories, along with their standard deviations and minimum and maximum values, were evaluated at the baseline of the target setting (2011), in 2013–2014, and in 2017.

Sodium changes varied between food subcategories, considering the measures of central tendency of sodium content of food products at baseline and at each data collection point (Table 2). Most food subcategories (except for corn snacks and mozzarella cheese) continually reduced both sodium means and medians over time, and statistically significant reductions were found for 65% of the subcategories from 2011 to 2017.

Table 2. Sodium content of food subcategories at baseline and at the first and second monitoring cycles, Brazil 2011–2017.

Food Categories	Sodium 2011 (mg/100 g)			Sodium 2013–2014 (mg/100 g)			Sodium 2017 (mg/100 g)			p*
	n	Mean ± SD	Median (Min–Max)	n	Mean ± SD	Median (Min–Max)	n	Mean ± SD	Median (Min–Max)	
Sliced bread	117	426.5 ± 107.1 [a,b]	432.0 (118.0–796.0)	87	380.3 ± 122.1 [a]	380.0 (126.0–870.0)	82	365.0 ± 87.6 [b]	380.0 (134.0–536.0)	<0.001
Buns	9	436.1 ± 121.4	462.0 (260.0–570.0)	8	388.5 ± 74.4	415.0 (270.0–462.0)	11	374.4 ± 59.4	372.0 (270.0–512.0)	0.359
Aerated cake mixes	125	372.3 ± 173.4 [a,b]	314.0 (166.7–1111.5)	201	309.6 ± 69.2 [a,c]	327.0 (117.0–474.0)	135	291.6 ± 92.6 [b,c]	293 (119.6–724.3)	<0.001
Creamy cake mixes	24	270.7 ± 75.6 [a]	280.0 (135.1–412.0)	33	250.5 ± 44.6	251.0 (69.0–333.0)	24	229.6 ± 82.1 [a]	226.2 (40.7–422.9)	0.047
Cakes without filling	64	335.7 ± 66.7 [a,b]	355.0 (188.3–462.9)	69	281.0 ± 85.9 [a,c]	300.0 (117.0–398.3)	68	241.1 ± 74.9 [b,c]	250.0 (101.7–355.0)	<0.001
Cakes with filling	41	249.9 ± 51.4 [a,b]	240.0 (107.0–330.0)	68	212.3 ± 47.0 [a,c]	224.0 (108.3–330.0)	48	185.8 ± 55.0 [b,c]	200.0 (80.0–255.0)	<0.001
Instant pastas	90	1960.0 ± 384.5 [a,b]	1993.5 (1104.9–2729.1)	97	1662.3 ± 265.7 [a]	1670.0 (1057.5–2548.6)	87	1598.6 ± 189.6 [b]	1607.1 (1057.5–2548.6)	<0.001
Corn snacks	25	831.9 ± 226.1	840.0 (351.0–1288.0)	39	753.9 ± 140.1	756.0 (352.0–1032.0)	40	827.4 ± 242.8	884.0 (348.0–1224.0)	0.067
Potato chips	22	547.6 ± 123.6	598.0 (305.0–720.0)	28	513.3 ± 130.7	516.0 (276.0–700.0)	30	475.4 ± 137.9	507.3 (200.0–748.0)	0.237
Mayonnaise	31	1063.3 ± 198.2 [a,b]	1058.3 (741.7–1566.7)	41	891.3 ± 157.9 [a]	925.0 (400.0–1075.0)	29	852.7 ± 194.9 [b]	933.3 (541.7–1075.0)	<0.001
Dairy spreads	80	659.5 ± 248.4 [a,b]	596.7 (314.0–1470.0)	80	524.4 ± 188.2 [a,c]	468.3 (300.0–1100.0)	45	434.5 ± 110.3 [b,c]	410.0 (300.0–670.0)	<0.001
Margarines	94	739.9 ± 363.6 [a]	730.0 (40.0–1660.0)	84	689.8 ± 351.4 [b]	710.0 (0.0–1660.0)	46	544.3 ± 207.3 [a,b]	600.0 (10.0–1070.0)	<0.001
Mozzarella cheese	26	600.2 ± 363.6 [a]	540.0 (350.0–160.0)	51	461.2 ± 132.2 [a]	486.7 (87.0–786.7)	28	517.2 ± 131.5	526.7 (86.7–796.7.0)	0.039
Rice condiments	5	31,425.1 ± 3009.7	32,120.0 (26.186.0–33,800.0)	4	29,530.0 ± 6140.7	32,370.0 (20,340.0–33,040.0)	5	28,505.1 ± 5237.6	31,260.0 (20,340.0–32,700.0)	0.325
Bouillon cubes and powders	41	1035.9 ± 94.4 [a]	1015.0 (900.0–1247.0)	26	985.2 ± 105.8 [b]	1019.0 (705.0–1183.0)	35	952.1 ± 88.2 [a,b]	967.0 (668.0–1057.0)	0.003
Paste condiments	14	33,494.5 ± 4054.4	33,450.0 (26,840.0–40,700.0)	14	32,900.0 ± 3173.6	33,850.0 (26,840.0–37,280.0)	14	31,845.7 ± 2615.9	32,220.0 (26,840.0–35,280.0)	0.303
Sweet biscuits	17	359.2 ± 81.3 [a,b]	386.7 (213.3–490.0)	45	318.2 ± 50.3 [a]	317.0 (236.7–416.0)	52	293.9 ± 72.4 [b]	306.7 (60.0–493.3)	0.019
Filled cookies	176	259.5 ± 66.0 [a,b]	251.7 (140.0–600.0)	198	242.6 ± 48.9 [a]	243.0 (127.0–390.0)	185	235.5 ± 57.3 [b]	240.0 (41.7–463.3)	0.006
Salted crackers	39	695.8 ± 260.8 [b]	686.7 (83.3–1220.0)	94	660.4 ± 147.1 [c]	633.0 (350.0–923.0)	84	590.9 ± 163.4 [b,c]	626.7 (150.0–1080.0)	0.031
Breakfast cereals	27	428.9 ± 141.8	430.0 (132.0–676.7)	21	406.7 ± 129.9	392.5 (195.0–679.3)	15	359.2 ± 69.5	390.0 (216.7–416.7)	0.209

* Kruskal–Wallis Test; [a, b, c] Dunn's Test: same letters in the same lines = p < 0.05.

For sliced bread, salted crackers, sweet biscuits, filled cookies, instant pastas, mayonnaise, cakes with and without filling, aerated and creamy cake mixes, margarines, dairy spreads and bouillons, there was a significant 8–34% reduction in mean sodium content between 2011 and 2017 (Table 3). The greatest sodium reductions occurred for cakes (25.7 to 28.0%), margarines (26.4%) and dairy spreads (28.0%). The speed of sodium reduction varied among the food subcategories between each monitoring cycle but most subcategories evidenced continual reduction of mean sodium content. Significant reductions in mean sodium content were achieved in nine subcategories between 2011 and 2013–2014 and in six subcategories in 2013–2014 and 2017. Four subcategories significantly reduced their mean sodium content in both periods (aerated cake mixes, cakes with and without filling and dairy spreads). Despite the reduction in mean sodium content for most subcategories in both periods, for mozzarella cheese and corn snacks, an initial reduction was followed an increase in overall mean sodium content. At this point, other studies pairing products from each period may for allow a better analysis about these different rates of sodium reduction. The distribution of sodium content varied highly between 2011 and 2017 amongst food subcategories and between time periods (Figures 1–5). The variability in sodium content within food subcategories declined for 70% (14) of the subcategories, converging towards the median sodium content (sliced breads, buns, creamy cake mixes, potato chips, bouillons, sweet cookies, filed cookies, salted crackers, breakfast cereals, dairy spreads, margarines, mozzarella cheese, instant pasta and paste condiments). The upper values of the interquartile ranges of all and the lower limits were also reduced for most categories.

Table 3. Reduction in mean sodium content of food subcategories, Brazil 2011−2017.

Food Categories	% Reduction in Mean Sodium		
	2011−2013/14	2013/14−2017	2011−2017
Loaf bread	10.8 *	3.9	14.3 *
Buns	11.0	3.6	14.2
Aerated cake mixes	16.9 *	5.8 *	21.8 *
Creamy cake mixes	7.4	8.4	15.2 *
Cakes without filling	16.1 *	14.2 *	28.0 *
Cakes with filling	14.8 *	12.7 *	25.7 *
Instant pastas	15.2 *	3.8	18.5 *
Corn snacks	9.4	−9.8	0.5
Potato chips	6.2	7.4	13.2
Mayonnaise	16.2 *	4.4	19.8 *
Dairy spreads	20.5 *	17.1 *	34.1 *
Margarines	6.8	21.0 *	26.4 *
Mozzarella cheese	23.2 *	−12.1	13.8
Rice condiments	6.0	3.5	9.3
Bouillon cubes and powders	4.8	3.3 *	8.0 *
Paste condiments	1.8	3.2	4.9
Sweet biscuits	11.4 *	7.9	18.4 *
Filled cookies	6.6 *	2.9	9.3 *
Salted crackers	5.0	10.4 *	15.0 *
Breakfast cereals	5.4	11.6	16.3

* $p < 0.05$.

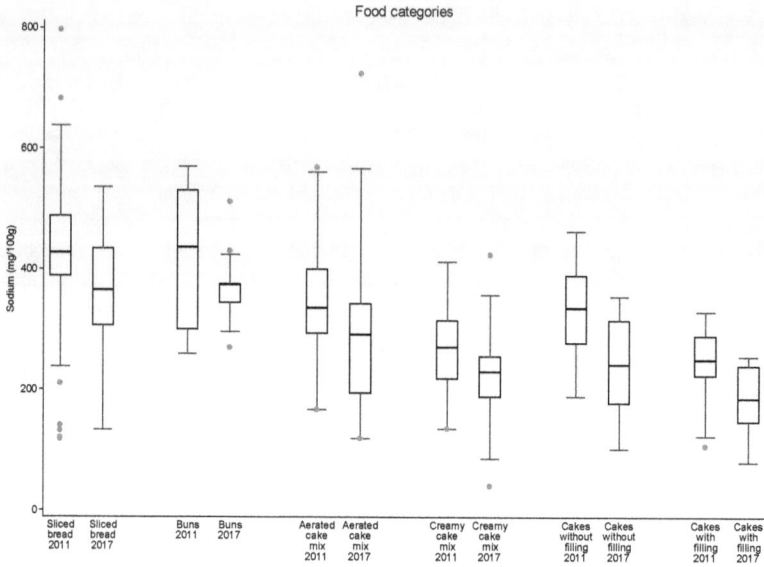

Figure 1. Distribution of sodium values from baseline to the second data collection for sliced bread, buns, aerated cake mixes, creamy cake mixes, cakes without filling and cakes with filling. The box displays the interquartile range and the median value is marked as a line within the box. The lines extending above and below the box indicate the most extreme value within the 75th percentile + 1.5x (interquartile range) and the 25th percentile − 1.5x (interquartile range), and additional values outside of this range are marked as grey circles.

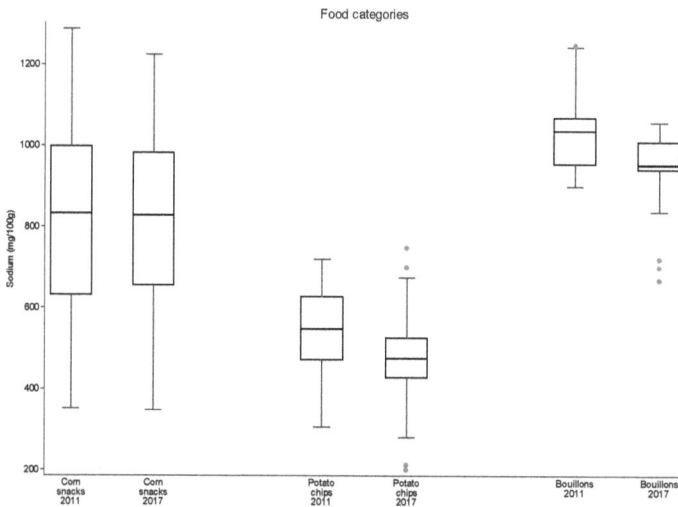

Figure 2. Distribution of sodium values from baseline to the second data collection for corn snacks, potato chips and bouillons. The box displays the interquartile range and the median value is marked as a line within the box. The lines extending above and below the box indicate the most extreme value within the 75th percentile + 1.5x (interquartile range) and the 25th percentile − 1.5x (interquartile range), and additional values outside of this range are marked as grey circles.

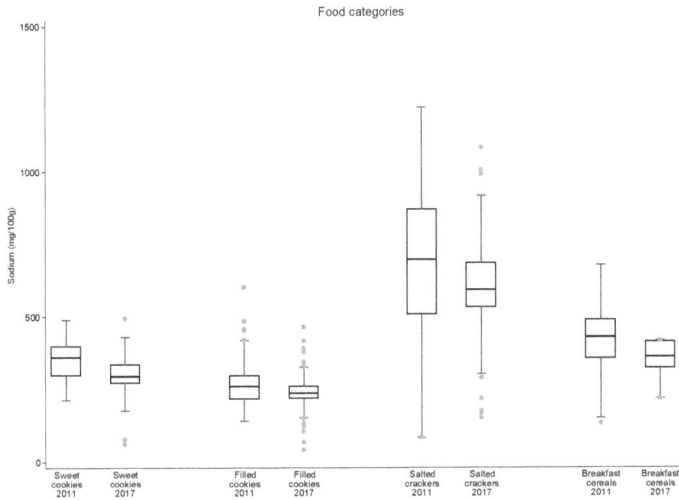

Figure 3. Distribution of sodium values from baseline to the second data collection for sweet cookies, filled cookies, salted crackers and breakfast cereals. The box displays the interquartile range and the median value is marked as a line within the box. The lines extending above and below the box indicate the most extreme value within the 75th percentile + 1.5x (interquartile range) and the 25th percentile − 1.5x (interquartile range), and additional values outside of this range are marked as grey circles.

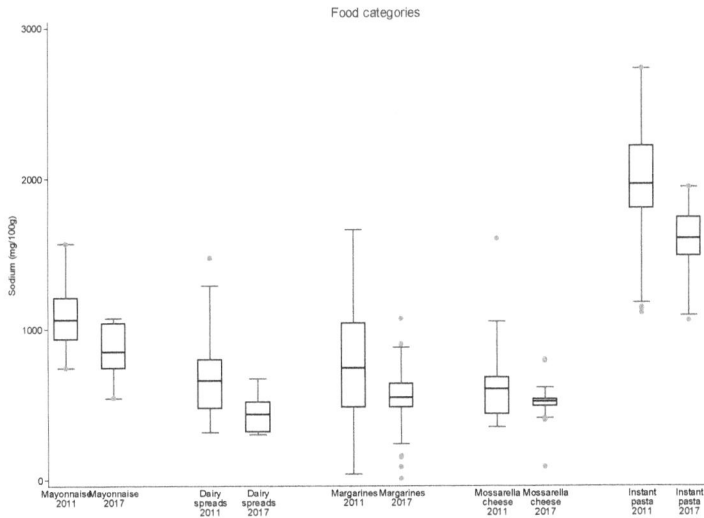

Figure 4. Distribution of sodium values from baseline to the second data collection for mayonnaise, dairy spreads, margarine, mozzarella cheese and instant pastas. The box displays the interquartile range and the median value is marked as a line within the box. The lines extending above and below the box indicate the most extreme value within the 75th percentile + 1.5x (interquartile range) and the 25th percentile − 1.5x (interquartile range), and additional values outside of this range are marked as grey circles.

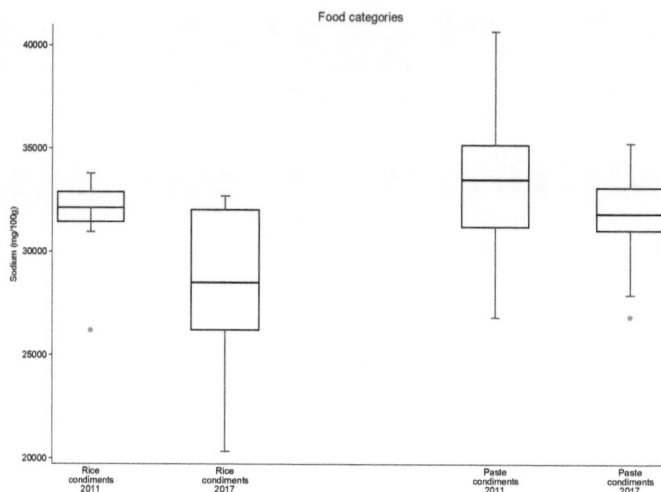

Figure 5. Distribution of sodium values from baseline to the second data collection for rice and paste condiments. The box displays the interquartile range and the median value is marked as a line within the box. The lines extending above and below the box indicate the most extreme value within the 75th percentile + 1.5*x* (interquartile range) and the 25th percentile − 1.5*x* (interquartile range), and additional values outside of this range are marked as grey circles.

4. Discussion

Brazil initiated the reduction of the sodium content of packaged foods in 2011 and has set biannual voluntary targets for food industries with respect to the maximum levels of sodium for the categories that contribute to over 90% of the sodium from industrialized foods. Therefore, the Brazilian sodium reduction strategy for processed foods relies on the commitment of the major food industry association in the country.

The extent of the impact of sodium reduction in processed foods has been questioned [34], but it must be considered part of the reduction of dietary sodium in Brazil and accurate results depend on updated food composition data to follow food reformulation. It is also important to consider that sodium reduction strategies include ready-to-eat foods and processed culinary ingredients, as bouillons and other salt-based condiments [35].

Reducing the dietary sodium intake of the Brazilian population from its current levels to the intended 2 g/day will require a combination of strategies to address all dietary sources of sodium. These strategies include the promotion of healthy diets (including awareness on the risks of excessive dietary sodium and the reduction of discretionary salt use), the promotion of healthy environments (especially schools, including restrictions to unhealthy foods), food regulation (for example front of pack information and other improvements in food labeling) and salt reduction in food services and restaurants.

Although national and international experiences have generally focused on single-nutrient approaches (especially for sodium), recent discussion of multi-nutrient profiling systems may provide broader reformulation strategies and more benefits to public health in the future through combined reduction of sodium, sugars and fats [36].

The data here presented provide an evaluation of the changes in sodium content of processed foods through voluntary sodium reduction targets in Brazil. Our results show overall progress in sodium reduction in most food subcategories, although it is apparent that some subcategories may not achieve the targets or may slow their reductions in the long term.

These results suggest that reformulation targets for sodium affect the upper limit of sodium content of food subcategories, as intended, and also induce changes in the subcategories as a whole by reducing the mean and median sodium content and by affecting the distribution of sodium content within each category.

The variation of sodium content in processed foods over four to six years in Brazil also suggests there may be category-specific issues and challenges that influence the extent of sodium reduction over time and amongst food categories. Nevertheless, it is likely that gradual reductions in sodium content allow food industries to develop the alternatives to reduce sodium more significantly and for consumers to adapt to foods with less sodium.

Sodium is important in processed foods for microbiologic protection, shelf life, sensorial characteristics (such as taste and crustiness), and performance of industrial processes, so these functional roles must be carefully considered in food reformulation [37]. Most food categories have met the PAHO regional targets for sodium reduction, although, considering the most stringent targets, many categories still need further sodium reduction.

Based on the comparison of Brazilian targets and the regional PAHO targets, it is also likely that the list of regional targets should be expanded and the existing inaugural targets may also need to be updated in order to advance in sodium reduction in the Americas.

These results contribute to the building of knowledge on voluntary and regulatory approaches to sodium reduction in packaged foods, such as the adoption of regulatory sodium targets by Argentina [38] and South Africa [24], while voluntary agreements with food industries have been adopted more frequently, based on successful experiences such as the one in the United Kingdom [38].

A key strength of this study is the completeness of data collection through accurate, updated and representative nutritional composition data and collection in food company websites. These data sources also allow systematic rounds of data collection for new assessments, including the introduction of new lower-sodium products and the discontinuity of other high-sodium products.

Our study also had several weaknesses. Firstly, food categories that had targets set after 2014 (meat products and soups) could not be included in this analysis because they did not complete two biannual rounds of data collection. Secondly, data collection and analysis only encompassed the products of companies that belonged to the Brazilian Association of Food Industries (ABIA) and did not include breads, cakes and other products from bakeries. Thirdly, we were also unable to assess food composition data using additional sources such as laboratory analysis, so the integrity of our nutritional data depended on the accuracy of food label information and the completeness and regular update of food product information on food company websites. Administrative reports by the National Health Surveillance Agency (ANVISA) suggest that food label information is generally accurate and reliable. Fourthly, all analyzes are based on simple means of sodium content, which do not consider the market share of each product. Sales-adjusted means, as used in Canada, the United States and the United Kingdom, express the actual contribution of each product to sodium consumption, although there is a reliance on access to very expensive market databases.

Future studies will allow a more complete understanding of the long-term impacts of voluntary strategies in Brazil, and assess the impact of these reductions on morbidity, mortality and costs of hypertension and cardiovascular disease and subsidized policy improvement. For example, in Argentina modeling studies of sodium reduction scenarios have contributed to the transition from voluntary to regulatory targets for sodium reduction [22].

5. Conclusions

The data here presented provide evidence that the voluntary approach to setting sodium reduction targets in Brazil is leading to a gradual reduction of sodium content in most food categories over time, and that these same monitoring results can be helpful for adjusting targets in the future in order to achieve maximum sodium reductions in 2020 or later. The continuous monitoring process to this point has revealed impacts comparable to regional references as well as the PAHO targets, although stronger enforcement by regulatory targets may be needed in the future with the help of policy-makers, health authorities and civil society in order to reach the overall food market and apply more stringent limits to sodium content in packaged foods.

Author Contributions: Nilson, E.A.F.; Spaniol, A.M.; and Gonçalves, V.S.S. designed the study and conducted the statistical analyses. Nilson, E.A.F. prepared the first draft of the manuscript. All authors were involved in the acquisition and/or interpretation of the data and made critical revisions to the manuscript for important intellectual content. Labbé, M. and Jaime, P.C. contributed material on monitoring approaches. All authors reviewed and approved the final draft.

Conflicts of Interest: All authors declare no conflicts of interest.

References

1. Brown, I.J.; Tzoulaki, I.; Candeias, V.; Elliott, P. Salt Intakes around the World: Implications for Public Health. *Int. J. Epidemiol.* **2009**, *38*, 791–813. Available online: https://academic.oup.com/ije/article-lookup/doi/10.1093/ije/dyp139 (accessed on 30 June 2017). [CrossRef] [PubMed]

2. World Health Organization. *Global Status Report on Noncommunicable Diseases 2014*; WHO: Geneva, Switzerland, 2014; Available online: http://apps.who.int/iris/bitstream/10665/148114/1/9789241564854eng.pdf?ua=1 (accessed on 30 June 2017).

3. Pan American Health Organization. *Salt Smart Americas: A Guide for Country—Level Action*; PAHO: Washington, DC, USA, 2013; Available online: http://www.paho.org/hq/index.php?option=com_docman&task=docdownload&gid=21554&Itemid=270&lang=en (accessed on 30 June 2017).

4. World Health Organization. *Scaling Up Action against Noncommunicable Diseases: How Much Will It Cost?* WHO: Geneva, Switzerland, 2011; Available online: http://whqlibdoc.who.int/publications/2011/9789241502313eng.pdf?ua=1 (accessed on 30 June 2017).

5. Webb, M.; Fahimi, S.; Saman, S.; Gitanjali, M.; Khatibzadeh, S.; Micha, R.; Powles, J. Cost Effectiveness of Government Supported Policy Strategy to Decrease Sodium Intake: Global Analysis across 183 Nations. *BMJ* **2017**, *356*. Available online: http://www.bmj.com/content/356/bmj.i6699.full.pdf (accessed on 30 June 2017). [CrossRef] [PubMed]

6. Ribeiro, L.; Duncan, B.; Brant, L.; Lotufo, P.; Mill, G.; Barreto, S. Cardiovascular Health in Brazil—Trends and Perspectives. *Circulation* **2016**, *133*, 422–433. Available online: http://circ.ahajournals.org/content/133/4/422 (accessed on 30 June 2017).

7. Ministério da Saúde. Saúde Brasil 2014. 2015. Available online: http://bvsms.saude.gov.br/bvs/publicacoes/saude_brasil_2014_analise_situacao.pdf (accessed on 30 June 2017).

8. Vigitel Brazil 2016: Surveillance of Risk and Protective Factors for Chronic Diseases by Telephone Survey: Estimates of Sociodemographic Frequency and Distribution of Risk and Protective Factors for Chronic Diseases in the Capitals of the 26 Brazilian States and the Federal District in 2016. 2017. Available online: http://portalsaude.saude.gov.br/images/pdf/2017/junho/07/vigitel_2016_jun17.pdf (accessed on 30 June 2017).

9. Ministério da Saúde. Plano de Ações Estratégicas Para o Enfrentamento Das Doenças Crônicas Não Transmissíveis (DCNT) no Brasil. 2011–2022. 2011. Available online: http://bvsms.saude.gov.br/bvs/publicacoes/plano_acoes_enfrent_dcnt_2011.pdf (accessed on 30 June 2017).

10. Louzada, M.L.C.; Martins, A.P.B.; Canella, D.S.; Baraldi, L.G.; Levy, R.B.; Claro, R.M.; Moubarac, J.C.; Cannon, G.; Monteiro, C.A. Alimentos Ultraprocessados e Perfil Nutricional da Dieta no Brasil. *Rev. Saúde Pública* **2015**, *49*. Available online: http://www.scielo.br/pdf/rsp/v49/0034-8910-rsp-S0034-89102015049006132.pdf (accessed on 30 June 2017).

11. Sarno, F.; Claro, R.M.; Levy, R.B.; Bandoni, D.H.; Monteiro, C.A. Estimated Sodium Intake for the Brazilian Population, 2008–2009. *Rev. Saude Publica* **2013**, *47*, 571–578. Available online: http://www.scielo.br/pdf/rsp/v47n3/en_0034-8910-rsp-47-03-0571.pdf (accessed on 30 June 2017). [CrossRef] [PubMed]

12. Martins, C.; De Sousa, A.; Veiros, M.; González-Chica, D.; Proença, R. Sodium Content and Labelling of Processed and Ultra-Processed Food Products Marketed in Brazil. *Public Health Nutr.* **2015**, *18*, 1206–1214. Available online: https://www.cambridge.org/core/services/aop-cambridge-core/content/view/5B78C17E59B2227DE7870981139A15DC/S1368980014001736a.pdf/sodium_content_and_labelling_of_processed_and_ultraprocessed_food_products_marketed_in_brazil.pdf (accessed on 30 June 2017). [CrossRef] [PubMed]

13. Rodrigues, V.M.; Rayner, M.; Fernandes, A.C.; de Oliveira, R.C.; Proença, R.P.C.; Fiates, G.M.R. Comparison of the Nutritional Content of Products, with and without Nutrient Claims, Targeted at Children in Brazil. *Br. J. Nutr.* **2016**, *115*, 2047–2056. Available online: http://nuppre.ufsc.br/files/2014/04/2016-Rodrigues-et-al.-Comparison-of-the-nutritional-content-of-products-with-and-without-nutrient-claims.pdf (accessed on 30 June 2017). [CrossRef] [PubMed]

14. Instituto Brasileiro de Geografia e Estatistica. Pesquisa de Orçamentos Familiares 2008–2009—Análise do Consumo Alimentar Pessoal. 2011. Available online: http://biblioteca.ibge.gov.br/visualizacao/livros/liv50063.pdf (accessed on 30 June 2017).

15. Oliveira, M.M.; Malta, D.C.; Santos, M.A.S.; Oliveira, T.P.; Nilson, E.A.F.; Claro, R.M. Self-Reported High Salt Intake in Adults: Data from the National Health Survey, Brazil, 2013. Epidemiol. *Serv. Saúde* **2015**, *24*, 249–256. Available online: http://www.scielo.br/pdf/ress/v24n2/en_2237-9622-ress-24-02-00249.pdf (accessed on 30 June 2017).

16. Hyseni, L.; Elliot-Green, A.; Lloyd-Williams, F.; Kypridemos, C.; O'Flaherty, M.; McGill, R.; Orton, L.; Bromley, H.; Cappuccio, F.P. Systematic Review of Dietary Salt Reduction Policies: Evidence for An Effectiveness Hierarchy? *PLoS ONE* **2017**, *12*. Available online: https://www.ncbi.nlm.nih.gov/pmc/articles/PMC5436672/pdf/pone.0177535.pdf (accessed on 30 June 2017). [CrossRef] [PubMed]

17. Hope, S.F.; Webster, J.; Trieu, K.; Pillay, A.; Ieremia, M.; Bell, C.; Moodie, M. A systematic review of economic evaluations of population-based sodium reduction interventions. *PLoS ONE* **2017**, *12*. Available online: https://www.ncbi.nlm.nih.gov/pmc/articles/PMC5371286/pdf/pone.0173600.pdf (accessed on 30 June 2017). [CrossRef] [PubMed]

18. Webster, J.; Trieu, K.; Dunford, E.; Hawkes, C. Target Salt 2025: A Global Overview of National Programs to Encourage the Food Industry to Reduce Salt in Foods. *Nutrients* **2014**, *6*, 3274–3287. Available online: https://www.ncbi.nlm.nih.gov/pmc/articles/PMC4145308/pdf/nutrients-06-03274.pdf (accessed on 30 June 2017). [CrossRef] [PubMed]

19. Campbell, N.; Legowski, B.; Legetic, B.; Ferrante, D.; Nilson, E.; Campbell, C.; L'Abbé, M. Targets and Timelines for Reducing Salt in Processed Food in the Americas. *J. Clin. Hypertens.* **2014**, *16*, 619–623. Available online: http://onlinelibrary.wiley.com/doi/10.1111/jch.12379/full (accessed on 30 June 2017). [CrossRef] [PubMed]

20. Wyness, L.A.; Butriss, J.L.; Stanner, S.A. Reducing the Population's Sodium Intake: The UK Food Standards Agency's Salt Reduction Programme. *Public Health Nutr.* **2011**, *15*, 254–261. Available online: https://www.cambridge.org/core/services/aop-cambridge-core/content/view/9289C9978849B50578E974F1F6BEA01E/S1368980011000966a.pdf/reducing-the-population-s-sodium-intake-the-uk-food-standards-agency-s-salt-reduction-programme.pdf (accessed on 30 June 2017). [CrossRef] [PubMed]

21. Trevena, H.; Neal, B.; Dunford, E.; Wu, J.H. An Evaluation of the Effects of the Australian Food and Health Dialogue Targets on the Sodium Content of Bread, Breakfast Cereals and Processed Meats. *Nutrients* **2014**, *6*, 3802–3817. Available online: http://www.mdpi.com/resolver?pii=nu6093802 (accessed on 30 June 2017). [CrossRef] [PubMed]

22. Zganiacz, F.; Wills, R.B.H.; Mukhopadhyay, S.P.; Arcot, J.; Greenfield, H. Changes in the Sodium Content of Australian Processed Foods between 1980 and 2013 Using Analytical Data. *Nutrients* **2017**, *9*. Available online: http://www.mdpi.com/resolver?pii=nu9050501 (accessed on 30 June 2017). [CrossRef] [PubMed]

23. Allemandi, L.; Tiscornia, M.V.; Ponce, M.; Castrouovo, L.; Dunford, E. Sodium content in processed foods in Argentina: Compliance with the national law. *Cardiovasc. Diagn. Ther.* **2015**, *5*, 197–206. Available online: https://www.ncbi.nlm.nih.gov/pmc/articles/PMC4451319/pdf/cdt-05-03-197.pdf (accessed on 30 June 2017). [PubMed]

24. Peters, S.; Dunford, E.; Ware, L.; Harris, T.; Walker, A.; Wicks, M.; Van Zyl, T.; Swanepoel, B.; Charlton, K.; Woodward, M.; et al. The Sodium Content of Processed Foods in South Africa during the Introduction of Mandatory Sodium Limits. *Nutrients* **2017**, *9*. Available online: http://www.mdpi.com/2072-6643/9/4/404/pdf (accessed on 30 June 2017). [CrossRef] [PubMed]

25. Nilson, E.A.F. The Strides to Reduce Salt Intake in Brazil: Have We Done Enough? *Cardiovasc. Diagn. Ther.* **2015**, *5*, 243–247. Available online: https://www.ncbi.nlm.nih.gov/pmc/articles/PMC4451315/pdf/cdt-05-03-243.pdf (accessed on 30 June 2017). [PubMed]

26. Brasil. Dietary Guidelines for the Brazilian Population. 2014. Available online: http://189.28.128.100/dab/docs/portaldab/publicacoes/guia_alimentar_populacao_ingles.pdf (accessed on 30 June 2017).

27. Nilson, E.A.F.; Jaime, P.C.; Resende, D.O. Iniciativas Desenvolvidas no Brasil Para a Redução do Teor de Sódio em Alimentos Processados. *Rev. Panam. Salud Pública* **2012**, *32*, 287–292. Available online: http://www.scielosp.org/pdf/rpsp/v32n4/en_07.pdf (accessed on 30 June 2017). [CrossRef] [PubMed]

28. Instituto Brasileiro de Geografia e Estatística. Pesquisa de Orçamentos Familiares 2008–2009—Aquisição Domiciliar Per Capita. Brasil, 2010. Available online: http://biblioteca.ibge.gov.br/visualizacao/livros/liv47307.pdf (accessed on 30 June 2017).

29. Campbell, N.; Legowski, B.; Legetic, B.; Nilson, E.; L'Abbé, M. Inaugural Maximum Values for Sodium in Processed Food Products in the Americas. *J. Clin. Hypertens.* **2015**, *17*, 611–613. Available online: http://onlinelibrary.wiley.com/doi/10.1111/jch.12553/full (accessed on 30 June 2017). [CrossRef] [PubMed]

30. Brasil. Ministério da Saúde. Termo de Compromisso com a Finalidade de Estabelecer Metas Nacionais Para a Redução do Teor de Sódio em Alimentos Processados no Brasil. Brasília, 2011. Available online: http://189.28.128.100/dab/docs/portaldab/documentos/termo_abia_abip_abima_abitrigo_2011.pdf (accessed on 30 June 2017).

31. Brasil. Ministério da Saúde. Termo de Compromisso com a Finalidade de Estabelecer Metas Nacionais Para a Redução do Teor de Sódio em Alimentos Processados no Brasil. Brasília, 2011. Available online: http://189.28.128.100/dab/docs/portaldab/documentos/termo_5_dez_2011.pdf (accessed on 30 June 2017).

32. Brasil. Ministério da Saúde. Termo de Compromisso com a Finalidade de Estabelecer Metas Nacionais Para a Redução do Teor de Sódio em Alimentos Processados no Brasil. Brasília, 2012. Available online: http://189.28.128.100/dab/docs/portaldab/documentos/termo_6_ago_2012.pdf (accessed on 30 June 2017).

33. Brasil. Ministério da Saúde. Termo de Compromisso com a Finalidade de Estabelecer Metas Nacionais Para a Redução do Teor de Sódio em Alimentos Processados no Brasil. Brasília, 2013. Available online: http://189.28.128.100/dab/docs/portaldab/documentos/termo_nov_2013.pdf (accessed on 30 June 2017).

34. De Moura Souza, A.; Nalin de Souza, B.; Bezerra, I.N.; Sichieri, R. The Impact of the Reduction of Sodium Content in Processed Foods in Salt Intake in Brazil. *Cad. Saúde Pública* **2016**, *32*, 1–7. Available online: http://www.scielo.br/pdf/csp/v32n2/en_0102-311x-csp-0102-311x00064615.pdf (accessed on 30 June 2017).

35. Nilson, E.A.F.; Spaniol, A.M.; Gonçalves, V.S.S. A Redução do Consumo de Sódio no Brasil. *Cad Saúde Pública* **2016**, *32*. Available online: http://www.scielosp.org/pdf/csp/v32n11/1678-4464-csp-32-11-e00102016.pdf (accessed on 30 June 2017). [CrossRef] [PubMed]

36. Combet, E.; Vlassopoulos, A.; Mölenberg, F.; Gressier, M.; Privet, L.; Wratten, C.; Sharif, S.; Vieux, F.; Lehmann, U.; Masset, G. Testing the Capacity of a Multi-Nutrient Profiling System to Guide Food and Beverage Reformulation: Results from Five National Food Composition Databases. *Nutrients* **2017**, *9*. Available online: https://www.ncbi.nlm.nih.gov/pmc/articles/PMC5409745/pdf/nutrients-09-00406.pdf (accessed on 30 June 2017). [CrossRef] [PubMed]

37. Konfino, J.; Mekonnen, T.A.; Coxson, P.G.; Ferrante, D.; Bibbins-Domingo. Projected Impact of a Sodium Consumption Reduction Initiative in Argentina: An Analysis from the CVD Policy Model—Argentina. *PLoS ONE* **2013**, *8*. Available online: http://journals.plos.org/plosone/article/file?id=10.1371/journal.pone.0073824&type=printable (accessed on 30 June 2017). [CrossRef] [PubMed]

38. Collins, M.; Mason, H.; O'Flaherty, M.; Guzman-Castillo, M.; Critchley, J.; Capewell, S. An Economic Evaluation of Salt Reduction Policies to Reduce Coronary Disease in England: A Policy Modeling Study. *Value Health* **2014**, *17*, 517–524. Available online: http://www.valueinhealthjournal.com/article/S1098-301501828-2/pdf (accessed on 30 June 2017). [CrossRef] [PubMed]

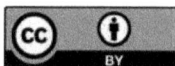

nutrients

MDPI

Article

Salt Reductions in Some Foods in The Netherlands: Monitoring of Food Composition and Salt Intake

Elisabeth H. M. Temme *, Marieke A. H. Hendriksen, Ivon E. J. Milder, Ido B. Toxopeus, Susanne Westenbrink, Henny A. M. Brants and Daphne L. van der A

National Institute for Public Health and the Environment (RIVM), 3720 BA Bilthoven, The Netherlands; Marieke.Hendriksen@rivm.nl (M.A.H.H.); Ivon.Milder@rivm.nl (I.E.J.M.); Ido.Toxopeus@rivm.nl (I.B.T.); Susanne.Westenbrink@rivm.nl (S.W.); Henny.Brants@rivm.nl (H.A.M.B.); Daphne.van.der.A@rivm.nl (D.L.v.d.A.)
* Correspondence: Liesbeth.Temme@RIVM.nl; Tel.: +31-30-274-2967

Received: 15 June 2017; Accepted: 19 July 2017; Published: 22 July 2017

Abstract: Background and objectives. High salt intake increases blood pressure and thereby the risk of chronic diseases. Food reformulation (or food product improvement) may lower the dietary intake of salt. This study describes the changes in salt contents of foods in the Dutch market over a five-year period (2011–2016) and differences in estimated salt intake over a 10-year period (2006–2015). Methods. To assess the salt contents of foods; we obtained recent data from chemical analyses and from food labels. Salt content of these foods in 2016 was compared to salt contents in the 2011 version Dutch Food Composition Database (NEVO, version 2011), and statistically tested with General Linear Models. To estimate the daily dietary salt intake in 2006, 2010, and 2015, men and women aged 19 to 70 years were recruited through random population sampling in Doetinchem, a small town located in a rural area in the eastern part of the Netherlands. The characteristics of the study population were in 2006: n = 317, mean age 49 years, 43% men, in 2010: n = 342, mean age 46 years, 45% men, and in 2015: n = 289, mean age 46 years, 47% men. Sodium and potassium excretion was measured in a single 24-h urine sample. All estimates were converted to a common metric: salt intake in grams per day by multiplication of sodium with a factor of 2.54. Results. In 2016 compared to 2011, the salt content in certain types of bread was on average 19 percent lower and certain types of sauce, soup, canned vegetables and legumes, and crisps had a 12 to 26 percent lower salt content. Salt content in other types of foods had not changed significantly. Between 2006, 2010 and 2015 the estimated salt intake among adults in Doetinchem remained unchanged. In 2015, the median estimated salt intake was 9.7 g per day for men and 7.4 g per day for women. As in 2006 and 2010, the estimated salt intake in 2015 exceeded the recommended maximum intake of 6 g per day set by the Dutch Health Council. Conclusion. In the Netherlands, the salt content of bread, certain sauces, soups, potato crisps, and processed legumes and vegetables have been reduced over the period 2011–2016. However, median salt intake in 2006 and 2015 remained well above the recommended intake of 6 g.

Keywords: sodium; salt; food reformulation; food composition; nutritional status; 24 h urine

---

1. Introduction

Dietary factors such as the intake of sodium (salt) and saturated fatty acids, and the related risk factors of a high systolic blood pressure are among the leading causes of non-communicable disease [1]. The World Health Organization (WHO) Member States have agreed on a voluntary global noncommunicable diseases (NCD) target for a 30% relative reduction in mean population intake of salt, with the aim of achieving a target of less than 5 g per day (approximately 2 g sodium) by 2025 [2]. The Dutch Health Council advises a maximum intake of 6 g (2.4 g sodium) per day [3]. Intake of salt in the Netherlands and most developed countries is well above these recommended intakes [4–7].

Major sources of salt are bread, cheese, meat and meat products (including meat cold cuts), savoury snacks, sauces, soups, and pastries [5,8,9]. Reformulation of these types of foods to reduce salt contents (or food product improvement/reformulation) is considered a promising strategy for lowering the dietary intake of salt [10]. To decrease salt intake of a certain population, large-scale structural efforts are needed to lower the salt content of food products at the time of production, as well as to initiate behavioural changes [11–13]. The WHO encourages a multisector approach, including partnerships between the public and private sectors to improve the composition of the food supply [10].

In the Netherlands, several initiatives focus on food product improvement related to salt (see Figure 1). The Federation of the Dutch Food and Grocery Industry initiated a Taskforce Salt Reduction in 2007. This taskforce, which included, e.g., producers of sauces and soups, cheese, snacks, and pastries, aimed at a reduction of salt levels in processed foods of 12% before 2010 [14]. The Dutch bakery sector has been an active player in the field of salt reduction via regulations laid down in the commodities act. The maximum level of salt in bread gradually decreased over the last decade [15]. In 2009, the maximum salt content per 100 g dry matter was 2.5%, in 2011 2.1%, and in 2012 1.9%. The latest amendment to the maximum level was on 1 January, 2013, at 1.8% per 100 g dry matter. Based on an average dry matter content of 64%, this is approximately 1.15 g per 100 g of bread (454 mg of sodium). Monitoring reports of the sector using analytical methods showed the expected reductions in salt contents of bread [16,17]. In 2014, the Agreement on Improvement of Product Composition: salt, saturated fat, and sugar (calories) was signed with four food sector parties under the supervision of the Dutch Ministry of Health, Welfare and Sport [18]. In this public-private agreement, several stakeholders involved in food production, hospitality, catering and retail were represented. Signing parties voluntarily agreed on a gradual reduction of the levels of salt, (saturated) fat and energy (from sugar and fat) in foods up to 2020. For salt, the ultimate goal is to reduce salt intake to 6 g/day by 2020, for diets complying with healthy dietary guidelines.

The National Institute of Public Health and the Environment (RIVM) is commissioned by the Ministry of Health, Welfare and Sport to monitor the changes in nutrient composition of foods sold in retail [8,19], as well as to monitor the effects on the intake in the population. Effects on daily dietary salt intake can be assessed by measuring salt excretion in 24 h urine. Estimation of salt intake from 24 h urinary sodium excretion is a more reliable method than dietary assessment because of the highly variable sodium content in recipes and the difficulty to quantify discretionary salt used in cooking and at the table.

This study has two objectives. First, it describes salt contents of foods in the Dutch market over a 5-year period (2011–2016) and secondly it reports on the results of monitoring salt intake in the Dutch population over a 10-year period (2006–2015 using 24 h urine collections).

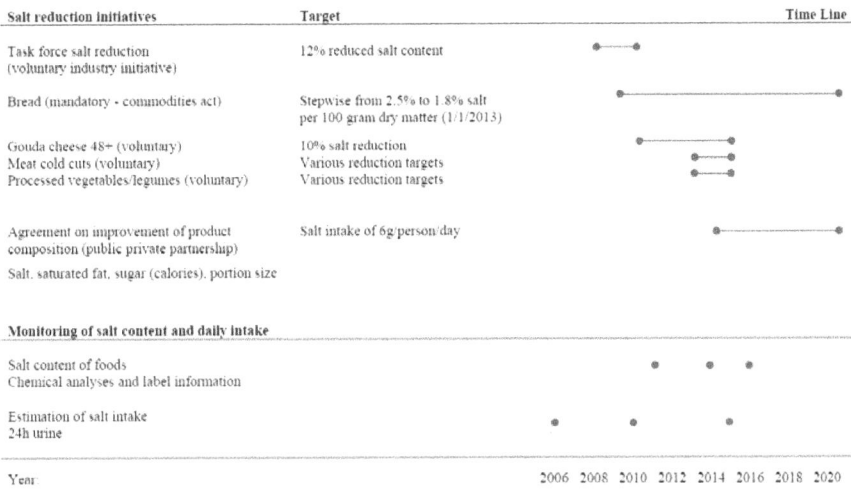

Figure 1. Overview of salt reduction targets and monitoring.

2. Materials and Methods

2.1. Evaluation of Salt Content of Foods

In this study, we evaluated the current salt content of foods compared to a reference. Food composition as provided in the Dutch Food Composition Database (NEVO, version 2011; [20]) was taken as a reference. New food composition data were collected until the end of June 2016. The average salt contents (as well as concentrations of saturated fatty acids and mono-and disaccharides) were calculated. Sodium levels (in grams) were multiplied by 2.54 to calculate the salt contents of foods (in grams). Salt contents include both naturally occurring as well as added salt. Two analyses were performed to evaluate the salt contents: one on the main food categories, and one on the foods with set salt maximum levels as defined in the Agreement on Improvement of Product Composition. This was done to evaluate whether achieved reductions for specific foods under the agreement also led to lower salt concentrations in the overall food category.

2.1.1. Selecting Major Processed Foods Contributing to Salt Intake

The major processed foods contributors to dietary salt intake were selected based on the salt content available in the Dutch Food Composition Database (NEVO), combined with consumed quantities of foods from the national Food Consumption Survey [5].

We included:

- Foods that can be reformulated for their salt content. For example, the food group "milk products" is excluded from the salt analyses, because the foods in this group do not contain added salt, and thus reformulation for salt is not feasible.
- Food groups that contributed at least 3% and food subgroups that contributed at least 0.5% to the daily intake of salt intake according to the Dutch National Food Consumption Survey for 7–69 year-olds (DNFCS 2007−2010); [5] and/or foods with a set maximum level for salt [21].
- Food groups with at least 10 comparable foods in the newly collected food composition data.

The food composition was compared for foods categorized in food groups. The food group categorization used consisted up to five hierarchical levels. The food group classification was based on the food group classification used in the Dutch food-based dietary guidelines (in Dutch: Wheel of Five in 2011) [22]. After consultation with the food industry, modifications were made to improve correspondence with food group classifications used by the food industry.

Foods were classified into food groups based on name and nutritional values by experienced dieticians.

The Dutch Food Composition Database (NEVO, version 2011; [20]) provided the reference values for the current comparison. The Dutch food composition database contains data, on an aggregated level, on the composition of foods and dishes eaten frequently by the Dutch population (based on the National Food Consumption Survey) and of major foods of importance for energy and/or selected nutrients. It provides food composition data for generic foods when possible. This means that data from comparable foods (for instance semi-skimmed milk of various brands) is aggregated to give a weighted mean value for the generic food (for instance 'semi-skimmed milk'). When aggregation is not possible, for instance for fortified foods, or foods listed under their brand name, the aggregated nutrient values are derived from chemical analyses, from label information, from recipe calculations, or other sources. For the reference dataset, we used (aggregated) nutrient values only when derived from (chemical) analyses and/or information obtained from the manufacturer. For food groups for which the food composition database contained insufficient data to construct a reference value, data were supplemented with data from the Innova database [23]. The Innova database contains label information on new foods on the market. A login account is needed to access the database.

2.1.2. Salt Content of Selected Processed Foods; New Data Collection and Selection

The salt contents referred to the unprepared products as sold; with the exception of some instant soups and instant sauces (sold as a dried powder). Thus, salt added during (home) preparation as well as at the table was not taken into account. For soups and sauces sold as dried powder, the salt content was calculated using the standard method of preparation.

New data collection took place until 1 July 2016. Data were mainly obtained from two sources, chemical analytical data by the Dutch Food Safety Authority (NVWA) and label information from the Food Label Database [24]. In addition, the Dutch Bakery Association provided chemical analytical data.

The NVWA carries out chemical analyses of salt in various foods. For this monitoring study commonly eaten foods were sampled (in total n = 1108 samples) in several major supermarkets (including private and national supermarket brands). The NVWA supplied data on for bread (n = 88), savoury snacks (n = 197), sauces (n = 88), soups (n = 102), confectionary and bakery ware (n = 92) and processed vegetables and legumes (n = 106) in 2015 [25]. In 2016 [26,27], salt contents of meats (n = 247), cheese (n = 98), sauces (including ketchup, curry and pasta sauces) (n = 10), and ready meals (n = 80) were sampled. Sodium contents were analysed by flame emission spectroscopy. For analysis, 350 mg ± 10 mg homogenized sample was weighed in a quartz vial insert. Three millilitres of nitric acid were added and the quartz vial was weighed without the cover (mass A). Then, the quartz insert keg was placed in a pressure vessel with 6 mL of 12.5% H_2O_2 solution. The pressure vessel was placed in a microwave with a PC-controlled temperature program (model Ethos one; Milestone Inc., Shelton, CT, USA) and digested according to the following program: 0 min, 20 °C; 0–15 min, 20–200 °C; 15–40 min, 200 °C; 40–60 min, 200–20 °C. The quartz insert keg was taken out of the pressure vessel by tweezers, cooled down by rinsing the outside with demineralised water, and dried with a tissue. Subsequently, the quartz keg was weighed and brought to mass A again with nitric acid. The digested sample was quantitatively transferred to a 50 mL plastic tube and made up to a final weight of 51.30 g (±0.05 g) with demineralised water. Two millilitres of the resulting solution was transferred to a plastic tube, diluted 10-fold with 18 mL of demineralised water, and thoroughly mixed prior to analysis. The solution was further diluted with a 0.39% nitric acid solution if necessary. Sodium was analysed by a flame photometer (Model 420 Flame Photometer; Sherwood Scientific Ltd., Cambridge, UK) with a propane/butane flame at a wavelength of 589 nm. Prior to analysis, the spectrophotometer was stabilized for 30 min with demineralised water. A calibration curve was built in the range 0.00–5.00 mg L^{-1} (six standard solutions). A 0.39% nitric acid solution was used as blank. The method was validated according to standard ISO 17025 guidelines with the following certified reference materials: LGC 7103 (sweet biscuits) and BCR 063R (skimmed milk powder). The method of performance characteristics were as follows: Recovery values: 102.1% for biscuits and 92.8% for skimmed milk powder; coefficient of variation of repeatability (RSDr): 3.0% for sweet biscuits and 0.4% for skimmed milk powder. Limit of detection (LOD): 0.23 g kg^{-1}; limit of quantification (LOQ): 0.46 g kg^{-1}. For the calculation of sodium chloride content, the amount of sodium was multiplied by 2.541×10^{-4} and the sodium chloride was expressed as g NaCl 100 g^{-1} (NaCl%). A single measurement was carried out in each sample.

The Dutch Bakery Association [16] supplied data from the seventh nationwide sample of bread, the average salt content in whole wheat bread (average of 93 breads), brown wheat bread (average of 91 breads), multi-grain bread (average of 91 breads), soft white bread buns (average of 48 buns), and soft brown bread buns (average of 19 buns). The average contents were weighted for the share industrial and artisan bread (80/20%).

New data label data was extracted from the Food Label Database [24] ($n = 3524$) (not open access) provided that the following criteria were met:

-	The name and/or description of the food was clear enough to allow categorization (based on expert judgement).
-	The food was aimed at individual consumers (contrary to foods for catering, clinical use, and bulk-sales).
-	Foods were unique (identical foods with different packaging size were included only once).
-	Data was available for on the amount of salt and/or sodium in the food.

To assess the (non)representativeness of the new data for main brands, the presence of supermarket and/or major private brands were evaluated and reported in the Table 1 To be assigned as not representative for supermarket brands (superscript a in Table 1) less than half of the major supermarkets brands (Albert Heijn, Jumbo, Aldi, Lidl, Plus, as well as at least one other supermarket brand within the Superunie purchasing organization (besides Plus) were available in the underlying data. To assess the main private brands within a food category, we listed the (up to 10) most commonly reported brands (excluding the supermarket brands) based on the national food consumption survey [5]. Presence in less than half of the intended brands was interpreted as an indication that the newly submitted data were not representative (in addition to the supermarket brands) of the product range within the relevant food category (superscript b in Table 1).

2.1.3. Statistical Analyses

For each included food group (see Table 1), as well as for foods with maximum set salt levels (see Table 2), we calculated the mean salt level, and their standard deviation. The mean values were compared in an analysis of variance ($p < 0.05$). When a significant difference was found post-hoc, least squares means tests were done. All analyses were performed for men and women separately. In addition, the analyses were adjusted for age, education, and day of the week (because of overrepresentation of weekend days).

All statistical analyses were performed with the GLM procedure in SAS 9.3®, SAS Institute Inc., Cary, NC, USA.

2.2. Estimation of Salt Intake Via 24 h Urinary Sodium Excretion

2.2.1. Study Population, Recruitment

In 2006, 2010 and 2015, monitoring surveys were carried out among adults aged 19−70 years in Doetinchem, a town in the eastern part of the Netherlands. The methodology of the surveys in 2006 and 2010 has been previously described in detail [4]. In 2015, a similar methodology was used.

In short, participants aged 50–70 years were recruited from an ongoing long-term monitoring study on chronic disease factors (Doetinchem Cohort Study; DCS)., and participants aged 19–49 years were recruited from the municipal register of Doetinchem (General Doetinchem Population Sample (GDPS)). Those participating in 2006 or 2010 were not invited to take part in the 2015 survey, to ensure independent study samples. Invitations were sent to a random sample of the populations, stratified for age. We aimed for equal sample size as in 2010 (n = 350) [4]. The current study was designed to detect a difference of at least 0.8 g (or 8%) in daily salt intake between 2015 and 2010, with 350 volunteers. Based on the response rates in 2010 (16% for the GDPS and 62% for the DCS) and power calculations, an estimation was made on the total number individuals needed to invite. For the random sample from the GDPS, depending on the age category, we expected a response rate between 5% and 20%. And for the random sample from the DCS, we expected a response rate between 30% and 65%.

In 2015, a total number of 2041 individuals were invited to participate (n = 1700 aged 19–49 years randomly drawn from the municipal register of Doetinchem, the general Doetinchem population sample (GDPS) and n = 341 aged 50–70 years from the Doetinchem cohort study (DCS)). The positive response rate (meaning those willing to participate) was 13% among individuals from the GDPS (n = 226) and 52% among DCS participants (n = 176). All 402 individuals were invited for one of the instruction meetings during the 3 weeks fieldwork in November 2015. Of those, 333 participants took part in a meeting and started 24-h collection. In total, 328 participants completed the study and handed in their 24-h urine jars at the study center. Upon collection of the jars, 3 individuals appeared to have misinterpreted the protocol (collected multiple days instead of 24-h) and were subsequently excluded from the study population. Furthermore, another 33 participants were excluded due to missing or over-collection of one urine void (based on recorded time of start and finish and completeness in a diary) and one person was excluded due to chronic kidney disease (self-reported in the questionnaire). Finally, two participants were excluded based on creatinine levels, resulting in a total number of 289 participants in the final study population. With this actual sample size of 289 participants, the difference in daily salt intake must have been around 1 g per day to be detected with 80% power.

The study was conducted according to the guidelines laid down in the Declaration of Helsinki. The study protocol was presented to the Medical Ethics Committee of the University Medical Centre Utrecht (15-447/C), who the decided a formal approval was not needed because of the non-invasive character of the study. Written informed consent was obtained from all participants. Participants received a gift voucher (of 30 €) for completing the study.

2.2.2. 24 hr Urine Collection and Assessment of Use of Discretionary Salt

Single 24 h urine collection took place in November 2015 and was performed using the same protocols and procedures as in 2006 and 2010. Participants were provided detailed written and oral instructions at the Municipal Health Centre in Doetinchem by trained researchers. Participants reported the time of start and finish of urine collection, as well as the completeness of the collection in a diary. In addition, a short questionnaire was administered, amongst others, to assess the use of discretionary salt (yes/no) in the week before the collection.

Urinary sodium and creatinine concentration (mmol/L) was determined in each specimen by indirect potentiometry using the Synchron LX system [28,29]. The concentrations (in mmol/L) were multiplied by the total volume of urine to estimate excretion in mmol/day. Conversion from sodium and creatinine in mmol/day to g/day was made by multiplying with the molar mass (Na = 23 g/mol; creatinine = 113 g/mol).

2.2.3. Statistical Analyses

Intake of sodium was calculated by multiplying the excretion with the factor 100/95, which reflects the estimated proportion of intake that is excreted via urine. Sodium intake was converted to salt intake by multiplication with a factor of 2.54.

Incomplete samples, defined as having creatinine excretion ≤5.0 mmol/day or ≤6.0 mmol/day both together with a urine volume of <1 L, and reported missing or overcollection of more than one urine void, were excluded from the analyses ($n = 38$), as well as one subject with chronic kidney disease.

Differences in salt intake between 2006, 2010 and 2015 were assessed by linear regression (using PROC MIXED in SAS 9.3®, SAS Institute Inc., Cary, NC, USA,), correcting for age, education and day of the week.

3. Results

3.1. Selecting Major Processed Foods Contributing to Salt Intake

Food groups that contributed at least 3% to salt intake and that can be reformulated were included: bread and cereal products, cheese, meat cold cuts and meat (preparations), savoury snacks, sauces, soups, and confectionary and bakery wares (see Figure 2). Together the selected food groups contributed 59% to daily salt intake.

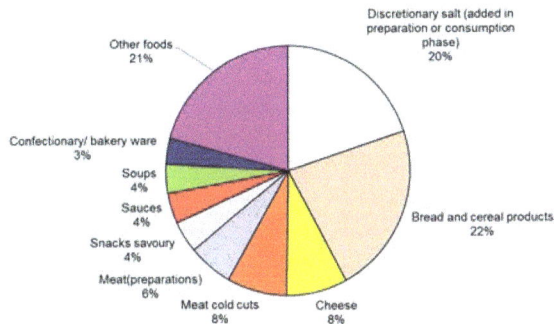

Figure 2. Food groups contributing to salt intake (including discretionary salt) in the Netherlands, food groups contributing more than 3% are included in this study.

3.2. Salt Content of Selected Processed Foods

Salt content of the selected food groups are shown in Table 1 comparing the new 2016 data to the reference in 2011. Table 2 shows the foods with maximum salt levels as set under the agreement of food product improvement and the percentages of compliant foods. Table 3 shows the salt content of foods with maximum salt levels.

The average salt content of "bread" in 2016 was 19% lower than in 2011 ($p < 0.05$; Table 1). From 2011 to 2013, the salt content of "bread" already declined, but since 2013, no further reduction was observed. The salt content of other types of "bread" or "bread replacements" or "breakfast cereal" in 2016 was not significantly different from 2011. The new data for "bread replacements" or "breakfast cereal" however were judged as not representative for major brands.

"Cheese (semi hard and hard-Gouda type)" and "cheese, melted and spreadable" contained less salt in 2016 compared to 2011 (respectively −9%, −13%). However, the differences were not statistically significant. In "meat cold cuts", in the main underlying subgroups and in "meat preparations" (such as bratwurst, roulades, burger and roast) salt contents in 2016 were not statistically different from 2011. In some selected "meat cold cuts" with set maximum salt levels, lower salt contents were observed. However, none of the changes were statistically significant. In "bacon" and other "meat cold cuts single prepared" (such as ham), the average salt content was respectively 12% and 6% lower in 2016 compared to contents in 2011 (see in Table 3). For "meat products composed prepared" (such as luncheon meat) the salt content was 5% lower, for "filet American" 21% lower. On the other hand for the other "Other cold meats composed raw smoked/dried", it was 5% higher compared to contents in 2011. Overall, 90% of "meat cold cuts" complied with agreed maximum salt levels (see in Table 2). Within the "savoury snacks" food group, salt contents did not change except for the subgroup "cut potato crisps". The salt content in this subgroup was 26% lower than in 2011 ($p < 0.05$).

In two of the five subgroups within the food category "sauces", salt contents were significantly lower. The salt content of "meal sauces on tomatoes/vegetables base" was 15% lower and "meal sauces with a binder" was 19% lower compared to contents in 2011. Although, the data for the latter were judged as not representative for major brands. For "pasta sauces", "ketchup" and "curry ketchup" maximum salt levels were formulated to be achieved in 2016. "Pasta sauces" contained 15% less salt and "ketchup" 41% less salt compared to 2011 (both $p < 0.05$). For another type of ketchup "curry ketchup", there was no change in the salt content, although 93% of this type of ketchup complies with current targets (Table 2). The salt content of the "soups sold as liquid" was statistically significantly lower (by 12%) in the newly submitted data compared to 2011. There was no statistically significant change observed in the salt content of "soups instant" (composition as prepared). For the entire group of "soups" (sold as liquid and instant), the salt content was 9% lower compared to 2011 ($p < 0.05$).

"Processed vegetable and legumes" contributed less than 3% to the average daily salt intake. The sector agreed on salt reduction targets. In the subgroup "green peas, carrots, peas/beans and carrots" the salt content was 25% lower than in 2011. This difference was statistically significant. In the group "butter beans, haricots, mushrooms"the salt content was 37% lower than in 2011, but this is not statistically significant. For the processed legumes the average salt content was significantly lower (42%) compared to 2011.

Table 1. Salt contents of foods (g/100 g) in 2016 compared to 2011, main food categories.

Food Group	Reference 2011-Salt Content				New Data 2016-Salt Content			Difference	
	N	Uval	AVG	SD	n	AVG	SD	(%)	
Bread and cereal products									
Bread ◇	25	82	1.29	0.24	194	1.04	0.13	−9%	¥
Bread luxury natural and sweet [b]	11	37	0.97	0.17	41	0.90	0.17	−7%	
Bread replacements [b]	21	2	1.23	0.59	61	1.23	0.60	0%	
Breakfast cereal [b]	24	2	0.60	0.54	76	0.51	0.48	−15%	
Cheese									
Cheese, semi hard and hard ◇	18	26	2.04	0.41	175	1.87	0.40	−9%	
Cheese, melted and spreadable [b]	12	2	1.52	0.52	73	1.33	0.49	−13%	
Meat cold cuts									
Single prepared ◇	13	8	2.54	0.58	153	2.36	0.55	−7%	
Composed prepared ◇	23	7	2.20	0.25	250	2.10	0.33	−5%	
Single raw smoked/dried [b]	5	9	3.92	0.87	44	3.96	1.36	1%	
Composed raw smoked/dried ◇	9	7	3.15	0.58	105	3.04	0.90	−4%	
Meat(preparations)									
Meat preparations unprepared	14	10	1.56	0.62	111	1.83	0.56	18%	
Snacks savoury									
Ragout snack ("kroket" type)	1	6	1.40		53	1.32	0.34	−6%	¥
Snacks savoury with meat	2	5	1.78	0.17	28	1.88	0.35	5%	
Cut potato crisps	8	7	1.75	0.49	37	1.29	0.28	−26%	
Pelleted crisps	9	5	2.18	0.85	91	2.06	0.79	−6%	
Salted biscuits	6	6	2.15	1.20	31	2.22	0.58	3%	
Sauces									
Tomato/vegetable meal sauces *◇	38	7	1.13	0.27	87	0.96	0.41	−15%	¥
Tomato/vegetable based cold sauces ◇	8	3	2.19	0.60	115	1.94	0.84	−11%	
Emulsion based sauces	15	4	1.53	0.37	121	1.40	0.56	−8%	
Sauces, peanut *	10	4	1.70	0.35	16	1.50	0.50	−12%	
Meal sauces with a binder *[b]	40	10	1.35	0.48	36	1.09	0.30	−19%	¥
Soups ◇									
Soups sold as liquid *	48	7	0.89	0.23	109	0.78	0.12	−12%	¥
Soups instant prepared *	28	7	0.90	0.24	52	0.87	0.17	−3%	
Confectionary and bakery ware									
Cakes [b]	4	4	0.79	0.44	51	0.75	0.35	−4%	
Biscuits [b]	28	3	0.57	0.28	24	0.77	0.18	36%	¥
Shortbreads	7	11	0.80	0.28	68	0.60	0.29	−25%	
Pies and pastries (sweet) [b]	9	8	0.44	0.17	70	0.35	0.21	−20%	

N = number of generic foods codes, UVal = average number of underlying values per generic food. n = number of new data points; ¥ Statistically significant difference (p < 0.05) between 2016 and 2011; * Food composition data are supplemented with Innova data on food composition; a: Information of less than 50% of supermarket brands is available in the new data; b: Information of less than 50% of other major brands (excluding supermarket brands) is available in the new data; ◇ Food with salt reduction targets (see Table 2).

Table 2. Foods with maximum salt levels agreed on via Agreement on Improvement of Product Composition.

Food Group	Food with Maximum Salt Targets	Maximum g/100 g	Start and End Date	<Max Salt Level % of Foods
Bread and cereal products			2010–01/01/2013	
Bread	White, brown, wholemeal, multigrain bread; both large and small and baguette	1, 8% ‡		n.a.
Cheese			2010–/12/2015	
Cheese	Gouda cheese 48+	−10% Π		
Meat cold cuts			06/2013–06/2015	90%
Single prepared	Bacon, grilled	2.80		
	Others	2.54		
Composed prepared		2.36		
Composed raw smoked/dried	Filet American	2.25		
	Others	3.20		
Sauces			01/01/2015–30/06/2016	
Tomato/vegetable meal sauces	Sauce for pasta	1.30		96%
Tomato/vegetable based cold sauces	Ketchup	2.49		87%
	Curry ketchup	2.06		93%
Soups			01/01/2015–30/06/2016	
Soups sold as liquid and instant prepared	Soups	0.89		79%
Processed vegetables and legumes			2011–2013	n.a.
Processed vegetables	Peas and/or carrots, bean	0.38		
	Butter beans, haricots, mushrooms	0.46		
Processed legumes	Legumes	0.51		

‡ The maximum 1.8% salt (based on dry matter), with an average bread moisture content of 64% which is around 1.15 g salt per 100 g bread; Π The target for cheese is 10% average reduced salt content, no maximum defined; n.a. not available; and percentage of foods below maximum in 2016 (adapted from reference [27]).

Table 3. Salt contents of foods with salt reduction targets (g/100 g) in 2016 compared to 2011.

Food Group	Food with Maximum Salt Targets	Reference 2011-Salt Content				New Data 2016-Salt			Difference	
		N	Uval	AVG	SD	n	AVG	SD	(%)	
Bread and cereal products										
Bread	White, brown, wholemeal, multigrain bread; both large and small and baguette	19	99	1.27	0.27	161	1.02	0.11	−21%	¥
Cheese										
Cheese	Gouda cheese 48+	7	58	2.09	0.35	80	1.89	0.35	−11%	
Meats cold cuts										
Single prepared	Bacon, grilled	2	3	2.76	1.41	26	2.46	0.83	−12%	¥
	Others	11	9	2.45	0.42	127	2.34	0.47	−6%	
Composed prepared		23	5	2.17	0.25	250	2.10	0.33	−5%	
Composed raw smoked/dried	Filet American	1	13	2.26	0.00	25	1.82	0.32	−21%	
	Others	8	7	3.21	0.51	80	3.42	0.64	5%	
Sauces										
Tomato/vegetable meal sauces	Sauce for pasta	38	7	1.12	0.26	87	0.96	0.41	−15%	¥
Tomato/vegetable based cold sauces	Ketchup	2	5	2.63	0.53	18 [a]	1.58	0.36	−41%	¥
	Curry ketchup	1	2	1.69	0.00	19	1.69	0.41	−1%	
Soups										
Soups sold as liquid and instant prepared		76		0.89	0.23	204	0.82	0.17	−9%	¥
Processed vegetables and legumes										
Processed vegetables	Peas and/or carrots, bean	4		0.47	0.12	44	0.35	0.10	−25%	¥
	Butter beans, haricots, mushrooms	2		0.64	0.02	17	0.41	0.16	−37%	
Processed legumes	Legumes	2	1	0.88	0.32	21	0.52	0.13	−42%	¥

N = number of generic foods codes, UVal = average number of underlying values per generic food. n = number of new data points; ¥ Statistically significant difference ($p < 0.05$) between 2016 and 2011; [a]: Exclusion of one ketchup because salt content was lower than 0.05 g/100 g.

3.3. Estimated Daily Salt Intake from 24 h Urinary Salt Excretion

The 24 h urinary salt excretion was similar in 2006, 2010 and 2015. In men, median estimated salt intake was 9.7 g/day in 2015. This was not different from 2006 (9.9 g/day; $p = 0.34$) and 2010 (10.0 g/day in 2010; $p = 0.46$). In women, median salt intake was 7.4 g/day in 2015. Compared to 2006 (7.9 g/day; $p = 0.23$) and 2010 (7.4 g/day; $p = 0.75$), see Figure 3.

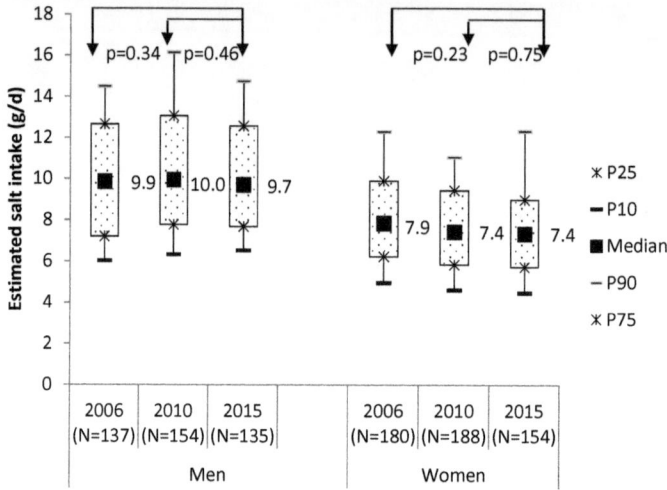

Figure 3. Salt intake (g per day) estimated from 24 h urine excretion in 2006, 2010 and 2015, correcting for age, education and day of the week. The proportion of participants reporting the use of discretionary salt was lower in 2010 as compared to 2006 (81% in 2010 versus 88% in 2006; $p = 0.009$). In 2015, the use of discretionary salt (83%) was not statistically significant different compared to 2010 ($p = 0.46$).

4. Discussion

This study showed that the salt content of certain foods in the Netherlands, such as bread, certain sauces, soups, potato crisps, and processed legumes and vegetables, has been reduced over the period 2011–2016. Significant salt reductions found ranged from −12% (some soups), to −19% (bread), and −42% (for processed legumes) in 2016 compared to 2011. In other food groups, such as meat cold cuts and cheese, the salt contents were not significantly different.

Salt reduction targets for foods can be voluntary or mandatory. In the Netherlands, mandatory maximum levels are set for bread (requested by the sector itself) and voluntary for other food categories without formal sanctioning. In some food categories, such as for processed vegetables/legumes and for ketchups, considerable salt reduction was achieved (for example −42% for processed legumes and −41% for ketchup) with the voluntary commitments. In other food categories, the voluntary set salt maximum levels showed limited ambitions and/or did not lead to significantly reduced salt contents. For example, in some of the meat cold cuts subcategories the observed changes were small and not statistically significant.

Globally, bread is the most targeted food for salt reduction, followed by foods such as other bakery products, processed meats, sauces and convenience meals [30]. The majority (81%) of national salt reduction strategies, like in the Netherlands, include industry engagement to reduce the salt content of foods [30]. To date there is little scientific knowledge concerning the factors that influence the effectiveness of public-private agreements to reach a certain societal goal. Bryden et al. [31] evaluated voluntary agreements between business and government trying to identify factors of success. They concluded that, if properly implemented and monitored, voluntary agreements can be effective and business can help to achieve public policy aims. Proper implementation includes realistic, but stretching, targets for businesses to achieve real changes [31]. In addition, substantial disincentives for non-participation and costly sanctions for non-compliance seem to improve the effectiveness of agreements [31]. Further research should evaluate whether these advices also apply to the field food product improvement.

The ultimate goal of lowering salt contents of foods is to reduce salt intake at the population level, and in this way improve health. To reach current salt intake reduction targets via food product improvement alone, all major salt contributing foods contributing need to be lowered by 30−40% [12]. Although this is an ambitious target, it might be possible for food categories such as bread, meat cold cuts, cheese, and soup as is shown via salt-reduced foods as used in experimental settings [32–34]. In these experiments, the participants consumed and liked the salt reduced foods similarly to the regular salted foods. However, in isolation, reformulation is unlikely to provide a complete solution to the challenge of improving eating patterns and nutrient provision, although it is a contributor [35]. More likely to be effective is a combination of strategies of food reformulation with changed food choice behaviour (e.g., more vegetables and less meat/cheese, choosing meat cold cuts with low salt contents, reducing discretionary salt) and/or reduction of portion sizes.

Athough we observed salt reduction in some food categories, median salt intake between 2006 and 2015 did not differ using 24 hr urinary analysis. Only a limited number of countries observed significant decreased salt intakes at the population level [11]. The significant decrease per day ranged from −1.15 (95% confidence interval (CI) −1.69 to −0.61) G/day in Finland [36], −0.9 G/day in the United Kingdom (UK) [37] to −0.35 (95% CI −0.52 to −0.18) G/day in Ireland [11]. The countries with successful salt reductions at the population level started at relatively high levels—11.8 g/day [36] in Finland and 9.5 g per day in UK [37], compared to 8.7 G/day in 2006 in our study population. In line with our own results, several countries, for example Austria and Switzerland, did not show a statistically significant change in salt intake (G/day) from pre- to post-intervention [11].

Recent reviews assessed the effectiveness of different types of population-level interventions implemented by governments for dietary salt reduction [11,30]. Especially, a multi-component approach is needed to reduce daily salt intakes, including more than one intervention activity [11]. In addition, incorporation of initiatives of a structural nature is needed (such as food product reformulation or the availability of low salt foods via public procurement). Seventy-five countries now have a national salt reduction strategy [30,38]. The majority of the strategies are to a certain extent multicomponent, as they include industry engagement to reformulate products (n = 61), establishment of salt content targets for foods (39), consumer education (71), front-of-pack labelling schemes (31), taxation on high-salt foods (3), and interventions in public institutions (54) [30]. The countries observing a statistically significant salt reduction had a multicomponent approach. In the UK, many activities were undertaken to lower salt intake from 2003 onwards. Efforts included public information/education campaigns, on-package nutrition information, restrictions on marketing to children, food procurement policy in specific settings, and food product reformulation [11,39]. Finland introduced mandatory warning labels on high salt foods in addition to food reformulation activities [40,41]. Furthermore, a long breath is needed to achieve salt reduction. In the UK it took more than 10 years, and in Finland 20 years, to achieve small steps in salt reduction in the population. In the Netherlands, the approach focusses on food reformulation activities and is ongoing. Additional product category agreements on salt reduction are planned for 2017, for example for meat products and breakfast cereals. The effect on daily salt intake is also dependent on food consumption patterns. Recent small changes in food consumption patterns in the Netherlands may either be in line with (e.g., lower meat consumption), or cancelling (e.g., more sauces consumption) the impact of recent modest reductions in the salt content of processed food [42].

Limitations and Strengths

The strength of our study is that we made a structured, comprehensive comparison of salt contents of foods, including the major contributors to daily intake. For many foods, data of independent chemical analyses were provided by the Dutch Food Safety Authority. The analytical data were complemented with nutritional label information. A representativeness check of our data with respect to the presence of major (private and supermarket) brands was carried out. Salt content stated on food labels may be calculated from food composition tables and differs from contents derived from chemical analyses. In most food categories, salt contents given on labels are higher than contents based on chemical analyses [26]. With increasing use of label information based on calculations from food composition tables, reduced salt content may be missed, because of circular reasoning. It therefore remains important that (a sample of) data are checked regularly by independent chemical analyses. To effectively monitor changes in food composition, researchers should ideally have access to food composition data of all individual foods sold in retail for multiple years. Examples of such a monitoring system exist from the USA [43,44] and France [45]. Food groups would a priori be comparable over subsequent years, as all foods (adjusted for marked share) are represented, and external validity is most likely higher than in the current study. Data quality needs to be taken into account, as indicated above. The use of generic food composition data (NEVO 2011) as a reference poses some issues. It is intrinsically difficult to compare generic foods with individual foods, as they are by definition different. The generic foods used as the reference were aggregated from food composition data of individual foods obtained over a period of several years, thus with less variation in salt contents than an analyses based on individual foods.

For the salt intake based on 24 hr urine, power calculations showed that this study had sufficient power to detect a reduction of around 1 g in daily salt intake in the total population between 2010 and 2015, given the sample size in 2015 of 289 subjects. To comply with the recommendations of 6 g a day 30–40% salt reduction is needed in major salt contributing foods. In order to detect smaller reductions (of 4–5%) in the mean population intake of salt, which were more likely given the current achievements, would have needed a larger sampling size. Thus, the fact that no changes in population intake were found despite salt reduction in some foods is not in contradiction with each other. Participants for the 24 hr urine study were sampled from a single town in the Netherlands and the participation rate was low; this limits the generalizability of the results from our study to the general population. Compared to the general Dutch population, participants were more likely to be non-smokers and were higher educated. However, as the study characteristics of the study populations over the three years were highly comparable, this study design may demonstrate a trend in salt intake.

5. Conclusions

In the Netherlands, the salt content of bread, certain sauces, soups, potato crisps, and processed legumes and vegetables has been reduced over the period 2011–2016. However, median salt intake in 2006 and 2015 using 24 hr urinary analysis remains well above the recommended intake of 6 g.

Acknowledgments: This research was funded by the Ministry of Health, Welfare and Sport. We thank the Dutch Food Safety Authority and the Dutch Nutrition Centre for their collaboration in the data collection, the Dutch Bakery Centre for providing analytical data and all manufacturers and retailers who provided food composition data. In addition, we thank all individuals that participated in the 24 hr urine study, as well as the field workers that contributed to the data collection.

Author Contributions: E.H.M.T., S.W., M.A.H.H. and D.L.v.d.A. designed the study; I.E.J.M., M.A.H.H., S.W., H.A.M.B.., D.L.v.d.A., E.H.M.T. collected and analyzed the data; E.H.M.T., M.A.H.H., I.B.T. and I.E.J.M. wrote the paper. All authors critically reviewed the paper. E.H.M.T. wrote the final version of the paper.

Conflicts of Interest: The authors declare no conflict of interest. The founding sponsors had no role in the design of the study; in the collection, analyses, or interpretation of data; in the writing of the manuscript, and in the decision to publish the results.

References

1. Global Burden of Disease, Risk Factors Collaborators. Global, regional, and national comparative risk assessment of 79 behavioural, environmental and occupational, and metabolic risks or clusters of risks in 188 countries, 1990–2013: A systematic analysis for the Global Burden of Disease Study 2013. *Lancet* **2015**, *386*, 2287–2323.

2. World Health Organization. *Global Action Plan for the Prevention and Control of Noncommunicable Diseases 2013–2020*; WHO: Geneva, Switzerland, 2013.

3. Kromhout, D.; Spaaij, C.J.; de Goede, J.; Weggemans, R.M. The 2015 Dutch food-based dietary guidelines. *Eur. J. Clin. Nutr.* **2016**, *70*, 869–878. [CrossRef] [PubMed]

4. Hendriksen, M.A.; van Raaij, J.M.; Geleijnse, J.M.; Wilson-van den Hooven, C.; Ocke, M.C.; van der A, D.L. Monitoring salt and iodine intakes in Dutch adults between 2006 and 2010 using 24 h urinary sodium and iodine excretions. *Public Health Nutr.* **2014**, *17*, 1431–1438. [CrossRef] [PubMed]

5. Van Rossum, C.T.M.; Fransen, H.P.; Verkaik-Kloosterman, J.; Buurma-Rethans, E.J.M.; Ocke, M.C. *Dutch National Food Consumption Survey 2007–2010. Diet of Children and Adults Aged 7 to 69 Years. RIVM Rapport 350050006*; National Institute for Public Health and the Environment: Bilthoven, The Netherlands, 2011.

6. Micha, R.; Khatibzadeh, S.; Shi, P.; Fahimi, S.; Lim, S.; Andrews, K.G.; Engell, R.E.; Powles, J.; Ezzati, M.; Mozaffarian, D. Global, regional, and national consumption levels of dietary fats and oils in 1990 and 2010: A systematic analysis including 266 country-specific nutrition surveys. *BMJ* **2014**, *348*, g2272. [CrossRef] [PubMed]

7. Powles, J.; Fahimi, S.; Micha, R.; Khatibzadeh, S.; Shi, P.; Ezzati, M.; Engell, R.E.; Lim, S.S.; Danaei, G.; Mozaffarian, D. Global, regional and national sodium intakes in 1990 and 2010: A systematic analysis of 24 h urinary sodium excretion and dietary surveys worldwide. *BMJ Open* **2013**, *3*, e003733. [CrossRef] [PubMed]

8. Temme, E.H.M.; Westenbrink, S.; Toxopeus, I.B.; Hendriksen, M.A.H.; Werkman, A.M.; Klostermann, V.L.C. *Natrium en Verzadigd Vet in Beeld [Sodium and Saturated Fat Content of Foods]. RIVM Briefrapport 350022002*; National Institute for Public Health and the Environment: Bilthoven, The Netherlands, 2013.

9. Auestad, N.; Hurley, J.S.; Fulgoni, V.L., 3rd; Schweitzer, C.M. Contribution of Food Groups to Energy and Nutrient Intakes in Five Developed Countries. *Nutrients* **2015**, *7*, 4593–4618. [CrossRef] [PubMed]

10. World Health Organisation. *Global Action Plan for the Prevention and Control of Noncommunicable Diseases 2013–2020*; World Health Organisation: Geneva, Switzerland, 2013.

11. McLaren, L.; Sumar, N.; Barberio, A.M.; Trieu, K.; Lorenzetti, D.L.; Tarasuk, V.; Webster, J.; Campbell, N.R. Population-level interventions in government jurisdictions for dietary sodium reduction. *Cochrane Database Syst. Rev.* **2016**, *9*, CD010166. [PubMed]

12. Hendriksen, M.A.; Verkaik-Kloosterman, J.; Noort, M.W.; van Raaij, J.M. Nutritional impact of sodium reduction strategies on sodium intake from processed foods. *Eur. J. Clin. Nutr.* **2015**, *69*, 805–810. [CrossRef] [PubMed]

13. McLaren, L.; McIntyre, L.; Kirkpatrick, S. Rose's population strategy of prevention need not increase social inequalities in health. *Int. J. Epidemiol.* **2010**, *39*, 372–377. [CrossRef] [PubMed]

14. Actieplan Zout in Levensmiddelen. Action Plan. In *Salt in Foods*; FNLI: Rijkwijk, The Netherlands, 2008.

15. Besluit van 15 november 2012, houdende wijziging van het Warenwetbesluit Meel en brood inzake het maximale zoutgehalte van brood. Staatsblad van het Koninkrijk der Nederlanden, nr 598, Den Haag, 2012. Commodities Act with Regulation on the Maximum Level of Salt in Bread. Available online: https://zoek.officielebekendmakingen.nl/stb-2012-598.html (accessed on 20 July 2017).

16. Vijfde Landelijke Steekproef Zoutgehalte in Brood, maart–mei 2013 (Fifth annual sampling of salt content of bread, March-May 2013). NBC (Netherlands Bakery Centre): Wageningen, The Netherlands.

17. Zesde Landelijke Steekproef Zoutgehalte in Brood, februari–april 2015 (Sixth annual sampling of salt content of bread, February-April 2015). NBC (Netherlands Bakery Centre): Wageningen, The Netherlands.

18. Akkoord Verbetering Productsamenstelling Zout, Verzadigd Vet, Suiker (Calorieën) (National agreement o Improve Product Composition: Salt, Saturated Fat, Sugar (Calories)). Supervisory committee of agreement: Den Haag, The Netherlands, 2014. Available online: http://www.akkoordverbeteringproductsamenstelling.nl/en (accessed on 20 July 2017).

19. Temme, E.H.M.; Milder, I.E.J.; Westenbrink, S.; Toxopeus, I.B.; Van den Bogaard, C.H.M.; Van Raaij, J.M.A. Monitoring Productsamenstelling Voor Zout, Verzadigd Vet en Suiker. RIVM Herformuleringsmonitor 2014.

RIVM Briefrapport 2015–0034 (Monitoring Product Composition for Salt, Saturated Fatty Acid and Sugar. RIVM Reformulation Monitor 2014, RIVM Letter Report 2015–0034). National Institute for Public Health and the Environment: Bilthoven, The Netherlands, 2015.

20. NEVO-online (Nederlands Voedingsstoffenbestand), NEVO-online versie 2011. (Dutch Food Composition Database NEVO-online version 2011). National institute for Public Health and the Environment: Bilthoven, The Netherlands, 2011.

21. Website Akkoord Verbetering Productsamenstelling (Website National Agreement to Improve Product Composition). Available online: http://www.akkoordverbeteringproductsamenstelling.nl (accessed on 20 July 2017).

22. Voedingscentrum. *Richtlijnen Voedselkeuze*; Voedingscentrum: Den Haag, Dutch, 2011.

23. Innova Innova's Food & Beverage Database. Available online: http://www.innovadatabase.com/home/index.rails (accessed on 1 May 2014).

24. Voedingscentrum Levensmiddelendatabank (LEDA) (Food Database LEDA). Dutch Nutrition Centre: Den Haag, The Netherlands. Available online: http://www.voedingscentrum.nl/professionals/productaanbod-en-levensmiddelendatabank.aspx (accessed on 13 July 2017).

25. Monitoring Van Het Gehalte Aan Keukenzout in Diverse Levensmiddelen 2015 (Monitoring the Content of Salt in Several Foods 2015). Dutch Food Safety Autority (NVWA): Utrecht, The Netherlands, 2016.

26. NVWA. *Monitoring Van Het Keukenzoutgehalte in Diverse Levensmiddelen 2016 (Monitoring the Content of Salt in Several Foods 2016)*; Dutch Food Safety Autority (NVWA): Utrecht, The Netherlands, 2017; Available online: https://www.nvwa.nl/documenten/communicatie/inspectieresultaten/eten-drinken/2017m/rapport-monitoring-van-het-gehalte-aan-keukenzout-in-diverse-levensmiddelen-2016 (accessed on 6 April 2017).

27. Monitoring Van Het Keukenzout- en Verzadigd Vetgehalte in Levensmiddelen Waarvoor Afspraken Zijn Gemaakt in Het Akkoord Verbetering Productsamenstelling 2016 (Monitoring the Content of Salt and Saturated Fatty Acids in Several Foods with Reduction Targets 2016). Dutch Food Safety Autority (NVWA): Utrecht, The Netherlands, 2017.

28. Chemistry Information Sheet CREm Creatinine. Beckman Coulter Synchron LX System(s). Available online: www.beckmancoulter.com (accessed on 20 July 2017).

29. Chemistry Information Sheet NA Sodium. Beckman Coulter Synchron LX System(s). Available online: www.beckmancoulter.com (accessed on 20 July 2017).

30. Trieu, K.; Neal, B.; Hawkes, C.; Dunford, E.; Campbell, N.; Rodriguez-Fernandez, R.; Legetic, B.; McLaren, L.; Barberio, A.; Webster, J. Salt Reduction Initiatives around the World—A Systematic Review of Progress towards the Global Target. *PLoS ONE* **2015**, *10*, e0130247. [CrossRef] [PubMed]

31. Bryden, A.; Petticrew, M.; Mays, N.; Eastmure, E.; Knai, C. Voluntary agreements between government and business—A scoping review of the literature with specific reference to the Public Health Responsibility Deal. *Health Policy* **2013**, *110*, 186–197. [CrossRef] [PubMed]

32. Willems, A.A.; van Hout, D.H.; Zijlstra, N.; Zandstra, E.H. Effects of salt labelling and repeated in-home consumption on long-term liking of reduced-salt soups. *Public Health Nutr.* **2014**, *17*, 1130–1137. [CrossRef] [PubMed]

33. Bolhuis, D.P.; Temme, E.H.; Koeman, F.T.; Noort, M.W.; Kremer, S.; Janssen, A.M. A salt reduction of 50% in bread does not decrease bread consumption or increase sodium intake by the choice of sandwich fillings. *J. Nutr.* **2011**, *141*, 2249–2255. [CrossRef] [PubMed]

34. Janssen, A.M.; Kremer, S.; van Stipriaan, W.L.; Noort, M.W.; de Vries, J.H.; Temme, E.H. Reduced-sodium lunches are well-accepted by uninformed consumers over a 3-week period and result in decreased daily dietary sodium intakes: A randomized controlled trial. *J. Acad. Nutr. Diet.* **2015**, *115*, 1614–1625. [CrossRef] [PubMed]

35. Buttriss, J.L. Food reformulation: The challenges to the food industry. *Proc. Nutr. Soc.* **2013**, *72*, 61–69. [CrossRef] [PubMed]

36. Laatikainen, T.; Pietinen, P.; Valsta, L.; Sundvall, J.; Reinivuo, H.; Tuomilehto, J. Sodium in the Finnish diet: 20-Year trends in urinary sodium excretion among the adult population. *Eur. J. Clin. Nutr.* **2006**, *60*, 965–970. [CrossRef] [PubMed]

37. Shankar, B.; Brambila-Macias, J.; Traill, B.; Mazzocchi, M.; Capacci, S. An evaluation of the UK Food Standards Agency's salt campaign. *Health Econ.* **2013**, *22*, 243–250. [CrossRef] [PubMed]

Nutrients **2017**, *9*, 791

38. Trieu, K.; McLean, R.; Johnson, C.; Santos, J.A.; Raj, T.S.; Campbell, N.R.C.; Webster, J. The Science of Salt: A Regularly Updated Systematic Review of the Implementation of Salt Reduction Interventions (November 2015 to February 2016). *J. Clin. Hypertens.* **2016**, *18*, 1194–1204. [CrossRef] [PubMed]

39. He, F.J.; Brinsden, H.C.; MacGregor, G.A. Salt reduction in the United Kingdom: A successful experiment in public health. *J. Hum. Hypertens.* **2014**, *28*, 345–352. [CrossRef] [PubMed]

40. Pietinen, P.; Valsta, L.M.; Hirvonen, T.; Sinkko, H. Labelling the salt content in foods: A useful tool in reducing sodium intake in Finland. *Public Health Nutr.* **2008**, *11*, 335–340. [CrossRef] [PubMed]

41. WHO. *Mapping Salt Reduction Initiatives in the WHO European Region*; World Health Organization, Regional Office for Europe: Copenhagen, Denmark, 2013.

42. Van Rossum, C.; Buurma-Rethans, E.; Vennemann, F.; Beukers, M.; Brants, H.; de Boer, E.; Ocké, M. *The Diet of the Dutch : Results of the First Two Years of the Dutch National Food Consumption Survey 2012–2016*; RIVM: Bilthoven, The Netherlands, 2016.

43. Gillespie, C.; Maalouf, J.; Yuan, K.; Cogswell, M.E.; Gunn, J.P.; Levings, J.; Moshfegh, A.; Ahuja, J.K.; Merritt, R. Sodium content in major brands of US packaged foods, 2009. *Am. J. Clin. Nutr.* **2015**, *101*, 344–353. [CrossRef] [PubMed]

44. Poti, J.M.; Dunford, E.K.; Popkin, B.M. Sodium reduction in US households' packaged food and beverage purchases, 2000 to 2014. *JAMA Intern. Med.* **2017**, *177*, 986–994. [CrossRef] [PubMed]

45. Menard, C.; Dumas, C.; Goglia, R.; Spiteri, M.; Gillot, N.; Combris, P.; Ireland, J.; Soler, L.G.; Volatier, J.L. OQALI: A French database on processed foods. *J. Food Compos. Anal.* **2011**, *24*, 744–749. [CrossRef]

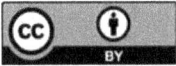

nutrients

MDPI

Article

Stages of Behavioral Change for Reducing Sodium Intake in Korean Consumers: Comparison of Characteristics Based on Social Cognitive Theory

So-hyun Ahn [1], Jong Sook Kwon [2], Kyungmin Kim [3] and Hye-Kyeong Kim [1,*]

[1] Department of Food Science and Nutrition, The Catholic University of Korea, Bucheon 14662, Korea;
    sohyunahn1123@nate.com
[2] Department of Food and Nutrition, Shingu College, Songnam 13174, Korea; jskwon@shingu.ac.kr
[3] Department of Food and Nutrition, Baewha Women's University, Seoul 03039, Korea;
    kyungmkim@baewha.ac.kr
*   Correspondence: hkyeong @catholic.ac.kr; Tel.: +82-2-2164-4314

Received: 18 June 2017; Accepted: 25 July 2017; Published: 27 July 2017

Abstract: High sodium intake increases the risk of cardiovascular disease. Given the importance of behavioral changes to reducing sodium intake, this study aims to investigate the stages of change and the differences in cognitive and behavioral characteristics by stage in Korean consumers. Adult participants (N = 3892) completed a questionnaire on the stages of behavioral change, recognition of social efforts, outcome expectancy, barriers to practice, nutrition knowledge and dietary behaviors, and self-efficiency related to reduced sodium intake. The numbers of participants in each stage of behavioral change for reducing sodium intake was 29.5% in the maintenance stage, 19.5% in the action stage, and 51.0% in the preaction stage that included the precontemplation, contemplation, and preparation stages. Multiple logistic regression showed that the factors differentiating the three stages were recognizing a supportive social environment, perceived barriers to the practice of reducing sodium intake, and self-efficacy to be conscious of sodium content and to request less salt when eating out. Purchasing experience of sodium-reduced products for salty foods, knowledge of the recommended intake of salt and the difference between sodium and salt, and improving dietary habits of eating salted fish, processed food, and salty snacks were factors for being in the action stage versus the preaction stage. These findings suggest that tailored intervention according to the characteristics of each stage is helpful in reducing sodium intake.

Keywords: stage of behavioral change; reducing sodium intake; consumer; social cognitive theory

1. Introduction

High dietary sodium intake is a major risk factor for hypertension that can induce cardiovascular disease and stroke [1,2] and is associated with an increased risk of renal disease, osteoporosis, and gastric cancer [3]. It has been reported that effective sodium-reduction programs not only improve public health, but are also cost effective [4,5]. In Korea, the food industry and government have made considerable efforts to develop sodium-reduced products and to raise public awareness through campaigns, public advertisements, and the labeling of sodium content in foods. Consequently, the average sodium intake in Korea has shown a decreasing trend since 2005. The average daily sodium intake was 3890 mg in 2014, which was reduced by 25% from 5256 mg in 2005, but it is still almost double the recommended daily intake [6].

Although public awareness is an important component of a successful salt-reduction initiative [7,8], awareness of the importance of sodium reduction is not always associated with behavioral change. The majority of dietary sodium in Korea is added to food during cooking and eating at the table [9], which suggests the importance of consumer education to change behavior to reach the recommended sodium-intake level. A transtheoretical model of behavioral change is useful to assess whether consumers are oriented toward change. According to the model, there are five stages of behavioral change that people move through in adopting a health-related behavior: precontemplation, contemplation, preparation, action, and maintenance [10].

Precontemplation is the stage in which people do not intend to change their behavior in the next six months and are not aware that their behavior is problematic [10]. People in the contemplation stage express an intention to make a change at some time but not soon; they are aware of the pros of changing and acutely aware of the cons. Preparation is the stage in which people intend to take action within the next month or may already have begun some significant steps toward behavioral change. The action stage is defined by consistent practice in the recent past, while the maintenance stage is typified as consistent practice for more than six months. Although this model has been applied to the individual for a variety of health behaviors [10,11], it can be used to assess the health behavior status of community members and to measure the effects of interventions [12]. A recent online survey conducted in eight countries reported that about one third of the population was not interested in reducing their salt intake (precontemplation stage), and only 39% of the population was in the action and maintenance stages [13]. However, there has been no report on the status of behavioral change with respect to reducing sodium intake in Korea.

Social cognitive theory is a comprehensive framework for understanding health-related behaviors and changing behaviors [14]. The theory proposes that behavior is a function of the aspects of the environment and of the person, all of which are in constant interaction. Personal factors for understanding behavior include skills and knowledge to perform the behavior, self-efficacy, and the outcome expectancy of the behavior. Environmental aspects influence the individual's behavior by providing appropriate modeling for learning the behavior and available materials to use [15]. It is necessary to understand the relationship between the stage of change and personal cognitive and behavioral characteristics to develop effective intervention for consumers. However, no previous studies have addressed the differences in reducing sodium intake by stages of behavioral change.

The objective of this study was to examine the status of behavioral change in reducing sodium intake and to describe the association between the stages of change and cognitive and behavioral factors in Korean consumers.

2. Subjects and Methods

2.1. Study Design and Participants

A nationwide cross-sectional survey was performed through a local network of the Korean National Council of Consumer Organizations. The regional distribution of the Korean population in 2011 was considered in the sampling. Participants aged at least 18 years were recruited through announcements to consumers using phone calls, e-mails, local newspaper advertisements, school newsletters, and Internet boards. All participants gave their informed consent for inclusion before they participated in the study. This study was conducted in accordance with the Declaration of Helsinki, and the protocol was approved by the Ethics Committee of the Catholic University of Korea (1040395-201705-02). The survey was conducted from 30 June 2011 to 31 October 2011.

2.2. Questionnaire

A self-administered questionnaire was developed based on previous studies [16–18], and face validity was established by experts. The questionnaire consisted of the following three sections: demographic information, questions for classifying the stage of behavioral change, and cognitive and behavioral factors related to reducing sodium intake (see in Supplementary Material).

2.2.1. Stage of Behavioral Change

The stage of behavioral change in reducing sodium intake was assessed by an algorithm with separate questions. Participants were asked, 'Are you currently practicing a low sodium diet? (a) yes, more than six months; (b) yes, but less than six months; (c) no'. Participants who responded '(a) yes, more than six months' were classified in the maintenance stage; those who responded '(b) yes, but less than six months' were classified in the action stage; and those who responded '(c) no' were asked an additional question to differentiate their stages. The question was 'Do you intend to make changes to reduce sodium intake in the near future or in the following month? (a) yes; (b) no, but in the next six months; (c) no, I haven't thought about it'. If they responded '(a) yes', they were classified in the preparation stage; if they responded '(b) no, but in the next six months', they were classified in the contemplation stag; and those who responded '(c) no, I haven't thought about it' were classified in the precontemplation stage.

2.2.2. Cognitive and Behavioral Factors

Consumer cognition related to reducing sodium intake was assessed according to four categories: recognition of supportive environment and experience in purchasing sodium-reduced foods, positive outcome expectancy and barriers to reducing sodium intake, perception and self-efficacy of reducing sodium intake, and nutrition knowledge. The list of positive outcome expectancy to low sodium intake was suggested, and participants were asked to select three main outcomes. The barriers to reducing sodium intake were suggested as follows: 'bad taste', 'hard to prepare and cook', 'limitation in choosing the food, menu, and restaurant', 'limited information, knowledge, and skills to practice', 'limitation to social relationship when dining with family or friends', 'preference for broth dishes (soup, stew)', and 'preference for kimchi, salted fish, and fermented sauces'. Perception and self-efficacy of reducing sodium intake were evaluated using eight questions, including consciousness of saltiness in food, willingness to select fresh food rather than processed or seasoned food, requesting less salt when eating out, and interest in low-sodium recipes. Nutrition knowledge was evaluated using 10 questions, including a conceptual understanding of sodium and salt, the health risks of excess sodium intake, the recommended daily intake of sodium, the physiological functions of sodium, the benefits of reducing sodium intake, high sodium foods, and nutrition labeling. In addition, dietary behavior related to sodium intake was assessed using 13 questions, including checking the sodium content in nutrition labeling, the frequency of eating out and eating high sodium foods, and habits of eating broth and adding salt to dishes. Participants were asked to respond 'yes', 'no', or 'I don't know' to the questions on nutritional knowledge. Barriers, perception and self-efficacy, and dietary behavior were rated with a five-point Likert scale, ranging from 1 (strongly disagree) to 5 (strongly agree). In the present study, Cronbach's alpha for barriers, perception and self-efficacy, nutrition knowledge, and dietary behavior ranged from 0.72 to 0.78, indicating good internal consistency in the responses.

2.3. Statistical Analysis

Data were analyzed using the SAS (version 9.3, SAS Institute, Inc., Cary, NC, USA) package program. Age, body mass index (BMI), and Likert scores were reported as means ± standard deviations. Means of the Likert scores were compared by analysis of covariance (ANCOVA) according to the stage of behavioral change. All categorized data were analyzed using chi-square tests. Multiple logistic regression was performed to examine the relationship between the stage of change and cognitive and behavioral factors in reducing sodium intake. A p-value of < 0.05 was considered statistically significant.

3. Results

3.1. Participant Demographics

A total of 3892 participants were included in the study after people who did not answer to the question to assess their stage of behavioral change were excluded (inclusion rate 89%). The general characteristics of the participants are shown in Table 1. The participants were aged 18 to 85 years, with a higher proportion in their 40s and 50s. Most of the participants were women (94.8%). Approximately 45% of the participants were college graduates or had higher levels of education.

When the participants were classified according to the stage of behavioral change, 29.5% were in the maintenance stage and 19.5% were in the action stage. The proportions of participants in the precontemplation stage, contemplation stage, and preparation stage were 23.3%, 24.0%, and 3.7%, respectively. These three groups were combined for analysis because there were relatively small numbers of participants in the preparation stage, and understanding the characteristics of those in the preaction stages is necessary to move forward to the action stage. Thus, five stages of behavioral change were reduced to three groups: maintenance (M), action (A), and preaction (P). Significant associations were found between demographic variables and an individual's stage of change. Thus, analyses of the association between cognitive and behavioral factors and the stages of change were adjusted by demographic variables such as age, gender, BMI, education level, and monthly income level.

3.2. Recognition of Supportive Environment and Experience of Purchasing Reduced Sodium Foods

The percentage of participants who recognized social efforts for reducing sodium intake through campaigns and nutritional education was 82.5% in the maintenance stage group; furthermore, the percentages were 74.9% and 54.7% in the action stage and preaction stage groups, respectively. Similarly, the largest proportions of participants recognizing sodium content labeling on processed food were in the order of the maintenance (74.4%), action (66.4%), and preaction (58.8%) stage groups. Recognizing social efforts and sodium content labeling on processed foods increased the odds of being in the action stage rather than the preaction stage by about 2.3 fold and 1.8 fold, respectively. Further, these two variables increased the odds of being in the maintenance stage versus the action stage significantly (Table 2).

The most frequently purchased reduced-sodium products were ham (36.7%), salt (32.8%), and cheese (26.7%). The experience rates of purchasing sodium-reduced foods were different among the three stage groups. Participants who had purchased low-sodium salt, sodium-reduced salted fish, low-sodium soy sauce, low-sodium ham, and low-sodium cheese had significantly higher odds of being in the action stage rather than the preaction stage. In addition, the purchasing experience of buying low-sodium cereal, low-sodium cheese, and low-sodium ramen increased the odds of being in the maintenance stage rather than the action stage (Table 2).

3.3. Positive Outcome Expectancy and Barriers to Reduce Sodium Intake

Table 3 presents the positive outcome expectancy and the barriers to reducing sodium intake that were statistically different among participants in the three stages of behavioral change. Participants perceived a decrease in blood pressure and an increase in the prevention of strokes and heart disease as the main benefits of reducing their sodium intake. Participants expecting a decrease in blood pressure as a reward for reducing their sodium intake had higher odds of being in the action stage versus the preaction stage. An expectation of cancer prevention was relatively low, but those who perceived the benefit had higher odds of being in the maintenance stage.

The proportions of participants who agreed to each barrier were the highest in the preaction stage followed, in order, by the action and maintenance stages. Having the following barriers reduced the odds of being in the action stage versus the preaction stage and the odds of being in the maintenance versus the action stage significantly: 'limited information, knowledge, and skills', 'bad taste', 'limitation to social relationship when dining with family or friends', and 'time-consuming and inconvenient process of cooking and preparing'. This result indicates that overcoming these barriers is important for individuals to take action. On the other hand, both 'preference for broth dishes' and 'preference for kimchi, salted fish, and fermented sauces' reduced the odds of being in the maintenance stage only by about half (0.46 and 0.45, respectively), which suggests that overcoming these two barriers are critical factors to reach sustained behavioral change for reducing sodium intake.

3.4. Perception and Self-Efficacy on Reducing Sodium Intake

All the questions on perception and self-efficacy related to reducing sodium intake showed significant differences between the three stages of change (Table 4). The scores were highest in the maintenance stage, followed by the action stage and the preaction stage. 'Willingness to buy fresh food rather than processed or instant food' got the highest score in all three groups, while 'unsatisfied feeling when eating foods with less salt' had the lowest score. This indicates that an 'unsatisfied feeling when eating foods with less salt' was the hardest barrier to overcome for respondents.

Table 1. Participants' demographics.

	M (N = 1151)	A (N = 758)	P (N = 1983)	Total (N = 3892)	p-Value
Stage of change (%)	29.6	19.5	50.9	100.0	
Age	52.7 ± 10.4 [1],a	52.2 ± 11.1 a	46.3 ± 11.8 b	49.3 ± 11.7	<0.0001
BMI (kg/m^2)	22.4 ± 2.5 b	22.6 ± 2.6 a	22.2 ± 2.6 b	22.3 ± 2.6	0.0032
Age					
18–29	19 (1.7%) [2]	18 (2.5%)	143 (8.1%)	190 (5.1%)	<0.0001
30–39	107 (9.8%)	82 (11.3%)	400 (20.8%)	589 (15.7%)	
40–49	259 (23.6%)	170 (23.5%)	614 (32.0%)	1043 (27.9%)	
50–59	427 (38.9%)	268 (37.0%)	497 (25.9%)	1192 (31.9%)	
60–69	229 (20.9%)	152 (21.0%)	206 (10.7%)	587 (15.7%)	
Over 70	56 (5.1%)	35 (4.8%)	49 (2.6%)	140 (3.8%)	
Gender					
Male	28 (2.5%)	26 (3.5%)	146 (7.5%)	200 (5.3%)	<0.0001
Female	1096 (97.5%)	719 (96.5%)	1797 (92.5%)	3612 (94.8%)	
Education level					
Middle school or less	148 (13.2%)	110 (15.0%)	186 (9.6%)	443 (11.7%)	<0.0001
High school	498 (44.4%)	395 (53.6%)	739 (38.2%)	1632 (43.0%)	
College or above	476 (42.5%)	232 (31.5%)	1009 (52.2%)	1717 (45.3%)	
Average monthly income					
Under $1000	116 (10.8%)	76 (11.3%)	141 (7.7%)	333 (9.3%)	0.0001
$1000~$2000	172 (16.0%)	127 (18.8%)	341 (18.6%)	640 (17.8%)	
$2000~$3000	252 (23.4%)	188 (27.9%)	456 (24.8%)	896 (25.0%)	
$3000~$4000	215 (20.0%)	141 (20.9%)	382 (20.8%)	738 (20.6%)	
$4000~$5000	171 (15.9%)	85 (12.6%)	316 (17.2%)	572 (15.9%)	
Over $5000	150 (13.9%)	58 (8.6%)	201 (10.9%)	409 (11.4%)	

M = Maintenance stage, A = Action stage, P = Preaction stage including the preparation, contemplation, and precontemplation stages, BMI = Body mass index. [1] Mean ± SD: Mean values with different superscripts are significantly different between the groups at α = 0.05 as determined by Duncan's multiple range test after one-way ANOVA; [2] N (%): by chi-square test among the groups according to the stage of change.

Table 2. Recognition of supportive environment and purchasing experience of reduced sodium foods.

	M	A	P	Total	p-Value [1]	A vs. P		M vs. A	
						OR [2]	95% CI	OR	95% CI
Recognition of social efforts for reducing sodium intake									
Yes	941 (82.5%) [3]	569 (74.9%)	1080 (54.7%)	2590 (66.8%)	<0.0001	2.25 *	1.83–2.77	1.58 *	1.24–2.02
Recognition of sodium labeling on processed foods									
Yes	741 (74.4%)	485 (66.4%)	1111 (58.8%)	2418 (64.9%)	<0.0001	1.83 *	1.49–2.24	1.35 *	1.08–1.70
Awareness of sodium labeling in restaurant or highway rest area									
Yes	263 (23.6%)	191 (25.6%)	355 (18.2%)	809 (21.2%)	<0.0001	1.56 *	1.24–1.96	0.93	0.74–1.19
Low-sodium food/goods ever used or purchased									
Low-sodium ham	444 (38.9%)	302 (41.0%)	618 (33.1%)	1364 (36.7%)	<0.0001	1.60 *	1.32–1.95	0.92	0.75–1.13
Low-sodium cereal	192 (17.2%)	90 (12.2%)	227 (12.2%)	509 (13.7%)	0.0002	1.22	0.91–1.62	1.41 *	1.06–1.89
Low-sodium ramen	261 (23.4%)	136 (18.5%)	334 (17.9%)	731 (19.7%)	0.0008	1.07	0.84–1.37	1.33 *	1.03–1.72
Sodium reduced salted fish	135 (12.1%)	114 (15.5%)	139 (7.5%)	388 (10.4%)	<0.0001	1.98 *	1.47–2.66	0.70	0.52–0.95
Sodium reduced kimchi	113 (10.1%)	77 (10.5%)	120 (6.4%)	310 (8.3%)	0.0001	1.38	0.98–1.94	0.96	0.68–1.35
Low-sodium cheese	371 (33.3%)	195 (26.5%)	428 (22.9%)	994 (26.7%)	<0.0001	1.30 *	1.05–1.62	1.33 *	1.06–1.66
Low-sodium soy sauce	307 (27.6%)	186 (25.3%)	273 (14.6%)	766 (10.6%)	<0.0001	1.77 *	1.39–2.23	1.11	0.88–1.40
Low-sodium salt	446 (40.0%)	279 (37.9%)	494 (25.5%)	1219 (32.8%)	<0.0001	2.07 *	1.69–2.54	1.01	0.82–1.24

M = Maintenance stage, A = Action stage, P = Preaction stage including the preparation, contemplation, and precontemplation stages. [1] *p* value from a chi-square test according to the stage of change group; [2] OR = Odds ratio; CI = Confidence interval. * Independently significant in multiple logistic regression models including age, sex, BMI, education level, income level (*p* < 0.05), reference is the response rate of 'yes' in each item; the pre-action stage is in A versus P, and the action stage is the reference group in M versus A; [3] *N* (%): the response rate of 'yes' to each item.

Table 3. Cognition of positive outcome expectancies and barriers to practicing according to the stages of change.

	M	A	P	Total	p-Value [1]	A vs. P		M vs. A	
						OR [2]	95% CI	OR	95% CI
Positive outcome expectancies									
Decrease of blood pressure	921 (80.0%) [3]	591 (78.0%)	1400 (70.6%)	2912 (74.8%)	<0.0001	1.35 *	1.09–1.69	1.11	0.86–1.41
Prevention to stroke and heart diseases	934 (81.2%)	580 (76.5%)	1439 (72.6%)	2953 (75.8%)	<0.0001	1.14	0.91–1.42	1.25	0.98–1.60
Reduction of swelling in body	324 (28.2%)	206 (27.2%)	656 (33.1%)	1186 (30.5%)	0.0014	0.79 *	0.64–0.97	1.00	0.80–1.25
Prevention to cancer	413 (35.9%)	234 (30.9%)	637 (32.1%)	1284 (33.0%)	0.0358	0.881	0.72–1.08	1.42 *	1.14–1.76
Barriers to practice									
Bad taste	653 (62.2%)	542 (74.5%)	1639 (83.7%)	2834 (75.7%)	<0.0001	0.56 *	0.44–0.70	0.56 *	0.44–0.70
Time-consuming and inconvenient process of cooking and preparing	351 (35.1%)	334 (46.6%)	1088 (56.1%)	1773 (48.1%)	<0.0001	0.70 *	0.58–0.85	0.59 *	0.48–0.73
Limitation in choosing the food, menu, and restaurant	855 (82.6%)	595 (82.9%)	1762 (90.5%)	3212 (86.8%)	<0.0001	0.61 *	0.46–0.80	0.91	0.69–1.21
Limited information, knowledge and skills to practice	634 (62.9%)	542 (76.7%)	1660 (86.3%)	2836 (77.9%)	<0.0001	0.55 *	0.43–0.69	0.51 *	0.40–0.64
Limitation to social relationships when dining with family or friends	824 (78.7%)	591 (82.3%)	1756 (90.6%)	3171 (85.6%)	<0.0001	0.57 *	0.43–0.76	0.70 *	0.53–0.91
Preference to broth dishes (soup, stew)	567 (53.9%)	516 (70.8%)	1466 (75.0%)	2549 (68.2%)	<0.0001	0.92	0.74–1.14	0.46 *	0.37–0.57
Preference to kimchi, salted fish, fermented sauces	498 (47.5%)	484 (66.2%)	1341 (68.6%)	2323 (62.2%)	<0.0001	0.91	0.74–1.11	0.45 *	0.37–0.56

M = Maintenance stage, A = Action stage, P = Preaction stage including the preparation, contemplation, and precontemplation stages. [1] p value from a chi-square test according to the stage of change group; [2] OR = Odds ratio; * Independently significant in multiple logistic regression models including age, sex, BMI, education level, and income level (p < 0.05), the reference is the response rate of 'yes' in each item. The pre-action stage is the reference group in A versus P, and the action stage is the reference group in M versus A; [3] N (%): the response rate of 'yes' to each item.

Table 4. Perceptions and self-efficacy of reducing sodium intake according to the stages of change.

	M	A	P	Total	p-Value [1]	A vs. P		M vs. A	
						OR [2]	95% CI	OR	95% CI
I feel unfulfilled or unsatisfied when eating foods with less salt. +	2.74 ± 0.85 a,[3]	2.42 ± 0.76 b	2.26 ± 0.66 c	2.43 ± 0.77	<0.0001	1.86 *	1.53–2.27	1.86 *	1.52–2.29
I usually recognize the sodium contents in food or dishes.	3.48 ± 0.86 a	3.08 ± 0.86 b	2.72 ± 0.88 c	3.02 ± 0.93	<0.0001	2.21 *	1.79–2.71	2.29 *	1.77–2.96
Practicing a low-sodium diet will improve my health status.	4.12 ± 0.69 a	3.87 ± 0.78 b	3.86 ± 0.70 b	3.94 ± 0.72	<0.0001	0.69	0.45–1.07	2.24 *	1.32–3.81
I will buy fresh food rather than processed or instant food.	4.15 ± 0.83 a	3.93 ± 0.86 a	3.90 ± 0.75 b	3.98 ± 0.81	<0.0001	0.70	0.45–1.07	1.13	0.72–1.76
I will ask to reduce the salt when eating-out.	3.46 ± 0.94 a	3.17 ± 0.93 b	2.93 ± 0.93 c	3.13 ± 0.96	<0.0001	1.76 *	1.41–2.19	1.50 *	1.16–1.95
I will choose dishes with natural flavor and taste rather than hot, salty, spicy ones.	3.91 ± 0.82 a	3.66 ± 0.84 b	3.56 ± 0.82 c	3.69 ± 0.84	<0.0001	1.26	0.91–1.75	1.24	0.85–1.81
I will have concern for low-sodium recipes.	4.08 ± 0.67 a	3.85 ± 0.75 b	3.66 ± 0.77 c	3.82 ± 0.76	<0.0001	1.51	0.97–2.34	1.74 *	1.00–3.05
I think that influence of consumers' sodium reduction can induce the change of social surroundings.	4.04 ± 0.72 a	3.85 ± 0.78 b	3.74 ± 0.78 c	3.85 ± 0.77	<0.0001	1.49	0.96–2.32	1.26	0.75–2.12

M = Maintenance stage, A = Action stage, P = Preaction stage including the preparation, contemplation, and precontemplation stages. [1] *p* value determined by a Duncan's multiple range test after one-way ANOVA. Different superscripts are significantly different between the groups at $\alpha = 0.05$. [2] OR = Odds ratio: The reference is <3 point score respondent; * independently significant in multiple logistic regression models including age, sex, BMI, education level, and income level ($p < 0.05$). The pre-action stage is the reference group is in A versus P, and the action stage is the reference group is in M versus A. [3] Mean ± SE: Mean values adjusted by age, sex, BMI, education level, and income level from ANCOVA analysis. Score 1 = strongly disagree, 2 = disagree, 3 = neither agree nor disagree, 4 = agree, 5 = strongly agree; a higher score means better perceptions and self-efficacy. (+ 5 = strongly disagree, 4 = disagree, 3 = neither agree nor disagree, 2 = agree, 1 = strongly agree).

'Recognizing sodium content', 'not feeling unsatisfied when eating foods with less salt', and 'requesting less salt when eating out' enhanced the odds of being in the action stage versus the preaction stage and the odds of being in the maintenance stage versus the action stage significantly. 'Recognizing the sodium content' enhanced the odds ratio by more than two fold for the action stage versus the preaction stage (odds ratio (OR); 2.2, 95% confidence interval (CI); 1.79–2.71) and for the maintenance stage versus the action stage (OR; 2.3, 95% CI; 1.77–2.96). On the other hand, the perception that 'practicing a low-sodium diet will improve my health status' was the only factor related to being in the maintenance stage rather than the action stage without differentiating between the preaction stage and the action stage. Participants with this perception had an odds ratio of 2.24 (95% CI; 1.32–3.81) for being in the maintenance stage versus the action stage.

3.5. Nutrition Knowledge Related to Sodium Intake

The rates of correct answers to most questions and the average scores of nutrition knowledge were the highest in the maintenance stage, followed by the action and preaction stages (Table 5). About 83% of participants knew that a sufficient intake of vegetables and fruits helps with sodium excretion. On the contrary, more than two thirds of participants did not know the difference between sodium and salt. Half the participants also did not know the recommended daily intake of sodium. The odds of being in the action stage were significantly enhanced when the participants knew the recommended daily intake of sodium and the difference between sodium and salt. This indicates that these concepts are important to taking action, although they are difficult. Notably, average scores of nutritional knowledge over six points enhanced the odds ratio of the maintenance stage versus the action stage without differentiating between the action stage and the preaction stage. Likewise, knowledge of the benefits of the sufficient intake of vegetables and fruits with regard to sodium excretion, using cooking methods to reduce sodium, the health risks of high sodium intake, the high sodium content in broth, and the physiological function of sodium was related to the enhanced odds of being in the maintenance stage.

3.6. Dietary Behavior Related to Sodium Intake

Table 6 presents the results of dietary behavior related to sodium intake that were statistically different among the three stages of behavioral change. Participants in higher stages of change showed more desirable dietary behavior in 11 out of 13 questions. Having good behavior in terms of checking the sodium content on nutritional labeling, not adding salt or sauce, the frequency of eating soup or stew, and a preference for grilled food over braised food with soy sauce enhanced the odds of being in the action stage versus the preaction stage and the odds of being in the maintenance stage versus the action stage significantly. On the other hand, improving dietary habits by not eating dried or salted fish, processed or instant food, salty snacks such as potato chips and crackers, and not frequently eating out was an important factor in being in the action stage rather than the preaction stage, without differentiating between the action stage and the maintenance stage. This was particularly true for participants avoiding processed or instant foods, who had an odds ratio of 1.93 (95% CI; 1.07–1.82) for being in the action stage versus the preaction stage. Eating plenty of fruits and vegetables was the only factor related to being in the maintenance stage rather than the action stage (OR; 1.99, 95% CI; 1.34–2.95) without differentiating between the preaction stage and the action stage.

Table 5. The percentage of correct answers and the nutritional knowledge scores related to sodium intake according to the stages of change.

	M	A	P	Total	p-Value[1]	A vs. P		M vs. A	
						OR[2]	95% CI	OR	95% CI
Excess intake of sodium can increase the risk of osteoporosis.	892 (79.4%)[3]	538 (72.0%)	1380 (70.6%)	2810 (73.5%)	<0.0001	1.11	0.90–1.37	1.38 *	1.09–1.75
The amount of sodium and the amount of salt are the same in the same food.	336 (30.0%)	247 (33.3%)	662 (33.9%)	1245 (32.7%)	0.0754	1.25 *	1.02–1.53	0.83	0.67–1.03
Two tablespoons of salt is the recommended goal intake of salt in a day.	646 (57.5%)	404 (54.7%)	870 (44.8%)	1920 (50.5%)	<0.0001	1.50 *	1.24–1.81	1.09	0.89–1.34
Sodium is necessary to keep the balance and equilibrium of body fluids.	813 (73.6%)	496 (67.6%)	1406 (72.4%)	2715 (71.8%)	0.0128	0.95	0.77–1.17	1.30 *	1.04–1.63
Sufficient intake of vegetables and fruits helps sodium excretion.	966 (86.6%)	593 (80.0%)	1591 (81.6%)	3150 (82.7%)	0.0002	0.95	0.74–1.20	1.58 *	1.20–2.09
Cooked fish with sauce contains much more salt than grilled fish in itself.	878 (79.0%)	517 (69.7%)	1412 (72.9%)	2807 (74.0%)	<0.0001	1.04	0.84–1.28	1.44 *	1.14–1.82
One tablespoon of salt contains the same amount of sodium as one tablespoon of soybean paste (miso).	588 (52.6%)	352 (47.4%)	906 (46.5%)	1846 (48.5%)	0.0048	1.10	0.91–1.33	1.17	0.96–1.44
The amount of sodium in the noodles themselves is more than that in the broth of ramen.	826 (73.3%)	495 (66.3%)	1346 (67.0%)	2667 (69.7%)	0.0031	1.06	0.87–1.30	1.33 *	1.06–1.66
Average score.	6.30 ± 0.07 [4]	6.03 ± 0.09	5.79 ± 0.05	5.98 ± 0.05	<0.0001	1.01 [5]	0.85–1.20	1.46 *	1.20–1.78

M = Maintenance stage, A = Action stage, P = Preaction stage including the preparation, contemplation, and precontemplation stages. [1] p-value from a chi-square test according to the stage of change group; [2] OR = Odds ratio: the reference is the correct answer in each item. * Independently significant in multiple logistic regression models including age, sex, BMI, education level, and income level ($p < 0.05$). The pre-action stage is the reference group is in A versus P, and the action stage is the reference group is in M versus A; [3] N (%); the rate of correct answer to each item. [4] Mean ± SE: Mean values adjusted by age, sex, BMI, education level, and income level from ANCOVA analysis; [5] Reference is respondent under a score of 6 (50th percentile of the average score).

Nutrients 2017, 9, 808

Table 6. Dietary behaviors related to sodium intake according to the stages of change.

	M	A	P	Total	p-Value[1]	A vs. P		M vs. A	
						OR[2]	95% CI	OR	95% CI
I often eat dried fish, salted and fermented fish, and salted mackerel	991 (87.4%) [3]	645 (86.5%)	1613 (82.1%)	3249 (84.5%)	0.0001	1.34 *	1.07–1.82	1.07	0.80–1.45
I often eat processed or instant food such as ramen, ham, and canned food.	1009 (89.9%)	654 (88.6%)	1534 (78.3%)	3197 (83.7%)	<0.0001	1.93 *	1.44–2.58	0.96	0.69–1.35
I add salt or sauces more when eating bland tasting dishes.	857 (75.7%)	471 (63.1%)	1073 (54.7%)	2401 (62.5%)	<0.0001	1.64 *	1.35–1.99	1.72 *	1.38–2.15
I eat all of the soup, stew, broth, or noodle liquid.	833 (73.7%)	518 (70.0%)	1236 (63.5%)	2587 (67.8%)	<0.0001	1.34 *	1.09–1.64	1.17	0.94–1.46
I frequently eat soy paste soup or other broth soups and stew (Jjigae, jeongol).	809 (71.8%)	502 (68.0%)	1169 (59.9%)	2480 (65.0%)	<0.0001	1.57 *	1.32–1.87	1.38 *	1.13–1.69
I eat out (including delivery foods) or have a dining meeting more than two or three times in a week.	903 (81.0%)	599 (81.4%)	1428 (73.1%)	2930 (77.0%)	<0.0001	1.38 *	1.09–1.74	0.97	0.75–1.26
I usually eat fried or pan-fried dishes and sliced raw fish with plenty of dipping sauces.	964 (85.8%)	602 (81.5%)	1430 (73.3%)	2996 (78.6%)	<0.0001	1.45 *	1.15–1.83	1.38 *	1.05–1.80
I prefer braised fish with soy sauce than fresh grilled fish.	864 (77.1%)	540 (73.3%)	1360 (69.6%)	2764 (72.5%)	<0.0001	1.23 *	1.00–1.53	1.26 *	1.00–1.56
I often eat plenty of fruits and vegetables. [+]	1055 (94.5%)	647 (89.0%)	1696 (87.3%)	3398 (89.8%)	<0.0001	1.32	0.97–1.80	1.99 *	1.34–2.95
I usually check the sodium content in nutrition labeling when eating-out or purchasing food. [+]	663 (58.9%)	361 (48.7%)	673 (34.5%)	1697 (44.5%)	<0.0001	1.87 *	1.54–2.26	1.45 *	1.19–1.78
I often eat potato chips or crackers as a snack.	1038 (92.1%)	671 (90.2%)	1646 (84.0%)	3355 (87.6%)	<0.0001	1.60 *	1.19–2.16	1.22	0.86–1.73
Average score.	893 (86.0%)	502 (18.6%)	1188 (63.8%)	2583 (72.5%)	<0.0001	1.60 *	1.28–1.99	1.96 *	1.50–2.56

M = Maintenance stage, A = Action stage, P = Preaction stage including the preparation, contemplation, and precontemplation stages. [1] p value from a chi-square test according to the stage of change group; [2] OR = Odds ratio; * Independently significant in multiple logistic regression models including age, sex, BMI, education level, and income level (p < 0.05). The pre-action stage is the reference group is in A versus P, and the action stage is the reference group is in M versus A. The reference is respondent over three points in each item; [3] N (%): the response rate is over three points (score range = 1–5; 5 = strongly disagree, 4 = disagree, 3 = neither agree nor disagree, 2 = agree, 1 = strongly agree); a higher score means better dietary pattern related sodium intake. ([+] 1 = strongly disagree, 2 = disagree, 3 = neither agree nor disagree, 4 = agree, 5 = strongly agree).

4. Discussion

This study provides the status of behavioral change in reducing sodium intake among Korean consumers. A recently performed an online survey in eight countries and showed that the percentages of people in each of the behavioral stages of salt reduction were 58% of the people in the preaction stage, 13% in the action stage, and 28% in the maintenance stage, although there was a significant difference across the countries in the distribution of the stages of change [13]. Koreans had higher proportions of people in the action and maintenance stages, potentially due to the recent nationwide sodium-reduction initiative. In addition, Koreans are open to sodium reduction compared with other people in the international study, considering that 23.3% of the participants of this study and 34% of the international study participants reported no intention to make changes in sodium intake (precontemplation stage) [13]. This indicates that it is time to change the strategy for moving from awareness to action for sodium reduction, although there is still a need to raise awareness and interest for those in the precontemplation stage.

This study examined cognitive and behavioral factors based on social cognitive theory according to the stages of behavioral change to assess the factors that were associated with taking action and maintaining the changes for reducing sodium intake. We classified responders into three categories for statistical analyses: the preaction, action, and maintenance stages. Multiple logistic regression analysis displayed meaningful factors differentiating the three stages. The comparison of participants in the action stage with those in the preaction stages was considered as determining the odds of 'taking action to reduce sodium intake', while the comparison of participants in the maintenance stage with those in the action stage reveals the odds of 'maintaining changes for reducing sodium intake'.

Many studies highlight that attitudes, knowledge of sodium intake, and health beliefs are important for changing sodium intake [19,20]. In addition to these factors, the perception of the social environment related to sodium intake seems to be important to changing behavior because the proportion of meals eaten outside of the home is continuously increasing as is the nationwide promotion of reducing sodium. The World Health Organization (WHO) recommends the development of supportive environments that promote healthy food choices to reduce the sodium consumption of the general population [21]. Recognizing social efforts and sodium labeling on processed foods were important factors for being in the action and maintenance stages. Further, participants who had purchased sodium-reduced foods, especially those recognized as salty foods such as ham, salt, soy sauce, and salted fish were more likely to be in the action stage. Previous studies have reported that most participants were capable of estimating the salt content of salty foods, but they were unaware of the salt content of the usual processed foods [20,22,23]. Thus, it is reasonable that consumers bought sodium-reduced products for salty foods first in the action stage and then began to consider less salty processed foods such as cereals and ramen in the maintenance stage. A supportive environment influences people to change by providing models for change and available foods for reduced sodium consumption [15].

Outcome expectancy is known as the primary motivational variable to elicit a change in behavior. It was reported that people who were aware that sodium intake was associated with increased blood pressure were more likely to practice sodium reduction than those who were not aware (OR = 2.17, 95% CI; 2.01–2.34) [24]. Our result is consistent with the previous study, although the odds ratio of being in the action stage is weaker. The result that the expectation of cancer prevention enhanced the likelihood of being in the maintenance stage indicates the need to educate the populace on the diverse health-related benefits of reducing their sodium intakes. Indeed, better knowledge about the relationship between sodium intake and osteoporosis was related to being in the maintenance stage, as shown in the results of the nutritional knowledge test. This study revealed that overcoming barriers to practicing was associated with the differentiation of the three stages, but 'preference for broth dishes' and 'preference for kimchi, salted fish, and fermented sauces' were hard to overcome in the early action stage. The majority of Koreans' sodium intake comes from fermented and salted traditional foods and soup-based meals [25]. These deeply rooted dietary habits are difficult to change but are critical to reaching the maintenance stage. Thus, more strategic intervention is needed such as developing various salt substitutes [26], fermentation technology to reduce sodium use, and reducing the size of the soup bowl.

Contrary to our expectations, the total nutritional knowledge score was not a differentiating factor between the preaction and action stages. Only knowledge on the recommended daily intake of salt and the difference between sodium and salt has a positive effect on the odds ratio of being in the action stage versus the preaction stage. The correct answer rate of these items was low, which is consistent with previous studies [13,19,27,28]. Lack of knowledge in these areas means that consumers are unlikely to be able to estimate their daily sodium intake and compare their intake with the recommended level. Indeed, it was reported that participants believed that their sodium intakes were equal to or less than the recommended level [24,29], despite strong evidence that the sodium intake of most populations exceeds the recommended level [30,31]. Therefore, it is evident that the recommended daily intake of sodium and the difference between sodium and salt should be focused on in the education of people in all the stages. The nutritional knowledge of the Korean consumer seems to be relatively high, considering a recent study that summarized the previous reports on the nutritional knowledge of the general population [32]. Detailed skills in practice are more effective for taking action in a situation in which the nutritional knowledge of the general population has reached a certain level. Actually, in our study, detailed dietary behaviors regarding low-sodium food selection and food preparation were different among the stages of change, and almost all of the desirable behaviors were associated with being in the action stage versus the preaction stage. It is known that behavioral change is a dynamic process that occurs in a sequential and cyclical order [33], which suggests the need for continuous education even for people in the action and maintenance stages.

In addition, self-efficacy is the primary resource for performing the behavior, considering that self-efficacy was more strongly related to intention to perform healthy eating practicing than was outcome expectancy [34]. Self-efficacy requires the ability to perform the behavior under a variety of circumstances, which suggests the need for nutrition education to improve skills and dietary behavior. Given the differences in cognition and behavior according to the stages, a tailored strategy, which is focused on motivating changes and raising self-efficacy, would be a promising approach. The results of this study suggest that educating individuals in detailed dietary behavior such as how to select low-sodium food would be more effective for those in the preaction stage, while it would be effective for those in the action stage to understand advanced nutritional knowledge such as the diverse health-related benefits of sodium reduction, tips to reduce sodium intake when cooking and eating, and the importance of a sufficient intake of fruits and vegetables.

This study has some limitations. We depended upon a self-administered questionnaire to obtain the results on the sample's dietary behavior related to sodium intake. Self-reports are likely to be biased to social expectation and difficult to verify. However, the results correspond to the differences in perception of barriers to reducing sodium intake according to the stages. We modified the five-stage model to three stages to simplify the analysis. This division may have masked factors associated with a readiness to make changes in sodium reduction, although our main interest was in taking action and maintenance. In addition, compared with the general Korean population, the participants were predominantly women and over-representative of the over 40 age group, who tend to be more health conscious. Nonetheless, this study provides a valid estimate because the recruitment of participants was nationwide with geographic distribution and the residential local size of population was taken into consideration.

In summary, the percentages of Korean consumers in each stage of behavioral change in order to reduce their sodium intake was 51.0% in the preaction stage, 19.5% in the action stage, and 29.5% in the maintenance stage. The factors associated with taking and maintaining action to reduce sodium intake were recognizing a supportive social environment, reducing barriers to practice, and enhancing self-efficacy. Therefore, campaigns that inform consumers of the health risks of high sodium intake and the establishment of a supportive environment, including sodium labeling, are effective for all consumers. In addition, there is a need for tailored education in purchasing, cooking, and eating according to the stages of behavioral change to reduce barriers and enhance self-efficacy.

5. Conclusions

The differences in cognitive and behavioral factors among the stages of behavioral change for reducing sodium intake in Korean consumers suggest the need of stage-matched intervention to reduce barriers and enhance self-efficacy for practicing low sodium diet, in addition to continual development of supportive social environment to raise public awareness.

Supplementary Material: The following are available online at www.mdpi.com/2072-6643/9/8/808/s1.

Acknowledgments: This research was supported by a grant from Korea Food and Drug Administration (11162Sobiyeon165) and the Catholic University of Korea, Research Fund 2015.

Author Contributions: Hye-Kyeong Kim and Jong Sook Kwon conceived and designed the overall study; So-hyun Ahn analyzed the data; Hye-Kyeong Kim and So-hyun Ahn wrote the manuscript; and Kyungmin Kim helped with the interpretation of the data and edited the manuscript.

Conflicts of Interest: The authors declare no conflict of interest.

References

1. He, F.J.; Li, J.; MacGregor, G.A. Effects of longer term modest salt reduction on blood pressure. Cochrane systematic review and meta-analysis of randomized trials. *BMJ* **2013**, *345*, f1325. [CrossRef] [PubMed]
2. Mozaffarian, D.; Fahimi, P.H.; Singh, G.M.; Micha, R.; Khatibzadeh, S.; Engell, R.E.; Lim, S.; Danaei, G.; Ezzati, M.; Powles, J. Global sodium consumption and death from cardiovascular causes. *N. Engl. J. Med.* **2014**, *371*, 624–634. [CrossRef] [PubMed]
3. Antonios, T.F.; MacGregor, G.A. Deleterious effects of salt intake other than effects on blood pressure. *Clin. Exp. Pharmacol. Physiol.* **1995**, *22*, 180–184. [CrossRef] [PubMed]
4. Webster, J.L.; Dunford, E.K.; Hawkes, C.; Neal, B. Salt reduction initiatives around the world. *J. Hypertens.* **2011**, *29*, 1043–1050. [CrossRef] [PubMed]
5. Asaria, P.; Chrisholm, D.; Mathers, C.; Ezzati, M.; Beaglehole, R. Chronic disease prevention: Health effects and financial costs of strategies to reduce salt intake and control tobacco use. *Lancet* **2007**, *370*, 2044–2053. [PubMed]
6. Ministry of Health and Welfare, Korea Centers for Disease Control and Prevention. *Korea Health Statistics 2014: Korea National Health and Nutrition Examination Survey (KNHANES V-2)*; Korea Centers for Disease Control and Prevention: Cheongwon, Korea, 2015.
7. Shankar, B.; Brambila-Macias, J.; Traill, B.; Mazzocchi, M.; Capacci, S. An evaluation of the UK Food Standards Agency's salt campaign. *Health Econ.* **2013**, *22*, 243–250. [PubMed]
8. Nissinen, A.; Kastarinen, M.; Tuomilehto, J. Community control of hypertension-experiences from Finland. *J. Hum. Hypertens.* **2004**, *18*, 553–556. [CrossRef] [PubMed]
9. Paik, H.Y. Nutritional review of salt. *J. Korean Soc. Food Sci. Nutr.* **1987**, *3*, 92–106.
10. Prohaska, J.O.; Velicer, W.F. The transtheoretical model of health behavior change. *Am. J. Health Promot.* **1997**, *12*, 38–48. [CrossRef]
11. Heather, N.; Rollnick, S.; Bell, A. Predictive validity of the readiness to change questionnaire. *Addiction* **1993**, *88*, 1667–1677. [CrossRef] [PubMed]
12. Prochaska, J.O.; Redding, C.A.; Harlow, L.L.; Rossi, J.S.; Velicer, W.F. The transtheoretical model of change and HIV prevention: A review. *Health Educ. Q.* **1994**, *21*, 471–486. [CrossRef] [PubMed]
13. Newson, R.S.; Elmadfa, I.; Biro, G.; Cheng, Y.; Prakash, V.; Rust, P.; Barna, M.; Lion, R.; Meijer, G.W.; Neufingeri, N.; et al. Barriers for progress in salt reduction in the general population. An international study. *Appetite* **2013**, *71*, 22–31. [CrossRef] [PubMed]
14. Baranowski, T.; Perry, C.L.; Parcel, G. How individuals, environments, and health behaviors interact: Social cognitive theory. In *Health Behavior and Health Education: Theory, Research and Practice*, 3rd ed.; Glanz, K., Rimer, B.K., Lewis, F.M., Eds.; Jossey-Bass: San Francisco, CA, USA, 2002; pp. 246–279.

15. Hearn, M.; Baranowski, T.; Baranowski, J.; Doyle, C.; Smith, M.; Lin, L.S.; Resnicow, K. Environmental influences on dietary behavior among children: Availability and accessibility of fruits and vegetables enable consumption. *J. Health Educ.* **1998**, *29*, 26–32. [CrossRef]

16. Jung, E.J.; Son, S.M.; Kwon, J.S. The effect of sodium reduction education program of a public health center on the blood pressure, blood biochemical profile and sodium intake of hypertensive adults. *Korean J. Community Nutr.* **2012**, *17*, 752–771. [CrossRef]

17. Son, S.M.; Lee, K.H.; Kim, K.W.; Lee, Y.K. *Nutrition Education and Counseling Practice*; Life Science Publishing Co.: Seoul, Korea, 2007; pp. 15–30.

18. Yim, K.S. The effects of a nutrition education program for hypertensive female elderly at the public health center. *Korean J. Community Nutr.* **2008**, *13*, 640–652.

19. Grimes, C.A.; Riddell, L.J.; Nowson, C.A. Consumer knowledge and attitudes to salt intake and labelled salt information. *Appetite* **2009**, *53*, 189–194. [CrossRef] [PubMed]

20. Kim, M.K.; Lopetcharat, K.; Gerard, P.D.; Drake, M.A. Consumer awareness of salt and sodium reduction and sodium labeling. *J. Food Sci.* **2012**, *77*, 307–313. [CrossRef] [PubMed]

21. World Health Organization. *Creating an Enabling Environment for Population-Based Salt Reduction Strategies: Report of a Joint Technical Meeting Held by WHO and the Food Standards Agency, United Kingdom, July 2010*; World Health Organization: Geneva, Switzerland, 2010. Available online: http://www.who.int/iris/handle/10665/44474 (accessed on 10 February 2017).

22. Kim, M.K.; Lee, K.G. Consumer awareness and interest toward sodium reduction trends in Korea. *J. Food Sci.* **2014**, *79*, S1416–S1423. [CrossRef] [PubMed]

23. Sarmugam, R.; Worsley, A.; Flood, V. Development and validation of a salt knowledge questionnaire. *Public Health Nutr.* **2014**, *17*, 1061–1068. [CrossRef] [PubMed]

24. Zhang, J.; Xu, A.Q.; Ma, J.X.; Shi, X.M.; Guo, X.L.; Engelgau, M.; Yan, L.X.; Li, Y.; Li, Y.C.; Wang, H.C.; et al. Dietary sodium intake: Knowledge, attitudes and practices in Shandong province, China, 2011. *PLoS ONE* **2013**, *8*, e58973. [CrossRef] [PubMed]

25. Yon, M.Y.; Lee, Y.N.; Kim, D.H.; Lee, J.Y.; Koh, E.M.; Nam, E.J.; Shin, H.H.; Kang, B.W.; Kim, K.W.; Heo, S.; et al. Major sources of sodium intake of the Korean population at prepared dish level -Based on the KNHANES 2008 & 2009. *Korean J. Community Nutr.* **2011**, *16*, 473–487.

26. Sultan, S.; Anjum, F.M.; Butt, M.S.; Huma, N.; Suleria, H.A. Concept of double salt fortification; a tool to curtail micronutrient deficiencies and improve health status. *J. Sci. Food Agric.* **2014**, *94*, 2830–2838. [CrossRef] [PubMed]

27. Marakis, G.; Tsigarida, E.; Mila, S.; Panagiotakos, D.B. Knowledge, attitudes and behaviour of Greek adults towards salt consumption: A Hellenic food authority project. *Public Health Nutr.* **2014**, *17*, 1877–1893. [CrossRef] [PubMed]

28. Webster, J.L.; Li, N.; Dunford, E.K.; Nowson, C.A.; Neal, B.C. Consumer awareness and self-reported behaviours related to salt consumption in Australia. *Asia Pac. J. Clin. Nutr.* **2010**, *19*, 550–554. [PubMed]

29. Land, M.A.; Webster, J.; Christoforou, A.; Johnson, C.; Trevena, H.; Hodgins, F.; Chalmers, J.; Woodward, M.; Barzi, F.; Smith, W.; et al. The association of knowledge, attitudes and behaviors related to salt with 24-hour urinary sodium excretion. *Int. J. Behav. Nutr. Phys. Act.* **2014**, *11*, 47. [CrossRef] [PubMed]

30. Okuda, N.; Stamler, J.; Brown, I.J.; Ueshima, H.; Miura, K.; Okayama, A.; Saitoh, S.; Nakagawa, H.; Sakata, K.; Yoshita, K.; et al. Individual efforts to reduce salt intake in China, Japan, UK, USA: What did people achieve? The INTERMAP Population Study. *J. Hypertens.* **2014**, *32*, 2385–2392. [CrossRef] [PubMed]

31. Ortega, R.M.; López-Sobaler, A.M.; Ballesteros, J.M.; Pérez-Farinós, N.; Rodriguez-Rodriguez, E.; Aparicio, A.; Perea, J.M.; Andrés, P. Estimation of salt intake by 24 h urinary sodium excretion in a representative sample of Spanish adults. *Br. J. Nutr.* **2011**, *105*, 787–794. [CrossRef] [PubMed]

32. Sarmugam, R.; Worsley, A. Current levels of salt knowledge: A review of the literature. *Nutrients* **2014**, *6*, 5534–5559. [CrossRef] [PubMed]

33. Diclemente, C.; Prohaska, J. Toward a comprehensive, transtheoretical model of change. In *Treating Addictive Behaviours*; Miller, W.R., Heather, N., Eds.; Plenum Press: New York, NY, USA, 1998; pp. 3–24.

34. Sheeshka, J.D.; Woolcott, D.M.; MacKinnon, N.J. Social cognitive theory as a framework to explain intentions to practice health eating behaviors. *J. Appl. Soc. Psychol.* **1993**, *23*, 1547–1573. [CrossRef]

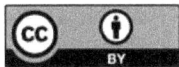

Article

Food Sources of Sodium Intake in an Adult Mexican Population: A Sub-Analysis of the SALMEX Study

Eloisa Colin-Ramirez [1,2,*], Ángeles Espinosa-Cuevas [3], Paola Vanessa Miranda-Alatriste [3], Verónica Ivette Tovar-Villegas [1], JoAnne Arcand [4] and Ricardo Correa-Rotter [3]

[1]   Sociomedical Research Department, Instituto Nacional de Cardiología 'Ignacio Chávez', Mexico City 14080, Mexico; veronicatovar92@hotmail.com
[2]   Consejo Nacional de Ciencia y Tecnología (CONACYT), Mexico City 03940, Mexico
[3]   Nephrology and Mineral Metabolism Department, Instituto Nacional de Ciencias Médicas y Nutrición Salvador Zubirán, Mexico City 14080, Mexico; angespinosac@gmail.com (Á.E.-C.); pvma2000@hotmail.com (P.V.M.-A.); correarotter@gmail.com (R.C.-R.)
[4]   Faculty of Health Sciences, University of Ontario Institute of Technology, Oshawa, ON L1H 7K4, Canada; joanne.arcand@uoit.ca
*   Correspondence: ecolinra@conacyt.mx; Tel.: +52-55-5573-2911 (ext. 1415)

Received: 15 June 2017; Accepted: 25 July 2017; Published: 27 July 2017

Abstract: Excessive dietary sodium intake increases blood pressure and cardiovascular risk. In Western diets, the majority of dietary sodium comes from packaged and prepared foods ($\approx$75%); however, in Mexico there is no available data on the main food sources of dietary sodium. The main objective of this study was to identify and characterize the major food sources of dietary sodium in a sample of the Mexican Salt and Mexico (SALMEX) cohort. Adult male and female participants of the SALMEX study who provided a complete and valid three-day food record during the baseline visit were included. Overall, 950 participants (mean age 38.6 $\pm$ 10.7 years) were analyzed to determine the total sodium contributed by the main food sources of sodium identified. Mean daily sodium intake estimated by three-day food records and 24-h urinary sodium excretion was 2647.2 $\pm$ 976.9 mg/day and 3497.2 $\pm$ 1393.0, in the overall population, respectively. Processed meat was the main contributor to daily sodium intake, representing 8% of total sodium intake per capita as measured by three-day food records. When savory bread (8%) and sweet bakery goods (8%) were considered together as bread products, these were the major contributor to daily sodium intake, accounting for the 16% of total sodium intake, followed by processed meat (8%), natural cheeses (5%), and tacos (5%). These results highlight the need for public health policies focused on reducing the sodium content of processed food in Mexico.

Keywords: salt; hypertension; processed foods

1. Introduction

Excessive dietary sodium intake increases blood pressure [1] and increases risk of hypertension, cardiovascular disease, stroke and chronic kidney disease [2–7]. Globally, it is estimated that 4.1 million deaths and 83 million years of disability were attributable to an excess dietary sodium intake in 2015 [8]. In Mexico, the prevalence of hypertension in those 20 years and older was 32.3% in men and 30.7% in women in 2012 [9]. Recently, mean dietary sodium intake in a healthy adult Mexican population was estimated to be 3150 mg/day (95% confidence interval: 3054, 3246 mg/day), being as high as 3735 mg/day among men, as measured by 24-h urinary sodium excretion [10]. These data show that sodium intake in Mexican population is higher than the World Health Organization (WHO) recommended intake of less than 2000 mg/sodium per day, a level set to reduce blood pressure and cardiovascular risk at the population level [11]. Together, these data highlight the need for population-based strategies in Mexico to achieve the WHO global target of reducing dietary sodium intake by 30% by 2025, for the prevention and control of non-communicable diseases [12].

Major sources of dietary sodium vary among different regions. In Western diets, the majority of dietary sodium comes from packaged and prepared foods ($\approx$75%), with a small contribution from discretionary salt that is added in cooking or at the table [13]. Conversely, in countries such as India [14], China [15] and Japan [16], discretionary use of salt remains a major source of dietary sodium. For example, in a Chinese population, it was found that 76% of dietary sodium came from salt added in home cooking, with a small contribution of processed foods [17]. In the Latin America region, Argentina reported that packaged and processed foods contributed between 65% and 70% to daily sodium intake [18]. In Mexico, there is no available data on the main food sources of dietary sodium. Knowledge of this information is key to identify targets and inform population-based strategies for sodium reduction at the population level. Thus, the main objective of this study was to identify and characterize the major food sources of dietary sodium in a sample of the Mexican Salt and Mexico (SALMEX) cohort. We also aimed to quantify the percentage of total sodium intake coming from different types of food, based on an analysis of food categories.

2. Materials and Methods

2.1. Study Population

This cross-sectional analysis was based on data from the Salt and Mexico (SALMEX) study. SALMEX was a cross-sectional study aimed at assessing the average salt, potassium, and iodine intake in an adult workers cohort from the National Institute of Medical Sciences and Nutrition Salvador Zubirán (INCMNSZ), in Mexico City, Mexico. One thousand and nine men and women between 18 and 65 years old were recruited in this cohort between 2010 and 2011. Participants of the SALMEX study were recruited from the INCMNSZ via an informative session on sodium intake and its role in human health that was delivered to the personnel from all the different areas and departments of this institution. At the end of these sessions, the SALMEX study was introduced to the attendees, who were invited to participate. Exclusion criteria were: history of heart failure, advanced kidney or liver disease, intestinal resection, diuretic drug initiation during the previous five days to enrolment, active infection, pregnancy, and lactation.

All subjects gave their informed consent for inclusion before they participated in the SALMEX study. The study was conducted in accordance with the Declaration of Helsinki, and the protocol was approved by the Health Research and Ethics Boards of the Instituto Nacional de Ciencias Médicas y Nutrición Salvador Zubirán (INCMNSZ) (REF. 191). Full results of the SALMEX study are currently being revised to be considered for publication, and have been published only as a conference abstract [19].

For the purposes of this sub-analysis of the SALMEX study, only participants with a complete and valid three-day food record were included.

2.2. Assessments

2.2.1. Anthropometric and Blood Pressure Measurements

Body weight and height were measured according to standard protocols [20]. Subjects wore light clothes and were barefoot. Body mass index (BMI) was calculated by dividing total body weight (kilograms) by height squared (square meters). Systolic and diastolic blood pressure were measured three times on the right arm, with the participants in a seated position and after a five-minute rest, using an Omron HEM-907XL automated sphygmomanometer (Omron Health Care, Inc., Vernon Hill, IL, USA).

2.2.2. Estimating Total Sodium Intake

As part of the SALMEX cohort, all included participants completed a three-day food record to estimate dietary sodium intake. Trained dietitians provided detailed instructions to the participants on how to fill out the food diaries. Subjects were asked to record all food and beverages consumed during the three days prior to the study visit, using standard household measures (e.g., cups and tablespoons) or commercial measures (e.g., weight of commercially packaged foods as given on the label or number of pieces consumed). All food records were reviewed by the study dietitian during an interview with the patient to identify any missing food items and to clarify food item descriptions and portion sizes using standardized food models.

Food records were analyzed by trained personnel to estimate total sodium intake by using a nutrient software program (Nutrikal®VO, V2, Consinfo, S.C., Mexico City, Mexico), which contains the nutritional composition of common Mexican foods. Additional food items were added to the Nutrikal database when none of the food items contained in the current database reflected the actual food consumed by the patient, or when sodium content for that specific food item was not reported in the database (e.g., panela cheese, some seasonings and sauces, etc.). Sodium content for food items added to the database was obtained from food labels or the Tables of Composition of Mexican Foods and Food Products [21]. A mean dietary intake from the three days was estimated for energy (kcal/day) and sodium (mg/day). Table salt was not considered for food record analysis due to the complexity of accurately estimating the amount of salt added in cooking or at the table, either at home or restaurants. Generic restaurant meals included in the Nutrikal database such as pizzas and hamburgers were considered for food record analysis; however, in the case of more specific restaurant meals not included in the database, such as meat or pasta dishes and salads, for which nutritional information was not available, ingredients, except for salt and salty seasonings, were considered separately for food record analysis.

Only participants with a complete and valid three-day food record were considered for analysis. A complete food record was defined as that with three days recorded; whilst a valid food record was considered that with a plausible energy intake reported (defined as $\geq$500 kcal/day and $\leq$4000 kcal/day) [22–24].

2.2.3. Identifying Food Sources of Sodium

Because the nutrient software program employed for food record analysis did not provide a break-down of dietary intake information to individual food items entered for analysis, and only provided the overall dietary intake information from the whole day or from the total amount of days recorded (e.g., total amount of sodium provided by all the foods entered from the three days), it was not feasible to sum up total sodium from all foods recorded within the food category to identify the main food sources of sodium, and thus we followed a food record-searching approach to search for relevant food sources of sodium in the food records. For this purpose, relevant food sources of sodium were identified prior to food record searching according to the following criteria:

(a)   To identify foods in the food supply that contain high amounts of sodium, the Nutrikal®VO (V2) nutrient software database, which contains the nutritional composition of common Mexican foods, was used. Database food items with a sodium content $\geq$480 mg/100 g of food product were identified. The cut-off of 480 mg of sodium/100 g of product as a means to identify potential food sources of sodium, was based on the rationale that a percent daily value (%DV) of 20% provided by a product-specific serving size is considered high by the U.S. Food and Drug Administration. Since the reference daily value was 2400 mg/sodium, 480 mg represented this 20% DV [25]. In Mexico, there is currently no a reference %DV to classify nutrient DVs reported on the food labels as high or low. Additionally, in this study, due to the complexity of determining product-specific serving sizes, we selected a standard portion of 100 g of product for all food items to identify a sodium content of 480 mg.

(b) To identify food sources of sodium not included in the Nutrikal®VO (V2) nutrient software database, an expert panel made up of two nutritional epidemiologists and one nutritionist scientist reviewed the Nutrikal®VO (V2) food list and developed a list of foods that were missing in the database, but are highly consumed by the Mexican population. The additional foods considered for inclusion were confirmed to have a sodium content ≥480 mg/100 g (e.g., carnitas and cecina tacos, panela cheese, chorizo, and some hot sauces and hot chili powder seasonings). Sodium content was obtained from food labels for packaged foods, and from the Tables of Composition of Mexican Foods and Food Products [21] in the case of tacos.

(c) To identify foods containing moderate amounts of sodium that are consumed highly frequently by the Mexican population, and thus cumulatively may contribute significant amounts of sodium, the same expert panel identified food items with sodium content >120 mg sodium/100 g of product. At this stage, foods such as Mexican street food [Mexican little whims (antojitos mexicanos)], cereal bars, some packaged cookies and bakery goods, and some type of chips, were included. Sodium content was obtained from the Nutrikal®VO (V2) nutrient software database, food labels, and the Tables of Composition of Mexican Foods and Food Products [21]. Based on the rationale that a 5% DV or less (equivalent to 120 mg/sodium or less according to a DV of 2400 mg/sodium) provided by a product-specific serving size is considered low [25], we also focused on products with sodium content >120 mg/100 g of product in order to ensure inclusion of moderate-sodium food items that may represent a relevant food source of sodium in this population.

All additional food items considered for inclusion as described in points b and c, were also considered for food record analysis to estimate total sodium intake. After food sources of sodium were identified (as previously described), these were intentionally searched in the food records by trained dietitians during the food record searching phase. The amount of sodium in mg provided by the total amount of each specific food item consumed per person during the three days and an average from the three days was recorded.

Similar to the food record analysis for estimating total sodium intake, and due to the complexity of accurately estimating the amount used, table salt was not considered during the food record searching phase, and in the case of specific restaurant meals not included in the database and for which there was no nutritional information available, such as meat or pasta dishes and salads, ingredients, except salt and salty seasonings, were considered separately. After the food record searching phase was completed, all food items (sources of sodium) identified in the food records were classified into 33 sodium-focused food categories based on Health Canada's Guidance for the Food Industry on Reducing Sodium in Processed Foods [26], and adapted for Mexican food, considering the raw material used for their elaboration, similar nutritional content, and culinary practices used.

2.2.4. Twenty-Four-Hour Urinary Sodium Excretion

One 24-h urine sample was collected from each participant during the last day of food recording. Participants were provided with detailed verbal and written instructions on how to collect the urine sample. They were asked to discard the first morning void and to collect all urine over the following 24 h, including the first void on the next morning. Participants were given a preservative-free container to collect the urine sample. Urinary sodium was determined by using the ion selective electrode method [27], and urinary creatinine was measured by Jaffe's colorimetric assay in automated analyzers (Synchron Cx5 PRO autoanalyser, Beckman Coulter Inc., Fullerton, CA, USA). Completeness of the 24-h urine samples was determined based on creatinine excretion by dividing total urinary creatinine by body weight in kilograms. Participants with urinary creatinine levels within the standard creatinine excretion rates (15–25 mg/kg/24-h for men and 10–20 mg/kg/24-h for women) [28] were considered for estimating 24-h urinary sodium excretion.

2.3. Statistical Analysis

Continuous variables were expressed as mean ± standard deviation, and categorical variables were presented as absolute (number of participants) and relative frequencies (percentages). For comparison of continuous variables, the Student's *t*-test for independent samples was employed, whilst the Pearson chi-square test or Fisher's exact test were used for categorical variables.

For each individual, the following parameters related to the sodium-focused food categories were estimated:

(a) an average daily sodium intake in mg from the three days recorded, provided by each food category; and

(b) the percentage that each food category contributed to total sodium intake, which was estimated by the three-day food record.

Since only one 24-h urine sample was collected and food sources of sodium were obtained from three days, percent of contribution to total sodium intake provided by each food category was based on total sodium intake estimated by the three-day food record instead of that estimated by the 24-h urinary sodium excretion.

The percent of the study population consuming at least one of the food items from each sodium-focused food category on at least one of the three days recorded was estimated, and it was considered the proportion of consumers for each food category. We conducted analyses for the entire study population, and then analyses considering only consumers of each food category.

Means [95% confidence intervals (CI)] in the entire study population (per capita) and among consumers were estimated for the two parameters listed above for all food categories, except for those with an overall consumer prevalence less than 5%, since estimates may be less precise in such small populations.

3. Results

Of the 1009 participants recruited in the SALMEX study, 979 provided a complete three-day food record, of which 950 were valid. Of these, 698 provided a complete 24-h urine sample. Overall, 950 participants with a complete and valid three-day food record were included for analysis of food sources of sodium, while only those with a complete 24-h urine sample (*n* = 698) were considered for estimating 24-h urinary sodium excretion. Characteristics of the study population by sex are shown in Table 1. Women were older and had lower systolic and diastolic blood pressure compared to men. Dietary sodium intake was 2647.2 ± 976.9 mg/day in the entire study population, observing a higher consumption among men (3018.2 ± 1091.9 mg/day) compared to women (2422.9 ± 823.6, *p* < 0.001), as measured by three-day food records. Twenty-four-hour urinary sodium excretion showed the same trend, with a higher excretion in men (4167.7 ± 1520.2 mg/day) than in women (3118.3 ± 1156.4, *p* < 0.001)

Table 1. Study population characteristics by sex [1].

Variable	Overall (*n* = 950)	Men (*n* = 358)	Women (*n* = 592)	*p* Value [2]
Age (years)	38.6 ± 10.7	37.6 ± 10.8	39.1 ± 10.6	0.04
Body mass index (kg/m²)	27.1 ± 4.8	27.3 ± 4.3	27.0 ± 5.0	0.30
Systolic blood pressure (mmHg) [3]	119.0 ± 14.0	125.2 ± 13.7	115.4 ± 12.8	<0.001
Diastolic blood pressure (mmHg) [3]	75.0 ± 9.3	77.5 ± 9.9	73.5 ± 8.6	<0.001
Dietary sodium intake (mg/day)	2647.2 ± 976.9	3018.2 ± 1091.9	2422.9 ± 823.6	<0.001
24-h urinary sodium excretion (mg/24 h) [4]	3497.2 ± 1393.0	4167.7 ± 1520.2	3118.3 ± 1156.4	<0.001

[1] Data are presented in mean ± standard deviation; [2] For comparison between men and women by using Student's *t*-test for independent samples; [3] Systolic and diastolic blood pressure measures were available for 885 of the 950 included participants (men *n* = 330, women *n* = 555); [4] Only subjects that provided a complete 24-h urine sample were considered for estimating 24-h urinary sodium excretion (overall *n* = 698, men *n* = 252, women *n* = 446).

Proportion of consumers for each sodium-focused group is shown in Table 2. In the overall population, savory bread (84%), processed meat (73%), natural cheeses (70%), sweet bakery goods (68%), salad dressings and mayonnaise (48%), cookies and cereal bars (39%), chips (28%), tacos (24%), breakfast cereal (22%), and canned peppers (19%), were the 10 food groups with the highest proportion of consumers; whilst chicken nuggets (2%), instant soups (1%), chocolate milk powder (1%), olives (0.7%), powdered milk (0.6%), hot cakes flour mix (0.6%), and peanut butter (0.1%), were the food groups with less than 5% of consumers. Additionally, natural cheeses (75% vs. 64%, $p < 0.001$), breakfast cereal (25% vs. 17%, $p = 0.004$), hot sauces and chamoy (bottled snack sauces) (11% vs. 7%, $p = 0.04$), and hot chili powder seasonings (7% vs. 3%, $p = 0.004$) showed a higher proportion of consumers among women compared to men; contrarily, there was a higher percentage of consumers of tacos (30% vs. 20%, $p = 0.001$) and hamburgers (9% vs. 5%, $p = 0.03$) in men than women.

Table 2. Population consuming at least one food of each food group (consumers) by sex [1].

Food Category	Overall (n = 950)	Men (n = 358)	Women (n = 592)	p Value [2]
Savory bread (bolillo, telera, baguette, sliced bread, hot dog buns, and others)	800 (84.2)	306 (85.5)	494 (83.4)	0.41
Processed meat (deli meat, sausages, bacon, chorizo, machaca and smoked pork chop)	692 (72.8)	268 (74.9)	424 (71.6)	0.28
Natural cheeses (Panela, Oaxaca, Goat, Parmesan, Brie, Camembert, Cheddar, Swiss, Gouda, Manchego, cream cheese, Provolone, etc.)	669 (70.4)	228 (63.7)	441 (74.5)	<0.001
Sweet bakery goods (packaged and unpackaged)	650 (68.4)	249 (69.6)	401 (67.7)	0.56
Salad dressings and mayonnaise	452 (47.6)	167 (46.6)	285 (48.1)	0.66
Cookies and cereal bars	369 (38.8)	125 (34.9)	244 (41.2)	0.054
Chips (potato, corn and wheat)	269 (28.3)	96 (26.8)	173 (29.2)	0.43
Tacos (assorted)	225 (23.7)	106 (29.6)	119 (20.1)	0.001
Breakfast cereal	206 (21.7)	60 (16.8)	146 (24.7)	0.004
Canned peppers (pickled and chipotle peppers)	176 (18.5)	67 (18.7)	109 (18.4)	0.91
Catsup and mustard	162 (17.1)	62 (17.3)	100 (16.9)	0.87
Tamales (assorted)	129 (13.6)	50 (14.0)	79 (13.3)	0.79
Margarine and butter	123 (12.9)	37 (10.3)	86 (14.5)	0.06
Mole	109 (11.5)	45 (12.6)	64 (10.8)	0.41
Canned fish (tuna and sardines)	104 (10.9)	39 (10.9)	65 (11.0)	0.97
Popcorn	99 (10.4)	29 (8.1)	70 (11.8)	0.07
Salty nuts and seeds	97 (10.2)	31 (8.7)	66 (11.1)	0.22
Wheat flour tortillas	96 (10.1)	38 (10.6)	58 (9.8)	0.69
Hot sauces and chamoy (bottled snack sauces)	91 (9.6)	25 (7.0)	66 (11.1)	0.04
Seasonings (seasoning sauces, salty seasoning powders and broth cubes)	84 (8.8)	32 (8.9)	52 (8.8)	0.94
Pizza	75 (7.9)	31 (8.7)	44 (7.4)	0.50
Crackers	72 (7.6)	24 (6.7)	48 (8.1)	0.43
Processed cheese [3]	69 (7.3)	29 (8.1)	40 (6.8)	0.44
Hamburgers	63 (6.6)	32 (8.9)	31 (5.2)	0.03
Hot chili powder seasonings	53 (5.6)	10 (2.8)	43 (7.3)	0.004
Canned beans	47 (4.9)	21 (5.9)	26 (4.4)	0.31
Chicken nuggets	21 (2.2)	9 (2.5)	12 (2.0)	0.62
Instant soups	13 (1.4)	5 (1.4)	8 (1.4)	1.0
Chocolate milk powder	12 (1.3)	5 (1.4)	7 (1.2)	0.77
Olives	7 (0.7)	4 (1.1)	3 (0.5)	0.44
Powdered milk	6 (0.6)	1 (0.3)	5 (0.8)	0.42
Hot cakes flour mix	6 (0.6)	1 (0.3)	5 (0.8)	0.42
Peanut butter	1 (0.1)	0 (0.0)	1 (0.2)	1.0

[1] Data are presented as n (%); [2] For comparison between men and women by using Pearson chi-square test or Fisher's exact test; [3] Processed cheese category included cheese products made from an emulsified blend of natural cheese. Includes spreads, blocks, and slices with or without added ingredients; e.g., American style cheese, spread, or melting slices.

Table 3 shows the total sodium contributed in mg by the top 26 food categories based on the prevalence of consumers for each food category, excluding those with a proportion of consumers less than 5%. Processed meat (223 mg/day), savory bread (209 mg/day), sweet bakery goods (178 mg/day), natural cheeses (118 mg/day) and tacos (114 mg/day) were the five leading categories in the overall population. This table also shows the percent of total sodium intake estimated by three-day food records attributed to each category; dietary sodium provided by these top 26 food categories accounted for the 52.7% of total sodium intake per person in this population, with bread products (savory bread and sweet bakery) representing a 16% of total sodium intake, followed by processed meat (8%), natural cheeses (5%) and tacos (5%).

Table 3. Total sodium contributed by the most frequently consumed food categories in the entire sample population (per capita) [1,2].

Food Category	Mg/Na/Day (*n* = 950)	% of Total Na Intake [3] (*n* = 950)
Processed meat (deli meat, sausages, bacon, chorizo, machaca and smoked pork chop)	223.4 (205.5, 241.3)	8.3 (7.6, 8.9)
Savory bread (bolillo, telera, baguette, sliced bread, hot dog buns, and others)	209.4 (198.2, 220.6)	8.3 (7.8, 8.7)
Sweet bakery goods (packaged and unpackaged)	178.2 (165.9, 190.4)	7.6 (7.0, 8.2)
Natural cheeses (Panela, Oaxaca, Goat, Parmesan, Brie, Camembert, Cheddar, Swiss, Gouda, Manchego, cream cheese, Provolone, etc.)	118.0 (108.5, 127.5)	5.0 (4.5, 5.4)
Tacos (assorted)	113.8 (89.2, 138.3)	5.2 (3.9, 6.5)
Breakfast cereal	52.7 (44.1, 61.2)	2.1 (1.7, 2.5)
Pizza	46.0 (33.2, 58.7)	1.6 (1.2, 2.1)
Tamales (assorted)	39.6 (32.3, 46.8)	1.8 (1.4, 2.3)
Chips (potato, corn and wheat)	31.8 (26.9, 36.6)	1.2 (1.0, 1.4)
Seasonings (seasoning sauces, salty seasoning powders and broth cubes)	31.5 (21.9, 41.0)	1.1 (0.8, 1.5)
Cookies and cereal bars	26.4 (22.6, 30.3)	1.1 (0.9, 1.3)
Canned fish (tuna and sardines)	26.3 (20.2, 32.3)	1.1 (0.8, 1.3)
Canned peppers (pickled and chipotle peppers)	25.2 (19.5, 30.9)	1.0 (0.7, 1.2)
Mole	24.9 (19.0, 30.8)	1.0 (0.7, 1.2)
Hamburger	22.6 (16.6, 28.5)	0.8 (0.6, 1.0)
Salad dressings and mayonnaise	20.5 (18.1, 23.0)	0.8 (0.7, 0.9)
Hot chili powder seasonings	19.5 (8.5, 30.6)	0.7 (0.3, 1.2)
Catsup and mustard	16.4 (13.0, 19.9)	0.6 (0.5, 0.7)
Wheat flour tortillas	15.9 (12.5, 19.4)	0.7 (0.5, 0.8)
Canned beans	12.7 (7.6, 17.7)	0.4 (0.3, 0.6)
Hot sauces and chamoy (bottled snack sauces)	12.7 (8.5, 16.8)	0.5 (0.3, 0.7)
Salty nuts and seeds	11.6 (7.2, 16.1)	0.4 (0.3, 0.6)
Processed cheese [4]	10.7 (7.9, 13.5)	0.4 (0.3, 0.5)
Crackers	9.9 (6.6, 13.2)	0.4 (0.3, 0.5)
Popcorn	8.4 (5.7, 11.1)	0.4 (0.3, 0.5)
Margarine and butter	5.5 (4.1, 7.0)	0.2 (0.2, 0.3)

[1] Data are presented as mean (95% CI); [2] Estimates are provided for food groups with a consumer prevalence greater than 5%; [3] Based on three-day food records; [4] Processed cheese category included cheese products made from an emulsified blend of natural cheese. Includes spreads, blocks, and slices with or without added ingredients; e.g., American style cheese, spread or melting slices.

When only individuals who consumed the foods (consumers) were included in the analysis, pizza (582 mg/day), tacos (480 mg/day), seasonings (356 mg/day), hot chili powder seasonings (350 mg/day), and hamburgers (340 mg/day) were identified as the top five contributors to daily sodium intake. Tacos provided nearly 22% of total sodium intake among tacos consumers, followed by pizza that represented a 21% of total sodium intake among tacos consumers (Table 4).

The top ten sodium-contributing food categories according to the percent of total sodium intake, as measured by three-day food records, attributed to each food category in the entire sample population (per capita) and among consumers, are summarizes in Figure 1.

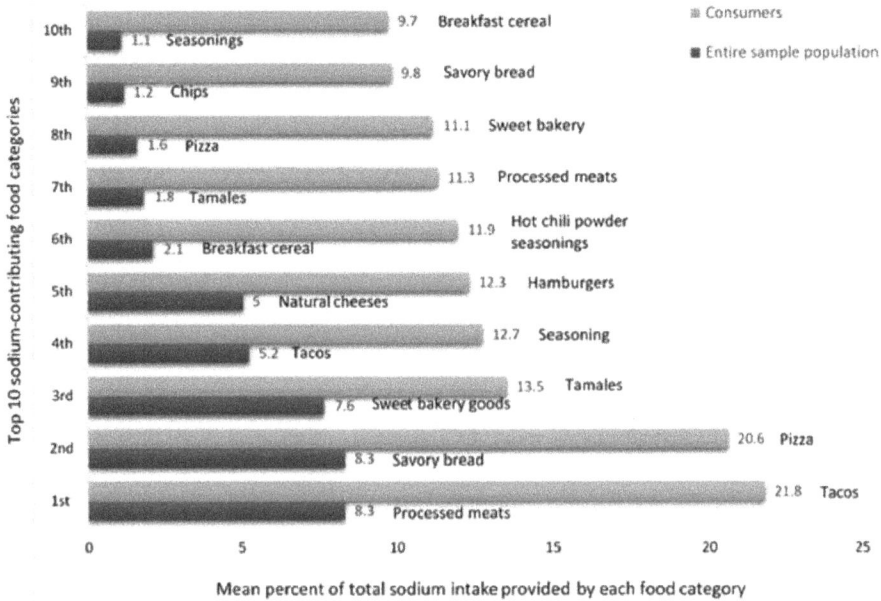

Figure 1. Top ten sodium-contributing food categories according to the percent of total sodium intake (as measured by three-day food records) attribute to each food category in the entire sample population (per capita) and among individuals who consumed the foods (consumers).

Table 4. Total sodium contributed by most frequently consumed food categories among individuals who consumed the foods (consumers) [1,2].

Food Category	Mg/Na/Day	% of Total Na Intake [3]
Pizza	582.1 (480.5, 683.7)	20.6 (17.2, 24.0)
Tacos (assorted)	480.2 (391.8, 568.7)	21.8 (16.9, 26.8)
Seasonings (seasoning sauces, salty seasoning powders and broth cubes)	355.8 (274.1, 437.5)	12.7 (9.6, 15.7)
Hot chili powder seasonings	350.3 (170.2, 530.4)	11.9 (6.0, 17.8)
Hamburgers	340.4 (301.9, 378.9)	12.3 (10.6, 13.9)
Processed meat (deli meat, sausages, bacon, chorizo, machaca and smoked pork chop)	306.7 (285.1, 328.2)	11.3 (10.6, 12.1)
Tamales (assorted)	291.5 (265.6, 317.4)	13.5 (10.9, 16.1)
Sweet bakery goods (packaged and unpackaged)	260.4 (246.5, 274.3)	11.1 (10.4, 11.9)
Canned beans	255.6 (180.1, 331.1)	8.4 (6.0, 10.8)
Breakfast cereal	243.0 (216.5, 269.4)	9.7 (8.5, 10.8)
Savory bread (bolillo, telera, baguette, sliced bread, hot dog buns, and others)	248.6 (237.2, 260.0)	9.8 (9.4, 10.3)
Canned fish (tuna and sardines)	240.0 (205.5, 274.4)	9.6 (7.9, 11.3)
Mole	216.7 (181.7, 251.7)	8.5 (6.7, 10.3)
Natural cheeses (Panela, Oaxaca, Goat, Parmesan, Brie, Camembert, Cheddar, Swiss, Gouda, Manchego, cream cheese, Provolone, etc.)	167.6 (156.0, 179.1)	7.0 (6.5, 7.6)
Wheat flour tortillas	157.8 (140.8, 174.7)	6.7 (5.7, 7.7)
Processed cheese [4]	147.5 (128.3, 166.6)	5.4 (4.7, 6.2)
Canned peppers (pickled and chipotle peppers)	135.8 (110.8, 160.9)	5.2 (4.1, 6.4)

Table 4. *Cont.*

Food Category	Mg/Na/Day	% of Total Na Intake [3]
Crackers	130.8 (98.2, 163.3)	4.6 (3.5, 5.8)
Hot sauces and chamoy (bottled snack sauces)	132.0 (96.7, 167.4)	5.1 (3.6, 6.5)
Salty nuts and seeds	113.7 (75.3, 152.2)	4.1 (3.0, 5.3)
Chips (potato, corn and wheat)	112.1 (99.1, 125.1)	4.4 (3.8, 4.9)
Catsup and mustard	96.3 (81.1, 111.5)	3.3 (2.8, 3.8)
Popcorn	80.6 (59.2, 102.0)	3.5 (2.5, 4.5)
Cookies and cereal bars	68.1 (59.8, 76.3)	2.9 (2.5, 3.3)
Salad dressings and mayonnaise	43.1 (38.8, 47.4)	1.6 (1.5, 1.8)
Margarine and butter	42.7 (34.2, 51.3)	1.9 (1.3, 2.4)

[1] Data are presented as mean (95% CI); [2] Estimates are provided for food groups with a consumer prevalence greater than 5%; [3] Based on three-day food records; [4] Processed cheese category included cheese products made from an emulsified blend of natural cheese. Includes spreads, blocks, and slices with or without added ingredients; e.g., American style cheese, spread or melting slices.

4. Discussion

This is the first study aimed at identifying major food sources of sodium in a sample of the Mexican population. Of the 33 sodium-focused food categories identified in the diet of this population, processed meat was the main contributor to daily sodium intake, representing 8% of total sodium intake per capita. However, if savory bread (8%) and sweet bakery (8%) are considered together as bread products, these were the major contributor to daily sodium intake accounting for the 16% of total sodium intake. Similar results have been reported across diverse occidental countries such as Costa Rica (48%, reported as cereal and cereal products among women) [29], United Kingdom (34.6%) [17], Colombia (30.5%) [30], France (24.2%) [31], and Canada (13.9%) [32], where bread products were found to be the major contributors for daily sodium intake, although the percentage of contribution varies across these countries. In the United States (19.5%, including breads, grains and cereals) [17] and Brazil (between 10% and 11% across age groups) [33], this food category was the second and third main source of total sodium intake, respectively. Thus, recognizing that bread products are relevant sources of dietary sodium in the western diet, some countries in the Americas region have set voluntary or regulated targets and timelines for reducing sodium content in bread, among other food products, as part of an initiative proposed by the Pan American Health Organization in 2013 to achieve the WHO global target of a 30% relative reduction in salt intake by 2025 [34]. For example, Argentina, where bread accounts for almost 25% of total salt in the diet [18], has achieved a 25% average reduction in sodium content of bread from 2011 to 2013 [35]. Similarly, Chile has reported an average decrease in sodium levels in bread from >830 mg/100 g to 479 mg/100 g [35]. Likewise, Mexico in 2012 set its voluntary food reformulation initiative with a bread category including sliced bread and bolillo (a product similar to baguette) to reduce their sodium content by 10% in five years. Average baseline sodium levels of these products were estimated at 520 mg/100 g [36]. Currently, monitoring studies of this initiative in Mexico have not been reported. Results of this study highlight the need of a collaborative effort to reduce the sodium content of processed foods, not only bread, but also processed meat, cheese and cereal products that were identified as relevant food sources of sodium in this population. Importantly, natural cheeses were listed in the top 10 sodium-contributing food categories, while processed chesses were not; this may be explained by the high prevalence of consumers of natural cheeses (70%) in this population, highlighting the need for initiatives to reduce the sodium content in these type of cheeses. Also, it is important to implement a monitoring plan to evaluate adherence to these initiatives.

In Asian countries, salt and salty condiments remain the main source of dietary sodium intake. Data from the INTERMAP Study revealed that in the Chinese population, most (76%) dietary sodium was from salt added in home cooking, followed by soy sauce (6%); while in the Japanese sample of this same study, the main food source of dietary sodium was soy sauce (20%) [17]. In a more recent study in Japanese population, it was reported that the contribution to daily sodium intake of seasonings such as salt or soya sauce may be as high as 62% in men and 63% in women [16].

In this Mexican population, within the combined contribution for total sodium intake of seasonings (1.1%), mole (1.0%), hot chili powder seasonings (0.7%), and hot sauces and chamoy (bottled snack sauces) (0.5%) represented 3.3% of the total sodium intake per person. However, estimation of sodium intake from table salt added in cooking at home or outside home was not feasible, due to the challenges of self-reporting the amount of salt used for cooking, especially if somebody else cooked; however, we believe that table salt added to meals in cooking represents an important contribution to total sodium intake, since home cooking remains a common practice and nearly 10% of Mexican population have their afternoon meal at local kitchens that serve homemade-style meals [37]. Importantly, seasonings and hot chili powdered seasonings represented 13% and 12% of total sodium intake, respectively, among consumers, highlighting the relevance of making people aware of the importance of reducing not only the use of table salt, but also salty seasonings, for the purpose of reducing dietary sodium intake, by providing alternatives to enhance the flavor of the food without adding salt or salty seasonings.

Additionally, in Mexico there is limited information on the nutritional content of restaurant foods, especially for sit-down restaurants, due to the lack of national policy on this regard; thus, salt and salty seasonings added to meals from sit-down restaurants were not taken into account in this analysis. Ingredients of these dishes were considered separately for food record analysis, except salt and salty seasonings, due to the complexity of accurately estimating the amount of salt and salty seasonings used in meal preparation. Initiatives to promote reporting on nutrient levels of restaurant foods are needed, to better inform the population on sodium content in foods eaten outside the home, and to help individuals make healthier choices.

Fast foods such as pizzas was found among the top 10 food sources of dietary sodium, and they were the second with the highest percent of total sodium intake among consumers. Local street-foods such as tacos and tamales were also identified as relevant food contributors for total sodium intake in this population; indeed, tacos and tamales were first and the third with the highest percent of total sodium intake among consumers. However, it is important to mention that other Mexican street foods such as sopes (fried corn tortilla topped with refried beans, fresh cheese, and salsa) and gorditas (snack food made of corn dough and filled with pork skin, fresh cheese, and salsa), when both combined, were found to be consumed by 8% of this population, but were not included in the analysis as a whole food, since there was no available information on their sodium content in the nutrient software database, or in the tables of nutrient composition of Mexican foods, and similar to restaurant meals, the ingredients of these Mexican street foods, except table salt, were considered separately for analysis.

Study Limitations

This study has three main limitations: (1) This analysis included foods for which sodium content was reported either in the nutrient software database, tables of nutrient composition of Mexican foods, or on food labels, possibly excluding relevant foods sources of sodium in the Mexican population for which there was no available information on sodium levels, such as restaurant dishes, and some Mexican street foods; (2) criteria to identified food sources of dietary sodium to be included in the analysis captured foods with a sodium density >120 mg sodium/100 g, which assured inclusion of moderate sodium content foods, but excluded low sodium density foods such as milk (approx. 44 mg of sodium in 100 g), that might represent certain percentages of total sodium intake in this population, especially when these low sodium foods are highly consumed by the population. Thus, the method used in this study to identify relevant food sources of sodium may have left out some other relevant sources of sodium that may explain, in part, the remaining 47% of total sodium intake not explained by the 26 food categories included in this analysis. However, we were able to identified processed foods with salt added and bread products (packaged and unpackaged) as main sources of dietary sodium intake and the main objective of product reformulation initiatives; (3) this study population included healthy volunteer workers from a health institution who enrolled in the study after attending an informative session on sodium intake and its role in human health, and thus they may be not comparable to the general population; additionally, these workers had access to a lunch service benefit (the institution provides lunch for free to all the personnel), thus eating patterns may not reflect sources of sodium in all segments of the Mexican population; (4) finally, the three-day food record method may have incorporated reporting bias to the dietary sodium estimates; however, in order to minimize this bias, all food records were reviewed by the study dietitian during an interview with the patient to identify any missing food items, and to clarify food item descriptions and portion sizes using standardized food models. Additionally, this dietary method included three days allowance to account for day-to-day variations in the eating patterns.

5. Conclusions

Overall, mean daily sodium intake estimated by three-day food records and 24-h urinary sodium excretion in this sample of the Mexican SALMEX cohort was 2647.2 mg/day and 3497.2 mg/day, respectively, which was higher than the 2000 mg/day intake recommended by the WHO. Bread products (savory bread and sweet bakery), processed meats, and cheeses were the top three contributors for total sodium intake, as measured by three-day food records in this study population, highlighting the need for public health policies focused on reducing the sodium content of processed food. Additionally, Mexican street foods such as tacos and tamales were found to be relevant food sources of sodium in this population. This data will raise awareness about the need for sensitizing the public about the contribution of these unpackaged foods (which have no food labels showing sodium levels) to total sodium intake. Also, it is important to set voluntary or regulated initiatives to report sodium levels in restaurant dishes that allow the public to make informed choices when eating out. Finally, further studies aimed at evaluating the contribution of table salt added during cooking in this population, and studies to establish sodium levels in diverse Mexican street foods are needed, to better understand the contribution of local eating patterns to the total dietary sodium intake in the Mexican population.

Acknowledgments: This work was supported by a National Council of Science and Technology (CONACYT) Research Grant No. SALUD-2016-C02-272561. Danone Institute provided a Research Grant to cover the cost of the materials and assays performed in the SALMEX study.

Author Contributions: E.C.-R. conceived and designed the study, analyzed the data and drafted the manuscript. A.E.-C., P.V.M.-A. and J.A. contributed to the design of the study, interpretation of the results and preparation of the manuscript. V.I.T.-V. contributed to the production and interpretation of the results and preparation of the manuscript. R.C.-R. contributed to interpretation of the results and preparation of the manuscript.

Conflicts of Interest: The authors declare no conflict of interest. The founding sponsors had no role in the design of the study; in the collection, analyses, or interpretation of data; in the writing of the manuscript, and in the decision to publish the results.

References

1. Farquhar, W.B.; Edwards, D.G.; Jurkovitz, C.T.; Weintraub, W.S. Dietary sodium and health: More than just blood pressure. *J. Am. Coll. Cardiol.* **2015**, *65*, 1042–1050. [CrossRef] [PubMed]
2. Aburto, N.J.; Ziolkovska, A.; Hooper, L.; Elliott, P.; Cappuccio, F.P.; Meerpohl, J.J. Effect of lower sodium intake on health: Systematic review and meta-analyses. *BMJ* **2013**, *346*, f1326. [CrossRef] [PubMed]
3. Graudal, N.A.; Hubeck-Graudal, T.; Jurgens, G. Effects of low sodium diet versus high sodium diet on blood pressure, renin, aldosterone, catecholamines, cholesterol, and triglyceride. *Cochrane Database Syst. Rev.* **2011**, *11*, CD004022.
4. He, F.J.; MacGregor, G.A. Effect of modest salt reduction on blood pressure: A meta-analysis of randomized trials. Implications for public health. *J. Hum. Hypertens.* **2002**, *16*, 761–770. [CrossRef] [PubMed]
5. He, J.; Gu, D.; Chen, J.; Jaquish, C.E.; Rao, D.C.; Hixson, J.E.; Chen, J.C.; Duan, X.; Huang, J.F.; Chen, C.S.; et al. Gender difference in blood pressure responses to dietary sodium intervention in the GenSalt study. *J. Hypertens.* **2009**, *27*, 48–54. [CrossRef] [PubMed]

6. He, F.J.; Li, J.; MacGregor, G.A. Effect of longer term modest salt reduction on blood pressure: Cochrane systematic review and meta-analysis of randomised trials. *BMJ* **2013**, *346*, f1325. [CrossRef] [PubMed]
7. Vollmer, W.M.; Sacks, F.M.; Ard, J.; Appel, L.J.; Bray, G.A.; Simons-Morton, D.G.; Conlin, P.R.; Svetkey, L.P.; Erlinger, T.P.; Moore, T.J.; et al. Effects of diet and sodium intake on blood pressure: Subgroup analysis of the DASH-sodium trial. *Ann. Intern. Med.* **2001**, *135*, 1019–1028. [CrossRef] [PubMed]
8. GBD 2015 Risk Factors Collaborators. Global, regional, and national comparative risk assessment of 79 behavioural, environmental and occupational, and metabolic risks or clusters of risks, 1990–2015: A systematic analysis for the Global Burden of Disease Study 2015. *Lancet* **2016**, *388*, 1659–1724.
9. Campos-Nonato, I.; Hernández-Barrera, L.; Rojas-Martínez, R.; Pedroza, A.; Medina-García, C.; Barquera-Cervera, S. Hypertension: Prevalence, early diagnosis, control and trends in Mexican adults. *Salud Publica Mex.* **2013**, *55*, S144–S150. [CrossRef] [PubMed]
10. Vallejo, M.; Colin-Ramirez, E.; Rivera, S.; Cartas, R.; Madero, M.; Infante, O.; Vargas-Barron, J. Assessment of sodium and potassium intake by 24-hour urinary excretion in a healthy Mexican population: The Tlalpan 2020 Cohort. *Arch. Med. Res.* **2017**, *48*, 195–202. [CrossRef] [PubMed]
11. World Health Organization. *Global Status Report on Noncommunicable Diseases 2014*; World Health Organization: Geneva, Switzerland, 2014.
12. World Health Organization. *Report of the Formal Meeting of Member States to Conclude the Work on the Comprehensive Global Monitoring Framework, Including Indicators, and a Set of Voluntary Global Targets for the Prevention and Control of Noncommunicable Diseases*; World Health Organization: Geneva, Switzerland, 2012.
13. Mattes, R.D.; Donnelly, D. Relative contributions of dietary sodium sources. *J. Am. Coll. Nutr.* **1991**, *10*, 383–393. [CrossRef] [PubMed]
14. Ravi, S.; Bermudez, O.I.; Harivanzan, V.; Kenneth Chui, K.H.; Vasudevan, P.; Must, A.; Thanikachalam, S.; Thanikachalam, M. Sodium intake, blood pressure, and dietary sources of sodium in an adult south indian population. *Ann. Glob. Health* **2016**, *82*, 234–242. [CrossRef] [PubMed]
15. Zhao, F.; Zhang, P.; Zhang, L.; Niu, W.; Gao, J.; Lu, L.; Liu, C.; Gao, X. Consumption and sources of dietary salt in family members in Beijing. *Nutrients* **2015**, *7*, 2719–2730. [CrossRef] [PubMed]
16. Asakura, K.; Uechi, K.; Masayasu, S.; Sasaki, S. Sodium sources in the Japanese diet: Difference between generations and sexes. *Public Health Nutr.* **2016**, *19*, 2011–2023. [CrossRef] [PubMed]
17. Anderson, C.A.; Appel, L.J.; Okuda, N.; Brown, I.J.; Chan, Q.; Zhao, L.; Ueshima, H.; Kesteloot, H.; Miura, K.; Curb, J.D.; et al. Dietary sources of sodium in China, Japan, the United Kingdom, and the United States, women and men aged 40 to 59 years: The INTERMAP study. *J. Am. Diet. Assoc.* **2010**, *110*, 736–745. [CrossRef] [PubMed]
18. Ferrante, D.; Apro, N.; Ferreira, V.; Virgolini, M.; Aguilar, V.; Sosa, M.; Perel, P.; Casas, J. Feasibility of salt reduction in processed foods in Argentina. *Rev. Panam. Salud Publica* **2011**, *29*, 69–75. [CrossRef] [PubMed]
19. Vega, O.; Mendoza, A.; Baeza, Y.; Rincón, R.; Espinosa-Cuevas, A.; Fonseca, J.; Nieves, I.; Herrero, B.; Correo, R. Asociación de la ingesta dietética de sal con hipertensión en trabajadores mexicanos: Estudio SALMEX. In *Conference Abstract Booklet, Proceedings of the LXI Annual Meeting of the Mexican Institute of Nephrology Research (Instituto Mexicano de Investigaciones Nefrológicas (IMIN)), Guadalajara, Mexico, 5–8 December 2012*; IMIN: Guadalajara, Mexico, 2012; p. 38.
20. Centers for Disease Control and Prevention; National Center for Health Statistics. *National Health and Nutrition Examination Survey (NHANES)*; Anthropometry Procedures Manual; Centers for Disease Control and Prevention: Atlanta, GA, USA, 2007. Available online: https://www.cdc.gov/nchs/data/nhanes/nhanes_07_08/manual_an.pdf (accessed on 14 June 2017).
21. Morales de León, J.C.; Bourges Rodríguez, H.; Camacho Parra, M.E. *Tablas de Composición de Alimentos y Productos Alimenticios Mexicanos (Versión Condesada 2015)*; Instituto Nacional de Ciencias Médicas y Nutrición Salvador Zubirán: México City, México, 2016; pp. 55–589.
22. Rhee, J.J.; Sampson, L.; Cho, E.; Hughes, M.D.; Hu, F.B.; Willett, W.C. Comparison of methods to account for implausible reporting of energy intake in epidemiologic studies. *Am. J. Epidemiol.* **2015**, *181*, 225–233. [CrossRef] [PubMed]
23. Yum, J.; Lee, S. Development and evaluation of a dish-based semiquantitative food frequency questionnaire for Korean adolescents. *Nutr. Res. Pract.* **2016**, *10*, 433–441. [CrossRef] [PubMed]

24. Teixeira, J.A.; Baggio, M.L.; Giuliano, A.R.; Fisberg, R.M.; Marchioni, D.M. Performance of the quantitative food frequency questionnaire used in the Brazilian center of the prospective study natural history of human papillomavirus infection in men: The HIM study. *J. Am. Diet. Assoc.* **2011**, *111*, 1045–1051. [CrossRef] [PubMed]

25. U.S. Food and Drug Administration. *How to Understand and Use the Nutrition Facts Label*; U.S. Food and Drug Administration: Silver Spring, MD, USA, 2016. Available online: https://www.fda.gov/food/ingredientspackaginglabeling/labelingnutrition/ucm274593.htm (accessed on 14 June 2017).

26. Health Canada, Bureau of Nutritional Sciences. *Guidance for the Food Industry on Reducing Sodium in Processed Foods*; Health Canada: Ottawa, ON, Canada, 2012.

27. Pelleg, A.; Levy, G.B. Determination of Na+ and K+ in urine with ion-selective electrodes in an automated analyzer. *Clin. Chem.* **1975**, *21*, 1572–1574. [PubMed]

28. Wielgosz, A.; Robinson, C.; Mao, Y.; Jiang, Y.; Campbell, N.R.; Muthuri, S.; Morrison, H. The impact of using different methods to assess completeness of 24-hour urine collection on estimating dietary sodium. *J. Clin. Hypertens. (Greenwich)* **2016**, *18*, 581–584. [CrossRef] [PubMed]

29. Carballo de la Espriella, M.; Morales Palma, G. Fuentes Alimentarias de sal/sodio en mujeres, Costa Rica. *Rev. Costarric. Salud Pública* **2011**, *20*, 90–96.

30. Gaitan Charry, D.A.; Estrada, A.; Argenor, L.G.; Manjarres, L.M. Food sources of sodium: Analysis based on a national survey in Colombia. *Nutr. Hosp.* **2015**, *32*, 2338–2345. [PubMed]

31. Meneton, P.; Lafay, L.; Tard, A.; Dufour, A.; Ireland, J.; Menard, J.; Volatier, J.L. Dietary sources and correlates of sodium and potassium intakes in the French general population. *Eur. J. Clin. Nutr.* **2009**, *63*, 1169–1175. [CrossRef] [PubMed]

32. Fischer, P.W.; Vigneault, M.; Huang, R.; Arvaniti, K.; Roach, P. Sodium food sources in the Canadian diet. *Appl. Physiol. Nutr. Metab.* **2009**, *34*, 884–892. [CrossRef] [PubMed]

33. De Moura, S.A.; Bezerra, I.N.; Pereira, R.A.; Peterson, K.E.; Sichieri, R. Dietary sources of sodium intake in Brazil in 2008–2009. *J. Acad. Nutr. Diet.* **2013**, *113*, 1359–1365. [CrossRef] [PubMed]

34. Campbell, N.; Legowski, B.; Legetic, B.; Ferrante, D.; Nilson, E.; Campbell, C.; L'Abbe, M. Targets and timelines for reducing salt in processed food in the Americas. *J. Clin. Hypertens. (Greenwich)* **2014**, *16*, 619–623. [CrossRef] [PubMed]

35. Campbell, N. Population Level Dietary Salt Reduction Initiative in the Americas. 2015. Available online: http://resources.cpha.ca/CPHA/Conf/Data/2015/A15-633e.pdf (accessed on 14 June 2017).

36. Secretaría de Gobernación. Acuerdo Por el Que se Recomienda la Disminución del Uso de Sal Común o Cloruro de Sodio en la Elaboración de Pan Como Una Medida de Prevención de Enfermedades Cardiovasculares, y Otras Crónico-Degenerativas. 2012. Available online: http://dof.gob.mx/nota_detalle.php?codigo=5256201&fecha=22/06/2012 (accessed on 14 June 2017).

37. García Urigüen, P. La Alimentación de los Mexicanos. In *Cambios Sociales y Económicos, y su Impacto en Los Hábitos Alimenticios*; Cámara Nacional de la Industria de Transformación: México City, Mexico, 2012. Available online: http://clubnutricion.com.mx/educacion_continua/La%20alimentaci%C3%B3n%20de%20los%20mexicanos%20%E2%80%94%20Estudio%20completo.pdf (accessed on 14 June 2017).

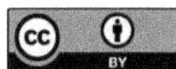

nutrients

MDPI

Article

Urinary Sodium and Potassium Excretion and Dietary Sources of Sodium in Maputo, Mozambique

Ana Queiroz [1], Albertino Damasceno [2,3], Neusa Jessen [2,4], Célia Novela [2], Pedro Moreira [1,4,5], Nuno Lunet [3,4] and Patrícia Padrão [1,4,*]

[1] Faculdade de Ciências da Nutrição e Alimentação da Universidade do Porto, Rua Dr. Roberto Frias, 4200-465 Porto, Portugal; anaqueiroz91@hotmail.com (A.Q.); pedromoreira@fcna.up.pt (P.M.)
[2] Faculdade de Medicina da Universidade Eduardo Mondlane, Avenida Salvador Allende, n° 702, 1111 Maputo, Mozambique; tino_7117@hotmail.com (A.D.); neusa.jessen@gmail.com (N.J.); celianovela@gmail.com (C.N.)
[3] Departamento de Ciências da Saúde Pública e Forenses e Educação Médica, Faculdade de Medicina da Universidade do Porto, Alameda Prof. Hernâni Monteiro, 4200-319 Porto, Portugal; nlunet@med.up.pt
[4] EPIUnit-Instituto de Saúde Pública, Universidade do Porto, Rua das Taipas, n° 135, 4050-600 Porto, Portugal
[5] Centro de Investigação em Atividade Física, Saúde e Lazer, Universidade do Porto, Rua Dr. Plácido da Costa, 4200-450 Porto, Portugal
*   Correspondence: patriciapadrao@fcna.up.pt; Tel.: +35-122-507-4320; Fax: +35-122-507-4329

Received: 10 June 2017; Accepted: 27 July 2017; Published: 3 August 2017

Abstract: This study aimed to evaluate the urinary excretion of sodium and potassium, and to estimate the main food sources of sodium in Maputo dwellers. A cross-sectional evaluation of a sample of 100 hospital workers was conducted between October 2012 and May 2013. Sodium and potassium urinary excretion was assessed in a 24-h urine sample; creatinine excretion was used to exclude unlikely urine values. Food intake in the same period of urine collection was assessed using a 24-h dietary recall. The Food Processor Plus® was used to estimate sodium intake corresponding to naturally occurring sodium and sodium added to processed foods (non-discretionary sodium). Salt added during culinary preparations (discretionary sodium) was computed as the difference between urinary sodium excretion and non-discretionary sodium. The mean (standard deviation) urinary sodium excretion was 4220 (1830) mg/day, and 92% of the participants were above the World Health Organization (WHO) recommendations. Discretionary sodium contributed 60.1% of total dietary sodium intake, followed by sodium from processed foods (29.0%) and naturally occurring sodium (10.9%). The mean (standard deviation) urinary potassium excretion was 1909 (778) mg/day, and 96% of the participants were below the WHO potassium intake recommendation. The mean (standard deviation) sodium to potassium molar ratio was 4.2 (2.4). Interventions to decrease sodium and increase potassium intake are needed in Mozambique.

Keywords: sodium; salt; urinary sodium; urinary potassium; Mozambique; Africa

1. Introduction

High sodium intake increases blood pressure (BP) and negatively affects endothelial and cardiovascular function, being positively associated with kidney disease, and cardiovascular morbidity and mortality [1–3]. Monitoring sodium intake at a population level, including the assessment of the contribution of different dietary sources of sodium to the overall consumption, are key aspects when designing interventions to control this risk factor.

The upper limit for sodium intake recommended by the World Health Organization (WHO) is two grams per day, corresponding to five grams of salt (sodium chloride)/day [4]. However, population-based data on sodium intake around the world shows that the intake far exceeds the recommendations [5]. In addition, potassium is another key nutrient that is inversely associated with blood pressure [6,7], and its relation with sodium intake should be taken into account when assessing the adequacy of sodium intake. Potassium increases urinary sodium excretion and reduces the risk of stroke and cardiovascular disease, attenuating sodium's negative effects [8,9]. In fact, the effects of high sodium and low potassium intake on BP levels have been regarded as synergic [10–12] The sodium sensitivity of blood pressure and, consequently, the risk of hypertension, have been shown to increase with diets low in potassium [13] and, also of note, a higher intake of potassium has even more benefits for those with a high intake of sodium [14].

The WHO recommends a minimum daily intake of 3510 mg of potassium per day, and that the ratio of sodium to potassium (Na/K ratio) should be one to one, which should be achievable if the WHO guidelines for those nutrients are attained. Otherwise, if the levels of consumption of sodium are high, the recommended level of potassium intake must be increased in order to maintain the ratio at one [15]. Urinary Na/K ratio is considered an important measure, since it has been shown to represent a stronger marker of the relation of sodium and blood pressure [16]. Consequently, it is a better predictor of incident hypertension and of outcomes of blood pressure than the isolated urinary excretion of sodium or potassium, as reported in several studies [17–20], particularly in hypertensive adult populations [21].

Previous studies evaluating worldwide sodium and potassium intakes revealed overall high sodium and low potassium consumption [16], with a few regions, including some African populations, presenting low sodium and high potassium consumption [22]. In most of the Sub-Saharan Africa (SSA) countries, the intake of sodium has been shown to be well above that recommended by WHO [23].

Despite the lack of data on sodium and potassium intake in Mozambique, the monitoring of these exposures is of the utmost importance in this setting, given the high prevalence of hypertension (25–64 years: 33.1% in 2005) [24] and the increasing public health impact of cardiovascular diseases (CVD) in the country [25,26].

In the last decades, a steep increase in urbanization has been observed in Mozambique [27]. This will expectedly promote dietary changes, mostly involving decreases in the consumption of foods rich in potassium, such as legumes, fruits, vegetables, and a more frequent intake of processed foods, which often are energy dense and rich in salt [28]. A previous study on the culinary practices of Maputo inhabitants, conducted with a sub-sample of the present study, reported a frequent use of processed food products, such as sugar-sweetened beverages and sodium-rich powdered chicken stocks [29], reflecting the nutrition transition occurring in Mozambique [30,31].

We aimed to (i) evaluate the urinary excretion of sodium, potassium and sodium to potassium ratio and (ii) to estimate the contribution of discretionary (sodium from salt added during culinary preparations) and non-discretionary sodium (naturally occurring sodium and sodium added to processed foods) to the total sodium intake in a sample of Maputo inhabitants.

2. Materials and Methods

This is a cross-sectional study, based on a convenience sample of 100 adults, assembled between October 2012 and May 2013. Participants were selected among the workers of the Maputo Central Hospital. The sample included both lay workers and health professionals; all participants were Maputo dwellers, belonging to different households, aged 25 to 64 years. An incentive of 200 meticais (equivalent to around $4 United States dollar) was given to participants, to cover transportation costs and thus ensure participation. Demographic characteristics, including sex, age, and education, and a 24-h dietary recall were obtained in a face-to-face interview. Anthropometric measurements were taken and a 24-h urine sample was collected.

2.1. 24-h Urine Collection

A container was supplied and participants were carefully instructed, through oral and written guidelines, to collect their urine over a 24-h period. They were taught to discard the first morning void and to collect all urine over the following 24 h, including the first void on the following morning, and to keep note of the time of the start and end of collection. This process occurred during weekdays and weekends, in periods not including any night shifts of the participants. Urine samples were analyzed for volume, creatinine, sodium and potassium. Sodium and potassium in urine were measured by flame photometry and creatinine by an automated validated enzymatic method.

To minimize systematic error due to incomplete urine collection, detailed instructions for a valid collection of urine were given orally and a leaflet was provided to each participant. In addition, a 3-L container was given to each participant to store the urine for 24 h, plus a 1-L plastic jug for each urine sample collection and a funnel to assist in both urine collection in the case of women, and in the transfer of urine from the jug to the 3-L container. Each participant was offered a backpack to facilitate the transportation of all this material when participants were away from home. Also, on the day of delivery of the 24-h urine participants were asked about the validity of their urine through the question, "How many times did you forget to pass urine sample in the counter during the 24 h". Participants were also questioned about the occurrence of any problem that may have compromised the validity of urine.

The urinary creatinine excretion was used to exclude samples unlikely to represent a 24-h urine collection, either by undersampling or oversampling. We used the 24-h urinary creatinine excretion in relation to body weight, that is, creatinine coefficient = creatinine (mg/day)/weight (kg). Coefficients between 14.4 to 33.6 in men and 10.8 to 25.2 in women were considered sufficient to ensure that the samples corresponded to a 24-h period as recommended [32]. This led to the exclusion of the samples from 18 participants, and a total of 82 were considered for data analysis.

2.2. Dietary Intake

A 24-h dietary recall referring to the day of urine collection was obtained by a trained interviewer. Participants were asked to report all foods and beverages consumed in the reference period, aided by a photographic book and household measures (spoons, plates, cups and glasses) to quantify portion sizes. Data was collected regarding the amount of different foods consumed, identifying those consumed outside home, and also detailed information on the amount of added fat, sugar, chicken powdered stocks, salt added at the table and during cooking, and the use of other seasonings, the brand of processed foods, recipes and culinary methods. Food Processor Plus® (Esha Research, Salem, OR, USA) was used to convert foods into nutrients; this software uses the U.S. Department of Agriculture food composition table, including raw and/or processed foods. Data referring to foods not available in the latter database was obtained from the Mozambican Food Composition Tables [33]. Data from the Brazilian Food Composition Table [34] was also used for foods not available in the Mozambican tables. For industrial food products, data from nutritional labels were used. Naturally occurring sodium and sodium added to processed foods (non-discretionary sodium), was then calculated and the salt added during culinary preparations (discretionary sodium) was estimated by the difference between urinary sodium excretion and non-discretionary sodium.

2.3. Anthropometric Measures

A SECA® (Seca GmbH, Hamburg, Germany) digital scale with an embedded stadiometer was used for weight and height measurements, to the nearest 0.1 km and 0.1 cm, respectively. The participants were evaluated lightly clothed, barefooted, positioned in the center of the scale and with the head positioned in the Frankfort plan, according to standard procedures [35]. Body mass index (BMI) was calculated as the weight (kg) divided by square of height (m) and WHO cutoffs were used to define underweight (<18.5 kg/m^2), normal weight (18.5–24.9 kg/m^2), overweight (25.0–29.9 kg/m^2) and obesity (≥ 30 kg/m^2) [36].

A constant tension tape was used to measure waist circumference, directly over the skin at the level of the midpoint between the inferior margin of the last rib and the iliac crest in the mid-axillary-line, to the nearest 0.1 cm. Abdominal obesity was considered present when waist circumference was >88 cm for women and >102 cm for men [37].

2.4. Statistical Analysis

For comparisons between men and women, we used the following statistical tests: (i) the independent samples t-test for continuous socio-demographic, anthropometric and urinary parameters; (ii) the Mann–Whitney U test for dietary intakes; (iii) the Chi-Square for categorical variables. Data analysis was conducted using the Statistical Package for Social Sciences, version 23 (IBM Corporation, New York, NY, USA).

2.5. Ethics

The study protocol was approved by the Mozambican National Bioethics Committee for Health and written informed consent was obtained from all participants. The ethic approval code is 236/CNBS/12.

3. Results

The participants' mean age was 40 years and approximately half reported more than primary school education. Just over half were classified as overweight or obese (Table 1).

Table 1. Characteristics of the study sample, overall and by sex.

	Total (*n* = 82)	Women (*n* = 39)	Men (*n* = 43)	*p*
Age (years), mean (SD)	39.9 (9.6)	41.8 (10.5)	38.1 (8.5)	0.082
Education level, *n* (%)				
Primary school not completed	17 (20.7)	11 (28.2)	6 (14.0)	
Primary school completed	43 (52.4)	18 (46.2)	25 (58.1)	
Secondary school completed	18 (22.0)	9 (23.1)	9 (20.9)	0.331
Post-secondary school	4 (4.9)	1 (2.6)	3 (7.0)	
BMI (kg/m^2), mean (SD)	26.7 (5.8)	29.6 (6.4)	24.1 (3.7)	<0.001
BMI categories, *n* (%)				
Thinness	1 (1.2)	0	1 (2.3)	
Normal weight	39 (47.6)	13 (33.3)	26 (60.5)	
Overweight	25 (30.5)	11 (28.2)	14 (32.6)	0.001
Obesity	17 (20.7)	15 (38.5)	2 (4.7)	
Waist circumference (cm), mean (SD)	89.2 (14.7)	93.8 (14.7)	85.0 (13.5)	0.007
Abdominal obesity, *n* (%)	27 (32.9)	24 (61.5)	3 (7.0)	<0.001

Standard deviation (SD); Body mass index (BMI).

As shown in Table 2, the most frequently consumed food groups in the previous 24 h (percentage of participants consuming, median intake among consumers) were cereal and cereal products (100%, 360 g), oils and fats (96%, 9 g) and vegetables (94%, 94 g).

A total of 90% of the participants consumed fruits and/or vegetables, from whom 26% met the recommended daily intake of at least 400 g [38].

Results from urine collection are shown in Table 3. Overall, the mean (standard deviation) urinary sodium excretion was 4220 (1830) mg/day and 92% of the participants did not meet the WHO recommendations for a maximum sodium intake of 2 g/day; in fact, almost half (56.4% of women and 41.9% of men) had a sodium intake above twice the recommended.

The mean (standard deviation) urinary potassium excretion was 1909 (778) mg/day, and 96% of the participants did not meet the WHO recommendations for minimum potassium intake. Mean (standard deviation) urinary sodium/potassium molar ratio was 4.7 (2.6) for women and 3.7 (2.1) for men (*p* = 0.06).

Sodium from salt added during culinary preparations was the most important contributor to total sodium intake (all participants, 60.1%; women, 66.5%; men, 54.2%), followed by salt from processed foods (all participants, 29.0%; women, 26.0%; men, 31.8%). Naturally occurring sodium accounted for 10.9% of the overall intake (7.4% in women and 14.0% in men) (Figure 1).

In this sample, 69.5% of participants used chicken stocks for cooking or seasoning food, 96.3% added salt when cooking and 35.4% used salt for salad seasoning.

Table 2. Dietary intake of the studied sample, overall and by sex.

Dietary Intake (g/Day) *	n [†]	Total	n [†]	Women	n [†]	Men	p
Cereal and cereal products	82	360 (63,1507)	39	322 (103, 1081)	43	407 (63, 1507)	0.072
Wheat Bread	66	200 (60, 700)	31	150 (60, 600)	35	300 (100, 700)	0.018
Rice	69	107 (27, 320)	33	107 (27, 320)	36	107 (27, 320)	0.804
Beans	26	94 (31, 250)	10	94 (31, 172)	16	94 (47, 250)	0.336
Meat products	51	125 (16, 500)	23	125 (16, 500)	28	89 (40, 375)	0.161
Fish and seafood dishes	38	94 (25, 375)	17	94 (63, 172)	21	94 (25, 375)	0.728
Eggs	23	55 (28, 110)	14	55 (28, 55)	9	55 (55, 110)	0.369
Milk and milk products	21	44 (8, 430)	6	47 (22, 430)	15	44 (8, 300)	0.622
Vegetables	77	94 (10, 361)	36	84 (13, 361)	41	102 (10, 294)	0.709
Fruits	49	188 (34, 1016)	25	188 (47, 1016)	24	188 (34, 958)	0.763
Oils and fats	79	9 (1, 105)	36	9 (1, 27)	43	9 (1, 105)	0.694
Sugars, preserves and confectionery	72	54 (1, 1837)	37	166 (1, 784)	35	21 (4, 1837)	0.016
Other foods	58	101 (9, 318)	27	101 (31, 203)	31	101 (9, 318)	0.656
Peanut	39	94 (34, 203)	19	94 (34, 205)	20	96 (45, 169)	0.857

* Results are presented as median (minimum, maximum); [†] Corresponds to the number of participants consuming each food item of food items from each group.

Table 3. Urinary data on sodium and potassium excretion, overall and by sex.

	Total	Women	Men	p
Sodium (mg/day), mean (SD)	4220 (1830)	4538 (2033)	3931 (1593)	0.135
Salt (g/day), mean (SD)	10.6 (4.6)	11.3 (5.1)	9.8 (4.0)	0.135
Compliance with recommendations, n (%) *	7 (8.5)	2 (5.1)	5 (11.6)	0.455
Potassium (mg/day), mean (SD)	1909 (778)	1841 (780)	1970 (779)	0.537
Compliance with recommendations, n (%) [†]	3 (3.7)	1 (2.6)	2 (4.7)	0.537
Ratio Na/K, mean (SD) [¥]	4.2 (2.4)	4.7 (2.6)	3.7 (2.1)	0.061

SD—standard deviation; * The upper limit for sodium intake recommended by the World Health Organization (WHO) is 2000 mg per day; [†] The WHO recommends a minimum daily intake of 3510 mg of potassium per day; [¥] Molar Ratio Na/K estimated taking into account the molar weight of sodium (23 g/mol) and potassium (39 g/mol).

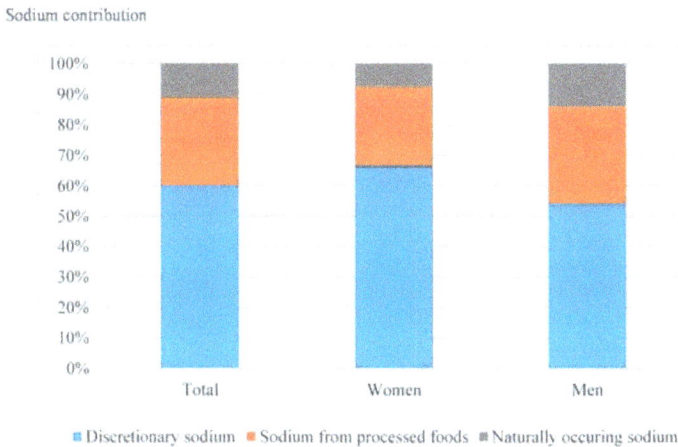

Figure 1. Mean sodium contribution (%) from discretionary salt use (added sodium during culinary preparations), salt added during processing (sodium from processed foods) and sodium intrinsic in food (naturally occurring sodium), overall and by sex.

4. Discussion

To the best of our knowledge, this is the first study on sodium intake in the Mozambican population using 24-h urinary sodium excretion. Our results showed that nine out of every 10 participants exceeded the recommended sodium consumption, and the mean intake was more than twice the recommended by the WHO [4]. Sodium from salt added during culinary preparations accounted for almost two thirds of the total sodium intake.

Data on sodium intakes in African countries is scarce and most of the available studies are older than 15 years, many of them dating back over 30 years. This data was used in recently published systematic reviews that revealed sodium intakes in adult populations from African countries above the WHO recommended maximum of 2 g/day [23,39], with lower values found in Sub-Saharan Africa (<3.3 g/day) than in other world regions [39]. Nevertheless, a recent study conducted in Benin, in urban and rural areas, revealed a mean dietary intake of 4.4 g/24 h of sodium and 1.8 g/24 h of potassium, which are in line with findings from the present study [40].

In a systematic review including data from several countries worldwide, mean sodium intake was always lower in women, with the difference between sexes ranging from 8.9% in South Asia to 10.7% in Western Europe [39]. In the latter study, estimated sodium intakes ranged from 2.18 g/day in Eastern Sub-Saharan Africa to 4.80 g/day in Asian regions [39]. Despite the fact that in our study, similarly to the situation described in other Sub-Saharan African countries [23], no significant differences between sexes were observed in sodium excretion, women presented a higher proportion of urinary sodium to potassium ratio than men. This finding may, at least partially, be explained by the reported significantly higher consumption of sugars, preserves and confectionery by women, as some foods in this group (e.g., cakes, biscuits and cookies) can be important sources of sodium and mostly are low in potassium. In addition, although not statistically significant, women, compared to men, reported a higher consumption of meat products which are also frequently high in sodium.

In our study, discretionary salt was the leading main source of sodium intake, as observed in other studies conducted in different countries [41,42] including South Africa [43], Japan and China [11,44]. Interestingly, besides the use of salt added at the table (35% of the participants) and during cooking (96% of the participants), using stock powder when cooking or adding it to prepared food and salads was shown to be frequent in the present sample of the Mozambican population (70% of the participants). As such, stock powder may be an important source of sodium intake by the Mozambican population, since many people probably do not look at labels and are not aware of sodium contents in these products, using them as additional seasoning. On the contrary, in European and North American countries sodium intake is dominated by sodium added by industry in processed/ultra-processed foods [45]. Yet an increase in the consumption of ultra-processed foods [46] may also be expected in Mozambique, along with globalization.

In addition to high sodium intake, a low intake of potassium, which is inversely related to blood pressure and to the risk of stroke [47], was also observed. Our data on urinary potassium excretion was well below the lower limit recommended by the WHO, which reflects the low consumption of potassium dietary sources such as fruit, vegetables and pulses.

The Na/K ratio was also calculated. In addition to being considered a stronger metric for the relation of sodium and blood pressure [16] than either sodium or potassium alone, the ratio may be an indicator of correction for completeness and correlated measurement errors that can occur during the 24-h period of urine collection [18,48]. Furthermore, since this ratio is independent of the total energy intake, unlike sodium and potassium intakes, which are strongly related to energy intake, it is a better index of sodium and potassium intake [49]. Additionally, as revealed by data from the INTERSALT study, there is a higher correlation of casual urinary Na/K ratio with 24-h urinary Na/K ratio than the correlation of casual urinary sodium or potassium and creatinine with 24-h urinary excretion of sodium or potassium, respectively. As such, the estimation of Na/K ratio in casual ("spot") urine may represent an alternative to the estimation in 24-h urine at a population level and, also, with repeated measurements, for individuals [50].

Higher sodium/potassium ratios are associated with higher blood pressure values. As such, monitoring this ratio over time can contribute to identify populations going through industrialization of diet and at high risk for nutrition-related chronic diseases [51] and increased risk of cardiovascular diseases [52]. We observed a mean sodium/potassium ratio far above the 1:1 ratio suggested by the WHO, which is considered beneficial for health [53]. Our results are consistent with the ones recently published about sodium and potassium intake in South Africa where 77% of the population exceeded the daily recommendation of 5 g salt, 93% of the population did not meet the potassium recommendations and median sodium to potassium ratio was 3.5, which is lower than the mean of our observations [54].

The 24-h urine collection, the major strength of our study, is considered to be the gold standard to assess sodium intake [41,55–58] since 90% of ingested sodium is excreted in the urine [57]. Besides rigorous validation through urinary creatinine excretion, which minimizes bias due to under- or over-collection, more than a single 24-h urine collection should have been obtained from each participant to decrease daily variability. The misclassification of the levels of sodium excretion in a one day only collection is expected to reflect mostly random error. However, the differences between the dietary intake of sodium in the days when participants collected the urine in relation with their usual intake, either random or due to real changes in intakes induced by the participation in the study, would be expectedly lower if urine collection covered a greater number of days. Nevertheless, the high levels of sodium excretion observed in our study are likely to be conservative estimates, as a Hawthorne effect-like bias would result in healthier behaviors.

Other limitations of the present study must be discussed. It was based on a non-representative sample, which limits the extrapolation of the obtained estimates to the overall Mozambican population. Although all the participants of the present study were from an urban setting, and employed, and around 50% had at least seven years of education, which could compromise the external validity of the results, inferences to the general population of Maputo may still be possible; in fact, according to the 2008/09 third national family budget survey [59], around 45% of the Mozambican population in the age group of 40 to 49 years had some degree of education, which is progressively increasing in the country, and the city of Maputo presents the best literacy indicators in the country. The prevalence of overweight and obesity in this sample suggest that the participants evaluated are similar to the population from Maputo city regarding this characteristics; a nationally representative survey conducted in 2005 found that one fifth of Mozambican adult population was overweight or obese, with a higher prevalence in women, urban areas and more literate people. The differences in energy intake between sexes were not statistically significant (2479 $\pm$ 852 Kcal in women and 2682 $\pm$ 1048 Kcal in men, $p = 0.347$), which may reflect limited statistical power, despite men presenting a greater intake.

The relatively small sample size also limits the precision of the estimates, but it does not compromise the validity of our findings. Also of note, the collection of urinary samples occurred during the warmer months of the year in Mozambique, when it is expected a lower proportion of urinary excretion of the ingested sodium [60]. Accordingly, the present estimates are expectedly lower than if the study had been conducted during the colder season.

The use of a 24-h dietary recall may also be associated with recall bias, although the short recall period (previous 24 h) allied to the use of memory aids (a photographic book and household measures) may have contributed to minimize it. Social desirability bias may also be present, although the interviewers were trained to help the participants in the process and instructed not to be judgmental. Additionally, underreporting of sodium consumption is commonly seen due to the correlation of sodium intake and total energy intake, which is underreported in dietary recall studies, particularly by women and overweight or obese people [57]. The "subtraction" method used to calculate discretionary sodium is not the gold standard recommendation and as some limitations due mainly to the difficulty in analyzing the sodium contents in the diverse foods. Even so, it represents an acceptable and more accessible way of obtaining discretionary salt intake [61].

Also of note, inferences on potassium intake based only in urinary excretions may be misleading as urinary measured potassium may not be representative of the dietary values, due to extra-renal losses, particularly fecal [62]. In the present study, analysis of 24-h dietary recall measures, which has been reported as highly correlated to actual potassium intake [62], showed mean (SD) potassium intake of 3097 (1222) mg for women and 3226 (1754) mg for men ($p = 0.705$), which are higher than the urinary measures. Therefore the compliance with the potassium recommendations were also higher when using the 24-h recall (35.9% in women and 34.9% in men). Accordingly, the mean (SD) ratios were lower than the estimates from urinary excretion, with Na/K of 3.0 (2.4) for women and 2.6 (1.8) for men ($p = 0.437$). Thus, we cannot rule out the possibility that, by using 24-h urinary data, the potassium intake was underestimated in the present study and thus the Na/K ratio may be overestimated. Even so, the Na/K ratio, either by urinary or dietary estimation, was above the recommended by WHO, indication of higher sodium and lower potassium intake in this sample of Mozambican population.

Sodium reduction is considered to be cost effective and one of the top 10 "best buys" interventions for preventing non-communicable diseases (NCDs) [63,64]. It was shown that a reduction of 2400 mg/day in sodium intake predicts a decrease of 5.8 mm Hg in systolic blood pressure after adjustment for age, ethnic group, and blood pressure status [65], which is expected to decrease stroke mortality, ischemic heart disease and other vascular diseases [66]. It is also important to note that the effects of sodium reduction on blood pressure tend to be greater in black people and in hypertensive subjects, which would be of great importance in Mozambique given the high proportion of hypertensive subjects not controlled [67].

In the WHO *Global Action Plan for the Prevention and Control of Non-Communicable Diseases 2013–2020*, one of the key target is to make a 30% relative reduction of mean sodium intake at the population level [68]. In Sub-Saharan countries, under epidemiological and nutritional transitions, this is particularly relevant, since it is expected that there will be a growth of globalization, which is frequently associated with dietary changes including the increase of sodium-rich and potassium-poor foods [69].

In a very recent systematic review about salt reduction initiatives around the world it was shown that the Eastern Mediterranean, South-East Asia and Africa are the three regions with the least salt reduction activity and where the NCDs are projected to increase the most [70]. Implementing a salt reduction program, such as the successful one in the United Kingdom (15% reduction in the average salt intake) and already followed by other countries, namely the United States, Canada and Australia, would expectedly represent an important step towards a healthier population and fewer socioeconomic losses [71]. Interventions on salt intake reduction in the Sub-Saharan Africa region were applied in South Africa (through legislation to make the food industry reduce the salt content of selected products) and in Mauritius (through salt reduction in bread) [42].

Our results present a first glimpse on the sodium and potassium consumption in Mozambique. Estimates in samples that are representative of the general population will be needed to confirm the findings from the present study in order to better identify population targets to prioritize interventions.

The sample of the Mozambican population evaluated in the present study revealed a high consumption on sodium, high Na/K ratio, and low potassium consumption in relation to the WHO recommendations. With the already high prevalence of hypertension in the country, future NCD prevention strategies should emphasize measures for population salt consumption control and enhancement of potassium intake. Besides consumer education, incentives for agricultural production of beans, nuts, fruits and vegetables, which are important food sources of potassium, the promotion of community and school gardens, as well as improvement of the transport network to facilitate the access of those foods, are measures that would promote an increase in potassium intake. According to a recently published revision of intervention strategies for reduction of salt consumption, although strategies involving multiple components, both upstream (regulatory and fiscal interventions, food labelling and media campaigns and population-wide policies such as mandatory reformulation) and downstream interventions (individually focused interventions like dietary counselling for individuals, worksites or communities), achieved the biggest population level reductions in salt consumption; the greater effects in population-wide salt consumption were observed with upstream, population-level strategies [72]. In a low-income country as Mozambique, where deprived groups more often consume foods high in salt, sugar and fat, inequalities may be widened by downstream interventions focused on individuals; upstream structural interventions are probably more indicated, as they may reduce inequalities and can be rapid, cost-effective and cost-saving. Further study on political feasibility and stakeholder influence are needed in order to set targets for population salt and potassium intake and develop a strategy, involving different stakeholders, namely the government and the food industries, to reduce sodium and increase potassium intakes.

5. Conclusions

In this convenience sample of Maputo inhabitants, less than one out of 10 participants met the recommended levels of sodium and potassium intakes, and the sodium-to-potassium ratio was far higher than the level recommended by WHO. Sodium from salt and stock powder added to culinary preparations was the most reported contributor for the total intake. This results suggest that population-level measures to modify the current patterns of consumption of sodium and potassium in the country are warranted towards the prevention of the farseeing additional burden to the health system. The main sources of sodium intake uncovered by this study should be further explored at a national level, if possible, to clarify their potential as targets for tailored interventions aiming to decrease salt intake towards the prevention of NCDs in Mozambique.

Acknowledgments: We gratefully thank to Vânia Silva and Sheinilla Karimo for their contribution in the analysis of the nutritional composition of foods.

Author Contributions: A.D., N.L., P.M. and P.P. conceived and designed the study. A.D. coordinated the study implementation. C.N. was responsible for data collection. A.Q., P.M., N.L. and P.P. analysed the data. A.Q., N.J., N.L. and P.P. drafted the manuscript. All authors critically revised the manuscript and approved the final version before submission.

Conflicts of Interest: The authors declare that they have no conflicts of interest.

References

1. Suckling, R.J.; He, F.J.; Macgregor, G.A. Altered dietary salt intake for preventing and treating diabetic kidney disease. *Cochrane Database Syst. Rev.* **2010**. [CrossRef]
2. Poggio, R.; Gutierrez, L.; Matta, M.G.; Elorriaga, N.; Irazola, V.; Rubinstein, A. Daily sodium consumption and cvd mortality in the general population: Systematic review and meta-analysis of prospective studies. *Public Health Nutr.* **2015**, *18*, 695–704. [CrossRef] [PubMed]
3. McMahon, E.J.; Campbell, K.L.; Bauer, J.D.; Mudge, D.W. Altered dietary salt intake for people with chronic kidney disease. *Cochrane Database Syst. Rev.* **2015**. [CrossRef]
4. World Health Organization (WHO). Guideline: Sodium Intake for Adults and Children. Available online: http://apps.who.int/iris/bitstream/10665/77985/1/9789241504836_eng.pdf?ua=1&ua=1 (accessed on 2 February 2017).
5. Brown, I.J.; Tzoulaki, I.; Candeias, V.; Elliott, P. Salt intakes around the world: Implications for public health. *Int. J. Epidemiol.* **2009**, *38*, 791–813. [CrossRef] [PubMed]
6. Whelton, P.K.; He, J.; Cutler, J.A.; Brancati, F.L.; Appel, L.J.; Follmann, D.; Klag, M.J. Effects of oral potassium on blood pressure: Meta-analysis of randomized controlled clinical trials. *JAMA* **1997**, *277*, 1624–1632. [CrossRef] [PubMed]
7. Geleijnse, J.M.; Kok, F.J.; Grobbee, D.E. Blood pressure response to changes in sodium and potassium intake: A metaregression analysis of randomised trials. *J. Hum. Hypertens.* **2003**, *17*, 471–480. [CrossRef] [PubMed]
8. Aaron, K.J.; Sanders, P.W. Role of dietary salt and potassium intake in cardiovascular health and disease: A review of the evidence. Mayo Clinic proceedings. *Mayo Clin.* **2013**, *88*, 987–995. [CrossRef] [PubMed]
9. Morris, R.C., Jr.; Schmidlin, O.; Frassetto, L.A.; Sebastian, A. Relationship and interaction between sodium and potassium. *J. Am. Coll. Nutr.* **2006**, *25*, 262s–270s. [CrossRef] [PubMed]

10. Geleijnse, J.M.; Witteman, J.C.M.; Stijnen, T.; Kloos, M.W.; Hofman, A.; Grobbee, D.E. Sodium and potassium intake and risk of cardiovascular events and all-cause mortality: The Rotterdam study. *Eur. J. Epidemiol.* **2007**, *22*, 763–770. [CrossRef] [PubMed]

11. Stamler, J.; Rose, G.; Stamler, R.; Elliott, P.; Dyer, A.; Marmot, M. Intersalt study findings. Public health and medical care implications. *Hypertension* **1989**, *14*, 570–577. [CrossRef] [PubMed]

12. Whelton, P.K. Sodium, potassium, blood pressure, and cardiovascular disease in humans. *Curr. Hypertens. Rep.* **2014**, *16*, 465. [CrossRef] [PubMed]

13. Kotchen, T.A.; Kotchen, J.M. Nutrition, diet, and hypertension. In *Modern Nutrition in Health and Disease*; Shils, M.E., Shike, M., Ross, A.C., Caballero, B., Cousins, R.J., Eds.; Lippincott Williams & Wilkins: Philadelphia, PA, USA, 2006; pp. 1095–1107.

14. Thornton, S.N. Salt in health and disease—A delicate balance. *N. Engl. J. Med.* **2013**, *368*, 2531. [CrossRef] [PubMed]

15. World Health Organization (WHO). Guideline: Potassium Intake for Adults and Children. Available online: http://www.who.int/nutrition/publications/guidelines/potassium_intake/en/ (accessed on 10 January 2017).

16. Rose, G.; Stamler, J.; Stamler, R.; Elliott, P.; Marmot, M.; Pyorala, K.; Kesteloot, H.; Joossens, J.; Hansson, L.; Mancia, G.; et al. Intersalt: An international study of electrolyte excretion and blood pressure. Results for 24 hour urinary sodium and potassium excretion. Intersalt cooperative research group. *Br. Med. J.* **1988**, *297*, 319–328.

17. Umesawa, M.; Iso, H.; Date, C.; Yamamoto, A.; Toyoshima, H.; Watanabe, Y.; Kikuchi, S.; Koizumi, A.; Kondo, T.; Inaba, Y.; et al. Relations between dietary sodium and potassium intakes and mortality from cardiovascular disease: The japan collaborative cohort study for evaluation of cancer risks. *Am. J. Clin. Nutr.* **2008**, *88*, 195–202. [PubMed]

18. Cook, N.R.; Obarzanek, E.; Cutler, J.A.; Buring, J.E.; Rexrode, K.M.; Kumanyika, S.K.; Appel, L.J.; Whelton, P.K.; Trials of Hypertension Prevention Collaborative Research Group. Joint effects of sodium and potassium intake on subsequent cardiovascular disease: The trials of hypertension prevention (TOHP) follow-up study. *Arch. Intern. Med.* **2009**, *169*, 32–40. [CrossRef] [PubMed]

19. Cook, N.R.; Kumanyika, S.K.; Cutler, J.A. Effect of change in sodium excretion on change in blood pressure corrected for measurement error: The trials of hypertension prevention, phase I. *Am. J. Epidemiol.* **1998**, *148*, 431–444. [CrossRef] [PubMed]

20. Khaw, K.T.; Barrett-Connor, E. The association between blood pressure, age, and dietary sodium and potassium: A population study. *Circulation* **1988**, *77*, 53–61. [CrossRef] [PubMed]

21. Perez, V.; Chang, E.T. Sodium-to-potassium ratio and blood pressure, hypertension, and related factors. *Adv. Nutr.* **2014**, *5*, 712–741. [CrossRef] [PubMed]

22. Carvalho, J.J.; Baruzzi, R.G.; Howard, P.F.; Poulter, N.; Alpers, M.P.; Franco, L.J.; Marcopito, L.F.; Spooner, V.J.; Dyer, A.R.; Elliott, P. Blood pressure in four remote populations in the INTERSALT Study. *Hypertension* **1989**, *14*, 238. [CrossRef] [PubMed]

23. Oyebode, O.; Oti, S.; Chen, Y.-F.; Lilford, R.J. Salt intakes in Sub-Saharan Africa: A systematic review and meta-regression. *Popul. Health Metr.* **2016**, *14*, 1. [CrossRef] [PubMed]

24. Damasceno, A.; Azevedo, A.; Silva-Matos, C.; Prista, A.; Diogo, D.; Lunet, N. Hypertension prevalence, awareness, treatment, and control in Mozambique: Urban/rural gap during epidemiological transition. *Hypertension* **2009**, *54*, 77–83. [CrossRef] [PubMed]

25. Damasceno, A.; Gomes, J.; Azevedo, A.; Carrilho, C.; Lobo, V.; Lopes, H.; Madede, T.; Pravinrai, P.; Silva-Matos, C.; Jalla, S.; et al. An epidemiological study of stroke hospitalizations in Maputo, Mozambique: A high burden of disease in a resource-poor country. *Stroke* **2010**, *41*, 2463–2469. [CrossRef] [PubMed]

26. Dgedge, M.; Novoa, A.; Macassa, G.; Sacarlal, J.; Black, J.; Michaud, C.; Cliff, J. The burden of disease in maputo city, Mozambique: Registered and autopsied deaths in 1994. *Bull. World Health Organ.* **2001**, *79*, 546–552. [PubMed]

27. The World Bank. Urban Population (% of Total). United Nations, World Urbanization Prospects. Available online: http://data.worldbank.org/indicator/SP.URB.TOTL.IN.ZS (accessed 20 September 2017).

28. Popkin, B.M. Contemporary nutritional transition: Determinants of diet and its impact on body composition. *Proc. Nutr. Soc.* **2011**, *70*, 82–91. [CrossRef] [PubMed]

29. Silva, V.; Santos, S.; Novela, C.; Padrão, P.; Moreira, P.; Lunet, N.; Damasceno, A. In Some observations on food consumption and culinary practices in Maputo, Mozambique. In Proceedings of the 8th International Conference on Culinary Arts and Sciences: Global, National and Local Perspectives, Porto, Portugal, 19–21 June 2013.

30. Gomes, A.; Damasceno, A.; Azevedo, A.; Prista, A.; Silva-Matos, C.; Saranga, S.; Lunet, N. Body mass index and waist circumference in Mozambique: Urban/rural gap during epidemiological transition. *Obes. Rev.* **2010**, *11*, 627–634. [CrossRef] [PubMed]

31. Gomes, J.; Damasceno, A.; Carrilho, C.; Lobo, V.; Lopes, H.; Madede, T.; Pravinrai, P.; Silva-Matos, C.; Diogo, D.; Azevedo, A.; et al. Determinants of early case-fatality among stroke patients in Maputo, Mozambique and impact of in-hospital complications. *Int. J. Stroke* **2013**, *8* (Suppl. A100), 69–75. [CrossRef] [PubMed]

32. WHO Regional Office for Europe. *Estimation of Sodium Intake and Output: Review of Methods and Recommendations for Epidemiological Studies*; Report on a Who Meeting by the Who Collaborating Center for Research and Training in Cardiovascular Diseases; World Health Organization: Geneva, Switzerland, 1984.

33. Korkalo, L.; Hauta-alus, H.; Mutanen, M. *Food Composition Tables for Mozambique*; University of Helsinki: Helsinki, Finland, 2011.

34. Giuntini, E.; Lajolo, F.; Menezes, E. Brazilian food composition table TBCA-USP (versions 3 and 4) in the international context. *Arch. Latinoam. Nutr.* **2006**, *56*, 366–374.

35. Lohman, T.; Roache, A.; Martorell, R. Anthropometric standardization reference manual. *Med. Sci. Sports Exerc.* **1992**, *24*, 952. [CrossRef]

36. World Health Organization (WHO). Body Mass Index-BMI. Available online: http://www.euro.who.int/en/health-topics/disease-prevention/nutrition/a-healthy-lifestyle/body-mass-index-bmi (accessed on 7 January 2017).

37. Expert Panel on Detection Evaluation and Treatment of High Blood Cholesterol in Adults. Executive summary of the third report of the national cholesterol education program (NCEP) expert panel on detection, evaluation, and treatment of high blood cholesterol in adults (adult treatment panel III). *JAMA* **2001**, *285*, 2486–2497. [CrossRef]

38. World Health Organization (WHO). Global Strategy on Diet, Physical Activity and Health. Promoting Fruit and Vegetable Consumption around the World. Available online: http://www.who.int/dietphysicalactivity/fruit/en/ (accessed on 20 March 2017).

39. Powles, J.; Fahimi, S.; Micha, R.; Khatibzadeh, S.; Shi, P.; Ezzati, M.; Engell, R.E.; Lim, S.S.; Danaei, G.; Mozaffarian, D.; et al. Global, regional and national sodium intakes in 1990 and 2010: A systematic analysis of 24 h urinary sodium excretion and dietary surveys worldwide. *BMJ Open* **2013**, *3*, e003733. [CrossRef] [PubMed]

40. Mizéhoun-Adissoda, C.; Houinato, D.; Houehanou, C.; Chianea, T.; Dalmay, F.; Bigot, A.; Aboyans, V.; Preux, P.-M.; Bovet, P.; Desport, J.-C. Dietary sodium and potassium intakes: Data from urban and rural areas. *Nutrition* **2017**, *33*, 35–41. [CrossRef] [PubMed]

41. Xu, J.; Wang, M.; Chen, Y.; Zhen, B.; Li, J.; Luan, W.; Ning, F.; Liu, H.; Ma, J.; Ma, G. Estimation of salt intake by 24-h urinary sodium excretion: A cross-sectional study in Yantai, china. *BMC Public Health* **2014**, *14*, 136. [CrossRef] [PubMed]

42. Sookram, C.; Munodawafa, D.; Phori, P.M.; Varenne, B.; Alisalad, A. Who's supported interventions on salt intake reduction in the Sub-Saharan Africa region. *Cardiovasc. Diagn. Ther.* **2015**, *5*, 186–190. [CrossRef] [PubMed]

43. Charlton, K.E.; Steyn, K.; Levitt, N.S.; Zulu, J.V.; Jonathan, D.; Veldman, F.J.; Nel, J.H. Diet and blood pressure in south Africa: Intake of foods containing sodium, potassium, calcium, and magnesium in three ethnic groups. *Nutrition* **2005**, *21*, 39–50. [CrossRef] [PubMed]

44. Stamler, J.; Elliott, P.; Dennis, B.; Dyer, A.R.; Kesteloot, H.; Liu, K.; Ueshima, H.; Zhou, B.F. Intermap: Background, aims, design, methods, and descriptive statistics (nondietary). *J. Hum. Hypertens.* **2003**, *17*, 591–608. [CrossRef] [PubMed]

45. Ni Mhurchu, C.; Capelin, C.; Dunford, E.K.; Webster, J.L.; Neal, B.C.; Jebb, S.A. Sodium content of processed foods in the united kingdom: Analysis of 44,000 foods purchased by 21,000 households. *Am. J. Clin. Nutr.* **2011**, *93*, 594–600. [CrossRef] [PubMed]

46. Monteiro, C.A.; Levy, R.B.; Claro, R.M.; de Castro, I.R.; Cannon, G. Increasing consumption of ultra-processed foods and likely impact on human health: Evidence from Brazil. *Public Health Nutr.* **2011**, *14*, 5–13. [CrossRef] [PubMed]

47. O'Donnell, M.; Mente, A.; Rangarajan, S.; McQueen, M.J.; Wang, X.; Liu, L.; Yan, H.; Lee, S.F.; Mony, P.; Devanath, A.; et al. Urinary sodium and potassium excretion, mortality, and cardiovascular events. *N. Engl. J. Med.* **2014**, *371*, 612–623. [CrossRef] [PubMed]

48. Espeland, M.A.; Kumanyika, S.; Wilson, A.C.; Reboussin, D.M.; Easter, L.; Self, M.; Robertson, J.; Brown, W.M.; McFarlane, M. Statistical issues in analyzing 24-h dietary recall and 24-h urine collection data for sodium and potassium intakes. *Am. J. Epidemiol.* **2001**, *153*, 996–1006. [CrossRef] [PubMed]

49. Cobb, L.K.; Anderson, C.A.; Elliott, P.; Hu, F.B.; Liu, K.; Neaton, J.D.; Whelton, P.K.; Woodward, M.; Appel, L.J. Methodological issues in cohort studies that relate sodium intake to cardiovascular disease outcomes: A science advisory from the American heart association. *Circulation* **2014**, *129*, 1173–1186. [CrossRef] [PubMed]

50. Iwahori, T.; Miura, K.; Ueshima, H.; Chan, Q.; Dyer, A.R.; Elliott, P.; Stamler, J.; INTERSALT Research Group. Estimating 24-h urinary sodium/potassium ratio from casual ('spot') urinary sodium/potassium ratio: The INTERSALT Study. *Int. J. Epidemiol.* **2016**. [CrossRef] [PubMed]

51. Hedayati, S.S.; Minhajuddin, A.T.; Ijaz, A.; Moe, O.W.; Elsayed, E.F.; Reilly, R.F.; Huang, C.L. Association of urinary sodium/potassium ratio with blood pressure: Sex and racial differences. *Clin. J. Am. Soc. Nephrol.* **2012**, *7*, 315–322. [CrossRef] [PubMed]

52. Yang, Q.; Liu, T.; Kuklina, E.V.; Flanders, W.D.; Hong, Y.; Gillespie, C.; Chang, M.H.; Gwinn, M.; Dowling, N.; Khoury, M.J.; et al. Sodium and potassium intake and mortality among us adults: Prospective data from the third national health and nutrition examination survey. *Arch. Intern. Med.* **2011**, *171*, 1183–1191. [CrossRef] [PubMed]

53. World Health Organization (WHO). Diet, Nutrition and the Prevention of Chronic Diseases. Report of the Joint Who/Fao Expert Consultation. Who Technical Report Series, No. 916 (Trs 916). Available online: http://www.who.int/dietphysicalactivity/publications/trs916/en/ (accessed on 12 March 2017).

54. Swanepoel, B.; Schutte, A.E.; Cockeran, M.; Steyn, K.; Wentzel-Viljoen, E. Sodium and potassium intake in south africa: An evaluation of 24-h urine collections in a white, black, and Indian population. *J. Am. Soc. Hypertens.* **2016**, *10*, 829–837. [CrossRef] [PubMed]

55. Ribič, C.H.; Zakotnik, J.M.; Vertnik, L.; Vegnuti, M.; Cappuccio, F.P. Salt intake of the Slovene population assessed by 24 h urinary sodium excretion. *Public Health Nutr.* **2010**, *13*, 1803–1809. [CrossRef] [PubMed]

56. Aparicio, A.; Rodriguez-Rodriguez, E.; Cuadrado-Soto, E.; Navia, B.; Lopez-Sobaler, A.M.; Ortega, R.M. Estimation of salt intake assessed by urinary excretion of sodium over 24 h in Spanish subjects aged 7–11 years. *Eur. J. Nutr.* **2017**, *56*, 171–178. [CrossRef] [PubMed]

57. McLean, R.M. Measuring population sodium intake: A review of methods. *Nutrients* **2014**, *6*, 4651–4662. [CrossRef] [PubMed]

58. Zhang, J.; Yan, L.; Tang, J.; Ma, J.; Guo, X.; Zhao, W.; Zhang, X.; Li, J.; Chu, J.; Bi, Z. Estimating daily salt intake based on 24 h urinary sodium excretion in adults aged 18–69 years in Shandong, china. *BMJ Open* **2014**, *4*. [CrossRef] [PubMed]

59. Khossa, D.; Macaringue, F.; Nassabe, J.; Ismael, M.; Nhantumbo, N.; Mandlate, T. Estatísticas e Indicadores Sociais, 2008–2010. Instituto Nacional de Estatística. Direcção de Estatísticas Demográficas Vitais e Sociais. Available online: www.ine.gov.mz (accessed on 20 March 2017).

60. Conkle, J.; van der Haar, F. The use and interpretation of sodium concentrations in casual (spot) urine collections for population surveillance and partitioning of dietary iodine intake sources. *Nutrients* **2017**, *9*, 7. [CrossRef] [PubMed]

61. Pan American Health Organization. Regional Expert Group for Cardiovascular Disease. Prevention through Population-Wide Dietary Salt Reduction. A Review of Methods to Determine the Main Sources of Salt in the Diet. 2011. Available online: http://www2.paho.org/hq/index.php?option=com_docman&task=doc_view&Itemid=270&gid=21491&lang=en (assessed on 16 July 2017).

62. Iwahori, T.; Miura, K.; Ueshima, H. Time to consider use of the sodium-to-potassium ratio for practical sodium reduction and potassium increase. *Nutrients* **2017**, *9*. [CrossRef] [PubMed]

63. Zarocostas, J. Who lists "best buys" for cutting deaths from non-communicable disease. *BMJ* **2011**, *342*. [CrossRef]

64. Eyles, H.; Shields, E.; Webster, J. Achieving the who sodium target: Estimation of reductions required in the sodium content of packaged foods and other sources of dietary sodium. *Am. J. Clin. Nutr.* **2016**, *104*, 470–479. [CrossRef] [PubMed]

65. He, F.J.; Li, J.; MacGregor, G.A. Effect of longer term modest salt reduction on blood pressure: Cochrane systematic review and meta-analysis of randomised trials. *BMJ* **2013**, *346*. [CrossRef] [PubMed]

66. Ettehad, D.; Emdin, C.A.; Kiran, A.; Anderson, S.G.; Callender, T.; Emberson, J.; Chalmers, J.; Rodgers, A.; Rahimi, K. Blood pressure lowering for prevention of cardiovascular disease and death: A systematic review and meta-analysis. *Lancet* **2016**, *387*, 957–967. [CrossRef]

67. Appel, L.J.; Brands, M.W.; Daniels, S.R.; Karanja, N.; Elmer, P.J.; Sacks, F.M. Dietary approaches to prevent and treat hypertension: A scientific statement from the American heart association. *Hypertension* **2006**, *47*, 296–308. [CrossRef] [PubMed]

68. World Health Organization (WHO). Global Action Plan for the Prevention and Control of NCDs 2013–2020. Available online: http://www.who.int/nmh/events/ncd_action_plan/en/ (accessed on 20 June 2017).

69. Popkin, B.M. The nutrition transition: An overview of world patterns of change. *Nutr. Rev.* **2004**, *62*, S140–S143. [CrossRef] [PubMed]

70. Trieu, K.; Neal, B.; Hawkes, C.; Dunford, E.; Campbell, N.; Rodriguez-Fernandez, R.; Legetic, B.; McLaren, L.; Barberio, A.; Webster, J. Salt reduction initiatives around the world-A systematic review of progress towards the global target. *PLoS ONE* **2015**, *10*, e0130247. [CrossRef] [PubMed]

71. He, F.J.; Brinsden, H.C.; MacGregor, G.A. Salt reduction in the United Kingdom: A successful experiment in public health. *J. Hum. Hypertens.* **2014**, *28*, 345–352. [CrossRef] [PubMed]

72. Hyseni, L.; Elliot-Green, A.; Lloyd-Williams, F.; Kypridemos, C.; O'Flaherty, M.; McGill, R.; Orton, L.; Bromley, H.; Cappuccio, F.P.; Capewell, S. Systematic review of dietary salt reduction policies: Evidence for an effectiveness hierarchy? *PLoS ONE* **2017**, *12*, e0177535. [CrossRef] [PubMed]

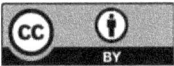

nutrients

MDPI

Article

Changes in Consumer Attitudes toward Broad-Based and Environment-Specific Sodium Policies—SummerStyles 2012 and 2015

Erika C. Odom [1,2,*], Corine Whittick [3,4], Xin Tong [1], Katherine A. John [1,5] and Mary E. Cogswell [1]

[1] Epidemiology and Surveillance Branch, Division for Heart Disease and Stroke Prevention, National Center for Chronic Disease Prevention and Health Promotion, Centers for Disease Control and Prevention, 4770 Buford Hwy NE, Atlanta, GA 30341, USA; fvx4@cdc.gov (X.T.); yfr6@cdc.gov (K.A.J.); mec0@cdc.gov (M.E.C.)
[2] United States Public Health Service, Commissioned Corps, Rockville, MD 20852, USA
[3] Mailman School of Public Health, Columbia University, New York, NY 10032, USA; corinewhittick@gmail.com
[4] Project IMHOTEP, Morehouse College, Atlanta, GA 30314, USA
[5] IHRC, Inc., Atlanta, GA 30346, USA
* Correspondence: iyo7@cdc.gov; Tel.: +1-770-488-8218

Received: 12 June 2017; Accepted: 27 July 2017; Published: 4 August 2017

Abstract: We examined temporal changes in consumer attitudes toward broad-based actions and environment-specific policies to limit sodium in restaurants, manufactured foods, and school and workplace cafeterias from the 2012 and 2015 SummerStyle surveys. We used two online, national research panel surveys to conduct a cross-sectional analysis of 7845 U.S. adults. Measures included self-reported agreement with broad-based actions and environment-specific policies to limit sodium in restaurants, manufactured foods, school cafeterias, workplace cafeterias, and quick-serve restaurants. Wald Chi-square tests were used to examine the difference between the two survey years and multivariate logistic regression was used to obtain odds ratios. Agreement with broad-based actions to limit sodium in restaurants (45.9% agreed in 2015) and manufactured foods (56.5% agreed in 2015) did not change between 2012 and 2015. From 2012 to 2015, there was a significant increase in respondents that supported environment-specific policies to lower sodium in school cafeterias (80.0% to 84.9%; $p < 0.0001$), workplace cafeterias (71.2% to 76.6%; $p < 0.0001$), and quick-serve restaurants (70.8% to 76.7%; $p < 0.0001$). Results suggest substantial agreement and support for actions to limit sodium in commercially-processed and prepared foods since 2012, with most consumers ready for actions to lower sodium in foods served in schools, workplaces, and quick-serve restaurants.

Keywords: attitudes; sodium reduction; policies; consumer

1. Introduction

Excessive consumption of dietary sodium is a major risk factor for hypertension, and subsequent heart disease and stroke, two of the leading causes of death in the United States. The average daily intake of sodium among U.S. adults is about 3500 mg/day [1], excluding salt added at the table, which far exceeds recommendations to limit sodium intake (<2300 mg/day) [2]. Although nearly half of adults report taking actions to reduce their sodium intake [3], voluntary initiatives that focused on individual sodium education and behaviors have not significantly lowered population sodium intake [4]. In fact, about 90% of U.S. adults still consume too much sodium [4]. Because most of the sodium consumed comes from commercially-processed and prepared foods [5], in 2010, the Institute of Medicine recommended government action to reduce sodium in the U.S. food supply. Reducing sodium calls for a multifaceted approach that includes the collaboration of food manufacturers, industry/vendors, and local policies [6–8]. Consumer agreement with such broad-based actions could suggest support for sodium reduction in manufactured and prepared foods.

In 2010, most respondents to a nationwide survey supported broad-based actions or environment-specific policies to limit sodium in manufactured foods (55.9%), restaurant food (47.0%), and food served in quick-serve restaurants (81.5%) [9]. Recent surveys from 2010 and 2012 suggests that at least 80% of U.S. adult consumers would support national standards that limit sodium in foods served in school cafeterias [10,11]. In a 2013 study, about half of respondents indicated support for policies increasing healthy food and drink options served in workplace cafeterias and vending machines [12]. Data also suggests that the promotion of low-sodium food options in the workplace may increase consumer's acceptance and willingness to choose healthier, low-sodium options while at work [13,14]. To better understand changes in consumer readiness for sodium-related policies, in this study we use data from the SummerStyles 2012 and 2015 surveys to (1) assess the percentage of adults who support broad-based actions and environment-specific policies to reduce sodium in restaurants, school and workplace cafeterias, and in manufactured foods, and (2) to determine if support has changed from 2012 and 2015, overall, and among population subgroups.

2. Materials and Methods

A cross-sectional study was conducted using data from two of Porter Novelli's online HealthStyles surveys. Data was collected by GfK's KnowledgePanel® (GfK North American Headquarters, New York, NY USA), an online national panel of noninstitutionalized U.S. participants. Panelists are randomly recruited by probability-based sampling (using random digit dial and addressed-based sampling methods) to reach respondents regardless of whether they have landline phones or Internet access, and are continuously replenished to maintain approximately 55,000 panelists. If needed, households are provided with a laptop computer and access to the Internet. The initial wave of SpringStyles was sent to a random sample of panelists ages 18 or older, while the second wave (SummerStyles) was sent to a random sample of panelists who completed the initial wave. Respondents could earn up to 20,000 cash-equivalent reward points (approximately $20) and were eligible to win an in-kind prize through a monthly sweepstakes if they participated in both waves. The Centers for Disease Control and Prevention (CDC) suggested potential questions to include, while Porter Novelli determined the final questionnaire content. CDC licensed the results (responses to the questions) from Porter Novelli. Licensed data provided did not include personally identifiable information and was determined exempt by CDC Institutional Review Board (IRB).

In total, 4170 panelists aged $\geq$18 years completed the 2012 SummerStyles survey, with a response rate of 65% (of respondents from the 2012 SpringStyles). In the 2015 SummerStyles survey, there were 4127 panelists aged $\geq$18 years, with a response rate of 67% (of respondents from the 2015 SpringStyles). In both surveys, the samples were weighted for age, gender, race, household income, education, census region, metropolitan status, and prior Internet access.

In this study, we excluded 268 participants (2012: N =122 and 2015: N =146) who had missing information on demographic and health characteristics and 184 participants (2012: N = 122 and 2015: N = 62) who had missing responses on sodium-related questions. The final sample included 7845 respondents; 3926 in 2012 and 3919 in 2015, respectively.

2.1. Measures

2.1.1. Consumer Agreement with or Support for Broad-Based Actions to Limit Sodium in Foods

To assess the level of consumer agreement with broad-based actions to limit sodium in restaurants and manufactured foods, participants were asked about agreement with the following statements: (1) "I think it's a good idea for the government to keep restaurants from putting too much salt in food" and (2) "I think it's a good idea for the government to keep food manufacturers from putting too much salt in food". A five-point Likert scale was used to record responses: 1 = strongly disagree;

2 = somewhat disagree; 3 = neither agree nor disagree; 4 = moderately agree; and 5 = strongly agree. Responses of strongly disagree, somewhat disagree, and neither agree nor disagree were grouped together and termed neutral/disagree. Responses of strongly agree and somewhat agree were grouped together and termed agree. To assess the level of consumer support for environment-specific policies to limit sodium in school cafeterias, workplace cafeterias, and quick-serve restaurants, participants were asked about level of support for the following: (1) "policies that lower sodium/salt content of foods in school cafeterias", (2) "policies to limit the amount of sodium/salt of foods in workplace cafeterias", and (3) "policies to limit the amount of sodium/salt in quick-serve restaurants". A four-point Likert scale was used to record responses: 1 = strongly oppose; 2 = slightly oppose; 3 = slightly support; 4 = strongly support. Responses of strongly oppose and slightly oppose were grouped together and termed neutral/not support, and responses of slightly support and strongly support were collapsed into support.

2.1.2. Demographic and Health Characteristics

Categorical variables were constructed for age (18–30 years, 31–50 years, and 51 years and older); sex; race-ethnicity (non-Hispanic White, non-Hispanic Black, Hispanic, and other); household income (<$15,000, $15,000–24,999, $25,000–39,999, $40,000–59,999 and ≥$60,000); education level (high school or less, some college, and college graduate or higher); and region (Northeast, Midwest, South, and West). Body mass index (BMI) was calculated from self-reported height and weight and categorized as normal (<25 kg/m^2), overweight (25–30 kg/m^2), and obese (≥30 kg/m^2). Self-reported hypertension status was determined by participant response to the question, "During the past year, have you had (or do you currently have) any of these health conditions: high blood pressure?"

2.1.3. Consumer Desire to Eat Less Sodium

Participants' level of agreement with the statement "I want to eat a diet that is low in sodium/salt" was assessed with a five-point Likert scale. Response categories were: 1 = strongly disagree; 2 = somewhat disagree; 3 = neither agree nor disagree; 4 = somewhat agree; 5 = strongly agree. Responses of strongly disagree and somewhat disagree were grouped together and termed, no. Responses of strongly agree and somewhat agree were grouped together and termed, yes, and neither agree nor disagree was termed neutral.

2.2. Statistical Analysis

Data were weighted to match the U.S. Current Population Survey (CPS) proportions, 2011 and 2014, using nine factors: sex, age, household income, race or ethnicity, household size, education, census region, metro status, and prior Internet access. Wald Chi-square tests were used to determine the differences between 2012 and 2015 in respondent attitudes toward broad-based actions or policies related to sodium reduction among various sociodemographic characteristics. After pooling the two years of data together, we performed a multivariate logistic regression analysis to examine the association between respondent characteristics and agreement or support for policies to limit sodium across all environments after controlling for survey year (2012, 2015), age, sex, race/ethnicity, household income, education level, BMI, hypertension status, and desire to eat a low-sodium diet. Adjusted odds ratios (aORs) and 95% confidence intervals (CI) were obtained, and a two-tailed p-value less than 0.05 was considered statistically significant. All statistical analyses were performed using SAS version 9.3 (SAS Institute Inc., Cary, NC, USA).

3. Results

Among the total 7845 respondents, 77.3% were 31 years or older, 51.2% were female, 67.0% were non-Hispanic white, 51.1% earned at least $60,000, 58.1% had more than a high school education, and 36.8% lived in the South (Table 1). There were no statistical differences on age, sex, race, household income, education level, region, BMI, or hypertension status between SummerStyles 2012 and 2015.

The percentage of respondents who responded "No" (2012: 15.8%, 2015: 12.0%) to wanting to eat a diet low in sodium decreased from 2012 to 2015 ($p = 0.0004$).

Table 1. Weighted percentage of respondents on selective demographic characteristics, SS2012 and SS2015.

Questionnaire and answers		Total	Year 2012	Year 2015	p-Value
			Sample N (Weighted %)		
Total Sample N		7845	3926	3919	
Age (years)					
	18–30	1187 (22.8)	616 (22.9)	571 (22.6)	
	31–50	2773 (34.2)	1471 (35.2)	1302 (33.1)	
	$\geq$51	3885 (43.1)	1839 (41.9)	2046 (44.3)	0.18
Gender					
	Male	3674 (48.8)	1843 (49.0)	1831 (48.6)	
	Female	4171 (51.2)	2083 (51.0)	2088 (51.4)	0.77
Race					
	White, non-Hispanic	5886 (67.0)	2939 (67.6)	2947 (66.3)	
	Black, non-Hispanic	738 (11.2)	374 (11.3)	364 (11.0)	
	Hispanic	808 (14.5)	390 (14.0)	418 (14.9)	
	Other, non-Hispanic	413 (7.4)	223 (7.1)	190 (7.7)	0.71
Household income					
	<$15,000	698 (9.1)	317 (9.4)	381 (8.8)	
	$15,000–$24,999	626 (9.1)	308 (9.2)	318 (9.0)	
	$25,000–$39,999	1230 (14.0)	562 (14.4)	668 (13.7)	
	$40,000–$59,999	1366 (16.7)	670 (16.8)	696 (16.7)	
	$\geq$60,000	3925 (51.1)	2069 (50.3)	1856 (51.8)	0.85
Education level					
	HS graduate or less	2691 (41.9)	1241 (42.0)	1450 (41.8)	
	Some college	2446 (28.9)	1264 (29.2)	1182 (28.5)	
	Bachelor's degree or higher	2708 (29.2)	1421 (28.8)	1287 (29.7)	0.76
Region					
	Northeast	1415 (18.0)	718 (17.7)	697 (18.4)	
	Midwest	1984 (21.7)	992 (22.1)	992 (21.4)	
	South	2712 (36.8)	1340 (36.8)	1372 (36.8)	
	West	1734 (23.4)	876 (23.4)	858 (23.4)	0.86
Body mass index (BMI)					
	<25	2774 (37.9)	1433 (38.7)	1341 (37.1)	
	25–30	2644 (32.2)	1324 (32.5)	1320 (32.0)	
	$\geq$30	2427 (29.9)	1169 (28.8)	1258 (30.9)	0.26
Hypertension Status					
	Yes	2162 (25.9)	1097 (27.1)	1065 (24.8)	
	No	5683 (74.1)	2829 (72.9)	2854 (75.2)	0.06
Want to eat a diet low in sodium					
	Yes	4550 (57.9)	2240 (57.3)	2310 (58.4)	
	Neutral	2217 (28.2)	1075 (26.9)	1142 (29.6)	
	No	1078 (13.9)	611 (15.8)	467 (12.0)	**0.0004**

HS, High school. SS, SummerStyles. Boldface signifies statistical significance (p-Value < 0.05).

Between 2012 and 2015, consumer agreement with broad-based actions to limit sodium in restaurant and manufactured foods did not change significantly. A little less than half of respondents (2012: 45.7%, 2015: 45.9%, Table 2) agreed with limiting sodium in restaurant foods, and more than half of respondents (56.5% for both 2012 and 2015) agreed with limiting sodium in manufactured foods. The lack of change between 2012 and 2015 was consistent across respondent characteristics, with a few exceptions. There was a decrease in consumer agreement to limit sodium in manufactured food among respondents that earned <$15,000 ($p = 0.04$) and who were neutral about eating a diet low in sodium ($p < 0.05$).

Table 2. Agreement with broad-based actions to limit sodium in restaurant and manufactured foods, SS2012 and SS2015.

Questionnaire and Answers	Agree to Limit Sodium in Restaurant Food			Agree to Limit Sodium in Manufactured Food		
	Year 2012	Year 2015	*p*-Value	Year 2012	Year 2015	*p*-Value
Total	45.7 (43.6–47.9)	45.9 (44.0–47.7)	0.94	56.5 (54.4–58.6)	56.5 (54.7–58.3)	0.99
Age (years)						
18–30	47.1 (42.1–52.2)	44.3 (39.8–48.8)	0.41	55.9 (50.9–60.9)	55.2 (50.7–59.7)	0.84
31–50	41.2 (37.6–44.7)	43.0 (39.8–46.3)	0.45	52.7 (49.2–56.3)	50.7 (47.4–53.9)	0.40
≥51	48.8 (45.8–51.9)	48.8 (46.3–51.2)	0.97	59.9 (56.9–62.9)	61.5 (59.1–63.8)	0.42
Gender						
Male	43.9 (40.8–47.0)	43.6 (40.9–46.2)	0.86	55.0 (51.9–58.1)	54.1 (51.4–56.8)	0.66
Female	47.5 (44.5–50.4)	48.0 (45.5–50.5)	0.78	57.9 (55.0–60.8)	58.7 (56.3–61.2)	0.65
Race						
White, non-Hispanic	43.0 (40.6–45.4)	41.8 (39.8–43.9)	0.46	54.7 (52.3–57.1)	52.9 (50.9–55.0)	0.27
Black, non-Hispanic	57.3 (50.4–64.2)	58.8 (53.1–64.5)	0.74	67.2 (60.5–74.0)	68.9 (63.6–74.2)	0.71
Hispanic	46.4 (39.8–53.0)	53.7 (48.2–59.1)	0.10	52.6 (46.0–59.2)	61.1 (55.7–66.4)	0.051
Other, non-Hispanic	52.0 (42.6–61.4)	46.5 (38.2–54.9)	0.40	63.8 (54.9–72.8)	60.3 (52.1–68.5)	0.57
Household income						
<$15,000	55.6 (47.9–63.4)	46.7 (40.7–52.6)	0.07	66.3 (59.0–73.6)	56.4 (50.5–62.3)	**0.04**
$15,000–$24,999	45.8 (38.3–53.2)	51.4 (44.9–57.9)	0.27	53.6 (46.2–61.1)	58.0 (51.5–64.4)	0.39
$25,000–$39,999	50.8 (45.1–56.4)	46.9 (42.5–51.4)	0.36	64.0 (58.6–69.4)	60.2 (55.9–64.5)	0.28
$40,000–$59,999	45.4 (40.2–50.5)	49.2 (44.8–53.6)	0.26	55.1 (50.0–60.3)	60.2 (55.9–64.4)	0.14
≥60,000	42.6 (39.7–45.5)	43.4 (40.8–46.0)	0.69	53.4 (50.5–56.4)	54.1 (51.4–56.7)	0.76
Education level						
HS graduate or less	49.5 (45.9–53.2)	46.6 (43.6–49.6)	0.23	58.5 (54.9–62.1)	56.2 (53.3–59.2)	0.34
Some college	44.3 (40.6–47.9)	47.6 (44.3–51.0)	0.18	54.6 (51.0–58.2)	58.3 (55.0–61.6)	0.14
Bachelor's degree or higher	41.7 (38.1–45.3)	43.0 (39.9–46.2)	0.59	55.4 (51.8–59.1)	55.1 (51.9–58.3)	0.89
Region						
Northeast	52.0 (47.0–56.9)	48.6 (44.3–52.9)	0.32	60.3 (55.5–65.1)	59.6 (55.4–63.9)	0.84
Midwest	41.7 (37.5–46.0)	46.3 (42.6–49.9)	0.11	54.2 (49.9–58.5)	56.1 (52.4–59.7)	0.51
South	45.9 (42.3–49.4)	45.8 (42.7–48.9)	0.97	57.3 (53.8–60.8)	56.9 (53.8–59.9)	0.84
West	44.6 (40.0–49.3)	43.4 (39.5–47.3)	0.69	54.4 (49.8–59.0)	53.8 (49.9–57.8)	0.85
BMI						
<25	44.6 (41.2–48.1)	45.9 (42.8–49.0)	0.60	55.1 (51.6–58.6)	55.7 (52.6–58.8)	0.79
25–30	44.1 (40.4–47.8)	45.2 (42.0–48.3)	0.67	55.5 (51.9–59.2)	55.8 (52.7–58.9)	0.91
≥30	49.1 (45.1–53.0)	46.5 (43.3–49.8)	0.33	59.4 (55.5–63.2)	58.1 (54.9–61.3)	0.61
Hypertension Status						
Yes	53.3 (49.2–57.3)	51.7 (48.3–55.2)	0.57	64.2 (60.3–68.1)	63.1 (59.8–66.4)	0.68
No	42.9 (40.4–45.4)	43.9 (41.8–46.1)	0.56	53.6 (51.1–56.1)	54.3 (52.2–56.5)	0.68
Want to eat a diet low in sodium						
Yes	60.3 (57.6–63.1)	59.9 (57.6–62.3)	0.84	70.9 (68.3–73.4)	71.7 (69.6–73.8)	0.63
Neutral	28.4 (24.7–32.2)	27.0 (23.9–30.0)	0.55	40.9 (36.9–44.9)	35.7 (32.4–38.9)	**0.05**
No	22.4 (17.8–27.0)	23.9 (19.3–28.4)	0.65	30.8 (25.9–35.7)	33.7 (28.7–38.6)	0.43

HS, High school. SS, SummerStyles. Boldface signifies statistical significance (*p*-Value < 0.05).

Between 2012 and 2015, support for environment–specific policies to reduce sodium in food prepared in school cafeterias (2012: 80.0%, 2015: 84.9%, Table 3), workplace cafeterias (2012: 71.2%, 2015: 76.6%), and quick-serve restaurants (2012: 70.8%, 2015: 76.7%) significantly increased. Overall, most respondents supported policies to reduce or limit sodium in these food outlets and the support increased between 2012 and 2015, but this increase was not statistically significant in all population subgroups. Increased support was seen among the following subgroups: those ≥31 years old, both males and females, non-Hispanic whites, those with a household income of ≥$40,000, those with some college education or higher, those who live in the Northeast, South, or Midwest, those who have a BMI <25 or ≥30 kg/m^2, non-hypertensives, or those who have a desire to eat a diet low in sodium. Among Hispanic respondents, there was an increased support specifically for policies limiting sodium in school cafeterias.

Nutrients **2017**, *9*, 836

Table 3. Support policies to limit sodium in foods prepared in schools, workplaces, and quick-serve restaurants, SS2012 and SS2015.

Questionnaire and Answers	School Cafeterias			Workplace Cafeterias			Quick-Serve Restaurants		
	Year 2012	Year 2015	p-value	Year 2012	Year 2015	p-Value	Year 2012	Year 2015	p-Value
Total	80.0 (78.3–81.8)	84.9 (83.5–86.2)	<0.0001	71.2 (69.3–73.1)	76.6 (75.1–78.2)	<0.0001	70.8 (68.9–72.7)	76.7 (75.2–78.3)	<0.0001
Age (years)									
18–30	79.0 (74.9–83.1)	81.2 (77.6–84.8)	0.42	68.1 (63.3–72.8)	73.8 (69.8–77.7)	0.07	67.6 (62.8–72.4)	73.5 (69.5–77.5)	0.06
31–50	79.6 (76.7–82.6)	84.0 (81.6–86.4)	**0.03**	70.0 (66.8–73.2)	74.4 (71.5–77.2)	**0.045**	68.7 (65.4–71.9)	73.6 (70.7–76.4)	**0.03**
≥51	81.0 (78.6–83.3)	87.4 (85.8–89.0)	**<0.001**	73.9 (71.3–76.5)	79.8 (77.8–81.7)	**0.0004**	74.3 (71.7–76.9)	80.7 (78.8–82.7)	**<0.0001**
Gender									
Male	77.5 (75.0–80.1)	83.0 (80.9–85.0)	**0.001**	67.4 (64.5–70.2)	73.6 (71.2–75.9)	**0.001**	66.7 (63.8–69.6)	73.4 (71.0–75.8)	**0.0005**
Female	82.5 (80.2–84.7)	86.7 (84.9–88.4)	**0.004**	74.9 (72.4–77.4)	79.5 (77.5–81.6)	**0.005**	74.7 (72.2–77.2)	79.9 (77.9–81.9)	**0.002**
Race									
White, non-Hispanic	78.2 (76.2–80.2)	83.1 (81.5–84.7)	**0.0002**	67.5 (65.3–69.8)	73.9 (72.0–75.7)	**<0.0001**	67.7 (65.5–69.9)	74.3 (72.5–76.1)	**<0.0001**
Black, non-Hispanic	89.6 (85.4–93.8)	90.0 (86.7–93.3)	0.88	83.8 (78.8–88.7)	85.5 (81.4–89.7)	0.59	82.7 (77.4–87.9)	86.2 (82.2–90.1)	0.30
Hispanic	80.6 (75.1–86.1)	88.5 (84.8–92.1)	**0.02**	73.5 (67.5–79.5)	80.3 (75.8–84.7)	0.08	73.0 (67.0–79.0)	80.0 (75.6–84.5)	0.07
Other, non-Hispanic	81.5 (74.4–88.6)	85.7 (79.8–91.5)	0.38	81.4 (74.5–88.3)	80.7 (74.2–87.1)	0.88	77.1 (69.3–84.9)	77.7 (70.7–84.7)	0.91
Household income									
<$15,000	79.8 (73.4–86.1)	80.1 (75.0–85.3)	0.93	72.7 (65.7–79.7)	77.0 (71.9–82.1)	0.33	70.2 (62.9–77.4)	75.0 (69.6–80.3)	0.30
$15,000–$24,999	80.4 (74.2–86.5)	86.3 (81.9–90.8)	0.13	73.9 (67.3–80.6)	77.9 (72.4–83.5)	0.37	74.8 (68.2–81.4)	79.5 (74.3–84.8)	0.28
$25,000–$39,999	83.7 (79.5–87.9)	86.0 (82.9–89.1)	0.40	78.0 (73.4–82.6)	79.3 (75.7–82.9)	0.65	77.7 (73.1–82.4)	80.7 (77.3–84.1)	0.31
$40,000–$59,999	77.3 (72.9–81.6)	87.5 (84.7–90.4)	**0.0001**	73.1 (68.7–77.5)	79.9 (76.5–83.4)	**0.02**	71.1 (66.5–75.7)	79.6 (76.0–83.2)	**0.004**
≥$60,000	79.9 (77.6–82.2)	84.3 (82.4–86.2)	**0.004**	67.8 (65.2–70.5)	74.6 (72.3–76.9)	**0.0002**	68.1 (65.4–70.8)	74.6 (72.3–76.8)	**0.0003**
Education level									
HS graduate or less	80.2 (77.2–83.1)	83.0 (80.7–85.3)	0.14	72.9 (69.7–76.2)	75.6 (72.9–78.2)	0.21	73.8 (70.6–77.1)	76.7 (74.1–79.3)	0.17
Some college	79.9 (77.1–82.8)	86.4 (84.2–88.7)	**0.0005**	72.6 (69.5–75.7)	78.7 (76.0–81.4)	**0.004**	72.5 (69.3–75.7)	78.1 (75.3–80.9)	**0.009**
Bachelor's degree or higher	80.0 (77.0–82.9)	86.0 (83.8–88.2)	**0.001**	67.2 (63.9–70.6)	76.1 (73.5–78.8)	**<0.0001**	64.6 (61.2–68.1)	75.4 (72.7–78.1)	**<0.0001**
Region									
Northeast	82.5 (78.8–86.2)	88.6 (85.8–91.4)	**0.01**	74.3 (70.1–78.5)	82.4 (79.2–85.7)	**0.003**	74.1 (69.9–78.4)	82.5 (79.3–85.7)	**0.002**
Midwest	79.6 (76.3–83.0)	82.8 (80.0–85.6)	0.15	69.4 (65.5–73.3)	75.1 (72.0–78.2)	**0.02**	68.5 (64.5–72.4)	75.4 (72.3–78.5)	**0.007**
South	78.4 (75.3–81.4)	85.0 (82.7–87.2)	**0.0006**	69.8 (66.5–73.1)	76.0 (73.3–78.6)	**0.004**	69.3 (66.0–72.6)	76.2 (73.6–78.9)	**0.001**
West	81.2 (77.7–84.8)	83.7 (80.7–86.7)	0.29	72.8 (68.7–76.8)	74.5 (71.0–78.0)	0.53	72.9 (68.8–76.9)	74.2 (70.6–77.7)	0.63
BMI									
<25	79.4 (76.5–82.2)	86.8 (84.6–89.0)	**<0.0001**	70.9 (67.8–74.0)	78.2 (75.6–80.9)	**0.0004**	70.3 (67.2–73.5)	79.0 (76.4–81.5)	**<0.0001**
25–30	80.6 (77.8–83.5)	81.9 (79.4–84.4)	0.51	71.1 (67.8–74.4)	73.6 (70.8–76.4)	0.25	70.3 (67.0–73.7)	73.4 (70.6–76.2)	0.17
≥30	80.3 (77.1–83.5)	85.6 (83.4–87.9)	**0.007**	71.7 (68.2–75.2)	77.8 (75.1–80.5)	**0.007**	71.9 (68.4–75.5)	77.5 (74.7–80.2)	**0.02**
Hypertension Status									
Yes	85.4 (82.6–88.3)	87.5 (85.3–89.8)	0.25	78.4 (75.1–81.7)	79.4 (76.6–82.2)	0.64	78.6 (75.4–81.9)	80.1 (77.3–82.8)	0.50
No	78.0 (76.0–80.1)	84.0 (82.4–85.6)	**<0.0001**	68.5 (66.2–70.8)	75.7 (73.9–77.6)	**<0.0001**	67.9 (65.6–70.2)	75.6 (73.8–77.5)	**<0.0001**
Want to eat a diet low in sodium									
Yes	88.8 (87.0–90.6)	92.6 (91.4–93.9)	**0.0007**	81.4 (79.3–83.6)	85.8 (84.2–87.5)	**0.002**	81.1 (78.9–83.3)	86.0 (84.4–87.7)	**0.005**
Neutral	74.3 (70.8–77.8)	77.8 (74.9–80.7)	0.13	64.8 (61.0–68.6)	68.8 (65.6–72.0)	0.11	64.0 (60.1–67.9)	68.5 (65.3–71.7)	0.08
No	58.1 (52.8–63.4)	64.5 (59.4–69.6)	0.09	45.0 (39.6–50.3)	51.1 (45.8–56.4)	0.11	45.0 (39.6–50.3)	51.6 (46.3–56.9)	0.08

HS, High school. SS, SummerStyles. Boldface signifies statistical significance (p-Value < 0.05).

Table 4. Adjusted odds ratios (aOR) [1] with 95% confidence intervals (CI) on outcome measures, SS2012 and SS2015.

Selected Characteristics		Agree to Limit Sodium in Restaurant Food	Agree to Limit Sodium in Manufactured Food	Support Policies to Limit Sodium in Foods Prepared in School, Workplace, and Quick-Serve Restaurants		
				School Cafeterias	Workplace Cafeterias	Quick-Serve Restaurants
Survey year						
	2012	Reference	Reference	Reference	Reference	Reference
	2015	0.98 (0.87, 1.11)	0.97 (0.86, 1.10)	**1.37 (1.18, 1.61)**	**1.30 (1.14, 1.49)**	**1.34 (1.17, 1.53)**
Age (years)						
	18–30	1.11 (0.93, 1.33)	1.03 (0.86, 1.24)	0.93 (0.74, 1.17)	0.84 (0.69, 1.03)	**0.79 (0.65, 0.97)**
	31–50	0.91 (0.79, 1.04)	**0.81 (0.70, 0.93)**	1.01 (0.84, 1.21)	0.89 (0.69, 1.03)	**0.84 (0.71, 0.98)**
	≥51	Reference	Reference	Reference	Reference	Reference
Gender						
	Male	Reference	Reference	Reference	Reference	Reference
	Female	1.08 (0.95, 1.22)	1.06 (0.94, 1.20)	**1.24 (1.06, 1.46)**	**1.34 (1.16, 1.53)**	**1.36 (1.18, 1.56)**
Race						
	White, non-Hispanic	Reference	Reference	Reference	Reference	Reference
	Black, non-Hispanic	**1.65 (1.33, 2.04)**	**1.59 (1.27, 2.00)**	**1.88 (1.36, 2.59)**	**2.00 (1.52, 2.62)**	**1.96 (1.48, 2.60)**
	Hispanic	**1.32 (1.08, 1.62)**	1.09 (0.90, 1.33)	**1.33 (1.01, 1.76)**	**1.36 (1.08, 1.72)**	**1.32 (1.05, 1.66)**
	Other, non-Hispanic	1.28 (0.97, 1.70)	**1.38 (1.03, 1.84)**	1.07 (0.75, 1.53)	**1.74 (1.24, 2.45)**	**1.41 (1.02, 1.94)**
Household income						
	<$15,000	**1.39 (1.10, 1.76)**	**1.47 (1.16, 1.88)**	0.89 (0.66, 1.21)	1.19 (0.91, 1.56)	0.97 (0.74, 1.26)
	$15,000–$24,999	1.16 (0.93, 146)	1.04 (0.83, 1.30)	1.09 (0.80, 1.49)	1.23 (0.94, 1.61)	1.25 (0.95, 1.64)
	$25,000–$39,999	1.19 (0.99, 1.44)	**1.44 (1.19, 1.73)**	1.27 (0.99, 1.62)	**1.51 (1.22, 1.86)**	**1.47 (1.19, 1.81)**
	$40,000–$59,999	1.17 (0.99, 1.40)	**1.20 (1.01, 1.43)**	1.04 (0.84, 1.29)	**1.33 (1.09, 1.61)**	1.19 (0.98, 1.44)
	≥60,000	Reference	Reference	Reference	Reference	Reference
Education level						
	HS graduate or less	**1.25 (1.07, 1.46)**	1.04 (0.89, 1.22)	0.94 (0.77, 1.14)	1.12 (0.95, 1.34)	**1.34 (1.12, 1.59)**
	Some college	1.14 (0.98, 1.33)	1.02 (0.88, 1.19)	1.02 (0.84, 1.29)	**1.25 (1.06, 1.47)**	**1.34 (1.12, 1.59)**
	Bachelor's degree or higher	Reference	Reference	Reference	Reference	Reference
BMI						
	<25	Reference	Reference	Reference	Reference	Reference
	25–30	0.96 (0.83, 1.11)	1.01 (0.87, 1.17)	0.84 (0.69, 1.02)	0.86 (0.73, 1.02)	**0.82 (0.70, 0.98)**
	≥30	0.97 (0.83, 1.14)	1.04 (0.89, 1.22)	0.85 (0.69, 1.04)	0.84 (0.71, 1.00)	**0.82 (0.69, 0.98)**
Hypertension Status						
	Yes	1.14 (0.99, 1.32)	1.14 (0.98, 1.33)	**1.25 (1.03, 1.53)**	1.16 (0.98, 1.37)	1.18 (0.995, 1.40)
	No	Reference	Reference	Reference	Reference	Reference
Want to eat a diet low in sodium						
	Yes	**5.04 (4.13, 6.15)**	**5.20 (4.33, 6.24)**	**5.91 (4.79, 7.29)**	**5.37 (4.45, 6.47)**	**5.35 (4.43, 6.45)**
	Neutral	**1.27 (1.02, 1.58)**	**1.31 (1.07, 1.59)**	**2.02 (1.65, 2.48)**	**2.20 (1.82, 2.67)**	**2.16 (1.78, 2.62)**
	No	Reference	Reference	Reference	Reference	Reference

[1] Covariates in the models were survey year, age, gender, race, household income, education, BMI, hypertension status, and want to eat a diet low in sodium. HS, High school. SS, SummerStyles. Boldface signifies statistical significance (p-Value < 0.05).

Multivariate logistic regression analyses showed that, in 2015, respondents were significantly more likely to support environment-specific policies limiting sodium in school cafeterias (aOR = 1.37, CI = 1.18–1.61, Table 4), workplace cafeterias (aOR = 1.30, CI = 1.14–1.49), and quick-serve restaurants (aOR = 1.34, CI = 1.17–1.53) than in 2012.

4. Discussion

Overall, while approximately half of consumers agree that it is a good idea to have broad-based actions limiting sodium in restaurants and in manufactured foods, attitudes did not differ between 2012 and 2015. Most consumers also support environment-specific policies that limit sodium in school cafeterias, workplace cafeterias, and quick-serve restaurants with a small, but statistically significant increase in agreement between 2012 and 2015. Consumer support for environment-specific policies limiting sodium in cafeterias and quick-serve restaurants were seen across a range of sociodemographic subgroups in both years, with the highest support observed among non-Hispanic blacks. Similarly, among Hispanic adults there was a high support for policies limiting sodium in school cafeterias, workplace cafeterias, and quick-serve restaurants, with a trend toward increased support between 2012 and 2015—though it did not reach statistical significance. A previous study suggests that non-Hispanic blacks and Hispanics are more likely to report taking action to reduce their sodium intake and are also more likely to report being told by a healthcare professional to do so [15], which may suggest an openness towards policies limiting sodium in the food supply.

Although the current findings show that there has been substantial agreement among consumers to limit sodium in commercially processed and prepared foods in various settings since 2012, the percent agreeing with "government actions" to limit sodium was up to 40 points lower than the percent agreeing to support environment-specific "policies" to limit sodium. It is possible that survey respondents might be more likely to agree with or support questions when framed as a general policy rather than when framed as actions of the government. Yet, almost all regions around the world have government or industry-led strategies aimed at sodium reduction through the reformulation of manufactured foods [16]. Consumers may be more open to policy changes in specific settings or environments. Among all of the settings evaluated in this study, agreement to limit sodium was lowest for restaurants; however, agreement to limit sodium in quick-serve restaurants was up to 30 percentage points higher than agreement to limit sodium in all restaurants. Similar findings from 2010 HealthStyles data suggest that respondents might be more supportive of policies regulating the sodium content of quick-serve foods or fast food rather than those regulating all restaurants [9]. Given that U.S. adults consume up to one-third of their daily energy from away-from-home sources [17], and that processed foods (i.e., restaurant and manufactured foods) compose a majority of consumer sodium intake in the U.S. [5], more studies are needed to determine how consumer education/communication on the sodium content of foods in these environments may change sentiments in favor of sodium reduction policies.

Previous studies also suggest consumer readiness for sodium reduction in cafeteria foods. In a 2010 survey of U.S. consumers, 90% of respondents supported policies to lower sodium content in school cafeterias [10]. Likewise, a majority of respondents suggested willingness to support healthy food options, including reduced sodium foods in worksite cafeterias [12,14,18]. Public support of nutrition policies can bolster the implementation of local educational programs and environmental interventions, including sodium reduction efforts in schools and worksites.

To our knowledge, no prior study has examined changes over time in U.S. consumers' attitudes about broad-based actions or policies to limit sodium across the range of food environments we examined. Most studies are limited to examinations at one point in time or include fewer food environments for addressing sodium reduction policies [9,13,19–22]. Our findings suggest increased support for environment-specific policies to lower sodium across most sociodemographic subgroups between 2012 and 2015, particularly those who were middle or older aged, non-Hispanic whites, earning ≥$40,000, college educated, not within normal BMI range, non-hypertensive, or who had a desire to eat a diet low in sodium. Although, some consumer groups appear ready to support policies to limit sodium in the food industry, the data from this study could be used to identify groups that could be targeted for interventional messaging and education on sodium reduction strategies from the medical community and public health agencies.

The findings presented in this study are subject to some limitations. The survey was not nationally representative of the U.S. population, although respondents were weighted to the general distribution of the U.S. population on age, sex, race/ethnicity, household income, household size, education, census region, metro status, and prior Internet access. Most of the respondents were middle or older aged, non-Hispanic whites, presenting an overrepresentation (in comparison to the general U.S. population), and had a household income $\geq$\$60,000, which may impact the generalizability of the findings. Second, the limited sample size may have decreased statistical power to find a difference in some respondent subgroups. For example, the difference observed among Hispanics (14% of the total sample) in the percent who support sodium reduction in workplace cafeterias is larger in percentage points (i.e., 6.8 percentage points) than the statistically significant difference among non-Hispanic whites (6.4 percentage points, 67% of the total sample). However, the relative difference is smaller. Third, self-reported height and weight, which were used to calculate respondents' BMI as well as hypertension status are subject to self-reporting bias. Respondents may have also provided socially desirable responses to questions on limiting sodium across various environments. Fourth, the results of the survey questions on limiting sodium which focus on "governmental actions" are not comparable to the questions that focus on "policies" due to the following: (1) participants' perception of these terms may have elicited differences in their responses; (2) the settings rated by consumers differed between the governmental actions questions and the policies questions; (3) the response categories for questions on governmental actions included a neutral category (i.e., neither agree nor disagree) that was combined with "disagree". A sensitivity analysis was conducted, combining neutral with agree; however, the direction of the findings showed that similar-support remained the same or was higher between 2012 and 2015. Finally, although a majority of the sample showed increased agreement and support for policies to limit sodium across all of the food environments examined between 2012 and 2015, there is very limited knowledge on whether consumers are willing to take action to have sodium reduced in processed foods [3,23].

5. Conclusions

The results of this study suggest that, since 2012, there has been substantial agreement and support for actions to limit sodium in commercially-processed and prepared foods, with most consumers ready for actions to lower sodium in foods served in schools, workplaces, and quick-serve restaurants. Moreover, consumer agreement with policies limiting sodium in these environments has increased between 2012 and 2015. In light of recently published sodium-reduction targets and recommendations to reduce sodium across the food industry [24], this analysis provides the public health community with a current view of consumer attitudes and suggests that there may be an increasing trend towards greater support for some of these policies. Future research could examine the role that clinicians and public health agencies play in educating consumers about the need to reduce sodium and how this knowledge may influence changes in consumer attitudes toward broad-based actions and environment-specific policies. It will also be important to understand whether increased support is associated with other changes in consumer behavior to limit sodium in their diet, such as consumer spending on low-sodium products.

Acknowledgments: This work was supported in part by Project IMHOTEP, an internship provided through a cooperative agreement with Morehouse College and the CDC.

Author Contributions: The findings and conclusions in this report are those of the author(s) and do not represent the official position of the Centers for Disease Control and Prevention. E.C.O., X.T., M.E.C. conceived and designed the study. X.T. analyzed the data. C.W. and E.C.O. wrote the paper. K.A.J. contributed to writing and formatting the paper.

Conflicts of Interest: The authors declare no conflict of interest.

References

1. U.S. Department of Agriculture. WWEIA Data Tables, 2013–2014. Available online: https://www.ars.usda. gov/ARSUserFiles/80400530/pdf/1314/Table_1_NIN_GEN_13.pdf (accessed on 30 January 2017).
2. U.S. Department of Agriculture; U.S. Department of Health and Human Services. Dietary Guidelines for Americans 2015–2020, 8th ed. Available online: https://health.gov/dietaryguidelines/2015/guidelines/ (accessed on 18 November 2016).
3. Patel, D.; Cogswell, M.E.; John, K.; Creel, S; Ayala, C. Knowledge, attitudes, and behaviors related to sodium intake and reduction among adult consumers in the United States. *Am. J. Health Promot.* **2017**, *31*, 9–18. [CrossRef] [PubMed]
4. Cogswell, M.E.; Zhang, Z.; Carriquiry, A.L.; Gunn, J.P.; Kuklina, E.V.; Saydah, S.H.; Yang, Q.; Moshfegh, A.J. Sodium and potassium intakes among US adults: NHANES 2003–2008. *Am. J. Clin. Nutr.* **2012**, *96*, 647–657. [CrossRef] [PubMed]
5. Harnack, L.J.; Cogswell, M.E.; Shikany, J.M.; Gardner, C.D.; Gillespie, C.; Loria, C.M.; Zhou, X.; Yuan, K.; Steffen, L.M. Sources of sodium in US adults from 3 geographic regions. *Circulation.* **2017**, *135*, 1775–1783. [CrossRef] [PubMed]
6. U.S. Department of Agriculture. School Meals, Healthy Hunger-Free Kids Act. Available online: https://www.fns.usda.gov/school-meals/healthy-hunger-free-kids-act (accessed on 30 January 2017).
7. General Services Administration/Health and Human Services. Health and Sustainability Guidelines for Federal Concessions and Vending Operations. Available online: https://www.gsa.gov/graphics/pbs/ Guidelines_for_Federal_Concessions_and_Vending_Operations.pdf (accessed on 30 January 2017).
8. Division for Heart Disease and Stroke Prevention, Sodium Reduction in Communities Program. Available online: https://www.cdc.gov/dhdsp/programs/sodium_reduction.htm (accessed on 30 January 2017).
9. Patel, S.M.; Gunn, J.P.; Tong, X.; Cogswell, M.E. Consumer sentiment on actions reducing sodium in processed and restaurant foods, ConsumerStyles 2010. *Am. J. Prev. Med.* **2014**, *46*, 516–524. [CrossRef] [PubMed]
10. Patel, S.M.; Gunn, J.P.; Merlo, C.L.; Tong, X.; Cogswell, M.E. Consumer support for policies to reduce the sodium content in school cafeterias. *J. Child. Nutr. Manag.* **2014**, *38*.
11. Kid's Safe & Healthful Foods Project, Poll Shows Strong Voter Support for Nutrition Standards for Food and Beverages Sold in School Vending Machines and a la Carte Lines. Available online: http://www. rwjf.org/content/dam/farm/communication_and_promotion/news_releases/2012/rwjf72628 (accessed on 22 June 2016).
12. Lee-Kwan, S.H.; Pan, L.; Kimmons, J.; Foltz, J.; Park, S. Support for food and beverage worksite wellness strategies and sugar–sweetened beverage intake among employed U.S. adults. *Am. J. Health Promot.* **2017**, *31*, 128–135. [CrossRef] [PubMed]
13. Donohoe Mather, C.M.; McGurk, M.D. Insights in Public Health: Promoting healthy snack and beverage choices in Hawai'i Worksites: The Choose Healthy Now! Project. *Hawaii J Med. Pub. Health* **2014**, *73*, 365–370.
14. Perlmutter, C.A.; Canter, D.D.; Gregoire, M.B. Profitability and accessibility of fat- and sodium-modified hot entrees in a worksite cafeteria. *J. Am. Diet. Assoc.* **1997**, *97*, 391–395. [CrossRef]
15. Jackson, S.L.; Coleman King, S.M.; Park, S.; Fang, J.; Odom, E.C.; Cogswell, M.E. Health professional advice and action to reduce sodium intake. *Am. J. Prev. Med.* **2016**, *50*, 30–39. [CrossRef] [PubMed]
16. Trieu, K.; Neal, B.; Hawkes, C.; Dunford, E.; Campbell, N.; Rodriguez–Fernandez, R.; Legetic, B.; McLaren, L.; Barberio, A.; Webster, J. Salt reduction initiatives around the World—A systematic review of progress towards the global target. *PLoS ONE* **2015**, *10*, e0130247. [CrossRef] [PubMed]
17. Smith, L.P.; Ng, S.W.; Popkin, B.M. Trends in US home food preparation and consumption: Analysis of national nutrition surveys and time use studies from 1965–1966 to 2007–2008. *Nutr. J.* **2013**, *12*, 1–10. [CrossRef] [PubMed]
18. Vanderlee, L.; Hammond, D. Does nutrition information on menus impact food choice? Comparisons across two hospital cafeterias. *Pub. Health Nutr.* **2014**, *38*, 1–10. [CrossRef] [PubMed]

19. Arcand, J.; Mendoza, J.; Qi, Y.; Henson, S.; Lou, W.; L'Abbe, M.R. Results of a national survey examining Canadians' concern, actions, barriers, and support for dietary sodium reduction initiatives. *Can. J. Cardiol.* **2013**, *29*, 628–631. [CrossRef] [PubMed]

20. Lee, J.; Park, S. Consumer attitudes, barriers, and meal satisfaction associated with sodium–reduced meal intake at worksite cafeterias. *Nutr. Res. Pract.* **2015**, *9*, 644–649. [CrossRef] [PubMed]

21. Mendoza, J.E.; Schram, G.A.; Arcand, J.; Henson, S.; L'Abbe, M. Assessment of consumers' level of engagement in following recommendations for lowering sodium intake. *Appetite* **2014**, *73*, 51–57. [CrossRef] [PubMed]

22. Roberto, C.A.; Bragg, M.A.; Schwartz, M.B.; Seamans, M.J.; Musicus, A.; Novak, N.; Brownell, K.D. Facts up front versus traffic light food labels: A randomized controlled trial. *Am. J. Prev. Med.* **2012**, *43*, 134–141. [CrossRef] [PubMed]

23. American Heart Association #BreakUpWithSalt, Sodium Reduction Initiative. Available online: https://act.sodiumbreakup.heart.org/dLkrLQb (accessed on 30 January 2017).

24. U.S. Food & Drug Administration. Draft Guidance for Industry: Voluntary Sodium Reduction Goals: Target Mean and Upper Bound Concentrations for Sodium in Commercially Processed, Packaged, and Prepared Foods. Available online: https://www.fda.gov/Food/GuidanceRegulation/GuidanceDocumentsRegulatoryInformation/ucm494732.htm (accessed on 25 April 2017).

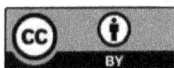

![nutrients logo] *nutrients*

MDPI

Article

The Healthy Eating Agenda in Australia. Is Salt a Priority for Manufacturers?

Rebecca Lindberg *, Tyler Nichols and Chrystal Yam

The Australian Health Policy Collaboration, College of Health and Biomedicine, Victoria University, 300 Queen St, Melbourne, VIC 3000, Australia; tyler.nichols1@vu.edu.au (T.N.); chrystalyam@yahoo.com.au (C.Y.)
* Correspondence: rebecca.lindberg@vu.edu.au

Received: 15 June 2017; Accepted: 10 August 2017; Published: 15 August 2017

Abstract: Many nation states have endorsed and acted on the World Health Organization's target of a 30% reduction in global salt consumption by 2025. In Australia, new government-led voluntary measures were initiated in 2009, consisting of public–private partnerships, front-of-pack labelling, and food reformulation targets (which include reduced salt). How Australia's private sector has responded to this healthy eating agenda has been investigated in a limited way, particularly with regards to manufacturers which produce processed foods considered significant sources of sodium. In this study we asked: have Australia's largest food manufacturers made " … positive (nutrition) changes to their product portfolios" as disclosed in their public policies, priorities, and communications? And, is salt reduction a priority for processed food manufacturers? A systematic search and critical content-analysis of grey literature published by food manufacturers was conducted. The results suggest half of the sample publically describe some salt reduction activities but the scale and efficacy of these changes is unclear from the available literature. The Australian Government's Healthy Food Partnership could capitalise on current documented activities in salt reduction, and implement a more comprehensive healthy eating agenda moving forward. In light of the increasing rates of hypertension, population salt consumption and diet-related disease, more could be done.

Keywords: salt; food policy; food reformulation; food industry

---

1. Introduction

Non-communicable diseases (NCDs), including cardiovascular and cerebrovascular disease, kill more people each year than all other causes combined [1]. The World Health Organization's (WHO) Global Action Plan for the prevention and control of NCDs [1] contains nine voluntary global prevention and reduction targets [1]. Two of the targets include a 30% reduction in salt intake and 25% reduction in raised blood pressure. These were set because of the known association between these risk factors and cardiovascular and cerebrovascular diseases, and other NCDs [2]. The Global Action Plan explicitly encourages collaborative partnerships between government, civil society and the private sector to achieve the targets by the year 2025.

Unfortunately, Australians are eating more salt than ever [3]. Almost one quarter of adults (23.1%) have high blood pressure and cardiovascular disease is Australia's most expensive disease group [3]. Adults consume an average of 9 g of salt per day—well above the WHO recommended daily intake of 5 g [4]. It is estimated that 75–80% of salt consumed is via "hidden salt" in processed foods [5]. These foods (Table 1) [6] include baked goods, cereal based products, processed meat, soup and sauces and may be prepared and consumed at home and/or sourced from quick service outlets and restaurants.

Table 1. Proportion of salt intake (%) from food groups using National Health Survey data 2014, adapted from [6]. Reproduced with permission from authors and organization.

Food Group	% Contribution to Overall Dietary Salt (Sodium) for All Persons
Cereal-based products and dishes (all)	24.8
Meat, poultry, game products and dishes (all)	18.3
Cereal and cereal products (all)	18.2
Sauces, dips and condiments (all)	5.9
Soup	4.5
Cheese	3.9

Reducing salt content in processed products is one of the most cost-effective preventative population health interventions [7]. Even modest reductions across the supply result in a substantial decrease in population intake and subsequently deliver health outcomes [8,9]. However, influencing and implementing food reformulation strategies is not without difficulty [5,10]. Consumer acceptance of reformulated products, manufacturing limitations, food safety, and quality and shelf-life trade-offs are all potential issues [10–12]. Despite these challenges, salt levels can be reduced by approximately 40% in breads and 70% in processed meat products without affecting consumer acceptability [12]. In fact most challenges can be mitigated or resolved and hence food reformulation is increasingly being supported by governments, advocated by civil society and considered and implemented by food industry.

1.1. International Policy Context

Influenced by the Global Action Plan and mounting evidence and advocacy on the need for changes in the food environment, over 80 countries have adopted national salt reduction strategies [13]. Of these strategies, 71 either include or plan to include, programs that engage food industry to achieve salt reduction at a population level [13]. In terms of high and middle-income countries, the United Kingdom (UK) was one of the first to adopt a national salt reduction strategy predating the Global Action Plan. Their 2003 strategy included voluntary reduction targets applied to more than 80 food categories, public awareness campaigns and mandatory labelling of high salt foods [13]. Despite the voluntary nature food manufacturers did, and continue to participate, with several publically disclosing their commitment and achievements in salt reduction [14–17]. The current targets are detailed within the Department of Health's "Public Health Responsibility Deal" [18]. Signatories to the "Deal" update their progress towards the targets on an online platform administered by Government [18]. Overall, in the last decade the UK has achieved a 15% reduction in population salt consumption [13]. Maintaining this progress requires ongoing monitoring, accountability and Governmental leadership [19].

Argentina and South Africa have displayed significant leadership by implementing mandatory maximum salt levels on a range of staple foods [13]. Food manufacturers have time frames in which they are required to comply, or face sanctions. Additionally, legislation in Argentina is applicable to the hospitality sector by setting maximum salt content in meals supplied in quick service and restaurants [13]. Mandatory targets may seem heavy-handed given the success of the voluntary system in the UK, but there is some evidence that even within the British food industry mandatory targets are preferable as they level the playing field [20,21].

1.2. Australian Policy Context

Australia has an international commitment to address noncommunicable diseases in line with the Global Action Plan. In Australia, a national collaboration of public health experts has adapted the Global Action Plan and the associated targets for the Australian setting [3]. This equates to reducing the average population salt intake to 6 g, and the proportion of the population affected by high blood pressure to 16.1%, by the year 2025 [3]. From 2009 to 2014 the Australian Food and Health Dialogue (FHD) was in operation as a public–private partnership to improve healthy eating. Its stated goals were admirable but the mechanism for implementation and accountability was criticised as weak [22–24].

Sodium (as a proxy for salt) was one of several reformulation action areas considered under the FHD [24]. Only 12 out of a possible 137 reformulation action areas had voluntary targets set for them over the duration of the FHD, nine of these regarding sodium [24]. While this indicates slow and disappointing progress in setting targets, it suggests that sodium reduction was a priority under the FHD. An evaluation of nine of the product groups (summarised in Table 2 [25]) shows good progress on food reformulation and compliance with the maximum sodium levels. However, these voluntary targets have been criticised as unambitious and likely to result in only minor effects to population intake [23].

Table 2. An evaluation of the FHD reformulation targets, adapted from [25]. Reproduced with permission from authors and organization.

Product Type		Agreed Sodium Reformulation Targets for the FHD	Proportion of Products Not Exceeding Maximum Sodium Target (at Baseline 2009–2012)	Proportion of Products Not Exceeding Maximum Sodium Target (2015)
Breads		Max. of 400 mg/100 g	28.0%	86.0%
Cheese	Cheddar and cheddar style	Max. of 710 mg/100 g	83.5%	86.4%
	Low moisture mozzarella	Max. of 550 mg/100 g	63.2%	68.4%
	Chilled processed	Max. of 1270 mg/100 mg	37.2%	43.2%
Processed meats	Bacon	Max. of 1090 mg/100 g	25.0%	59.0%
	Ham and other cured meats		46.9%	79.7%
	Emulsified luncheon meats	Max. of 830 mg/100 g	22.7%	44.4%
Potato/Corn/Extruded Snacks (PCES)	Cereal-based snacks	Max. of 700 mg/100 g	88.4%	92.3%
	Potato chips	Max. of 800 mg/100 g	92.5%	91.8%
	Extruded snacks	Max. of 1250 mg/100 g	95.5%	93.5%
	Salt & vinegar products	Max. of 1100 mg/100 g	52.9%	78.3%
Ready-to-eat breakfast cereals		15% reduction across products with sodium levels exceeding 400 mg/100 g	54.5%	83.2%
Simmer sauces	Asian style	15% reduction across sauces with sodium levels exceeding 680 mg/100 g	41.0%	59.3%
	Indian style	15% reduction in across sauces with sodium levels exceeding 420 mg/100 g	40.0%	68.0%
	Pasta		33.3%	75.8%
	Simmer (other)		25.0%	45.5%
Savoury crackers	Plain crackers (flour-based)	Max. of 850 mg/100 g	76.8%	87.2%
	Flavoured crackers (flour based)	Max. of 1000 mg/100 g	72.3%	78.6%
	Flavoured rice/corn cakes/crackers	Max. of 850 mg/100 g	70.0%	75.7%
Savoury Pies	Wet	10% reduction across those with sodium levels exceeding 400 mg/100 g	28.4%	51.2%
	Dry	10% reduction across those with sodium levels exceeding 500 mg/100 g	36.6%	27.6%
Soups	Wet/condensed soup products	Max. of 300 mg/100 g	75%	80.0%
	Dry soup products	Max. of 290 mg/100 g	27.2%	77.9%

Due to a change in national governments, the FHD was inactive for a 1–2 years period [24] and re-emerged as the Healthy Food Partnership (The Partnership) in November 2015. The Partnership continues to support the voluntary front-of-pack labelling Health Star Rating scheme [24] and in 2016 appointed a food reformulation working group to review the existing targets and explore expansion of the voluntary targets (including sodium) to other food categories [26]. The Partnership website [26] states:

The Australian Government, food industry bodies and public health groups have agreed to cooperatively tackle obesity, encourage healthy eating and empower food manufacturers to make positive changes to their product portfolios.

1.3. Study Aim and Research Questions

At this mid-point between setting the Global Action Plan and the year 2025, it is timely to assess the adequacy of the Australian government's action on salt reduction and NCDs to date. Comprehensive accountability for nutrition action typically involves gathering information, monitoring and measuring financial or institutional performance against the mandatory or voluntary standards, and utilising this intelligence to improve performance [27]. Gathering information for this purpose can include a range of methods and analysis, including an investigation of food and beverage manufacturers' policies, practices and disclosure of their contributions to improving nutrition [28].

In this study we sought to contribute to accountability and answer the research questions:

- Have Australia's largest food manufacturers made " … positive (nutrition) changes to their product portfolios" as disclosed in their public policies, priorities, and communications?
- And, is salt reduction a priority for processed food manufacturers?

2. Materials and Methods

In order to answer the research questions, we critically appraised Australia's largest food manufacturer's public priorities and reported actions in relation to healthy eating and salt reduction in processed foods. A systematic search of grey literature published by food manufacturers was designed and conducted to appraise stated priorities and achievements. Grey literature (such website content, policies, media releases) from 2010 to 2017 was sought to coincide with the Global Action Plan, the FHD and the Partnership.

2.1. Search Strategy

The largest food manufacturers (as defined by the company's net profit in the 2015–2016 financial year) were identified via the Ibisworld "Australia's Top 100 Food and Drink Manufacturers" publication [29]. The list was appraised by the first and second authors to include Australian manufacturers of relevant products (i.e., processed foods described in Tables 1 and 2). Manufacturers that exclusively produced or processed alcoholic beverages, fresh meat/abattoirs, or fruit and vegetables, were excluded. Importers without Australian production capacity were also excluded as we prioritised Australian-made products to assess the Australian Government-led healthy eating agenda.

Each inclusion/exclusion decision was recorded. Discrepancies were discussed between the first two authors and resolved, recording the outcome. For example, one author may have located a manufacturer that produced well-known products in the Australian market, whereas the second author may have correctly identified that the company imports these goods. The final included list was checked by the third author.

After initial screening, the websites of included manufacturers were further investigated and searched for descriptions of the company's commitment or activities relevant to healthy eating and salt or sodium reduction. The search occurred February–May 2017. Where possible, within website search boxes were used, applying the following terms:

- Health
- Nutrition
- Salt
- Sodium
- Reformulation

If the website did not have a search box function, the first and second authors manually reviewed the website home page and sub-pages including nutrition sections, corporate social responsibility sections, annual reports and media sections. The title of media releases, statements on the website, nutrition policies, corporate social responsibility plans or any other content that was returned in the search was reviewed. Based on the titles relevant grey literature were saved. The "about us" (or similar) section of each website was also downloaded, as was each manufacturers most recent annual report (2016) and/or corporate responsibility report (2016 or 2017). Manufacturers that produced several brands were noted, and the branded website was also searched. For international companies, the Australian version of their site was searched.

Included manufacturers were contacted via email/online enquiry forms, to provide them with the opportunity to add additional published material. All grey literature were added to EndNote and used for content analysis.

2.2. Synthesis and Analysis

The included grey literature were read in full by the first author and the content for each manufacturer was manually inductively analysed, colour coding the literature. Evidence of food reformulation, participation in voluntary measures including the Health Star Rating and/or the Partnership, introduction of new healthier product lines and targets for reduced sodium content were recorded. Nutrition priorities such as action or policies that restrict marketing to children, support reductions in energy content, serving sizes, sugar and saturated/trans-fats and/or increased fibre, new healthier product lines, manufacturing of healthy nutritious foods and consumer information were also recorded. Other priorities were noted including local production, philanthropy, and environment as these themes often overlapped and were communicated alongside manufacturer's nutrition priorities.

The results were summarised in a table and audited by the second and third authors to triangulate the findings and resolve any discrepancies. The authors then focussed on the manufacturers where salt/sodium was included in their public communications and attempted to document the extent of the commitment, progress made and transparency in goals. Data immersion occurred by reading and re-reading the content, discussing emergent ideas and subsequently co-analysing and co-coding the data to agree on themes relevant to the research questions.

3. Results and Discussion

Thirty-three of Australia's 100 largest manufacturers make product lines of relevance to salt-reduction and therefore, were included in the study (Table 3). One-hundred and forty three grey literature were reviewed to extract data on manufacturers, including website content, media releases, policies, annual reports and emails from company representatives.

This study found that over half ($n = 17$) of the 33 manufactures disclosed that they were reducing salt in at least some of their food products (see Table 3). All of the manufacturers provided some evidence of nutrition and healthy eating as a part of company's policies, protocols and priorities (see Table 4). Interestingly the content included in the inductive analysis suggested that most manufacturers also reported the environment and sustainability as a part of their priorities and this emergent theme will be briefly discussed further below (Section 3.3). Other priorities for manufacturers include quality control and food safety, community development and philanthropy, gender diversity and workplace culture, regulatory compliance, commitment to Australian made and local jobs, and expansion into Asia and abroad.

The main themes relevant to the research questions will be expanded on below and potential reasons for these findings will be discussed. The implications for policy and practice will also be considered.

3.1. Salt Reduction in Manufacturers' Product Portfolios

Manufacturer's policies and priorities on salt reduction could be categorized in three main ways: those with "no evidence", those with "some evidence" and those with "considerable evidence".

This study found that 16 out of 33 companies that produce processed foods in the Australian market that are considered significant sources of sodium, provide no evidence or documentation of reducing salt in their products (see Table 3). These manufacturers may be reducing salt and not disclose this, or may have no commitment to reformulation or salt reduction. Cheese, processed meat products such as hamburgers, pies and chicken nuggets, pasta and pasta sauces, crackers and snack foods had voluntary sodium reformulation targets during the FHD from 2010 to 2014 and the adoption and/or maintenance of these targets is not evident among these manufacturers' publically available documents. The Healthy Food Partnership has not yet endorsed the continuation or expansion of the targets although this was due February 2017 [30]. Technical, financial or consumer-based barriers may be real or perceived challenges to reformulation by these manufacturers [5,10].

Of the 17 manufacturers that disclosed some action on salt-reduction, by investigating the literature to identify the extent of the commitment, progress made and transparency in goals, it appears that most manufacturers had broad aspirations or achievements for their products (Table 3). For example Coca-Cola Amatil report they " ... reduced salt and sugar in key tomato products helping Australians eat healthier" [31]. Similar statements about tonnes of salt removed from the food supply, "reduced salt" product lines, and participation in front-of-pack labelling schemes imply that companies are aware of the high levels of population salt intake, the government-led agenda and/or the consumer demand for reduced salt and are therefore making positive changes to their portfolio. The scale and efficacy of these changes is unclear from the publically available literature.

Manufacturers such as Mondelez, Nestle and Unilever are among the largest multinational food companies in the world and they appear to be, in comparison to the rest of the sample, more transparent and provide considerable documentation of their achievements and aspirations for food reformulation. Both Mondelez and Unilever have corporate responsibility progress reports that describe their salt-reduction (and other) priorities, progress against targets and partnerships to help achieve the targets [32,33]. Mondelez's 2015 report [32] notes the target of a 10% reduction across all product lines by 2020 and significant progress in food-reformulation in Latin American Oreo biscuits and Ritz crackers in the UK. Interestingly these are the regions where the company also participates in the Pan-American Sodium Consortium and the UK Responsibility Deal, suggesting public–private partnerships can trigger progress on healthier products. Oreo and Ritz biscuits are international products and those sold in Latin America and the UK respectively are lower in salt than in Australia. Mondelez states these reductions in these markets is a significant achievement [32]. This implies the reductions have been achieved without reducing consumer acceptability.

Nestle and Unilever state that they have adopted the WHO recommended upper intake level of 5 g salt per day and formulated their products to help consumers to not exceed this level [33,34]. The Unilever website includes a table of their nutrition criteria for maximum level of salt in a range of product groups, a position statement on salt reduction and progress, by country, towards their 2020 target. In Australia 68% of products sold by Unilever meet levels to enable 5 g/daily [33]. These companies appear to undertake the research and development, partnership, and monitoring that enables reporting and food reformulation. There is evidence of the leadership from senior levels within the company of food reformulation and public accountability as demonstrated in the stated responsibilities expected of the Board of Directors [35]. These companies may offer a model for other manufacturers.

The results suggest that of 33 Australian food manufacturers included in this study approximately half document salt-reduction efforts in their publically available literature. Participation in government-led measures and/or salt reduction was outlined in greatest detail by the multi-national food companies. The efficacy and scale of the "positive (nutrition) changes" is unclear from the content included in this study and regular independent monitoring of food reformulation activities in Australia would be preferable.

3.2. Salt and Other Nutrition Priorities

There was documentation of nutrition activities and policies for all of the included manufacturers (see Table 4) but the scope, validity of claims and effect of these activities is unclear from the available literature. Several included manufacturers make nutritious foods consistent with national dietary guidelines including dairy, poultry and cereals. It was common to find grey literature that educated the consumer about the nutritional benefits of products and/or how to interpret food labels using nutrition information panels, daily intake guides and the Health Star Rating system. George Weston Foods, for example, reports in their corporate responsibility document that they are a member of the GoScan "app" program. On their Tip Top (bread manufacturer) website [36], the frequently asked questions section provides information on ingredients, the benefits of fibre and the function of salt as an ingredient in bread. Several manufacturers employed dietitians to blog, provide recipes and information.

Some manufacturers (see Table 4) also described reformulating foods to reduce saturated and trans fats, sugar, energy and increase fibre and protein. Snack food companies also disclosed their compliance with responsible marketing to children initiatives [37,38] and several mentioned compliance with school canteen guidelines [39,40]. In comparison to other risk-associated macro or micro-nutrients, salt received no more or less attention.

It is commonly understood that websites and public documents are designed to create brand loyalty and provide consumers and investors with information. Therefore enabling consumers to " . . . access trusted product information" [41] to benefit their nutrition and health, is not out of the ordinary. However, it also reinforces the common expectation of individual responsibility for dietary choices and behavior, and could be considered as a way to distance corporations from responsibility for the nutrition of their food products.

In answer the first research question, it is unclear from industry's public priorities and policies if " . . . positive (nutrition) changes to . . . product portfolios" are comprehensively occurring in the Australian food supply, despite the reported nutrition activities. Therefore, it is also uncertain if the Partnership is achieving its goals after 18 months of work. In answer to the second research question, salt reduction appears to be one of several nutrition and healthy-eating priorities for most processed food manufacturers. It is encouraging that half of the sample report some activity to reduce salt and now more can be done to comprehensively reduce population sodium consumption.

3.3. Manufacturers Responsibilities

The inductive analysis suggests that some, mainly the large and multinational companies disclose three, four or five "responsibilities" that they implement and aspire to [31,40,41]. Community and philanthropy is typically one, the environment is another and healthier and higher quality products for consumers is often the third. These triple-bottom line principles appear well enshrined in the corporate culture of large multinational food manufacturers, although evidence of food companies not behaving responsibly also exists [42].

Table 3. Priorities and actions publically reported by Australian food manufacturers—salt.

Company Name Major Relevant Australian-Made Brands	Example Relevant Products	Documentation of Salt Reduction	Example Priorities or Actions
Arnotts Campbells	Crackers, savoury biscuits, canned soups	✓	"Campbell Arnott's … have undertaken a stepwise reduction of sodium in order to meet the Tick's sodium criteria for soups. In 2004, only 33% of Campbell's soups met the Tick's sodium criteria of 300 mg/100 g or less. By 2009, approximately 83% of all Campbell's soups met the sodium criteria". Source: Personal communication from Arnotts (28 May 2017)
Baiada Poultry Steggles, Lilydale	Chicken nuggets, kievs, schnitzels	✓	Steggles supplies products that are compliant with the Australian School Canteen association's nutrition bodies, which stipulate products must have: "450 mg or less of sodium per 100 g". Source: "Healthy Chicken for Kids" section of Steggles website (visited 22 May 2017)
Bega Cheese	Cheese		
Bellamy's Organic	Toddler snacks, pasta		
Burra Foods	Cheese		
Cerebos Asian Home Gourmet, Fountain & Gravox	Gravies, sauces, ready meals	✓	Fountain has created a healthier range of sauces, which include: "25% less added salt than Fountain regular tomato and barbeque 500 mL squeeze sauces" Source: Fountain sauces website (visited 18 May 2017)
Coca-Cola Amatil SPC, Ardmona	Baked beans, tinned spaghetti	✓	In 2014 "Reduced salt and sugar in key tomato products helping Australians eat healthier". Source: 90 year history section of SPC Ardmona website (visited 18 May 2017)
Cordina Chicken Farms	Schnitzel, nibbles, burgers		
Devondale Murray Goulburn	Cheese, cream cheese, butter		
Freedom Foods Group Freedom Foods	Cereals, snacks, spreads	✓	"At Freedom Foods … You won't find any that have more than 600 mg of sodium per 100 g". Source: "Salt" section of Freedom Foods website (visited 18 May 2017)
General Mills Holding (Australia) Latina Fresh, Nature Valley, Old El Paso, Pasta Master	Pasta sauce, snacks tacos	✓	Old El Paso offers a "reduced salt taco spice mix", also "healthy fiesta" burrito kit packet with the Heart Foundation tick. Source: Old El Paso website (visited 18 May 2017)
George Weston Foods Tip Top, Don, KR Castlemaine, Mauri ANZ	Bread, small goods, bread-making products	✓	"Reducing salt GWF is one of Australia's first companies to establish a sodium criteria as part of the National Heart Foundation Heart Tick program and Voluntary Sodium Reduction Roundtable initiative. Since 2007, we've reduced salt across our breads and small goods, contributing to the removal of more than 340 tonnes of salt from Australian diets." Source: "Corporate Responsibility at GWF" document, GWF website (visited 11 April 2017)

Nutrients **2017**, *9*, 881

Table 3. *Cont.*

Company Name *Major Relevant Australian-Made Brands*	Example Relevant Products	Documentation of Salt Reduction	Example Priorities or Actions
Goodman Fielder *Country Life, Golden Canola, Helgas, Holbrooks, Irvines, La Famiglia Kitchen, Lawsons, Logicol, Meadowlea, MacKenzie, Mighty Soft, Molenberg, Olive Grove, Praise, White Wings, Wonder White*	Bread, pastry, cheese, sauces, spreads, cake mixes	✓	Helgas wraps advertised as salt-reduced wraps: "40% less salt than the market leader". Source: Helgas website (visited 11 May 2017)
Green's Foods *Waterthins, Poppin, Roccas Deli*	Crackers, popcorn		
Heinz	Baked beans, canned tomatoes, sauces	✓	"At Heinz we're always interested in discovering new way to make our products even more nutritious and appealing—from ... to our growing section of reduced sugar and salt products". Source: Health section, Heinz website (visited 1 May 2017)
Ingham's	Nuggets		
Kellogg Australia Holdings	Cereal, snack bars	✓	"2012—We announced that we'd reduced the salt levels in Corn Flakes and Rice Bubbles cereals in Australia by 20%. This reduction meant that since 1997, we'd reduced salt levels across our cereals by up to 59%—that equates to approximately 276 metric tonnes, or more than 4.9 m salt shakers (60 g) removed from Australian diets every year." Source: Our history section of Kellogg's website (visited 26 May 2017)
Mars *Dolmio, KanTong, Master foods, Uncle Bens*	Sauces, spreads and rice-based ready meals	✓	"We have been progressively reducing salt across our total portfolio in line with our commitment to the Department of Health and Ageing salt reduction targets, and many of our products now carry the National Heart Foundation Tick ... " Source: "Food" section of Mars Australia website (visited 17 April 2017)
McCain Foods	Ready-meals, pizzas		
Mondelez Australia *Vegemite*	Crackers, spread	✓	"Reduced Salt VEGEMITE is best enjoyed by the many Australians consciously reducing their salt intake for health and wellbeing reasons. Older Australians and parents wishing to choose lower salt options for the family will love Reduced Salt VEGEMITE ... " Source: Vegemite website (visited 3 April 2017)
Nestle *Maggi, Milo, Uncle Toby's*	Breakfast cereal, bars, drink, noodles, stock	✓	" ... The foundation members of the Healthier Australia Commitment ... have voluntarily agreed to the following collective targets for reductions ... by 2015: Reduce sodium in products by 25 per cent—equivalent to over 270,000 kilograms of sodium removed from the food supply ... " Source: Nestle media release 2012, on website (visited 28 April 2017)
Norco Co-Op	Butter, cheese		
Parmalat Australia *Lemnos, President*	Cheese		

Table 3. *Cont.*

Company Name Major Relevant Brands *Australian-Made Brands*	Example Relevant Products	Documentation of Salt Reduction	Example Priorities or Actions
Patties Foods *Four'N'Twenty, Herbert Adams, Nanna's*	Pies, pastries, sausage rolls		
Pepsico Australia & New Zealand *Doritos Corn Chips, Nobby's Nuts, Red Rock Deli, Parker's Pretzels, Sakata Rice Crackers, Smith's Chips, Sunbites, Twisties*	Breakfast cereal, snack foods	✓	"The reduction in saturated fat follows Smith's previous commitment of a 25% reduction in salt content across its product range by 2012. Forty products have thus far been reformulated." Source: Media release "Smiths—Australia's favourite chip now has 75% less saturated fat" available on Smiths website (visited 26 April 2017)
Sanitarium	Breakfast cereal	✓	Health Star Rating salt standards have set the agenda for their product reformulation work—previously they had their own internal nutrition standards, but the new initiative has superseded this. Source: Personal email (received 30 May 2017)
San Remo	Pasta and sauces		
Scalzo Food Industries	Snacks		
Simplot Australia *Birds Eye, Leggos, Edgell, Lean Cuisine, Harvest, Chiko, I&J, Top Cut, Five Tastes, Simply Great Meals*	Frozen snacks, ready-meals, meal kits, meat, small goods	✓	"We are proud to report that 29 tonnes of salt has been removed from our Leggo's pasta sauce range as a direct result of [the Food and Health Dialogue] … " Source: Nutrition news section "reducing sodium for better health" dated 10 October 2016 (visited 11 May 2017)
Sunrice	Rice, snacks		
Thomas Foods International	Burgers, meatballs, sausages		
Unilever Australia *Bertoli, Continental, Flora*	Margarine, pasta, sauces, stock, soup	✓	Unilever reports their global progress, but also their progress by nation state. In Australia in 2016 68% of the foods in their portfolio met the salt levels they devised to reach the WHO 5 g per day target. Source: Performance against the USLP global nutrition targets in key countries report (2016)
Warrnambool Cheese & Butter	Cheese, butter		

Table Key: Obtained a tick (Reformulation concerning any salt/sodium nutrients; Reduced-salt product lines; Described participation in Food and Health Dialogue, Heart Foundation Tick program, the Healthy Food Partnership, Industry reformulation activities); Did not obtain a tick (Reformulation concerning other nutrients; No evidence of Australian product lines reducing salt/sodium).

Table 4. Priorities and actions publically reported by Australian foodmanufacturers—nutrition.

Company Name	Documentation of Nutrition as a Priority/Activity	Example Priorities or Actions
Arnotts	✓	"We welcomed the development of the Australian Food and Grocery Council's (AFGC) Responsible Children's Marketing Initiative and have pledged its commitment to marketing communications to children under 12 years of age only when it will further the goal of promoting healthy dietary choices and healthy lifestyles in accordance with the core principles set out below . . ." Source: "Our commitment" section of Arnott's website (visited 26 April 2017)
Baiada Poultry	✓	Steggles supplies products that are compliant with the Australian School Canteen association's nutrition bodies, which stipulate products must have: "1000 kJ of energy or less per 1000 g; 4 g or less of saturated fat per 100 g". Source: "Healthy Chicken for Kids" section of Steggles website (visited 22 May 2017)
Bega Cheese	✓	Manufactures cheese, a nutritious food consistent with the Australian Dietary Guidelines Source: Bega website (visited 7 April 2017)
Bellamy's Organic	✓	Bellamy's website hosts a blog from Paediatric Dietitian and Nutritionist Susie Burrell. The "Top Five Nutrients Your Toddler Needs" blog entry provides consumers information to increase healthy eating in children Source: Blog 12 September 2016, on Bellamy website (visited 28 February 2017)
Burra Foods	✓	Manufactures milk and other dairy products consistent with the Australian Guide to Healthy Eating Source: Burra website (visited 7 April 2017)
Cerebos	✓	Fountain "No Added Sugar" Tomato and BBQ Sauces were launched in 2013 and are sweetened using the natural sweetener, Natvia. Source: Personal communication, email (received 18 May 2017)
Coca-Cola Amatil	✓	"Why aren't Australians eating enough legumes? On average Australians eat 18.5 g of legumes, or a quarter of one serve, per week. But this average is deceptive because actually most people are not eating any legumes . . . " Source: SPC media release 6 August 2012, SPC website (visited 9 April 2017)
Cordina Chicken Farms	✓	Manufactures chicken breast, thigh and other minimally processed poultry products consistent with the Australian Guide to Healthy Eating Source: Cordina website (visited 7 April 2017)
Devondale Murray Goulburn	✓	Infographic on the benefits of dairy products Source: Dairy goodness section, Murray Goulburn website (visited 19 May 2017)
Freedom Foods Group	✓	Provides consumers with information on allergens and food composition in their products. In addition, sections on body mass index and weight management, nutrition and cardiovascular health and mental health. Source: "Your Health and Wellbeing" section, Freedom Foods website (visited 15 April 2017)
General Mills Holding (Australia)	✓	"Australia: Compliance with the Responsible Child Marketing Initiatives of the Australian Food and Grocery Council" Source: General Mills Global Responsibility 2017 report, p. 28
George Weston Foods	✓	"Helping consumers make healthy choices: GWF is a member of the GoScan program, which helps consumers access trusted product information from their mobile phone". Source: "Our quality promise", Corporate responsibility at GWF, website (visited 11 April 2017)
Goodman Fielder	✓	Wonder White bread products displayed online with information on their composition and associated nutrition claims. Source: "Health and Nutrition", Wonder White website (visited 18 April 2017)
Green's Foods	✓	Removed trans-fats in popcorn "Poppin" products Source: Personal communication (11 April 2017)

Table 4. *Cont.*

Company Name	Documentation of Nutrition as a Priority/Activity	Example Priorities or Actions
Heinz	✓	Heinz infant feeding advisory service. Source: Heinz for baby website (visited 4 May 2017)
Ingham's	✓	Manufactures chicken breast, thigh and other minimally processed poultry products consistent with the Australian Guide to Healthy Eating Source: Ingham website (visited 7 April 2017)
Kellogg Australia Holdings	✓	Kellogg's one of the first manufacturers to employ dietician and continues to employ and utilise this skill set. Source: Nutrition at its best, Kellogg's website (26 May 2017)
Mars	✓	"To help our consumers make informed choices, we've renovated our products and introduced more nutritional information. Now it's easier than ever to be aware and compare". Source: Mars "Making Chocolate Better Program", Mars chocolate website (11 April 2017)
McCain Foods	✓	"Healthy Choice" prepared meals product line Source: McCains website (visited 29 March 2017)
Mondelez Australia	✓	The "Call for Wellbeing" report includes their targets for increasing whole grain content, reducing portion sizes, reducing saturated fat content and displaying front of pack labelling, and progress against these targets Source: "The Call for Well-being" 2015 Progress report, available on Mondelez website (visited 11 April 2017)
Nestle	✓	Development of the "together counts" website to " … educate the community about the concept of energy balance, promoting healthy eating and physical activity..." Source: Media release "Food industry commits to reduce salt, saturated fat and energy", 10 October 2012
Norco Co-Op	✓	Manufactures milk, a nutritious food consistent with the Australian Dietary Guidelines Source: Norco website (visited 7 April 2017)
Parmalat Australia	✓	Manufactures milk, a nutritious food consistent with the Australian Dietary Guidelines Source: Parmalat website (visited 7 April 2017)
Patties Foods	✓	Patties pies display the voluntary front of pack labelling; the Health Star Rating system Source: Patties website (19 April 2017)
Pepsico Australia & New Zealand	✓	"With new nutritional goals informed by the latest guidelines from the World Health Organization and others, we plan to further reduce added sugar, sodium and saturated fat levels, while growing our "Everyday Nutrition" brands faster than the balance of our portfolio". Source: Pepsico Annual report 2016, p. 7
Sanitarium	✓	Manufactures breakfast cereals consistent with the Australian Dietary Guidelines Source: Sanitarium website (visited 7 May 2017)
San Remo	✓	Introduction of new product line—pulse pasta. "Pulse Pasta is 100% Lentils, Peas, Borlotti Beans and Chickpeas. Pulses are a good source of protein to keep you fuller for longer, rich in soluble fibre for digestion and some are also a great source of iron for plenty of energy to fuel your body. … it is also Gluten Free and Vegan friendly and you can use it just like normal pasta!" Source: San Remo website (visited 24 May 2017)
Scalzo Food Industries	✓	Manufactures nut-products, consistent with the Australian Dietary Guidelines Source: Scalzo website (visited 17 May 2017)

Table 4. *Cont.*

Company Name	Documentation of Nutrition as a Priority/Activity	Example Priorities or Actions
Simplot Australia	✓	"Simplot has taken the initiative to include the HSR icon on all Simplot branded food products available via retail outlets at your local supermarket". Source: Nutrition commitment section Simplot website (visited 25 May 2017)
Sunrice	✓	Consumer information on nutritional benefits of rice, dietary recommendations regarding serves of cereals and information on low-glycemic index foods Source: Sunrice website (visited 7 May 2017)
Thomas Foods International	✓	Manufactures meat products consistent with the Australian Dietary Guidelines Source: Thomas Foods website (visited 7 May 2017)
Unilever Australia	✓	Unilever nutrition targets Source: Performance against the USLP global nutrition targets in key countries report 2016.
Warrnambool Cheese & Butter	✓	Manufactures cheese, a nutritious food consistent with the Australian Dietary Guidelines Source: WCB website (visited 7 April 2017)

Table Key: Obtained a tick (Reformulation concerning nutrients, not including sodium, such as fat, sugar, kilojoules, protein, fibre, vitamins, minerals; Development of healthier-product lines; Providing consumer nutrition information, including participation in the Health Star Rating; Producing a core food "healthy" product consistent with the Australian Dietary Guidelines; Marketing standards (i.e., advertising to children)); Did not obtain a tick (Food safety, quality assurance and allergen compliance; Reformulation concerning non-nutrient components (i.e., artificial colours/flavours, organic health claims); Manufactured only discretionary foods).

The environment was a common publically articulated priority by manufacturers in this sample. The Australian Packaging Covenant [43], and compliance with waste, water and pollution standards were often reported. So called "greenwashing" has been identified in food [44] and other companies but innovation to benefit the environment by the private sector also occurs. McCain foods, which reports no action on salt and provided limited evidence of nutrition policies, stipulates that they " ... regard compliance with the law as a minimum standard to be achieved. Our aim is to continuously improve our environmental performance ... " [45]. To deliver on this they describe measuring their current impacts, setting environmental targets for improvement and monitoring progress against these targets. This company and several others [46–53] are making contributions to planetary health (or at least report that they are) and this could be coupled with human health in order to increase manufacturer's action in line with the healthy eating agenda.

4. Implications

This study found Australia's food manufacturers, with few exceptions, do not appear to be making significant "positive (nutrition) changes" to their product portfolios, although half document at least some salt-reduction activities. In light of the increasing rates of hypertension [3] and population salt consumption [4], more could be done.

In terms of the policy ramifications, the Australian Government's Healthy Food Partnership has the opportunity to endorse the continuation of voluntary targets for food reformulation, set time frames, expand the included products and settings (retail, quick-service, and restaurants) and transparently monitor and report on progress. At this mid-point between the WHO Global Action Plan and the 2025 salt reduction target, there is significant opportunity for Australia to achieve what the UK Responsibility Deal and the Pan-Pacific Sodium Consortium have achieved. Introducing regulatory scaffolding around sodium reduction targets has been suggested as a proactive approach for the Australian government to adopt in order to increase participation in voluntary measures [54].

In the Australian political context, bi-partisan support for food reformulation measures that address public health concerns would be appropriate. With or without bi-partisan commitment, or government support, key stakeholders in the Australian food supply such as food manufacturers, distributors and retailers could proactively respond to international leadership and public health concerns. Some food manufacturing companies are already showing significant innovation and progress.

Similarly, direct engagement of public health organisations with industry on developing and delivering on triple-bottom line policies and priorities has merit. The potential for company directors to bear responsibility for the health effects of company products, such as occurred for producers of tobacco products, lead and asbestos, could benefit from engagement with public health experts.

Manufacturers' willingness to dedicate sections of their websites, reports and media content to environmental responsibility could provide a platform to support nutrition responsibility too. Significant research on the inter-linked challenges and opportunities for human and planet health via food production and consumption could be used, and relevant stakeholders across the food system could be engaged, to increase the health of the planet and people [42].

Study Limitations

This study only included publically available information relevant to salt and nutrition and when invited to provide further information, several company's declined stating it was commercially confidential and many did not reply at all. This means that highly relevant material demonstrating commitment to public health may not have been discoverable. Websites typically include current material and the search may not have located achievements or policies in the past that were relevant in the 2010–2017 period. The content analysis reported themes, however did not objectively assess the validity of claims made by companies. Green washing and corporate irresponsibility by food manufacturers has been identified elsewhere in the literature [42,44,55] and further research could reveal the extent to which this was or is occurring in the Australian food manufacturing sector. The findings should be interpreted with this in mind. Finally, whilst this is only a study of Australian food manufacturers, the method could be easily adopted elsewhere and findings are likely to be applicable considering the high levels of salt consumption from processed foods in contemporary world-wide food supply chains [56].

5. Conclusions

This study found Australia's food manufacturers, with few exceptions, do not appear to be making significant and comprehensive "positive (nutrition) changes" in relation to salt or healthier food products. More could be done to capitalise on current nutrition activities, mobilise manufacturers and support product reformulation to improve the nutrition profile of processed foods. The Healthy Food Partnership is yet to develop a high-level ambitious strategy and implementation plan to improve and accelerate reformulation progress by 2025 and beyond, in response to the significant and rising levels of diet-related diseases in Australia. Comprehensive salt reduction targets and independent monitoring, combined with strong leadership through the Partnership, increased investment and strategic oversight by the Australian government would help manufacturers to reformulate products and reduce population salt intake.

Acknowledgments: Thank you to Lyndal Bond and Maria Duggan and Rosemary Calder for reading this work and providing critical feedback. Thanks also to Jacqui Webster, Graham MacGregor and Rosemary Calder for assistance with the early concept.

Author Contributions: R.L. conceived and designed the study and was involved in all phases, including the principal authoring of the paper; T.N. performed the initial literature review, assisted in data collection and analysis and authoring the final paper; C.Y. provided strategic insight on the design, checked final included sample and assisted with the analysis and authoring the final paper.

Conflicts of Interest: The authors declare no conflict of interest. C.Y. has no conflicts of interest to declare however wishes to stipulate that the work and views in the paper are her own. All other authors declare no conflict of interest. The founding sponsors had no role in the design of the study; in the collection, analyses, or interpretation of data; in the writing of the manuscript, and in the decision to publish the results.

References

1. World Health Organization (WHO). *Global Action Plan for the Prevention and Control of Noncommunicable Diseases 2013–2020*; WHO: Geneva, Switzerland, 2012.
2. Ha, S.K. Dietary salt intake and hypertension. *Electrolyte Blood Press.* **2014**, *12*, 7–18. [CrossRef] [PubMed]
3. McNamara, K.; Knight, A.; Livingston, M.; Kypri, K.; Malo, J.; Roberts, L.; Stanley, S.; Grimes, C.; Bolam, B.; Gooey, M.; et al. *Targets and Indicators for Chronic Disease Prevention in Australia*; Australian Health Policy Collaboration Technical Paper No. 2015-08; AHPC: Melbourne, Australia, 2015; ISBN 978-0-9944893-0-2.
4. Santos, J.A.; Webster, J.; Land, M.-A.; Flood, V.; Chalmers, J.; Woodward, M.; Neal, B.; Petersen, K.S. Dietary salt intake in the Australian population. *Public Health Nutr.* **2017**, *20*, 1–8. [CrossRef] [PubMed]
5. Webster, J.; Trieu, K.; Dunford, E.; Nowson, C.; Jolly, K.A.; Greenland, R.; Reimers, J.; Bolam, B. Salt reduction in Australia: From advocacy to action. *Cardiovasc. Diagn. Ther.* **2015**, *5*, 207–218. [CrossRef] [PubMed]
6. VicHealth. *The State of Salt: The Case for Salt Reduction in Victoria Supporting Evidence Document*; The Victorian Health Promotion Foundation (VicHealth): Melbourne, Australia, 2015. Available online: https://www.vichealth.vic.gov.au/media-and-resources/publications/state-of-salt (accessed on 7 April 2017).
7. Cobiac, L.J.; Magnus, A.; Lim, S.; Barendregt, J.J.; Carter, R.; Vos, T. Which interventions offer best value for money in primary prevention of cardiovascular disease? *PLoS ONE* **2012**, *7*, e41842. [CrossRef] [PubMed]
8. Magnusson, R.; Reeve, B. "Steering" private regulation? A new strategy for reducing population salt intake in Australia. *Sydney Law Rev.* **2014**, *36*, 255–289.
9. Goodall, S.; Gallego, G.; Norman, R. *Scenario Modelling of Potential Health Benefits Subsequent to the Introduction of the Proposed Standard for Nutrition, Health and Related Claims*; Centre for Health Economics Research and Evaluation, University of Technology Sydney: Sydney, Australia, 2008; pp. 26–31.
10. Dötsch, M.; Busch, J.; Batenburg, M.; Liem, G.; Tareilus, E.; Mueller, R.; Meijer, G. Strategies to reduce sodium consumption: A food industry perspective. *Crit. Rev. Food Sci. Nutr.* **2009**, *49*, 841–851. [CrossRef] [PubMed]

11. Cobcroft, M.; Tikellis, K.; Busch, J. Salt reduction: A technical overview. *Food Aust.* **2008**, *60*, 83–86.
12. Jaenke, R.; Barzi, F.; McMahon, E.; Webster, J.; Brimblecombe, J. Consumer acceptance of reformulated food products: A systematic review and meta-analysis of salt-reduced foods. *Crit. Rev. Food Sci. Nutr.* **2016**, *57*, 3357–3372. [CrossRef] [PubMed]
13. Webster, J.; Trieu, K.; Dunford, E.; Hawkes, C. Target salt 2025: A global overview of national programs to encourage the food industry to reduce salt in foods. *Nutrients* **2014**, *6*, 3274–3287. [CrossRef] [PubMed]
14. Federation of Bakers. Why Does Bread Contain Salt? Available online: https://www.fob.uk.com/nutrition-and-health/bread-contain-salt/ (accessed on 23 March 2017).
15. Heinz. Is It True That There Is a Lot of Salt in Some Heinz Products? Available online: http://www.heinz.co.uk/FAQs (accessed on 22 March 2017).
16. Premier Foods. Encouraging Healthier Choices. Available online: http://www.premierfoods.co.uk/-responsibility/Encouraging-healthier-choices (accessed on 2 April 2017).
17. Brakes Group. Brakes Commitments to Health and Wellbeing—Salt. Available online: https://www.brake.co.uk/your-business/health-nutrition/healthier-eating (accessed on 1 June 2017).
18. Department of Health (UK). About the Public Health Responsibility Deal. Available online: https://responsibilitydeal.dh.gov.uk/about/ (accessed on 1 June 2017).
19. Consensus Action on Salt and Health (CASH). CASH Warns of Thousands of Unnecessary Deaths from Salt—And Urges Public Health England to Take Immediate Action. Available online: http://www.actiononsalt.org.uk/news/surveys/2017/SAW%202017/193773.html (accessed on 18 May 2017).
20. Cappuccio, F.; Capewell, S.; Lincoln, P.; McPherson, K. Policy options to reduce population salt intake. *BMJ* **2011**, *343*. [CrossRef] [PubMed]
21. Consensus Action on Salt and Health (CASH). Salt Reduction in the UK. Available online: http://www.actiononsalt.org.uk/UK%20Salt%20Reduction%20Programme/145617.html (accessed on 11 April 2017).
22. Elliott, T.; Trevena, H.; Sacks, G.; Dunford, E.; Martin, J.; Webster, J.; Swinburn, B.; Moodie, R.; Wilson, A.; Neal, B. A systematic interim assessment of the Australian Government's Food and Health Dialogue. *Med. J. Aust.* **2014**, *200*, 92–95. [CrossRef] [PubMed]
23. Trevena, H.; Dunford, E.; Neal, B.; Webster, J. The Australian Food and Health Dialogue—The implications of the sodium recommendation for pasta sauces. *Public Health Nutr.* **2014**, *17*, 1647–1653. [CrossRef] [PubMed]
24. Jones, A.; Magnusson, R.; Swinburn, B.; Webster, J.; Wood, A.; Sacks, G.; Neal, B. Designing a Healthy Food Partnership: Lessons from the Australian Food and Health Dialogue. *BMC Public Health* **2016**, *16*, 651. [CrossRef] [PubMed]
25. National Heart Foundation of Australia. *Report on the Evaluation of the Nine Food Categories for Which Reformulation Targets Were Set under the Food and Health Dialogue*; National Heart Foundation of Australia: Melbourne, Australia, 2016.
26. Australian Government Department of Health. Healthy Food Partnership. Available online: http://www.health.gov.au/internet/main/publishing.nsf/Content/-reformulation (accessed on 16 March 2017).
27. Kraak, V.I.; Swinburn, B.; Lawrence, M.; Harrison, P. An accountability framework to promote healthy food environments. *Public Health Nutr.* **2014**, *17*, 2467–2483. [CrossRef] [PubMed]
28. Access to Nutrition Foundation (ATNF). *Access to Nutrition—Global Index 2016*; ATNF: Utrecht, The Netherlands, 2016.
29. IBISWorld. *Australia's Top 100 Food and Drink Companies*; IBISWorld: Surry Hills, Australia, 2016.
30. Healthy Food Partnership Reformulation Working Group. Work Plan for Reformulation Working Group: October 2016–December 2017. Available online: http://www.health.gov.au/internet/main/publishing.nsf/Content/9BD46D97B65A6209CA257FAD00823957/$File/HFP%20Reformulation%20Working%20Group%20work%20plan.pdf (accessed on 23 March 2017).
31. Coca-Cola Amatil. Coca-Cola Amatil Website. Available online: https://www.ccamatil.com/ (accessed on 7 March 2017).
32. Mondelez International. The Call for Well-Being. 2015. Available online: http://www.mondelezinternational.com/~/media/MondelezCorporate/uploads/downloads/CFWB2014ProgressReport.pdf (accessed on 6 April 2017).
33. Unilever. Performance against the USLP Global Nutrition Targets in Key Countries 2016. Available online: https://www.unilever.com/Images/progress-2016-in-key-countries-final_tcm244-501118_en.pdf (accessed on 6 April 2017).

34. Nestle. Media Release: New Nestle Collaboration Seeks Alternatives to Salt. Available online: http://www.nestle.com.au/media/pressreleases/new-neslte-collaboration-seeks-alternatives-to-salt (accessed on 1 March 2017).
35. Mondelez International. Governance, Membership and Public Affairs Committee Charter. Available online: http://www.mondelezinternational.com/~/media/Mondelez-Corporate/uploads/downloads/7%20%20GovernancemembershipandPACcharter.pdf (accessed on 13 April 2017).
36. Tip Top. Tip Top Website. Available online: http://www.tiptop.com.au/ (accessed on 17 April 2017).
37. Mars. Mars Responsible Marketing Code. Available online: http://www.mars.com/global/-about-us/policies-and-practices/marketing-code (accessed on 22 March 2017).
38. Simplot Australia. Simplot Australia Website. Available online: https://www.simplot.com.au/ (accessed on 10 April 2017).
39. Arnotts. Arnotts Website. Available online: http://www.arnotts.com.au/ (accessed on 21 March 2017).
40. Nestle. Nestle Website. Available online: http://www.nestle.com.au/ (accessed on 11 April 2017).
41. George Weston Foods. George Weston Foods Website. Available online: http://www.georgewestonfoods.com.au (accessed on 27 April 2017).
42. Lang, T.; Heasman, M. *Food Wars: The Global Battle for Mouths, Minds and Markets*; Routledge: Abingdo, UK, 2015.
43. Australian Packaging Covenant. *A Commitment by Governments and Industry to the Sustainable Design, Use and Recovery of Packaging*; Australian Packaging Covenant: Sydney, Australia, 2010. Available online: http://www.packagingcovenant.org.au/data/Resources/Aust_Packaging_Covenant_amended_10_October_2011.pdf (accessed on 9 May 2017).
44. Bancerz, M. New CSR in the food system: Industry and non-traditional corporate food interests. *Can. Food Stud.* **2016**, *3*, 127–144. [CrossRef]
45. McCain Foods. Mccain Foods Website. Available online: http://mccain.com.au/ (accessed on 6 April 2017).
46. Burra Foods. Burra Foods Website. Available online: http://www.burrafoods.com.au/ (accessed on 6 April 2017).
47. Bega Cheese. Bega Website. Available online: http://www.begacheese.com.au/ (accessed on 4 April 2017).
48. Green's Foods. Green's Foods Website. Available online: http://www.greens.com.au/ (accessed on 21 March 2017).
49. Ingham's. Ingham's Website. Available online: http://inghams.com.au/ (accessed on 30 March 2017).
50. Norco. Norco Website. Available online: http://www.norco.com.au/ (accessed on 21 April 2017).
51. Patties Foods. Patties Foods Website. Available online: http://pattiesfoods.com.au/ (accessed on 27 April 2017).
52. San Remo. San remo Website. Available online: http://sanremo.com.au/ (accessed on 13 April 2017).
53. Thomas Foods International. Thomas Foods International Website. Available online: http://thomasfoods.com/ (accessed on 24 April 2017).
54. Magnusson, R.; Reeve, B. Food reformulation, responsive regulation, and "regulatory scaffolding": Strengthening performance of salt reduction programs in Australia and the United Kingdom. *Nutrients* **2015**, *7*, 5281–5308. [CrossRef] [PubMed]
55. Ban, Z. Delineating responsibility, decisions and compromises: A frame analysis of the fast food industry's online csr communication. *J. Appl. Commun. Res.* **2016**, *44*, 296–315. [CrossRef]
56. Trieu, K.; Neal, B.; Hawkes, C.; Dunford, E.; Campbell, N.; Rodriguez-Fernandez, R.; Legetic, B.; McLaren, L.; Barberio, A.; Webster, J. Salt reduction initiatives around the world—A systematic review of progress towards the global target. *PLoS ONE* **2015**, *10*. [CrossRef] [PubMed]

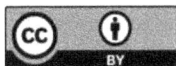

nutrients

MDPI

Article

Characterization of Breakfast Cereals Available in the Mexican Market: Sodium and Sugar Content

Claudia Nieto [1], Sofia Rincon-Gallardo Patiño [2], Lizbeth Tolentino-Mayo [1,*], Angela Carriedo [3] and Simón Barquera [1]

[1] Instituto Nacional de Salud Pública, Av. Universidad 655, Col. Santa María Ahuacatitlán, Cuernavaca C.P 62100, Morelos, Mexico; claudia.nieto@insp.mx (C.N.); sbarquera@insp.mx (S.B.)
[2] Virginia Tech, 223 Wallace Hall, Blacksburg, VA 24061, USA; sofiargp@vt.edu
[3] London School of Hygiene & Tropical Medicine, Keppel St, Bloomsbury, London WC1E 7HT, UK; angela.carriedo@lshtm.ac.uk
* Correspondence: mltolentino@insp.mx; Tel.: +52-5487-1000

Received: 9 June 2017; Accepted: 3 August 2017; Published: 16 August 2017

Abstract: Preschool Mexican children consume 7% of their total energy intake from processed breakfast cereals. This study characterized the nutritional quality and labelling (claims and Guideline Daily Amount (GDA)) of the packaged breakfast cereals available in the Mexican market. Photographs of all breakfast cereals available in the 9 main food retail chains in the country were taken. The nutrition quality of cereals was assessed using the United Kingdom Nutrient Profiling Model (UKNPM). Claims were classified using the International Network for Food and Obesity/non-communicable Diseases Research, Monitoring and Action Support (INFORMAS) taxonomy and the GDA was defined according to the Mexican regulation, NOM-051. Overall, a total of 371 different breakfast cereals were analysed. The nutritional profile showed that 68.7% were classified as "less healthy". GDAs and claims were displayed more frequently on the "less healthy" cereals. Breakfast cereals within the "less healthy" category had significantly higher content of energy, sugar and sodium ($p < 0.001$). Most of the claims were displayed in the "less healthy" cereals ($n = 313$). This study has shown that there is a lack of consistency between the labelling on the front of the pack and the nutritional quality of breakfast cereals.

Keywords: breakfast cereals; edible grain; nutrition labelling; claims

1. Introduction

The consumption of ultra-processed foods has become a common practice in the whole world [1–3], with this consumption pattern also occurring in Latin America and Mexico [3,4]. In Mexico, the second highest contribution to total energy intake has come from products that are high in saturated fat, added sugar and sodium [4]. A total of 58% of the calories consumed by Mexicans came from packaged foods and beverages [5]. Breakfast cereals, ready-to-eat cereals or sweetened cereals are considered ultra-processed food products with high amounts of energy, saturated fat, sugar and sodium [6–8]. Evidence suggests that an excessive intake of calories and added sugars from packaged food and sweetened beverages has contributed to the rapid growth of obesity worldwide [9]. The proportion of obese adults and children has increased in both developed and developing countries [10]. The latest Mexican National Health and Nutrition Survey states that the prevalence of being overweight and obese reached 72.5% in adults, while the combined prevalence is 33.2% for children [11].

In a similar way, consuming too much sodium contributes to a range of adverse health outcomes [12–14]. Excessive sodium intake is a dietary risk factor that contributes to hypertension, cardiovascular diseases and death [12–15]. In 2013, the World Health Organization Global Action Plan of for the Prevention and Control of Non-Communicable Diseases [16] set a target to reduce the mean population intake of sodium by 30%. Some studies [17–20] have reported that most processed foods have a high sodium content. Another study has suggested that one of the key actions to reduce the total population's salt intake is a 54% reduction in the sodium content of ready-to-eat breakfast cereals, along with other reductions, such reducing the sodium content in other processed foods, reducing sodium in foods consumed away from home, and reducing discretionary salt use. All of these changes would result in the achievement of the WHO sodium target [21].

One of the main dietary patterns for breakfast among Mexican children consists of cereal with milk; 6% of Mexican children exclusively consume ready-to-eat cereals with milk for breakfast [22]. The Mexican National Health and Nutrition Survey of 2012 indicates that between 42% and 49% of children aged <2 years consumed sweetened cereals [23]. Another study mentioned that the highest dietary energy contribution (33%) came from minimally processed cereals [24]. An observational study reported that 7% of the total energy intake of preschool Mexican children was from processed breakfast cereals [25]. Therefore, breakfast cereals substantially contribute to the daily energy and nutrient intakes of the Mexican population. An international survey estimated that Mexican breakfast cereals provided at least 600 mg sodium/100 g [26], which is 1.5 times the UK maximum target for breakfast cereals (the average target is 235 mg) [27]. Furthermore, whilst there is no recent nationally representative study, a 1998 study in a small sample of the normotensive population in the northern region of Mexico estimated the consumption of salt was 9.4 g [28]. A more recent study [29] in 2017 showed that 20% of the population adds salt to their meals. The same population was reported to add salt five days a week, twice a day. A contribution of 44% of the sodium consumed in the country came from breads, meats, pizzas, soups, sandwiches, cheese and snacks. A study conducted in healthy participants that evaluated 24-h urinary excretion reported that the sodium intake was higher than the WHO recommendations [30].

A systematic review concluded that consuming ready-to-eat cereals is associated with a higher sugar intake [31]. In an experimental study, high-sugar cereals were found to increase the total sugar consumption of children and decrease the nutrition quality of their breakfast [8]. Breakfast cereals have typically been marketed as healthy products. Nevertheless, it has been documented that such products feature nutritional or health claims, promotional characters and/or premium offers as a marketing strategy, which are frequently oriented towards children [32,33]. In Australia, breakfast cereals are among the food categories with the highest percentage of products (54%) carrying health or nutritional claims [34]. According to Dixon et al. [35], nutrient content claims and sports celebrity endorsements influence preferences towards energy-dense and nutrient-poor food products displaying these claims and endorsements.

Several strategies to tackle obesity have been recognized worldwide that aim to improve diets. The front of package labelling (FOPL) system for food products is a tool that informs consumers about the nutritional content of foods in an easy and simple way [36,37]. These systems are being regulated by governments as a public health strategy to influence the population into adopting healthier diets, such as Bolivia, Chile, Ecuador, United Kingdom, Mexico, New Zealand and Australia [38,39].

Context of Front of Package Labelling Regulation in Mexico

Before the FOPL became mandatory in 2014, the largest consortium of food manufacturers in Mexico decided to place a voluntary FOPL system called the GDA (Guideline Daily Amount) on packaged foods as a means of self-regulation. However, evidence has found that this type of FOPL system is not well understood by Mexican consumers [40,41]. Such labelling had reference values higher than the WHO recommendations on certain nutrients, including sugar and sodium. The current mandatory food labelling launched in 2014 is regulated by the Official Mexican Norm 051 [42], which provides manufacturers with the needed information to place the front of package labels on their food products. Other regulations have been implemented in Mexico since 1988. The Official Mexican Norm

086 [43] (NOM-086 by their initials in Spanish) regulates the presence of claims in the front of the package. Therefore, all nutritional declarations should be submitted to the NOM-086.

Given the significant contribution of breakfast cereals to the Mexican diet as well as the lack of strong policies for claims and food promotion, it is important to assess the quality of breakfast cereals and to identify current practices of package labelling. The aim of this study was to characterize the nutritional quality of breakfast cereals using the Nutrient Profiling Model of the United Kingdom (UKNPM) [44] and to characterize the labelling (use of claims and GDA) in such products.

2. Materials and Methods

2.1. Sampling

This is a cross-sectional study conducted in four different cities of Mexico from November 2013 until December 2014. Data were collected with photos of breakfast cereals (n = 434) taken from the eight main food retail chains in the country. A two-staged sampling design was used to select the stores from which to collect breakfast cereal data from in order to have a variety of food-retailer stores from different socio-economic areas in four cities in Mexico. The stores were mapped using a geo-reference system to determine the AGEB (Area Geoestadísticas Básicas-basic geo-statistical area) of these locations. AGEBs are delineated urban areas with 25,000 inhabitants or more, which are used to locate specific socio-demographic circumstances, such as living conditions, use of the land and so on. They are proxy estimations of the socio-demographic characteristics of areas in each city. The supermarkets in each AGEB were randomly selected to be proportional to the distribution of the three levels of marginalization defined by the National Institutes of Statistics and Geography on a scale of low, middle and high. To cover a broad sample of breakfast cereals, we included different retailers from urban areas of each city. Fieldworkers visited a total of 9 stores and in each store, photos were captured of every different cereal product on the shelf at the time of the visit. The sampling strategy for cereals was for convenience, but it allowed an extensive coverage of the stocked cereals in Mexico.

2.2. Ethical Approval

This study was evaluated and approved by the Research, Ethics and Biosafety Committees of the National Institute of Public Health of Mexico (ethical approval number: 1153). Before conducting the study, the research team asked for permission from the supermarket's manager to access the stores and take photos of available breakfast cereals in the country.

2.3. Data Collection

Data from all available breakfast cereals in the selected supermarkets were collected. Trained nutritionists took photographs of available cereals in supermarkets using a smartphone. Six photographs of each breakfast cereal were taken (front of package, back of package, GDA, price, nutrient content and promotion; if applicable). Duplicated products or products with missing data and illegible photographs were not analysed (n = 63). Therefore, we analysed the information of (n = 371) breakfast cereals. To create the variables, data were directly obtained from the photographs of the cereal package and transcribed to an excel spreadsheet. The personnel who captured the data followed a standardized operation procedure created by the researchers of the Mexican National Institute of Public Health. We included information, such as product name, brand, price, GDA, claims, serving size, nutrition content and location of the supermarket. The GDA was defined according to the Mexican regulation, NOM-051 [42], which states that a food product must display nutritional information on the front of the package. The nutrients of concern are those nutrients that may pose a substantial public health concern due to overconsumption. These include energy, saturated fat, sugar and sodium [45].

2.4. Nutrition Quality of Breakfast Cereals

Nutrient content was analysed per 100 g of each product. The analysed nutrients were energy (kcal), saturated fat (g), sugar (g), sodium (mg), fibre (g) and protein (g). The nutrition quality of cereals was assessed using the United Kingdom Nutrient Profiling Model (UKNPM) [44]. The model uses a simple scoring system where points are allocated based on the nutrient content of 100 g of a food or drink. Points are awarded for 'A' nutrients (energy, saturated fat, total sugar and sodium) and for 'C' nutrients (fruit, vegetables and nut content, fibre and protein). The score for 'C' nutrients is then subtracted from the score for 'A' nutrients to give the final nutrient profile score [44]. This model provides an assessment of the overall nutrition composition. Products with a score greater or equal than four were considered "less healthy", while a score less than four were considered "healthy" products. This categorization was used for the sample of breakfast cereals to categorize the quality of such products available for consumers in different areas of the country.

2.5. Claims

Claims are defined as any representation which states, suggests or implies that a food has particular characteristics relating to its origin, nutritional properties, nature, production, processing, composition and any other quality [46]. In order to categorize the claims, the exact text displayed in the front of the package of cereals was typed into the database. Claims were coded and classified using the International Network for Food and Obesity/non-communicable Diseases Research, Monitoring and Action Support (INFORMAS) taxonomy [47], which is shown in Table 1. Claims were divided into three main categories and their subcategories: (1) nutritional claims (health-related claim and nutrient claim); (2) health claims (general health claim, nutrient and other function claim as well as reduction of disease risk claim); and (3) other claims (environment-related claim and other health-related claims). A single food product could display several types of claims. The format of the claim was considered, including whether it was written text, numerical or symbolic. Products with a combination of numerical and written text formats within the same claim were coded as a numerical format.

Table 1. INFORMAS taxonomy about main categories and subcategories of claims [47].

Categories of Claim	Description	Subcategories and *Example*
Nutrition claims	Any representation which states, suggests or implies that a food has particular nutritional properties including but not limited to the energy value and to the content of protein, fat and carbohydrates as well as the content of vitamins and minerals.	Health-related claim *100% plant (goodness)* Nutrient claim *90 calories per serving*
Health claims	Any representation that states, suggests or implies that a relationship exists between a food or a constituent of that food and health	General health claim *Healthy eating* Nutrient and other function claim *Includes calcium, which helps build stronger teeth and bones* Reduction of disease risk claim *Lowers your blood pressure*
Other claims	Two sub claim categories have been created under the category 'other claims' to address claims that are not specifically related to nutrient or disease but are still heath related	Environment-related claim *Rainforest Alliance Certified* Other health-related claims *Genetically modified organism (GMOs)*

2.6. Statistical Analysis

Proportions, medians and standard deviations (SD) were used to summarize descriptive data for the nutritional content of the products. Nutrient values were standardized by the amount per 100 g of product. The prevalence ratio was calculated to find out how more likely is to find FOP labels and claims in less healthy products. Products were categorized into two categories: "healthy" and "less healthy". This categorization was based in the UKNPM. Mann–Whitney U Tests was used to compare nutritional content of the two categories as well as to make comparisons between the labelling of the packages (products carrying a claim and products without claims; in addition to products carrying a GDA and products without GDA). A Chi^2 test was used to assess differences between the UKNPM scores for individual nutrients. A p less than 0.05 was considered statistically significant. Data were analysed using the Statistical Package STATA (Version 12.0).

3. Results

A total of 371 breakfast cereals were analysed, which represented a total of 84 brands. The nutritional profile showed that 31.3% of the cereals were under the "healthy" classification, while 68.7% were classified as "less healthy". The average energy content in the sample of breakfast cereals was 374.4 ± 122.2 kcal. These cereals had on average 1 ± 1.7 g of saturated fat, 26.6 ± 14.1 g of sugar and 450 ± 225.5 mg of sodium.

GDAs in FOPL were displayed more frequently in "less healthy" cereals compared to "healthy cereals". From the sample, 23% of the GDAs were displayed on "healthy" cereals, while 77% were displayed on "less healthy" cereals. Similarly, the claims were displayed more frequently in "less healthy" cereals (68%). Table 2 displays the mean UKNPM score of the nutrients of interest (energy, saturated fat, sugar and sodium). Significant differences between "healthy" and "less healthy" cereals were found for energy ($p = 0.02$), sugar ($p < 0.001$) and sodium ($p < 0.001$).

Table 2. Comparison of the nutritional content of breakfast cereals available in the Mexican market ($n = 371$).

Nutrients	Healthy ($n = 116$) [†] Median (p25–p75)	Less Healthy ($n = 255$) [†] Median (p25–p75)	p Value
Energy (kcal/100 g)	362.7 (343–378.3)	380 (366.6–400)	<0.001
Saturated Fat (g)	1 (0.5–1.6)	0.8 (0–1.7)	0.81
Sugar (g)	16.6 (0.3–21.4)	30.6 (24.6–37)	<0.001
Sodium (mg)	148.3 (16.6–383.3)	473.3 (393.3–600)	<0.001
UKNPM Score	0 (0–2)	9 (6–13)	<0.001
Nutrients	Claims ($n = 282$) [§] Median (p25–p75)	No-Claims ($n = 89$) Median (p25–p75)	p Value
Energy (kcal/100 g)	373.3 (360–397.9)	376.6 (366.6–400)	0.02
Saturated Fat (g)	1 (0–1.7)	0.7 (0–1.6)	0.50
Sugar (g)	25.4 (17.5–33.3)	30 (16.6–34.5)	0.11
Sodium (mg)	446.6 (300–533)	450 (200–566)	0.92
UKNPM Score	6 (2–11)	8 (3–11)	0.056
Nutrients	GDA ($n = 228$) [*] Median (p25–p75)	No-GDA ($n = 143$) Median (p25–p75)	p Value
Energy (kcal/100 g)	370 (361.7–390)	388.8 (361.1–406)	<0.001
Saturated Fat (g)	1 (0.03–1.7)	1 (0–1.9)	0.21
Sugar (g)	29.6 (20–34.5)	23.2 (6.7–33.3)	0.004
Sodium (mg)	466.7 (366.7–570)	350 (83.3–466.7)	<0.001
UKNPM Score	8 (4–11.5)	5 (0–9)	<0.001

All values measured per 100 g per product; [†] "Healthy" and "less healthy" cereals were determined by the United Kingdom Nutrient Profiling Model; [§] We considered a claim according to the Codex Alimentarius definition; and [*] GDA: Guideline Daily Amounts.

Breakfast cereals under the "less healthy" category had a significantly higher content of energy, sugar and sodium ($p < 0.001$). In addition, the median number of calories in the "healthy" category was lower compared to the median number in "less healthy" cereals ($p < 0.001$). When comparing the nutritional content of cereals with claims and no-claims, there were significant differences in energy content ($p = 0.02$). For other nutrients, such as saturated fat, sugar and sodium, the nutritional content was almost the same with no significant differences. In Figure 1, "less healthy" cereals have mean scores of sugar (6.3) and sodium (4.9) that were almost double those for the "healthy" cereals.

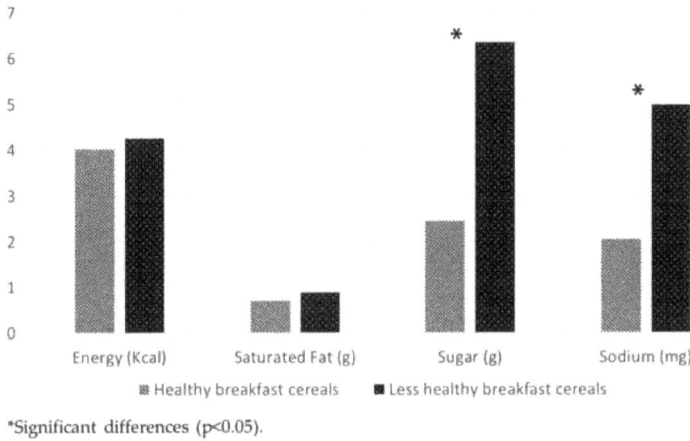

*Significant differences (p<0.05).

Figure 1. United Kingdom Nutrient Profiling Model scores of breakfast cereals in the Mexican market.

3.1. Labelling of the Breakfast Cereals (GDAs and Claims in the Front of Package Labelling)

Breakfast cereals with GDA in the FOPL are 1.4 times more likely to be classified as 'less healthy' in comparison to cereals with no GDA in the label (95% CI = 1.19–1.65). Cereals that displayed the GDA in the front of the package had a higher content of sugar ($p < 0.004$) and sodium ($p < 0.001$) as well as a higher UKNPM score ($p = 0.001$). However, cereals that displayed GDA had less calories ($p = 0.001$) compared to cereals that did not displayed any GDA (Table 2). Not all of the sample of breakfast cereals displayed the GDA system, with only ($n = 228$) breakfast cereals displaying the GDA on the front of the package. The "less healthy" category of cereals displayed the GDA more frequently ($n = 176, 77.2\%$), while healthy cereals displayed the GDA less frequently ($n = 52, 23\%$) (Table 3).

3.2. Displayed Claims on Breakfast Cereals

A total of 282 (76%) breakfast cereals displayed 587 claims, with an average of 2 claims per package. Furthermore, a single product could display up to 9 different claims on the front of the package. From the overall claims displayed in breakfast cereals, nutritional claims represented 86%, while health claims comprised 4% and other claims were on 10% (Table 3). We found that most of the nutritional content claims were commonly about antioxidants/vitamins/minerals (55%), followed by fibre (19%) and fats (10%). We found only two claims about sodium (1%). Claims about cholesterol (3.3%) and energy (1.4%) were mostly displayed on the "less healthy" cereals. The breakfast cereals categorized as "healthy" displayed health-related ingredient claims (22.7%), nutrient content claims (70.7%) and nutrient comparative claims (6.7%). However, none of the cereals under the healthy category displayed claims about having more calcium or more fibre in the package. We found a higher proportion of health-related ingredient claims and nutritional content claims on the "less healthy" category of cereals. For the "less healthy" cereals, 70.5% featured nutrient content claims, 25.9% featured health-related ingredient claims and 3.6% featured nutrient comparative claims. For the nutrient comparative claims, over 68% were made about antioxidants/vitamins/minerals (e.g., fortified with vitamins and minerals; as well as great source of iron). Most of the claims were presented in the written text format (71%), followed by numerical (26%) and symbolic (2%) types of claims. All the symbolic format of claims ($n = 14$) were displayed on the healthy category of cereals.

Table 3. Types and format of claims displayed in breakfast cereals (*n* = 586) [†,‡].

Type of Claim [§]	Total of Claims (*n* = 586) (%)	Displayed Claims in "Healthy Cereals" (*n* = 274) (%)	Displayed Claims in "Less Healthy Cereals" (*n* = 313) (%)
Nutrition claims (*n* = 503)	86	82.1	88.8
Health-related ingredient claim (*n* = 123)	24	22.7	25.9
Wholegrain (n = 54)	44	60.8	31.9
Fruits/nuts/honey (n = 15)	12	9.8	13.9
Grains/seeds (n = 26)	21	19.6	22.2
Cereals (n = 26)	21	5.9	31.9
Probiotics (n = 2)	2	3.9	0.0
Nutrient content claim (*n* = 355)	71	70.7	70.5
Fiber (n = 66)	19	27.0	11.7
Energy (n = 5)	1	0.0	2.6
Antioxidants/vitamins/minerals (n = 195)	55	39.0	67.9
Fats (n = 34)	10	8.2	10.7
Sugar (n = 11)	3	6.3	0.5
Calcium (n = 3)	1	1.9	0.0
Protein (n = 24)	7	13.8	1.0
Salt (n = 2)	1	1.3	0.0
Cholesterol (n = 12)	3	1.3	5.1
Omega 3 (n = 3)	1	1.3	0.5
Nutrient comparative claim (*n* = 25)	5	6.7	3.6
More calcium (n = 1)	4	0.0	10.0
Reduced sugar (n = 7)	28	13.3	50.0
More fiber (n = 3)	12	0.0	30.0
Splenda sweetened (n = 14)	56	86.7	10.0
Health claims (*n* = 23)	4	4.4	3.5
General health claim (*n* = 11)	48	33.3	63.6
General/healthy (n = 11)	100	100.0	100.0
Nutrient and other function claim (*n* = 7)	30	25.0	36.4
Calcium or Vitamin D for bone (n = 6)	86	100.0	75.0
Nutrient+digestion (n = 1)	14	0.0	25.0
Reduction of disease risk claim (*n* = 5)	22	41.7	0.0
Heart-related (n = 2)	40	40.0	0.0
Cholesterol absorption (n = 3)	60	60.0	0.0
Other claims (*n* = 61)	10.4	13.5	7.7
Other health related claim (*n* = 55)	90.2	83.8	100.0
Environment claim (*n* = 6)	9.8	16.2	0.0
Format of claim			
Numerical (*n* = 155)	26.4	26.6	26.2
Written text (*n* = 418)	71.2	68.2	73.8
Symbolic (*n* = 14)	2.4	5.1	0.0
GDA *		22.8	77.2

[†] Total (*n* = 371) cereals. [‡] each product could carry more than one claim. [§] We stratified the claims according to the INFORMAS taxonomy. * GDA: Guideline Daily Amounts.

4. Discussion

This cross-sectional study is the first study that explores the nutritional quality, labelling and different types of claims displayed on breakfast cereals in the Mexican market. Approximately 69% of the cereals in the Mexican market fall into the category of being "less healthy". However, this information is not easy to interpret on the food label and is frequently not available to consumers. Many "less healthy" cereals carried nutritional or health messages. Nevertheless, the nutritional content of breakfast cereals was significantly higher for the nutrients of concern, such as energy, sugar and sodium, compared to those cereals categorised as "healthy".

As national data revealed one of the most important breakfast food patterns includes the intake of ready to eat cereal with milk [22], overconsumption of cereals filled with nutrients of interest might represent a risk for obesity, diabetes, hypertension and cardiovascular diseases. The Nutrient Intake Recommendations for the Mexican population estimates that the breakfast intake for preschool children should be around 325 calories [48]. However, a single serving of 100 g of breakfast cereal contributes an average of 362.8 calories, which is higher than the breakfast recommendation.

Some studies have found that breakfast cereals contributed to nutritional requirements, which is explained by food fortification [49,50]. Nevertheless, some researchers consider ready-to-eat cereals as a discretionary food. In the dietary supplement of the Mexican National Health and Nutrition Survey of 2012, ready-to-eat cereals have been considered a high saturated fat and/or added sugar (HSFAS) product, herein referred to as discretionary foods that should be sparingly consumed because of their high caloric content and low concentration of essential nutrients [4,51]. Another study mentioned that ready-to-eat cereals, among other processed foods, significantly contribute to the mean intake of added sugar in the Mexican diet [52]. Despite the fact that breakfast cereals are fortified, Mexican dietary guidelines do not recommend the consumption of refined cereals due the excess of possibly dangerous nutrients, such as sugar and sodium [48,53].

A longitudinal cohort study suggested that the consumption of whole-grain breakfast cereals decreased the risk of hypertension in male adults [54]. However, this study did not evaluate the consumption of processed cereals with added sugar and sodium, which might increase the risk of obesity, hypertension and other cardiovascular diseases. Furthermore, the results of Figure 1 show that the "less healthy" cereals, which are the most widely available in the Mexican market, doubled the content of added sugar and sodium compared to "healthy cereals". The results of this study are consistent with two studies that showed that Mexican cereals are amongst the highest in sugar and sodium [26,55].

Our study revealed that there is a high content of added sodium in the Mexican national sample of breakfast cereals available in supermarkets (median 450 mg/100 g (SD 225.5 mg/100 g)) when using the cut-off points of the UK traffic light labelling system [56]. The United Kingdom's sodium target for 2017 is 235 mg/100 g [57]. Australia's target for cereals with more than 400 mg/100 g sodium is a reduction of 15% [58]. Current salt reduction strategies in Mexico are focused on reducing sodium in canned products and meats. Nevertheless, they have not considered the significant amount of sodium in breakfast cereals. Therefore, our results might urge the government to set sodium targets specifically for breakfast cereals.

In 2013, the prevalence of hypertension in Mexico reached 31.5% [59]. Therefore, the local government of Mexico City launched the campaign "Less salt, more health" to remove saltshakers from the tables of restaurants. By the end of the year, 5179 restaurants followed the campaign aiming to reduce sodium intake [60]. Additionally, the government should implement strategies to encourage the food industry to reduce sodium in processed foods.

Our study demonstrated that products displaying claims or GDAs on the front of the package do not necessarily reflect the nutritional quality of the product. Furthermore, such labelling could mislead consumers at the time of purchase. This is consistent with literature that indicates that labelling might confuse consumers when buying a product [33,41,61]. In Mexico, a single study revealed that the GDA format was found to be confusing even for dietitian students, who were unable to correctly read the labelling information on food products [40]. An understandable FOPL system such as the traffic light or a summary indicator might be an important strategy to help consumers when choosing healthier products with less dangerous nutrients [37–41].

Cereals that displayed a GDA tended to have higher content of possibly dangerous nutrients. This might be explained by the fact that, at the time we conducted our research (2013–2014), the presented GDA was the result of the industry's voluntary scheme, which used their own cut-off points. Moreover, the results of the study suggest that claims and GDAs on food packages might be used by food industries as marketing strategies to gain the attention of consumers. Some cereals (*n* = 143) did not have the GDA on the front of the package at the time of data collection, as the front of package labelling regulation had not yet been implemented by the government at that time (2013).

Since 2014, the Mexican government has introduced a mandatory FOPL strategy. The strategy consisted of placing the GDA on the front of the package. At this time, the cut-off points were established by the Ministry of Health (MoH) [62]. Despite great efforts to regulate the labelling in all food products, the cut-off points were not in line with the WHO recommendations. The cut-off points established by the MoH use 2 g of sodium as reference; moreover, they do not consider that the total intake of the population comes not only from processed foods that display labels; that non-processed foods also contribute to the sodium intake.

Claims do not reflect the healthiness of the products. This is consistent with two studies [7,63], which showed that cereals with nutritional claims did not have better nutritional profiles than cereals without these claims. It is important to mention that all the symbolic format of claims (*n* = 14) were displayed only on "healthy cereals" category. As most of the symbolic formats are logos endorsed by the "Association of Cardiology", this might mean that they are checking the nutritional content of their endorsed food products.

These data might suggest the need for stronger standards in the FOPL to enable consumers to identify healthy food products, using adequate cut-off points for nutrients of interest (energy, sugar and sodium). A higher proportion of nutritional claims displayed on "less healthy" breakfast cereals suggest that stricter regulations about food labelling are needed. Mexico has the national act, NOM 086 [43], which regulates any types of claims allowed in food products. Nevertheless, compliance with this regulation is not regularly monitored. This result is consistent with other studies [64,65]. Since advertising techniques on the front of the package of food products have heavily increased, this study can set the example for other Latin-American countries to assess their food products.

Limitations of the Study and Research Needs

This study was limited to data taken from the packaging of breakfast cereals, and does not evaluate individual consumption. Moreover, it is hard to prove the contribution of breakfast cereals to habitual nutritional intake [66,67]. It is known that individuals and populations do not consume isolated nutrients or foods as they eat combinations and food patterns determined by social, cultural and economic factors [9,22]. Another limitation of the current study was that researchers did not have the opportunity to assess the reliability of the personnel who collected the data. An interrater reliability test would have been ideal. Nevertheless, all fieldworkers were trained nutritionists, who collected the nutritional information from the packages of food products. We did not analyse the promotions and the use of characters in the package, although it is known that such factors influence the decision-making of consumers. There was possible bias when capturing the data from the photographs taken in the supermarkets. In order to decrease this possible bias, the research team established cut-off points of plausible values to eliminate outliers. Further research is needed to inform policy makers about the hazards of misleading claims, which might influence food selection and thus, could affect health. Further information is needed, as the world population is consuming higher amounts of processed foods. Research is also needed to evaluate the consumption of breakfast cereals and the nutritional quality of these cereals at the population level.

5. Conclusions

This study has shown that there is a lack of consistency between the labelling on the front of the pack and the nutritional quality of breakfast cereals. Mexico has taken the first steps by implementing a mandatory FOPL system for all processed foods. Nevertheless, the presence and use of a broader range of claims presents a new challenge. The current government should monitor the use of claims, set sodium targets on breakfast cereals and improve the current FOPL in addition to encouraging the food industry to follow the Mexican Regulations on labelling.

Acknowledgments: The authors would like to acknowledge PhD. Alejandra Moreno-Altamirano for providing insight for discussion and MSc. Amy Fuller for her English editing. The financial support of this study was founded by the International Development Research Centre (IDRC), and Bloomberg Philanthropies.

Author Contributions: C.N. suggested the research idea, did the bibliographical research, analysed data, interpreted the results, edited and wrote the manuscript. S.R.G. contributed to drafting the manuscript, analysing the data and interpreting the results. L.T.M. was the coordinator of the data collection, completed the bibliographical research as well as providing insight for methods, results and discussion. A.C. was involved with the methodology in addition to providing insight for methods, results and discussion. S.B. was responsible for the data acquisition and contributed to the writing of the manuscript. All authors read and approved the final version of the manuscript.

Conflicts of Interest: The authors declare no conflicts of interest. The founding sponsors had no role in the design of the study; in the collection, analyses, or interpretation of data; in the writing of the manuscript; and in the decision to publish the results.

References

1. Martínez Steele, E.; Baraldi, L.G.; da Louzada, M.L.C.; Moubarac, J.-C.; Mozaffarian, D.; Monteiro, C.A. Ultra-processed foods and added sugars in the US diet: Evidence from a nationally representative cross-sectional study. *BMJ Open* **2016**, *6*, e009892. [CrossRef] [PubMed]
2. Monteiro, C.A.; Cannon, G.; Moubarac, J.-C.; Martins, A.P.B.; Martins, C.A.; Garzillo, J.; Canella, D.S.; Baraldi, L.G.; Barciotte, M.; Louzada, M.L.; et al. Dietary guidelines to nourish humanity and the planet in the twenty-first century. A blueprint from Brazil. *Public Health Nutr.* **2015**, *18*, 2311–2322. [CrossRef] [PubMed]
3. Moubarac, J.-C. *Ultra-Processed Food and Drink Products in Latin America: Trends, Impact on Obesity, Policy Implications*; Pan American Health Organization World Health Organization: Washington, DC, USA, 2015; pp. 1–58.
4. Aburto, T.C.; Pedraza, L.S.; Sanchez-Pimienta, T.G.; Batis, C.; Rivera, J.A. Discretionary Foods Have a High Contribution and Fruit, Vegetables, and Legumes Have a Low Contribution to the Total Energy Intake of the Mexican Population. *J. Nutr.* **2016**, *146*, 1881S–1887S. [CrossRef] [PubMed]
5. Popkin, B.M. Nutrition, agriculture and the global food system in low and middle income countries. *Food Policy* **2014**, *47*, 91–96. [CrossRef] [PubMed]
6. Wiles, N.L. The nutritional quality of South African ready-to-eat breakfast cereals. *S. Afr. J. Clin. Nutr.* **2017**, *30*, 93–100. [CrossRef]
7. Schwartz, M.B.; Vartanian, L.R.; Wharton, C.M.; Brownell, K.D. Examining the Nutritional Quality of Breakfast Cereals Marketed to Children. *J. Am. Diet. Assoc.* **2008**, *108*, 702–705. [CrossRef] [PubMed]
8. Harris, J.L.; Schwartz, M.B.; Ustjanauskas, A.; Ohri-Vachaspati, P.; Brownell, K.D. Effects of serving high-sugar cereals on children's breakfast-eating behavior. *Pediatrics* **2011**, *127*, 71–76. [CrossRef] [PubMed]
9. Popkin, B.M.; Hawkes, C. Sweetening of the global diet, particularly beverages: Patterns, trends, and policy responses. *Lancet Diabetes Endocrinol.* **2016**, *4*, 174–186. [CrossRef]
10. Ng, M.; Fleming, T.; Robinson, M.; Thomson, B.; Graetz, N.; Margono, C.; Mullany, E.C.; Biryukov, S.; Abbafati, C.; Abera, S.F.; et al. Global, regional, and national prevalence of overweight and obesity in children and adults during 1980–2013: A systematic analysis for the Global Burden of Disease Study 2013. *Lancet* **2014**, *384*, 766–781. [CrossRef]
11. Hernández, M.; Rivera, J.; Shamah, T.; Cuevas, L.; Gómez, L.; Gaona, E.; Romero, M.; Méndez, I.; Saturno, P.; Villalpando, S.; et al. *Encuesta Nacional de Salud y Nutrición de Medio Camino 2016*; Instituto Nacional de Salud Pública: Cuernavaca, Mexico, 2016.
12. He, F.J.; MacGregor, G.A. Salt and sugar: Their effects on blood pressure. *Pflug. Arch. Eur. J. Physiol.* **2015**, *467*, 577–586. [CrossRef] [PubMed]
13. Mozaffarian, D.; Fahimi, S.; Singh, G.M.; Micha, R.; Khatibzadeh, S.; Engell, R.E.; Lim, S.; Danaei, G.; Ezzati, M.; Powles, J. Global Sodium Consumption and Death from Cardiovascular Causes. *N. Engl. J. Med.* **2014**, *371*, 624–634. [CrossRef] [PubMed]
14. Johnson, C.; Raj, T.S.; Trudeau, L.; Bacon, S.L.; Padwal, R.; Webster, J.; Campbell, N. The Science of Salt: A Systematic Review of Clinical Salt Studies 2013 to 2014 Search Strategy and Selection Criteria. *J. Clin. Hypertens* **2015**, *17*, 401–411. [CrossRef] [PubMed]
15. Watkins, D.A.; Olson, Z.D.; Verguet, S.; Nugent, R.A.; Jamison, D.T. Cardiovascular disease and impoverishment averted due to a salt reduction policy in South Africa: An extended cost-effectiveness analysis. *Health Policy Plan.* **2016**, *31*, 75–82. [CrossRef] [PubMed]
16. World Health Organization. Global Action Plan for the Prevention and Control of Noncommunicable Diseases 2013–2020. [Internet]. World Health Organization. 2013. Available online: http://apps.who.int/iris/bitstream/10665/94384/1/9789241506236_eng.pdf (accessed on 5 August 2017).
17. Peters, S.A.E.; Dunford, E.; Ware, L.J.; Harris, T.; Walker, A.; Wicks, M.; van Zyl, T.; Swanepoel, B.; Charlton, K.E.; Woodward, M.; et al. The sodium content of processed foods in South Africa during the introduction of mandatory sodium limits. *Nutrients* **2017**, *9*, 404. [CrossRef] [PubMed]
18. Allemandi, L.; Tiscornia, M.V.; Ponce, M.; Castronuovo, L.; Dunford, E.; Schoj, V. Sodium content in processed foods in Argentina: Compliance with the national law. *Cardiovasc Diagn Ther.* **2015**, *5*, 197–206. [PubMed]
19. Dos Kraemer, M.V.S.; de Oliveira, R.C.; Gonzalez-Chica, D.A.; da Proença, R.P.C. Sodium content on processed foods for snacks. *Public Health Nutr.* **2016**, *19*, 967–975. [CrossRef] [PubMed]

20. Martins, C.A.; de Sousa, A.A.; Veiros, M.B.; González-Chica, D.A.; da Proença, R.P.C. Sodium content and labelling of processed and ultra-processed food products marketed in Brazil. *Public Health Nutr.* **2015**, *18*, 1206–1214. [CrossRef] [PubMed]

21. Eyles, H.; Shields, E.; Webster, J.; Mhurchu, C.N. Achieving the WHO sodium target: Estimation of reductions required in the sodium content of packaged foods and other sources of dietary sodium. *Am. J. Clin. Nutr.* **2016**, *104*, 470–479. [CrossRef] [PubMed]

22. Afeiche, M.C.; Taillie, L.S.; Hopkins, S.; Eldridge, A.L.; Popkin, B.M. Breakfast Dietary Patterns among Mexican Children Are Related to Total-Day Diet Quality. *J. Nutr.* **2017**, *147*, 239780. [CrossRef] [PubMed]

23. Gutierrez, J.P. *Encuesta Nacional de Salud y Nutrición 2012 (ENSANUT. 2012)*; Instituto Nacional de Salud Pública: Cuernavaca, Mexico, 2012; pp. 1–200.

24. Rivera, J.A.; Pedraza, L.S.; Aburto, T.C.; Batis, C.; Sánchez-Pimienta, T.G.; González-Cossío, T.; López-Olmed, N.; Pedroza-Tobías, A. Overview of the Dietary Intakes of the Mexican Population: Results from the National Health. *J. Nutr.* **2016**, *146*, 1S–5S. [CrossRef] [PubMed]

25. González-Castell, D.; González-Cossío, T.; Barquera, S.; Rivera, J.A. Alimentos industrializados en la dieta de los preescolares mexicanos. *Salud Publica Mex.* **2007**, *49*, 345–356. [CrossRef] [PubMed]

26. World Action on Salt and Health. International Breakfast Cereal Survey [Internet]. 2016. Available online: http://www.worldactiononsalt.com/less/surveys/2016/190129.html (accessed on 5 August 2017).

27. Foods Standards Agency. Salt Targets. Available online: https://www.food.gov.uk/northern-ireland/nutritionni/salt-ni/salt-targets (accessed on 24 July 2017).

28. Ballesteros-Vásquez, M.; Cabrera-Pacheco, R.M.; Saucedo-Tamayo, M.; Grijalva-Haro, M.I. Consumo de fibra dietética, sodio, potasio y calcio y su relación con la presión arterial en hombres adultos normotensos. *Salud Publica Mex.* **1998**, *40*, 241–247. [CrossRef] [PubMed]

29. León-Estrada, S.; Pedroza, A.; Quezada, A.; Flores-Aldana, M.; Barquera, S. *Fuentes Dietéticas que Aportan Mayor Contenido de Sodio a la Dieta de los Adultos Mexicanos y Patrones Asociados: Análisis de la ENSANUT 2012*; Instituto Nacional de Salud Pública: Cuernavaca, Mexico, 2014; pp. 2–28.

30. Vallejo, M.; Colín-Ramírez, E.; Rivera, S.; Cartas Rosado, R.; Madero, M.; Infante Vázquez, O.; Varqas-Barrón, J. Assessment of Sodium and Potassium Intake by 24 h Urinary Excretion in a Healthy Mexican Cohort. *Arch. Med. Res.* **2017**, *48*, 195–202. [CrossRef] [PubMed]

31. Priebe, M.G.; McMonagle, J.R. Effects of Ready-to-Eat-Cereals on Key Nutritional and Health Outcomes: A Systematic Review. *PLoS ONE* **2016**, *11*, e0164931. [CrossRef] [PubMed]

32. Harris, J.; Schwartz, M.; Brownell, K.; Sarda, V.; Dembek, C.; Munsell, C. *Cereal FACTS 2012: Limited Progress in the Nutrition Quality and Marketing of Children's Cereals*; Yale Rudd Center Food Policy & Obesity: Hartford, CT, USA, 2012; 70p.

33. Soo, J.; Letona, P.; Chacon, V.; Barnoya, J.; Roberto, C.A. Nutritional quality and child-oriented marketing of breakfast cereals in Guatemala. *Int. J. Obes.* **2016**, *40*, 39–44. [CrossRef] [PubMed]

34. Williams, P.; Yeatman, H.; Ridges, L.; Houston, A.; Rafferty, J.; Ridqes, A.; Roesler, L.; Sobierajski, M.; Spratt, B. Nutrition function, health and related claims on packaged Australian food products—Prevalence and compliance with regulations. *Asia Pac. J. Clin. Nutr.* **2006**, *15*, 10–20. [PubMed]

35. Dixon, H.; Scully, M.; Niven, P.; Kelly, B.; Chapman, K.; Donovan, R.; Martin, J.; Baur, L.A.; Crawford, D.; Wakefield, M. Effects of nutrient content claims, sports celebrity endorsements and premium offers on pre-adolescent children's food preferences: Experimental research. *Pediatr Obes.* **2014**, *9*, e47–e57. [CrossRef] [PubMed]

36. Organisation for Economic Co-operation and Development (OECD). Promoting Sustainable Consumption: Good Practices in OECD Countries. *J. Urban Health Bull. N. Y. Acad. Med.* **2010**, *87*, 1–62.

37. Cecchini, M.; Warin, L. Impact of food labelling systems on food choices and eating behaviours: A systematic review and meta-analysis of randomized studies. *Obes. Rev.* **2016**, *17*, 201–210. [CrossRef] [PubMed]

38. Freire, W.B.; Waters, W.F.; Rivas-Mariño, G.; Nguyen, T.; Rivas, P.; Krug, E.G. A qualitative study of consumer perceptions and use of traffic light food labelling in Ecuador. *Public Health Nutr.* **2016**, *387*, 1–9. [CrossRef] [PubMed]

39. Corvalán, C.; Reyes, M.; Garmendia, M.L.; Uauy, R. Structural responses to the obesity and non-communicable diseases epidemic: The Chilean Law of Food Labeling and Advertising. *Obes. Rev.* **2013**, *14*, 79–87. [CrossRef] [PubMed]

40. Stern, D.; Tolentino, L.; Barquera, S. Revisión del etiquetado frontal: Análisis de las Guías Diarias de Alimentación (GDA) y su comprensión por estudiantes de nutrición en México. *Inst. Nac. Salud Publica* **2013**, *53*, 37.

41. Rincón-Gallardo, P.S.; Carriedo, A.; Tolentino-Mayo, L.; Allemandi, L.; Tiscornia, V.; Araneda, J.; Murillo, A. *Review of Current Labelling Regulations and Practices for Food and Beverage Targeting Children and Adolescents in Latin America Countries (Mexico, Chile, Costa Rica and Argentina) and Recommendations for Facilitating Consumer*; United Nations Children's Fund (UNICEF): Hong Kong, China, 2016.

42. Diario Oficial de la Federación. NORMA Oficial Mexicana NOM-051-SCFI/SSA1-2010. Especificaciones Generales de Etiquetado Para Alimentos y Bebidas no Alcohólicas Preenvasados-Información Comercial y Sanitaria. 2010. pp. 1–31. Available online: http://dof.gob.mx/nota_detalle.php?codigo=5137518&fecha=05/04/2010 (accessed on 5 August 2017).

43. Diario Oficial de la Federación. NORMA Oficial Mexicana NOM-086-SSA1-1994, Bienes y Servicios—Alimentos y Bebidas no Alcohólicas con Modificaciones en su Composición. Especificaciones Nutrimentales. 1996. Available online: http://www.salud.gob.mx/unidades/cdi/nom/086ssa14.html (accessed on 5 August 2017).

44. Rayner, M.; Scarborough, P.; Boxer, A.S.L. *Nutrient Profiles: Development of Final Model*; Food Standards Agency: London, UK, 2005.

45. U.S. Department of Agriculture. *Scientific Report of the 2015 Dietary Guidelines Advisory Committee. Advisory Report to the Secretary of Health and Human Services and the Secretary of Agriculture*; U.S. Department of Agriculture (USDA): Washington, DC, USA, 2015. [Internet]. Available online: http://health.gov/dietaryguidelines/2015-scien-tific-report/pdfs/scientific-report-of (accessed on 5 August 2017).

46. Codex Alimentarius Commission. *Guidelines for Use of Nutrition and Health Claims*; CAC/GL 23-1997; Codex Alimentarius Commission: Rome, Italy, 1997.

47. Rayner, M.; Wood, A.; Lawrence, M.; Mhurchu, C.N.; Albert, J.; Barquera, S.; Friel, S.; Hawkes, C.; Kelly, B.; Kumanyika, S.; et al. Monitoring the health-related labelling of foods and non-alcoholic beverages in retail settings. *Obes. Rev.* **2013**, *14*, 70–81. [CrossRef] [PubMed]

48. Academia Nacional de Medicina. Guías Alimentarias y de Actividad Física [Internet]. 2015. pp. 1–188. Available online: https://ods.od.nih.gov/pubs/2015_DGAC_Scientific_Report_ODS_Compiled_DS_Statements.pdf (accessed on 5 August 2017).

49. Rampersaud, G.C. Benefits of Breakfast for Children and Adolescents: Update and Recommendations for Practitioners. *Am. J. Lifestyle Med.* **2008**, *3*, 86–103. [CrossRef]

50. Michels, N.; De Henauw, S.; Breidenassel, C.; Censi, L.; Cuenca-Garcí, M.; Gonzalez-Gross, M.; Gottrand, F.; Hallstrom, L.; Kafatos, A.; Kersting, M.; et al. European adolescent ready-to-eat-cereal (RTEC) consumers have a healthier dietary intake and body composition compared with non-RTEC consumers. *Eur. J. Nutr.* **2015**, *54*, 653–664. [CrossRef] [PubMed]

51. Batis, C.; Rodríguez-Ramírez, S.; Ariza, A.C.; Rivera, J.A. Intakes of Energy and Discretionary Food in Mexico Are Associated with the Context of Eating: Mealtime, Activity, and Place. *J. Nutr.* **2016**, *146*, 1907S–1915S. [CrossRef] [PubMed]

52. Sánchez-Pimienta, T.; Batis, C.; Lutter, C.K.; Rivera, J.A. Sugar-Sweetened Beverages Are the Main Sources of Added Sugar Intake in the Mexican. *J. Nutr.* **2016**, *146*, 1888S–1896S. [CrossRef] [PubMed]

53. Perez-Escamilla, R. The Mexican Dietary and Physical Activity Guidelines: Moving Public Nutrition Forward in a Globalized World. *J. Nutr.* **2016**, *146*, 1924. [CrossRef] [PubMed]

54. Kochar, J.; Gaziano, J.M.; Djoussé, L. Breakfast cereals and risk of hypertension in the Physicians' Health Study I. *Clin Nutr.* **2012**, *31*, 89–92. [CrossRef] [PubMed]

55. Rincón-Gallardo Patiño, S.; Tolentino-Mayo, L.; Flores Monterrubio, E.A.; Harris, J.L.; Vandevijvere, S.; Rivera, J.A.; Barqera, S. Nutritional quality of foods and non-alcoholic beverages advertised on Mexican television according to three nutrient profile models. *BMC Public Health* **2016**, *16*, 733. [CrossRef] [PubMed]

56. FSA. Guide to Creating a Front of Pack (FoP) Nutrition Label for Pre-packed Products Sold through Retail Outlets. Food Stand Agency [Internet]. Available online: http://www.dh.gsi.gov.uk (accessed on 27 June 2013).

57. He, F.; Brinsden, H.; MacGregor, G. Salt reduction in the United Kingdom: A successful experiment in public health. *J. Hum. Hypertens.* **2014**, *28*, 345–352. [CrossRef] [PubMed]

58. Trevena, H.; Neal, B.; Dunford, E.; Wu, J.H.Y. An evaluation of the effects of the australian food and health dialogue targets on the sodium content of bread, Breakfast cereals and processed meats. *Nutrients* **2014**, *6*, 3802–3817. [CrossRef] [PubMed]

59. Campos-Nonato, I.; Hernández-Barrera, L.; Rojas-Martínez, R.; Pedroza-Tobías, A.; Medina-García, C.; Barquera, S. Hipertensión arterial: Prevalencia, diagnóstico oportuno, control y tendencias en adultos mexicanos. *Salud Publica Mex.* **2013**, *55*, 144–150. [CrossRef]

60. Boletin Menos Sal, Más Salud. [Internet]. 2013. Available online: http://www.salud.cdmx.gob.mx/campanas/menos-sal-mas-salud (accessed on 10 July 2017).

61. Wells, L.E.; Farley, H.; Armstrong, G.A. The importance of packaging design for own-label food brands. *Int. J. Retail. Distrib. Manag.* **2007**, *35*, 677–690. [CrossRef]

62. De Secretaría Salud, D.R. Estrategia Nacional Para la Prevención y el Control del Sobrepeso, la Obesidad y la Diabetes. Secr Salud [Internet]. 2013. p. 105. Available online: http://www.gob.mx/cms/uploads/attachment/file/40477/EstrategiaNacionalSobrepeso.pdf (accessed on 5 August 2017).

63. Maschkowski, G.; Hartmann, M.; Hoffmann, J. Health-related on-pack communication and nutritional value of ready-to-eat breakfast cereals evaluated against five nutrient profiling schemes. *BMC Public Health* **2014**, *14*, 1178. [CrossRef] [PubMed]

64. Schaefer, D.; Hooker, N.H.; Stanton, J.L. Are Front of Pack Claims Indicators of Nutrition Quality? Evidence from 2 Product Categories. *J. Food Sci.* **2016**, *81*, H223–H234. [CrossRef] [PubMed]

65. Al-Ani, H.H.; Devi, A.; Eyles, H.; Swinburn, B.; Vandevijvere, S. Nutrition and health claims on healthy and less-healthy packaged food products in New Zealand. *Br. J. Nutr.* **2016**, *116*, 1087–1094. [CrossRef] [PubMed]

66. Eyles, H.; Neal, B.; Jiang, Y.; Ni Mhurchu, C. Estimating population food and nutrient exposure: A comparison of store survey data with household panel food purchases. *Br. J. Nutr.* **2016**, *115*, 1835–1842. [CrossRef] [PubMed]

67. Potischman, N.; Freudenheim, J.L. Biomarkers of Nutritional Exposure and Nutritional Status Biomarkers of Nutritional Exposure and Nutritional Status: An Overview. *J. Nutr.* **2003**, 873–874.

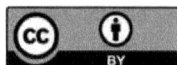

nutrients

MDPI

Review

Applying a Consumer Behavior Lens to Salt Reduction Initiatives

Áine Regan [1,*], Monique Potvin Kent [2], Monique M. Raats [3], Áine McConnon [4], Patrick Wall [1] and Lise Dubois [2]

[1] School of Public Health, Physiotherapy and Sports Science, University College Dublin, Dublin 4, Ireland; patrick.wall@ucd.ie
[2] School of Epidemiology and Public Health, Faculty of Medicine, 600 Peter Morand Crescent, University of Ottawa, Ottawa, ON K1G 5Z3, Canada; Monique.PotvinKent@uottawa.ca (M.P.K.); ldubois@uottawa.ca (L.D.)
[3] Food, Consumer Behaviour and Health Research Centre, University of Surrey, Guildford GU2 7XH, UK; m.raats@surrey.ac.uk
[4] Avila Research, Cabinteely, Dublin 18, Ireland; aine.mcconnon@gmail.com
* Correspondence: aine.regan@teagasc.ie; Tel.: +353-1-8059764

Received: 15 June 2017; Accepted: 16 August 2017; Published: 18 August 2017

Abstract: Reformulation of food products to reduce salt content has been a central strategy for achieving population level salt reduction. In this paper, we reflect on current reformulation strategies and consider how consumer behavior determines the ultimate success of these strategies. We consider the merits of adopting a 'health by stealth', silent approach to reformulation compared to implementing a communications strategy which draws on labeling initiatives in tandem with reformulation efforts. We end this paper by calling for a multi-actor approach which utilizes co-design, participatory tools to facilitate the involvement of all stakeholders, including, and especially, consumers, in making decisions around how best to achieve population-level salt reduction.

Keywords: consumer behavior; multi-actor; reformulation; salt reduction

1. Introduction

Across the globe, governments have adopted healthy eating strategies to reduce the incidence of diet-related non-communicable diseases [1]. The reduction of population-level salt intake has been singled out as a 'best buy' feasible and cost-effective public health initiative by the World Health Organisation (WHO). There is consistent evidence showing that reductions in population salt intake leads to reductions in blood pressure which subsequently lowers the risk for cardiovascular disease [2–4]. Debate over this relationship has been amplified through recent media reporting of conflicting science; however, the evidence in favor of salt reduction remains convincing (see Webster et al. 2017 for a comprehensive review on this topic). In 2013, WHO member states agreed on a global target of a 30% reduction in mean population intake of salt by 2025 [5]. Achieving this target will require a multi-actor approach combining many different elements and strategies.

As of 2014, 75 countries were identified as having national salt reduction strategies, representing a 50% increase from 2010 [3]. Of these strategies, 80% incorporated some element of food industry engagement, and reformulation of food products to reduce salt in particular was a common strategy [6]. Food reformulation has been identified as a key pillar for achieving population level salt reduction [7], particularly in industrialized countries where processed and restaurant foods are the largest contributor of total individual dietary sodium intake [6]. In contrast, reformulation efforts are not prioritized in countries such as China and Japan, where salt added during cooking/at the table is a larger contributor to sodium in the diet than processed foods [6]. For those countries engaging the food industry in salt reduction efforts, a voluntary and collaborative reformulation approach has been favored. This generally involves the publication of reduction benchmarks to guide food manufacturers in reducing levels of unhealthy target nutrients voluntarily. In some countries, reformulation efforts are accompanied by a coordinated monitoring and evaluation program, with the goal of holding the food industry accountable for achieving reformulation targets [8]. That said, an increasing number of countries are opting for legislative means to limit the salt levels in foods, for example, through mandating maximum levels of sodium content in specific foods, taxing high-sodium products and mandatory food labeling schemes [3]. Modeling studies suggest that legislative measures are more effective than voluntary reformulation programs in reducing consumers' salt intake [9]. At the same time, there is evidence to suggest that the voluntary approach is also making progress. Across several countries with voluntary programs, significant reductions have been made in the salt content of commonly consumed foods [6]. For example, in the UK, a comparison between 2006 and 2011 showed a 7% reduction in the overall mean sodium content of foods measured [10]. Across government and industry, there has been relatively widespread stakeholder acceptance of reformulation as a feasible and cost-effective strategy for reducing population level salt intake.

With processed foods identified as contributing between 75–80% of total sodium intake in many industrialized countries, reformulation as a strategy to reduce population-level salt intake has resulted in part from a belief that consumers are unable to adequately monitor or change their own salt intake [11]. Indeed, recent research highlights that, while consumers are aware of high levels of salt content in processed food, they may still underestimate the extent of those salt levels [12]. By adopting a strategy of making changes to the environment as opposed to trying to change the behavior of the individual, reformulation attempts to overcome the well-acknowledged difficulty of achieving positive behavior change amongst consumers who are aware of the negative impact of salt on health, but who often fail to take action [13]. Reformulation strategies predominantly focus on changing the food environment rather than consumer behavior; in this paper, we argue that understanding and accounting for consumer behavior remains central to the success of reformulation strategies and salt reduction initiatives more broadly. We also argue the merits of having consumers more centrally involved in designing and implementing salt reduction initiatives to ensure that factors which shape consumer behavior are identified and addressed from the outset.

2. Accounting for Consumer Behavior in Salt Reduction Initiatives

Even though a salt reduction initiative such as reformulation is not primarily focused on changing consumer behavior, consumer behavior still has an important role in determining the ultimate success of that initiative. Whether a consumer decides to accept or reject a reformulated product will ultimately determine the success of reformulation strategies. Significant attention within the area of reformulation has been given to the technical food science and technology developments required to reformulate foods and to the regulations which need to be considered [14]. Reformulation efforts are heavily underpinned by an evidence base of food and sensory science research to ensure the technical quality and safety of the reformulated products [15]. However, without consumer acceptance, these efforts are futile. In the following section, we consider how reformulation strategies can be impacted by consumer behavior and what we can learn from this to ensure the future success of salt reduction initiatives.

A key challenge for reformulation efforts is determining the best strategy to introduce reformulated products onto the market; anticipating how consumers will react to reformulated foods is critical to this issue. Some argue that foods should be reformulated gradually without making the consumer aware of such activity, adopting the argument that population taste will adjust in line with this gradual reformulation effort [15]. To be successful in shifting population tastes and maintaining consumer acceptance, a principle of progressive, incremental change is usually followed. There is consistent evidence to suggest that preference for dietary salt can be adapted following reduction in the salt content over a period of time [11,16]. This reduction can be achieved through modest, sequential reductions over a relatively short period of time, even as little as six weeks [17]. Often, industry stakeholders prefer to make these changes without informing consumers, a strategy commonly referred to as 'health by stealth' [13]. Reformulation of a product is not actively promoted in the belief that this will prevent consumers from rejecting products based on the perceived attributes of the product (e.g., perceiving that a reformulated product is of reduced taste or lower quality) [1]. Food manufacturers are concerned that if consumers are made aware that a product has been reformulated to include less salt, they may assume that it will have inferior sensory properties because they psychologically associate 'low salt' with poor taste or quality.

The stealth approach is not without its challenges. Eventually, the food industry will reach a point at which 'stealth' reformulation will no longer be a viable option; on the one hand, technical challenges will be faced whereby further salt reduction could compromise the safety of the product and on the other hand, consumers will reach a threshold where they will begin to notice a sensory change in the product [13,18]. The latter in particular is a concern for the food industry. This was evident in relation to the highly-publicized 2011 Campbell's Select Harvest Soup range, where the company announced that they were going to renege on reformulation commitments and add salt back into their soup formulations in an effort to boost declining sales [15]. While further research in the area of sensory science and food technology can help to address these concerns to some extent, user-led research could also offer significant value to reformulation efforts [19]. For example, co-design approaches with consumers to decide what category of foods are acceptable to target for further reformulation could be of particular interest; for example, food with a currently healthy image may be more acceptable for reformulation than unhealthy foods [20]. Co-design approaches would help to elucidate the likely future success of further reformulation efforts as well as the preference amongst consumers for replacement ingredients and consumer acceptance of food technology processes used to replace sodium in foods. This is a particularly salient point as behavioral research has demonstrated consumer aversion towards perceived 'unnatural' technology processes and a demand for 'clean labels'—foods with minimal and natural ingredients lists [21].

To adjust and 'train' consumer palates for a low-salt diet, widespread buy-in from all members of the food industry is required such that widespread salt reduction efforts exist within similar-product categories and across different-product categories. For example, if only some food manufacturers reduce the amount of salt in, for example, bread, and other higher-salt content breads are still available on the market, then it will be difficult for consumers to adjust their sensory acceptance of low-salt bread [13]. However, even where salt reductions are made simultaneously across all products in a certain food category, this will still not be sufficient to achieve change. A whole-of-industry approach is required to ensure that consumers' overall diets are substantially lower in salt; reducing salt content in one category of foods will have little impact unless salt reductions occur across a sufficiently large number of different product categories [15,18]. If such a scenario is ever to be realized, consumer demand for a low-salt food value chain is necessary—product supply needs to align with consumer demand. For example, there is evidence to suggest that reducing salt in commercial food could simply lead to consumers adopting compensatory behavior and adding it back in through discretionary salt use at preparation and consumption [22]. In contrast, if efforts are made to encourage the consumer to seek a low-salt 'way of life', this would lead to more successful reformulation efforts: previous research has found that consumers who are motivated to reduce their own dietary salt intake are then more accepting of actual reductions in the salt content of food products [15]. Reformulation efforts need to be coupled with strategies to motivate and facilitate individual consumer behavior change.

There has been much attention focused on nudging consumers towards healthier food choices via food labeling [13]. In their audit of food labeling across five European countries, Hieke et al. [23] identified that 26% of the products sampled displayed a nutrition or health claim or a symbol identifying products as healthier options for consumers. Such claims and symbols play a key role in influencing consumers' perceptions and expectations not only about the product, but also about the manufacturer. Labels allow manufacturers to promote the positive nutritional characteristics of food products and to demonstrate to the consumer a commitment and willingness to be transparent in their reformulation efforts [24]. It is common for reformulation strategies to be carried out in tandem with front-of-pack (FOP) labeling, mandatory nutrition labeling, and/or social marketing campaigns to encourage consumer demand for healthier food products [25,26]. Although sensory attributes drive much of the food industry's approach to food reformulation, and undoubtedly are primary indicators of acceptability of a reformulated food product, food selection and consumption is also influenced by non-sensory factors such as an individual's health and dietary needs, social relationships and their general attitudes towards health and wellness [27]. Many food manufacturers have tapped into the increasing market demand for more healthful food products; product reformulation is viewed as giving them a competitive advantage as it allows them to market their products as healthier [25,26]. It has been reported that the turning point in the salt reduction campaign in the UK was when salt actually became a competitive marketing issue between companies [28].

Nutrition claims are the labels which bear most relevance for food reformulation efforts, as they allow food manufacturers to market their food products as healthier versions of the original product. Nutrition claims can take the form of a content claim that describes the level of the nutrient contained in the food or a comparative claim, where the label compares the nutrient levels and/or energy value of two or more similar foods [20]. It is these latter claims which make it explicit to the consumer that reformulation has taken place (e.g., '30% less sodium' or 'reduced salt'). The ability to promote their reformulation efforts via comparative claims may act as an incentive for food manufacturers to engage in reformulation—but it is not always straightforward. For example, Buttriss [21] relates the point that under European regulations, manufacturers must achieve at least a 30% reduction in salt to enable them to make comparative nutrition claims on product labeling, which is a substantial change and would significantly alter the product, potentially losing consumers—even those who are motivated to seek out low-salt products. Comparative claims can also give the impression to the consumer that the salt level of the product was much too high to begin with, calling into question the overall healthiness of the food product [29]. Indeed, the impact of comparative claims on consumers' perceptions and behaviors has been found to have undesirable effects: research shows that when exposed to products with 'reduced salt' labeling, consumers revealed immediate negative taste perceptions and engaged in compensatory salt use, adding additional salt to the meal [30]. Comparative claims, although a seemingly attractive option for marketing industry reformulation efforts, also may have unintended negative behavioral effects.

There is also a moral argument as to whether it is appropriate for inherently unhealthy foods to be labeled and marketed as 'low salt' or 'reduced salt'. Evidence suggests that such labels could lead to a halo effect whereby the consumer assumes the food to be, on the whole, a healthier choice than it actually is, in essence, allowing consumers to interpret such labels as a license to (over)indulge [31,32]. Rather than focusing on individual nutrient content, labeling which communicates at the level of the healthiness of the overall food through simplified nutrition labels and symbols on the front of the pack may be more desirable. Labeling systems which interpret the nutrient profile of the whole food have been implemented in different countries including the Dutch Choices logo, 'Pick the Tick' and the 'Health Star Rating' in Australia and New Zealand, and the American Heart Association's heart-check mark [33,34]. To be allowed to carry such health logos/labels, the food must have a nutrient composition which complies with criteria for maximum levels of different nutrients including saturated fat, sugar and sodium. In order to meet these criteria for processed foods and obtain a better overall nutrition profile, reformulation may be required, thus, these symbols can act as a motivator for industry to reformulate [35,36]. Warning labels can also act as an incentive for industry to reformulate; for example, New York City adopted a mandatory sodium warning label policy on restaurant menus whereby a warning symbol had to accompany a meal which had more than 2300 mg of sodium [37].

In choosing different labeling options to accompany reformulation strategies, assumptions are being made about how people view food and make decisions related to health. In particular, an assumption is being made about whether consumers consider healthfulness of food at the individual nutrient level (e.g., salt) or whether they make decisions based on the overall perceived healthiness of the product, bringing many different attributes to bear on their decision. It is vital to reflect on how consumers process labeling information and their preferred formats for receiving nutrition information. Evidence suggests that inconsistencies in labeling across a variety of different schemes can leave consumers confused about what particular figures or symbols represent, or the recommended daily intake for specific nutrients [38]. Having to compare food products which vary in their levels of unhealthy nutrients can also challenge consumers' information processing capabilities [39]. When it comes to making purchasing decisions, consumers tend to engage in heuristic information processing which involves 'skimming' the available information in a situation and using cues (prior experience, familiar brand) for quick judgments [40]. Interpreting food labeling is often viewed as difficult and time-consuming and it is often the case that consumers will only engage with food labeling information when there is a particular motivation to do so [41,42]. Labeling can act as a motivator and facilitator for some consumers to purchase healthier food products. It can also incentivize reformulation amongst food manufacturers. However, we cannot depend on consumers to pay attention to labeling in every situation; thus, it alone is not sufficient to supplement reformulation efforts. Both initiatives need to be coupled with wider policy incentives and supports, and importantly, there is a need to ensure that the views and voices of consumers are considered at each step of policy development.

3. Future Directions and Conclusions

Significant action has been taken to reduce population-level salt intake; however, the recommended global intake level of less than five grams of salt per day has not yet been achieved [29] and meeting the global target of a 30% reduction in mean population intake of salt by 2025 will require more action [5]. Reformulation has been identified as a key pillar for achieving these targets [7]. However, its potential impact should be contextualized. For example, a number of Asian countries have the highest global sodium intakes but the primary dietary source is not processed foods, rather salt added during cooking [43,44]; coupled with the size of the population in this region, to achieve a reduction in global salt intake, initiatives which reach beyond reformulation efforts will be necessary. At the same time, in industrialized countries, behavioral research shows that we cannot focus only on making changes to the food environment—we also need to account for how the consumer will adapt and react to those changes. In order to reach set targets, a multi-faceted approach towards salt reduction is recommended [6]. As laid out in this paper, this approach should be executed with careful consideration of how the consumer will respond and react to salt reduction initiatives. In the current paper, we have referred to relevant behavioral research to support the presented arguments; however, we have not carried out a systematic review of the literature. Therefore, our paper does not reflect the full breadth of work in this field and some relevant literature may not have been included. Future research would be well placed to undertake a systematic review of the available literature to further support, clarify or contest the arguments laid out in the current paper.

Reaching global salt reduction targets will require a multi-actor approach comprising of government, public health agencies, the food manufacturing industry, the restaurant and catering industry, scientists, health care professionals, and consumers working together [13]. Future research is needed to better understand the different viewpoints which drive the reformulation agenda and more broadly, the process through which salt reduction policies and strategies are developed [45,46]. In so doing, this will help to build a better understanding of the extent to which current strategies are being developed to meet the needs of consumers and whether more can be done to ensure that the voice of the consumer is being accounted for during the policy-making process. Greater engagement of consumers in policy development can help to build mutual trust and reflexivity. There has been much discussion on the introduction of healthy eating policies by governments. In the UK, the Responsibility Deal has generated debate over the appropriate role of government in encouraging food environment changes. Consumers may not be as receptive to public health initiatives as we might anticipate—concerns over restricted food choices and 'nanny-state' sentiments have been evident in the past [47,48]. A recent study with Irish consumers found that a large majority of the respondents were, at least in principle, supportive of reformulation strategies to reduce salt intake—however, as policies became more restrictive, support declined [45]. Including consumers in the design of initiatives could be a mechanism for ensuring that salt reduction strategies have consumer buy-in, whilst also ensuring fairness and transparency—key principles for good governance [49]. There is significant merit in considering how we can better involve the consumer at an earlier stage of policy development with regard to salt reduction strategies. Co-design and participatory approaches and tools can help to facilitate the involvement of all stakeholders, including, and especially, consumers, in the design and implementation of salt reduction strategies.

Through reformulation, significant reductions to the salt content of commonly-consumed foods have already taken place, although further reductions are required. However, reformulation alone will not suffice; ultimately, future success will require a concerted effort by all stakeholders along the value chain. There is a need to strengthen accountability structures so that key stakeholders shoulder an appropriate level of responsibility for taking action to reduce salt intake. The food industry needs to continue in their efforts to lower the salt content of food products and to adopt responsible and transparent labeling; consumers need to be encouraged to reduce their discretionary use of salt and to purchase products that are low in salt; policy-makers need to implement policies which target the range of determinants contributing to a high salt diet including individual and environmental factors; public health agencies and health care professionals need to continue their efforts in driving and supporting consumer behavior change. Actions by stakeholders across the value chain will need to be implemented at a regional and national level in a manner that is culturally appropriate and that seeks and anticipates the views and responses of the end user: the consumer.

Acknowledgments: This paper was written with the financial support of (1) the European Commission under the International Network on Early Childhood Health Development (INECHD) Marie Curie Research Exchange Programme (Project No. 247551) and (2) the Department of Agriculture, Food and the Marine in Ireland under the Food Institutional Research Measures programme (Project No.: 13 F 460).

Author Contributions: Á.R. drafted and led the writing of the manuscript. All authors commented on drafts of the manuscript and contributed to revisions of the manuscript.

Conflicts of Interest: The authors declare no conflict of interest.

References

1. Savio, S.; Mehta, K.; Udell, T.; Coveney, J. A survey of the reformulation of Australian child-oriented food products. *BMC Public Health* **2013**, *13*, 836. [CrossRef] [PubMed]
2. Charlton, K.E.; Webster, J.; Kowal, P. To legislate or not to legislate? A comparison of the UK and South African approaches to the development and implementation of salt reduction programs. *Nutrients* **2014**, *6*, 3672–3695. [CrossRef] [PubMed]
3. Trieu, K.; Neal, B.; Hawkes, C.; Dunford, E.; Campbell, N.; Rodriguez-Fernandez, R.; Legetic, B.; McLaren, L.; Barberio, A.; Webster, J. Salt reduction initatives around the world—A systematic review of progress towards the global target. *PLoS ONE* **2015**, *10*, e0130247. [CrossRef] [PubMed]
4. Webster, J.; Waqanivalu, T.; Arcand, J.; Trieu, K.; Cappuccio, F.P.; Appel, L.J.; Woodward, M.; Campbell, N.R.; McLean, R. Understanding the science that supports population-wide salt reduction programs. *J. Clin. Hypertens.* **2017**, *19*, 569–576. [CrossRef] [PubMed]
5. World Health Organisation. *Global Action Plan for the Prevention and Control of Noncommunicable Diseases 2013–2020*; World Health Organisation: Geneva, Switzerland, 2013.
6. Webster, J.; Trieu, K.; Dunford, E.; Hawkes, C. Target Salt 2025: A global overview of national programs to encourage the food industry to reduce salt in foods. *Nutrients* **2014**, *6*, 3274–3287. [CrossRef] [PubMed]
7. World Health Organisation. *Reducing Salt Intake in Populations: Report of a WHO Forum and Technical Meeting*; WHO: Geneva, Switzerland, 2007.
8. Arcand, J.; Mendoza, J.; Qi, Y.; Henson, S.; Lou, W.; L'Abbe, M.R. Results of a national survey examining canadians' concern, actions, barriers, and support for dietary sodium reduction interventions. *Can. J. Cardiol.* **2013**, *29*, 628–631. [CrossRef] [PubMed]

9.   Cobiac, L.J.; Vos, T.; Veerman, J.L. Cost-effectiveness of interventions to reduce dietary salt intake. *Heart* **2010**, *96*, 1920–1925. [CrossRef] [PubMed]

10. Eyles, H.; Webster, J.; Jebb, C.; Capelin, C.; Neal, B.; Mhurchu, C.N. Impact of the UK voluntary sodium reduction targets on the sodium content of processed foods from 2006 to 2011: Analysis of household consumer panel data. *Prev. Med.* **2013**, *57*, 555–560. [CrossRef] [PubMed]

11. Antunez, L.; Gimenez, A.; Ares, G. A consumer-based approach to salt reduction: Case study with bread. *Food Res. Int.* **2016**, *90*, 66–72. [CrossRef]

12. Grimes, C.A.; Kelley, S.; Stanley, S.; Bolam, B.; Webster, J.; Khokhar, D.; Nowson, C.A. Knowledge, attitudes and behaviours related to dietary salt among adults in the state of Victoria, Australia 2015. *BMC Public Health* **2017**, *17*, 532. [CrossRef] [PubMed]

13. Zandstra, E.H.; Lion, R.; Newson, R.S. Salt reduction: Moving from consumer awareness to action. *Food Qual. Prefer.* **2016**, *48*, 376–381. [CrossRef]

14. Grasso, S.; Brunton, N.P.; Lyng, J.G.; Lalor, F.; Monahan, F.J. Healthy processed meat products: Regulatory, reformulation and consumer challenges. *Trends Food Sci. Technol.* **2014**, *39*, 4–17. [CrossRef]

15. Bobowski, N.; Rendahl, A.; Vickers, Z. A longitudinal comparison of two salt reduction strategies: Acceptability of a low sodium food depends on the consumer. *Food Qual. Prefer.* **2015**, *40*, 270–278. [CrossRef]

16. Levings, J.L.; Cogswell, M.E.; Gunn, J.P. Are reductions in population sodium intake achievable? *Nutrients* **2014**, *6*, 4354–4361. [CrossRef] [PubMed]

17. National Heart Foundation of Australia. *Rapid Review of the Evidence: Effectiveness of Food Reformulation as a Strategy to Improve Population Health*; National Heart Foundation of Australia: West Melbourne, Australia, 2012.

18. Jaenke, R.; Barzi, F.; McMahon, E.; Webster, J.; Brimblecombe, J. Consumer acceptance of reformulated food products: A systematic review and meta-analysis of salt-reduced foods. *Crit. Rev. Food Sci. Nutr.* **2017**, *57*, 3357–3372. [CrossRef] [PubMed]

19. Khan, S.S.; Timotijevic, L.; Newton, R.; Coutinho, D.; Llerena, J.L.; Ortega, S.; Benighaus, L.; Hofmaier, C.; Xhaferri, Z.; de Boer, A. The framing of innovation among European research funding actors: Assessing the potential for 'responsible research and innovation' in the food and health domain. *Food Policy* **2014**, *62*, 78–87. [CrossRef]

20. Dean, M.; Lahteenmaki, L.; Shepherd, R. Getting balanced nutrition messages across nutrition communication: Consumer perceptions and predicting intentions. *Proc. Nutr. Soc.* **2011**, *70*, 19–25. [CrossRef] [PubMed]

21. Buttriss, J.L. Food reformulation: The challenges to the food industry. *Proc. Nutr. Soc.* **2012**, *72*, 61–69. [CrossRef] [PubMed]

22. De Kock, H.L.; Zandstra, E.H.; Sayed, N.; Wentzel-Viljoen, E. Liking, salt taste perception and use of table salt when consuming reduced-salt chicken stew in light of South Africa's new salt regulations. *Appetite* **2016**, *96*, 383–390. [CrossRef] [PubMed]

23. Hieke, S.; Kuljanic, N.; Pravst, I.; Miklavec, K.; Kaur, A.; Brown, K.A.; Egan, B.M.; Pfeifer, K.; Gracia, A.; Rayner, M. Prevalence of nutrition and health-related claims on pre-packaged foods: A five-country study in Europe. *Nutrients* **2016**, *8*, 137. [CrossRef] [PubMed]

24. Hodgkins, C.; Barnett, J.; Wasowicz-Kirylo, G.; Stysko-Kunkowska, M.; Gulcan, Y.; Kustepeli, Y.; Akgungor, S.; Chryssochoidis, G.; Fernández-Celemin, L.; genannt Bonsmann, S.S. Understanding how consumers categorise nutritional labels: A consumer derived typology for front-of-pack nutrition labelling. *Appetite* **2012**, *59*, 806–817. [CrossRef] [PubMed]

25. Williams, P.; McMahon, A.; Boustead, R. A case study of sodium reduction in breakfast cereals and the impact of the *Pick the Tick* food information program in Australia. *Health Promot. Int.* **2003**, *18*, 51–56. [CrossRef] [PubMed]

26. Young, L.; Swinburn, B. Impact of the *Pick the Tick* food information programme on the salt content of food in New Zealand. *Health Promot. Int.* **2002**, *17*, 13–19. [CrossRef] [PubMed]

27. Dickson-Spillmann, M.; Siegrist, M.; Keller, C. Development and validation of a short, consumer-oriented nutrition knowledge questionnaire. *Appetite* **2011**, *56*, 617–620. [CrossRef] [PubMed]

28. European Commission. *Working Paper on Product Reformulation and Portion Size*; European Commission: Brussels, Belgium, 2009.

29. Kloss, L.; Meyer, J.D.; Graeve, L.; Vetter, W. Sodium intake and its reduction by food reformulation in the European Union–A review. *NFS J.* **2015**, *1*, 9–19. [CrossRef]

30. Liem, G.; Miremadi, F.; Zandstra, E.H.; Keast, S.J. Health labelling can influence taste perception and use of table salt for reduced-sodium products. *Public Health Nutr.* **2012**, *15*, 2340–2347. [CrossRef] [PubMed]

31. Chandon, P. How package design and packaged-based marketing claims lead to overeating. *Appl. Econ. Perspect. Policy* **2013**, *35*, 7–31. [CrossRef]

32. Faulkner, G.P.; Pourshahidi, L.K.; Wallace, J.M.W.; Kerr, M.A.; McCaffrey, T.A.; Livingstone, M.B.E. Perceived 'healthiness' of foods can influence consumers' estimations of energy density and appropriate portion size. *Int. J. Obes.* **2014**, *38*, 106–112. [CrossRef] [PubMed]

33. Lobstein, T.; Davies, S. Defining and labelling 'healthy' and 'unhealthy' food. *Public Health Nutr.* **2008**, *12*, 331–340. [CrossRef] [PubMed]

34. Temme, E.H.M.; van der Voet, H.; Roodenburg, A.J.C.; Bulder, A.; van Donkersgoed, G.; van Klaveren, J. Impact of foods with health logo on saturated fat, sodium and sugar intake of young Dutch adults. *Public Health Nutr.* **2010**, *14*, 635–644. [CrossRef] [PubMed]

35. Traill, W.B.; Bech-Larsen, T.; Gennaro, L.; Koziol-Kozakowska, A.; Kuhn, S.; Wills, J. Reformulation for healthier food: A qualitative assessment of alternative approaches. In Proceedings of the 2012 AAEA/EAAE Food Environment Symposium, Boston, MA, USA, 30–31 May 2012.

36. Vyth, E.L.; Steenhuis, I.H.M.; Roodenburg, A.J.C.; Brug, J.; Seidell, J.C. Front-of-pack nutrition label stimulates healthier product development: A quantitative analysis. *Int. J. Behav. Nutr. Phys. Act.* **2010**, *7*, 65. [CrossRef] [PubMed]

37. Downs, S.; Bloem, M.; Graziose, M.M. Salt and the city: A preliminary examination of New York City's sodium warning labels. *FASEB J.* **2017**, *31*, 302.

38. Gilbert, P.A.; Heiser, G. Salt and health: The CASH and BPA perspective. *Nutr. Bull.* **2005**, *30*, 62–69. [CrossRef]

39. Traill, W.B. Economic perspectives on nutrition policy evaluation. *J. Agric. Econ.* **2012**, *63*, 505–527. [CrossRef]

40. Chaiken, S. Heuristic versus systematic information processing and the use of source versus message cues in persuasion. *J. Pers. Soc. Psychol.* **1980**, *39*, 752–766. [CrossRef]

41. Marotta, G.; Simeone, M.; Nazzaro, C. Product reformulation in the food system to improve food safety. Evaluation of policy interventions. *Appetite* **2014**, *74*, 107–115. [CrossRef] [PubMed]

42. Enwright, G.; Good, H.; Williams, N. Qualitative Research to Explore People's Use of Food Labelling Information. Prepared for the Social Science Research Unit, Food Standards Agency. 2010. Available online: http://www.food.gov.uk/multimedia/pdfs/qualilabelres.pdf (accessed on 4 May 2017).

43. Powles, J.; Fahimi, S.; Micha, R.; Khatibzadeh, S.; Shi, P.; Ezzati, M.; Engell, R.E.; Lim, S.S.; Danaei, G.; Mozaffarian, D. Global, regional and national sodium intakes in 1990 and 2010: A systematic analysis of 24 h urinary sodium excretion and dietary surveys worldwide. *BMJ Open* **2013**, *3*, e003733. [CrossRef] [PubMed]

44. Anderson, C.A.; Appel, L.J.; Okuda, N.; Brown, I.J.; Chan, Q.; Zhao, L.; Ueshima, H.; Kesteloot, H.; Miura, K.; Curb, J.D. Dietary sources of sodium in China, Japan, the United Kingdom, and the United States, women and men aged 40 to 59 years: The INTERMAP study. *J. Am. Diet. Assoc.* **2010**, *110*, 736–745. [CrossRef] [PubMed]

45. Kraak, V.I.; Swinburn, B.; Lawrence, M.; Harrison, P. A Q methodology study of stakeholders' views about accountability for promoting healthy food environments in England through the Responsibility Deal Food Network. *Food Policy* **2014**, *49*, 207–218. [CrossRef]

46. Regan, A.; Shan, L.; Wall, P.; McConnon, A. Perspectives of the public on reducing population salt intake in Ireland. *Public Health Nutr.* **2016**, *19*, 1327–1335. [CrossRef] [PubMed]

47. Patel, S.M.; Gunn, J.P.; Tong, X.; Cogswell, M.E. Consumer sentiment on actions reducing sodium in processed and restaurant foods, ConsumerStyles 2010. *Am. J. Prev. Med.* **2014**, *46*, 516–524. [CrossRef] [PubMed]

48. Reeve, B.; Magnusson, R. Food reformulation and the (neo)-liberal state: New strategies for strengthening voluntary salt reduction programs in the UK and USA. *Public Health* **2015**, *129*, 1061–1073. [CrossRef] [PubMed]

49. Graham, J.; Amos, B.; Plumptre, T. *Principles for Good Governance in the 21st Century, Policy Brief No. 15*; Institute of Governance: Ottawa, ON, Canada, 2003.

nutrients

MDPI

Article

Dietary Sources of High Sodium Intake in Turkey: SALTURK II

Yunus Erdem [1], Tekin Akpolat [2], Ülver Derici [3], Şule Şengül [4], Şehsuvar Ertürk [4], Şükrü Ulusoy [5], Bülent Altun [1] and Mustafa Arıcı [1,*]

[1] Department of Internal Medicine, Division of Nephrology, Hacettepe University Faculty of Medicine, Ankara 06230, Turkey; yerdem@hacettepe.edu.tr (Y.E.); baltun@hacettepe.edu.tr (B.A.)

[2] Department of Internal Medicine, Division of Nephrology, Istinye University Liv Hospital, Istanbul 34510, Turkey; tekinakpolat@yahoo.com

[3] Department of Internal Medicine, Division of Nephrology, Gazi University Faculty of Medicine, Ankara 06560, Turkey; ulver@gazi.edu.tr

[4] Department of Internal Medicine, Division of Nephrology, Ankara University Faculty of Medicine, Ankara 06100, Turkey; sule.sengul@medicine.ankara.edu.tr (Ş.Ş.); sehsuvarerturk@yahoo.com (Ş.E.)

[5] Department of Internal Medicine, Karadeniz Teknik University Faculty of Medicine, Trabzon 61080, Turkey; sulusoy2002@yahoo.com

* Correspondence: marici@hacettepe.edu.tr; Tel.: +90-31-2305-1710; Fax: +90-31-2311-3958

Received: 14 June 2017; Accepted: 16 August 2017; Published: 24 August 2017

Abstract: Previous research has shown daily salt intakes in Turkey to be far above the recommended limits. Knowing the sources of dietary salt could form a basis for preventive strategies aimed towards salt reduction. This study aimed to investigate dietary sources of salt in Turkey. A sub-group ($n = 657$) was selected from the PatenT2 study population, which represented the urban and rural areas of 4 major cities (Ankara, Istanbul, Izmir, and Konya). A questionnaire inquiring about sociodemographic characteristics, medical histories, detailed histories of diet, and salt consumption was completed. Participants were asked to collect a 24-h urine sample and to record their food intake (dietary recall) on the same day. Of 925 participants selected, 657 (71%) provided accurate 24-h urine collections, based on creatinine excretion data. The mean daily 24-h urinary sodium excretion was 252.0 ± 92.2 mmol/day, equal to daily salt intake of 14.8 ± 5.4 g. Of the 657 participants with accurate 24-h urine collections, 464 (70%) provided fully completed dietary recalls. Among these 464 participants, there was a significant difference between the 24-h urinary sodium excretion-based salt intake estimation (14.5 ± 5.1 g/day) and the dietary recall-based salt intake estimation (12.0 ± 7.0 g/day) ($p < 0.001$). On the other hand, a positive correlation was obtained between the dietary recall-based daily salt intake and 24-h urinary sodium excretion-based daily salt intake ($r = 0.277$, $p < 0.001$). Bread was the main source of salt (34%) followed by salt added during cooking and preparing food before serving (30%), salt from various processed foods (21%), and salt added at the table during food consumption (11%). Conclusively, this study confirmed a very high salt intake of the adult population in four major cities in Turkey. The present findings support the emerging salt reduction strategy in Turkey by promoting lower salt content in baked bread, and less salt use in habitual food preparation and during food consumption in the home.

Keywords: blood pressure; epidemiology; hypertension; salt intake; urinary sodium; dietary sodium

1. Introduction

The relationship between hypertension and dietary salt is well known, and has been documented in experimental, observational, and clinical studies [1–4]. It is also known that the amount of daily salt consumption is above the recommended limits in many countries [2,5]. Strategies focusing on decreasing dietary salt would decrease the prevalence of hypertension and the incidence of cardiovascular events [2,6]. In Finland and the United Kingdom, population-level reductions in salt intake have been associated with declines in rates of cardiovascular diseases [7,8]. A recent modelling study of preventable risk factors for coronary heart disease (CHD) in Turkey reported that dietary changes (i.e., less saturated fat, less salt and higher fruit/vegetable consumption) can make the greatest contribution in reducing the CHD burden, with salt reduction alone saving 17,000 lives/year and 28,000 lives/year by 2025 at salt intake levels of 10 g and 5 g per day, respectively [9]. In light of these data, determining the sources of dietary salt by examining eating habits of societies and raising awareness on this issue appear to be an important preventive measure for cardiovascular diseases. In developed countries, salt-restriction strategies are being established by revealing the main sources of dietary salt. Unfortunately, studies on the sources of dietary salt are limited in number in low- and middle-income countries with high burdens of hypertension and cardiovascular diseases. In Turkey, which is an upper-middle income country, cardiovascular risk is high and hypertension is prevalent. In a previous study, we showed that daily salt intake in Turkey was too high (18.01 g/day) [10]. The present study aimed to investigate dietary sources of such high salt consumption in Turkey, as knowing the sources of dietary salt will form the basis for preventive strategies aimed towards salt reduction.

2. Materials and Methods

This study was conducted on a sub-group selected from the population of the PatenT2 study [11] in 2012, which was representative of Turkey and conducted to determine the rates of prevalence, awareness, and control of hypertension in adults. The exclusion criteria for this study were as follows: being pregnant, using diuretics, fasting for the last 24 h before enrollment, and having cardiac failure, renal failure, chronic liver disease, or diabetes mellitus. The present study was designed to represent the adult population in the urban and rural areas of four major cities (Ankara, Istanbul, Izmir, and Konya). These four cities account for 1/3 of the country's population, have a population distribution across urban and rural areas similar to that of country, and have a variety of dietary habits.

Sociodemographic characteristics and medical histories of all participants, as well as detailed records and histories of diet (content and amount) and salt consumption, were recorded via a questionnaire and a detailed face-to-face interview. A 24-h urine sample was collected from all participants within the period of February–March 2012 for the analysis of sodium, potassium, urea, and creatinine levels. An explanatory leaflet, along with the necessary equipment, was given to all participants, and they were instructed carefully about the method of urine collection. Beginning from the first urine sample of the day (in the morning), urine was collected over 24 h and was transferred into the urine container. Participants were instructed to keep urine samples in a cool and dark place. At the end of the collection period, healthcare workers measured the urine volume. The urine samples were then placed into cooler bags (4 °C) (Igloo Products Corporation, Katy, TX, USA) and within 24 h, they were sent to the central laboratory, where analyses were performed immediately. Participants who had 24-h urinary creatinine excretion within the predetermined limits of 10–30 mg/kg [12] were included in the analysis. Daily salt intake was estimated based on calculation of 24-h urinary sodium excretion on the assumption that all sodium ingested was in the form of sodium chloride. Salt intake was calculated using the equation of 1 g salt = 17.1 mmol of sodium in 24-h urine.

Each participant was instructed to record his/her food intake in detail (dietary recall) on the day (any day in a week) that he/she collected the 24-h urine sample. On the next day, the interviewers, who were trained for this study, visited the participants' houses to collect the 24-h urine samples, checked the diet recalls, asked the participants to complete any omissions, and clarified any details as required. Thereafter, they questioned the participants about how many times and how much they eat a day; the amount of salt and tomato paste (which includes significant salt and is used in almost all home-made foods in Turkey) added during the meal preparation; and were also asked as to the household member preparing the meals. The accuracy of the forms tried to be achieved by a double check in the study. After the interviewers checked the forms, they marked some forms as inaccurate. Then, the researchers evaluated the dietary recall forms of the participants without knowing the interviewers' interpretation. The researchers controlled whether the forms were adequately completed or not and they also marked some forms as inaccurate. Then, in the final check, all forms marked as inaccurate by the interviewers or researchers were excluded from the analysis.

In order to determine the amount of salt added during food consumption, a pre-estimation method was derived by the researchers. In this estimation, 12 different saltshakers were used, and the number and size of holes of each saltshaker were measured. These saltshakers were given to 12 individuals, and they were asked to add a sprinkle of salt using their saltshakers as they always do while eating. The amount of salt sprinkled on from each saltshaker was then measured in grams. The average amount of salt was calculated and this was accepted as the amount of salt consumed when a participant adds salt once during the meal. All participants reported how many times they added salt to each meal and the amount of salt consumed was calculated according to these estimates. All participants were also asked to record how much bread they ate (number and size of slices) and the amount of salt consumed from bread was calculated according to the estimation by Akpolat et al. [13]. The amount (grams per serving) of food eaten was coded from the Food and Nutrition Photograph Catalog [14]. The group of each food item recorded in the dietary recall of the participants was identified and, accordingly, the salt content of each food was estimated in grams per 100 g of food using the United States Department of Agriculture National Nutrient Database [15].

2.1. Sample Size

In the sample size calculation, inclusion of 249 participants was found to be adequate, with the assumption that the precision of the amount of salt calculated from the amount of sodium estimated from 24-h urine samples was 1 g and that the estimated standard deviation was ± 8 with a two-sided 95% confidence interval at a significance level of 0.05. Since there was a difference between male and female participants in terms of eating habits, inclusion of 498 (2×249) participants was found to be adequate for two different clusters. Additionally, assuming a 30% loss related to the dietary recall assessment forms that were not fully completed, inclusion of 711 ($249 \times 2/0.7$) participants was found to be adequate in the present study.

2.2. Statistical Analysis

All statistical analyses were performed using the Predictive Analytics Software (PASW 18.00; SPSS Inc., Chicago, IL, USA). In the comparison of normally distributed numeric and categorical variables, Student's t-test and chi-square test were used, respectively. The correlation analysis for the relationship between the salt intake calculated by 24-h urinary sodium and the salt intake estimated by dietary recall was performed using Spearman's rho test. The Bland-Altman method was also used to assess the agreement between salt intake calculated from the dietary recall and 24-h urine measurement [16]. All tests were evaluated at 5% type-I error level to infer statistical significance.

3. Results

Among 925 participants enrolled, data from 657 participants who had 24-h urinary creatinine excretion within the predetermined limits were analyzed. Of the participants, 53.1% were female and 46.9% were male. Demographic and clinical characteristics of the participants are presented in Table 1. The amount of 24-h urinary sodium excretion was 252.0 ± 92.2 mmol/day. The corresponding mean daily salt intake was 14.8 ± 5.4 g/day with a significant difference between males and females (15.7 ± 5.5 g/day and 14.0 ± 5.2 g/day, respectively; $p < 0.001$). Daily salt intake was higher in those living in the rural areas ($n = 144$ (22%)) compared with those living in urban areas ($n = 513$ (78%)) (16.0 ± 5.5 g/day vs. 14.5 ± 5.4 g/day, $p = 0.001$). There were no significant differences between urban and rural areas in terms of age ($47.5 + 15.5$ years vs. $48.1 + 14.7$ years, $p = 0.799$), male/female ratio

(231/282 vs. 77/67, $p = 0.073$), and body mass index (BMI) (28.8 + 5.9 kg/m^2 vs. 29.2 + 5.3 kg/m^2, $p = 0.293$).

Table 1. Demographic and clinical characteristics of the 657 participants with accurate 24 h urine samples.

Variable	Male ($n = 308$)	Female ($n = 349$)	Total ($n = 657$)	p
Age, years, mean ± SD	48.7 ± 16.1	46.7 ± 14.6	47.6 ± 15.3	0.073
Age groups, years, n (%)				
18–35	75 (24.4)	90 (25.8)	165 (25.1)	0.308
36–64	187 (60.7)	221 (63.3)	408 (62.1)	
≥65	46 (14.9)	38 (10.9)	84 (12.8)	
BMI, kg/m^2, mean ± SD	27.9 ± 4.6	29.8 ± 6.5	28.9 ± 5.7	0.001
BMI groups, n (%)				
Normal weight (<24.9 kg/m^2)	84 (27.2)	102 (29.2)	186 (28.3)	<0.001
Overweight (25–29.9 kg/m^2)	125 (40.6)	92 (26.4)	217 (33.0)	
Obese (≥30 kg/m^2)	99 (32.1)	155 (44.4)	254 (38.7)	
Hypertension, n (%)				
Absent	184 (59.7)	218 (62.5)	402 (61.2)	0.475
Present	124 (40.3)	131 (37.5)	255 (38.8)	
BP, mmHg, mean ± SD				
Systolic BP	131.0 ± 19.5	123.2 ± 19.2	126.9 ± 19.7	<0.001
Diastolic BP	75.4 ± 11.5	72.1 ± 10.8	73.7 ± 11.2	<0.001
Laboratory parameters, mean ± SD				
24-h urinary sodium, mmol/day	267.4 ± 94.2	238.4 ± 88.3	252.0 ± 92.2	<0.001
Urinary creatinine, mg/day	1746.9 ± 486.2	1373.5 ± 407.3	1548.5 ± 483.1	<0.001

SD, standard deviation; BMI, body mass index; BP, blood pressure.

There were 464 (70.6%) participants with fully completed dietary assessment forms. These participants were compared with the remaining 193 participants who did not record their diet correctly regarding age, gender, and BMI. There was no significant differences between the groups in terms of gender and BMI. The mean age of the participants correctly recording their dietary recall was higher (49 ± 15 vs. 44 ± 16, $p = 0.001$).

The mean estimated daily salt intake according to the dietary recall data was 12.0 ± 7.0 g/day (Table 2). While the dietary recall-based salt intake was similar in males and females (11.9 ± 6.6 and 12.2 ± 7.3, respectively; $p = 0.950$), salt intake was higher in those living in the rural areas, compared with those living in the urban areas (14.5 ± 8.1 and 11.3 ± 6.4, respectively; $p = 0.001$).

Table 2. Salt intake in a subset of 464 participants with fully completed dietary assessment forms and a valid 24-h urine collection.

	Male ($n = 210$)	Female ($n = 254$)	Total ($n = 464$)
24-h urinary sodium, mmol/day	256.4 ± 85.6	237.0 ± 87.4	245.8 ± 87.0
Salt intake estimated from 24-h urinary sodium, g/day	15.1 ± 5.0	13.9 ± 5.1	14.5 ± 5.1
Salt intake estimated from dietary recall, g/day	11.9 ± 6.6	12.2 ± 7.3	12.0 ± 7.0

The absolute difference between the 24-h urinary sodium excretion-based salt intake estimation (14.5 ± 5.1 g/day) and the dietary recall-based salt intake estimation (12.0 ± 7.0 g/day) was about 2.5 g; the difference was statistically significant ($p < 0.001$). There was a positive correlation between the dietary recall-based salt intake estimation and the 24-h urinary sodium excretion-based salt intake estimation ($r = 0.277$, $p < 0.001$) in the participants with reliable dietary assessments, as well as both in males ($r = 0.238$, $p < 0.001$) and females ($r = 0.310$, $p < 0.001$) separately.

Evaluation of the sources of salt in dietary recall revealed that the majority of salt consumed was from bread (34%) and salt added during food preparation (30%) followed by processed foods (21%) and salt added during food consumption (11%) (Table 3, Figure 1). Food items belonging to processed foods are also presented in Table 3. There were significant differences both between males and females (4.6 + 4.0 g/day vs. 3.7 + 4.0 g/day, $p < 0.001$) and between urban and rural areas (3.5 + 2.9 g/day vs. 6.3 + 6.1 g/day, $p < 0.001$) in terms of the amount of salt intake from bread.

Table 3. Estimated dietary salt intake (g/day) and distribution of major food sources of salt.

Food Items	Estimated Salt Intake (g/Day, Mean ± SD)
Bread	4.1 ± 4.1
Salt added during cooking and preparing food before serving	3.6 ± 4.5
Salt from various processed foods	2.5 ± 2.5
	Distribution of processed foods (%)
Breakfast foods (cheese, olive, butter, eggs, etc.)	62%
Pickle	16%
Meat-poultry-fish and meat products	10%
Dried nuts and fruits	4%
Biscuits and crackers	3%
Others *	6%
	Estimated Salt Intake (g/day, Mean ± SD)
Salt added at the table during food consumption	1.4 ± 2.5
Foods that contain salt in nature (e.g., some vegetables, etc.)	0.5 ± 0.8

SD, standard deviation; * Frozen food products and ready-to-eat food products.

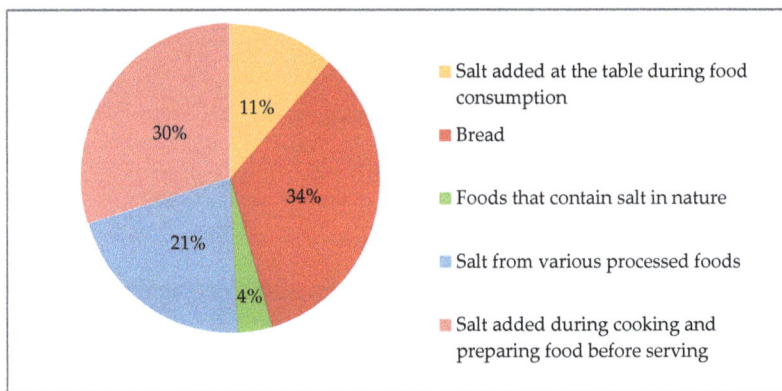

Figure 1. Sources of dietary salt.

The limits of agreement for the difference were calculated as −16.579 g/day to 11.750 g/day using the Bland-Altman method (Figure 2). The mean difference and its 95% confidence intervals were −2.414 g/day (Confidence interval: −3.060 g/day to −1.768 g/day).

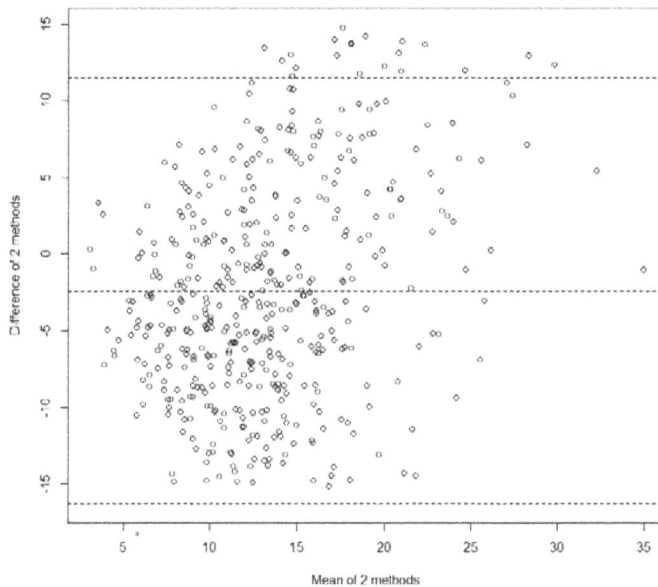

Figure 2. The Bland-Altman plot.

4. Discussion

It is already known that salt consumption is very high in Turkey. The present study determined once more that salt consumption was still high (14.8 salt g/day) even though it was lower than our finding of 18.0 g/day in 2007, reported in the previous study [10]. The present study also determined the sources of dietary salt in Turkey. It was found that bread was the main source (34%, 4.1 ± 4.1 g/day), followed by salt added during food preparation (30%, 3.6 ± 4.5 g/day), processed foods (21%, 2.5 ± 2.5 g/day), and salt added during food consumption (11%, 1.4 ± 2.5 g/day). The most striking point of this distribution is that salt intake was lower from processed foods, but higher from bread and traditional cooking style, compared to in developed countries [17,18].

Various methods can be used to determine the amount and sources of salt intake [19–22]. Collecting a 24-h urine sample is the gold standard method of determining the amount of salt intake for population surveys. The present study estimated the mean salt intake of the subgroup as 14.5 ± 5.1 g/day based on a single accurate 24-h urine collection. Dietary recall, which is used both to estimate the amount and to determine the sources of salt consumption, was also used in the present study and the salt consumption of the subgroup determined using dietary recall was 12.0 ± 7.0 g/day. However, there was a significant difference between daily salt intake estimated by the dietary recall and by the 24-h urinary sodium excretion ($p < 0.001$). This difference might be attributed to using a non-validated dietary recall questionnaire. However, the positive correlation obtained between the dietary recall-based salt intake estimation and the 24-h urinary sodium excretion-based salt intake estimation ($r = 0.277$, $p < 0.001$) in this study might suggest relative reliability of the data on the sources of salt determined based on the dietary recall. Some previous studies have also reported similar results [23]. Accordingly, the data of dietary recall assessments were used for the subgroup analysis of the food items in the present study.

Sources of dietary salt vary among countries. In the USA, nearly half (44%) of dietary sodium was obtained from 10 different categories of foods: bread and rolls, cold cuts/cured meats, pizza, poultry, soups, sandwiches, cheese, pasta mixed dishes, meat mixed dishes, and savory snacks [17]. A large-scale study from the USA evaluating 24-h diet in children, adolescents, and adults reported that approximately 1/3 of daily salt consumption was obtained from foods eaten outside the home; therefore, supermarkets, restaurants, and schools also had a role in reducing dietary salt [24]. In the present study, the main source of salt intake was bread (34%), followed by salt added during food preparation (30%) and salt intake from processed foods (21%). The main source of salt in South India was found to be salt added to the foods prepared with pulses, rice, vegetables, fruits, and milk and dairy products [25]. To our knowledge, data on sources of salt consumption from underdeveloped countries are limited.

In Turkey, bread (34%) was found to be the main source of dietary salt. In a review evaluating salt intake in Europe, bread contribution to total salt intake was reported as 25.9% in Ireland, 24.8% in Belgium, 24.2% in France, 19.1% in Spain, and 19% in the UK [26]. In another study from Portugal, the bread contribution to daily salt intake was reported to be 20–27% [27]. One potential reason for this difference may be the variance in the amount of salt in bread (502 mg/100 g bread in Spain, 708 mg/100 g bread in France, and 397 mg/100 g bread in the UK [26]) and the amount of bread consumed daily. According to a study by Akpolat et al. [13], the amount of salt (approximately 1800 mg) in 100 g bread and the daily average bread consumption (about 400 g/day/person) are very high in Turkey compared to other countries, for example, 186 g/day/person in Ireland, 129 g/day/person in Belgium, 137 g/day/person in France, 126 g/day/person in Spain, and 101 g/day/person in the UK [26]. Bread is the main source of dietary salt and it is suggested that a reduction in bread salt would have a significant impact on global health [28]. However, as salt is an important component of bread baking, salt reduction has some dimensions that could affect both producers and consumers, such as taste, volume, quality, and shelf-life [28]. Bread is a widely used nutritional element, particularly in middle-income countries. For this reason, the development of country-specific policies for reducing bread consumption and reducing salt in bread is necessary. Within this context, according to the regulations of the Republic of Turkey Ministry of Food, Agriculture and Livestock, the recommended salt content of bread in Turkey was changed in 2012 from 1.75 g/100 g bread to 1.5 g/100 g bread as part of a salt-reduction health initiative [29]. Even the food industry has not developed an action plan to reduce salt in bread; the government has planned to follow up this regulation, and has made attempts to inspect bread bakeries with respect to the amount of salt in bread. Although the average salt level of bread in the UK is lower than in Turkey, attempts to reduce the amount of salt in 100g of bread are ongoing; as a result, there was a reduction of approximately 20% between 2001 (1.23 ± 0.19 g/100 g) and 2011 (0.98 ± 0.13 g/100 g) in the UK [30]. Moreover, in the comprehensive overview of national initiatives for salt reduction by Webster et al. [31], attempts to reduce salt in bread were reported in many countries, such as a reduction by 26% in Spain between 2005 and 2009, a reduction by 18% in Ireland between 2003 and 2013, a reduction by 12% in France between 2008 and 2011, and a reduction by 6% in Belgium between 1990 and 2009. In the systematic review and meta-analysis by Jaenke et al. [32], the authors concluded that salt could be substantially reduced in bread, which was one of the highest contributors to population salt intake, without jeopardizing consumer acceptability.

The percentage of salt intake from processed foods (21%) was lower in the present study than for developed countries. Among the processed foods consumed in Turkey, foods for breakfast (62%), pickles (16%), and meat-poultry-fish and meat products (10%) were determined to be the main sources of salt. Frozen food products and prepared foods are not consumed widely in Turkey. However, consumption of frozen food products will increase with the increasing developmental level of the country, leading to an increased risk for future generations.

In various countries, ongoing efforts are being made to determine strategies and to develop nationally applicable models for popularizing salt restriction in order to reduce the amount of daily salt intake within the limits defined by the World Health Organization [33–35]. To achieve the intended goals, it would be necessary to know the current status of salt intake and the sources of salt depending on the eating habits of each population. For instance, data from the USA has revealed that the amount of salt intake from processed foods is very high (>80%); thus, what needs to be done in the USA is

Nutrients **2017**, *9*, 933

a reduction in salt in processed foods and in restaurants. Whereas in Turkey, reducing salt in bread and salt added in traditional cooking methods would be a more effective strategy for a nationwide salt reduction policy. Following the previous epidemiological study on salt consumption in Turkey [10], the Republic of Turkey Ministry of Health started a strategy program for salt reduction in 2011 [29,36]. In this action plan, firstly the salt contents of bread, pastrami, olives, cheese, and tomato paste were reduced. Secondly, saltshakers were removed from the tables of public cafeterias. Lastly, public service announcements were broadcast on television and regulations were developed for school canteens [36]. However, it has yet to be found whether government regulations are applied by the food industry and local bakeries. Moreover, there is a need to investigate the potential health impacts of this reduction at the population level. Currently, the Republic of Turkey Ministry of Health has announced the second term of the action plan covering the years 2017–2021. This plan has the aims for monitoring whether the salt content of bread and other food items have been reduced across the country. The health implications of salt reduction will also be evaluated during this action plan.

The strength of the present study was the inclusion of an adequate number of participants with accurate 24-h urinary samples and fully completed dietary recall assessment forms. However, collecting 24-h urinary sample and dietary recall data from the participants only once was the main limitation of the present study. Another limitation was not using a validated dietary recall questionnaire. We observed that the difference between the daily salt intake estimated by the dietary recall and estimated by the 24-h urinary sodium excretion was large, which was also a limitation of the present study. Thus, one should consider that the distribution of dietary salt sources presented is valid with the assumption of a non-selective discordance for the different sources of salt between the two measurements. Bearing this in mind, we still believe that this distribution at a minimum correctly describes the relative dominance of bread and added salt during food preparation as the commonly preferred sources. In further field studies, it would be beneficial to collect 24-h urinary samples more than once at different times, as well as to use a validated dietary recall questionnaire at the day 24-h urinary samples will be collected.

5. Conclusions

In conclusion, mean adult daily salt consumption is far above recommendations in Turkish cities, as it is in many regions of the world. Moreover, relatively high bread consumption and the corresponding high salt intake in Turkey were remarkable outcomes of the present study. Each country needs to plan and take strategical measures appropriate for their own eating habits. For this purpose, health authorities, legislators, and food producers should collaborate and develop models appropriate for their countries. The findings of this study of the main sources of dietary salt will help further developments of salt reduction strategies in Turkey.

Acknowledgments: The study was funded by the Turkish Society of Hypertension and Renal Diseases. The funding sponsor has no role in the design of the study; in the collection, analyses or interpretation of data; in the writing of the manuscript, or in the decision to publish the results. The field study, training, and control of the field healthcare workers, transportation of the samples to laboratory and data collection were carried out by OMEGA Contract Research Organization in Turkey. The epidemiologist Mutlu Hayran, MD, PhD, made a substantial contribution to the statistical analyses of the whole data set. The laboratory studies were carried out by Duzen Laboratories Group, Biological Sciences Research, Development and Production Inc. in Turkey.

Author Contributions: Y.E., T.A., S.U., B.A. and M.A. conceived and designed the study, drafted the first manuscript and provided final oversight; U.D., S.S. and S.E. analyzed and interpreted the data.

Conflicts of Interest: The authors declare that there are no conflicts of interest.

References

1. Altun, B.; Arici, M. Salt and blood pressure: Time to challenge. *Cardiology* **2006**, *105*, 9–16. [CrossRef] [PubMed]
2. World Health Organization. *WHO Guideline: Sodium Intakes for Adults and Children*; WHO Press: Geneva, Switzerland, 2012.
3. Chen, J.; Gu, D.; Huang, J.; Rao, D.C.; Jaquish, C.E.; Hixson, J.E.; Chen, C.S.; Chen, J.; Lu, F.; Hu, D.; et al. Metabolic syndrome and salt sensitivity of blood pressure in non-diabetic people in China: A dietary intervention study. *Lancet* **2009**, *373*, 829–835. [CrossRef]
4. Polonia, J.; Martins, L.; Pinto, F.; Nazare, J. Prevalence, awareness, treatment and control of hypertension and salt intake in Portugal: Changes over a decade. The PHYSA study. *J. Hypertens.* **2014**, *32*, 1211–1221. [CrossRef] [PubMed]
5. Brown, I.J.; Tzoulaki, I.; Candeias, V.; Elliott, P. Salt intakes around the world: Implications for public health. *Int. J. Epidemiol.* **2009**, *38*, 791–813. [CrossRef] [PubMed]
6. Martikainen, J.A.; Soini, E.J.; Laaksonen, D.E.; Niskanen, L. Health economic consequences of reducing salt intake and replacing saturated fat with polyunsaturated fat in the adult Finnish population: Estimates based on the FINRISK and FINDIET studies. *Eur. J. Clin. Nutr.* **2011**, *65*, 1148–1155. [CrossRef] [PubMed]
7. Tuomilehto, J.; Jousilahti, P.; Rastenyte, D.; Moltchanov, V.; Tanskanen, A.; Pietinen, P.; Nissinen, A. Urinary sodium excretion and cardiovascular mortality in Finland: A prospective study. *Lancet* **2001**, *357*, 848–851. [CrossRef]
8. He, F.J.; Pombo-Rodrigues, S.; Macgregor, G.A. Salt reduction in England from 2003 to 2011: Its relationship to blood pressure, stroke, and ischaemic heart disease mortality. *BMJ Open* **2014**, *4*, e004549. [CrossRef] [PubMed]
9. Sahan, C.; Sozmen, K.; Unal, B.; O'Flaherty, M.; Critchley, J. Potential benefits of healthy food and lifestyle policies for reducing coronary heart disease mortality in Turkish adults by 2025: A modelling study. *BMJ Open* **2016**, *6*, E011217. [CrossRef] [PubMed]
10. Erdem, Y.; Arici, M.; Altun, B.; Turgan, C.; Sindel, S.; Erbay, B.; Derici, U.; Karatan, O.; Hasanoglu, E.; Caglar, S. The relationship between hypertension and salt intake in Turkish population: SALTURK study. *Blood Press.* **2010**, *19*, 313–318. [CrossRef] [PubMed]
11. Sengul, S.; Akpolat, T.; Erdem, Y.; Derici, U.; Arici, M.; Sindel, S.; Karatan, O.; Turgan, C.; Hasanoglu, E.; Caglar, S.; et al. Changes in hypertension prevalence, awareness, treatment, and control rates in Turkey from 2003 to 2012. *J. Hypertens.* **2016**, *34*, 1208–1217. [CrossRef] [PubMed]
12. Arici, M. Clinical assessment of a patient with chronic kidney disease. In *Management of Chronic Kidney Disease*; Arici, M., Ed.; Springer: Berlin/Heidelberg, Germany, 2014; pp. 15–28.
13. Akpolat, T.; Kadi, R.; Utas, C. Hypertension, salt, and bread. *Am. J. Kidney Dis.* **2009**, *53*, 1103. [CrossRef] [PubMed]
14. Rakıcıoglu, N.; Tek, N.; Ayaz, A.; Pekcan, G. *Yemek ve Besin Fotoğraf Kataloğu. Ölçü ve Miktarlar*, 2nd ed.; Hacettepe Üniversitesi Sağlık Bilimleri Fakültesi Beslenme ve Diyetetik Bölümü: Ankara, Turkey, 2009.
15. United States Department of Agriculture Agricultural Research Service. USDA Food Composition Databases. Available online: https://ndb.nal.usda.gov/ndb/ (accessed on 9 June 2017).
16. Bland, J.M.; Altman, D.G. Statistical methods for assessing agreement between two methods of clinical measurement. *Lancet* **1986**, *1*, 307–310. [CrossRef]
17. Centers for Disease Control and Prevention (CDC). Vital signs: Food categories contributing the most to sodium consumption—United States, 2007–2008. *MMWR* **2012**, *61*, 92–98.
18. Fischer, P.W.; Vigneault, M.; Huang, R.; Arvaniti, K.; Roach, P. Sodium food sources in the Canadian diet. *Appl. Physiol. Nutr. Metab.* **2009**, *34*, 884–892. [CrossRef] [PubMed]
19. Zhang, L.; Zhao, F.; Zhang, P.; Gao, J.; Liu, C.; He, F.J.; Lin, C.P. A pilot study to validate a standardized one-week salt estimation method evaluating salt intake and its sources for family members in China. *Nutrients* **2015**, *7*, 751–763. [CrossRef] [PubMed]
20. Zhao, F.; Zhang, P.; Zhang, L.; Niu, W.; Gao, J.; Lu, L.; Liu, C.; Gao, X. Consumption and sources of dietary salt in family members in Beijing. *Nutrients* **2015**, *7*, 2719–2730. [CrossRef] [PubMed]
21. Rumpler, W.V.; Kramer, M.; Rhodes, D.G.; Moshfegh, A.J.; Paul, D.R. Identifying sources of reporting error using measured food intake. *Eur. J. Clin. Nutr.* **2008**, *62*, 544–552. [CrossRef] [PubMed]

22. Conway, J.M.; Ingwersen, L.A.; Moshfegh, A.J. Accuracy of dietary recall using the USDA five-step multiple-pass method in men: An observational validation study. *J. Am. Diet. Assoc.* **2004**, *104*, 595–603. [CrossRef] [PubMed]

23. Freedman, L.S.; Commins, J.M.; Moler, J.E.; Willett, W.; Tinker, L.F.; Subar, A.F.; Spiegelman, D.; Rhodes, D.; Potischman, N.; Neuhouser, M.L.; et al. Pooled results from 5 validation studies of dietary self-report instruments using recovery biomarkers for potassium and sodium intake. *Am. J. Epidemiol.* **2015**, *181*, 473–487. [CrossRef] [PubMed]

24. Drewnowski, A.; Rehm, C.D. Sodium intakes of US children and adults from foods and beverages by location of origin and by specific food source. *Nutrients* **2013**, *5*, 1840–1855. [CrossRef] [PubMed]

25. Ravi, S.; Bermudez, O.I.; Harivanzan, V.; Kenneth Chui, K.H.; Vasudevan, P.; Must, A.; Thanikachalam, S.; Thanikachalam, M. Sodium intake, blood pressure, and dietary sources of sodium in an adult South Indian population. *Ann. Glob. Health* **2016**, *82*, 234–242. [CrossRef] [PubMed]

26. Quilez, J.; Salas Salvado, J. Salt in bread in Europe: Potential benefits of reduction. *Nutr. Rev.* **2012**, *70*, 666–678. [CrossRef] [PubMed]

27. Polonia, J.J.; Magalhaes, M.T.; Senra, D.; Barbosa, L.; Silva, J.A.; Ribeiro, S.M. Association of 24-h urinary salt excretion with central haemodynamics and assessment of food categories contributing to salt consumption in Portuguese patients with hypertension. *Blood Press. Monit.* **2013**, *18*, 303–310. [CrossRef] [PubMed]

28. Belz, M.C.; Ryan, L.A.; Arendt, E.K. The impact of salt reduction in bread: A review. *Crit. Rev. Food Sci. Nutr.* **2012**, *52*, 514–524. [CrossRef] [PubMed]

29. Resmi Gazete. Gıda, Tarım ve Hayvancılık Bakanlığı. Türk Gıda Kodeksi Ekmek ve Ekmek Çeşitleri Tebliği. Tebliğ No: 2012/2. Sayı: 28163. Available online: http://www.resmigazete.gov.tr/eskiler/2012/01/20120104-6.htm (accessed on 9 June 2017).

30. Brinsden, H.C.; He, F.J.; Jenner, K.H.; Macgregor, G.A. Surveys of the salt content in UK bread: Progress made and further reductions possible. *BMJ Open* **2013**, *3*, E002936. [CrossRef] [PubMed]

31. Webster, J.; Trieu, K.; Dunford, E.; Hawkes, C. Target salt 2025: A global overview of national programs to encourage the food industry to reduce salt in foods. *Nutrients* **2014**, *6*, 3274–3287. [CrossRef] [PubMed]

32. Jaenke, R.; Barzi, F.; McMahon, E.; Webster, J.; Brimblecombe, J. Consumer acceptance of reformulated food products: A systematic review and meta-analysis of salt-reduced foods. *Crit. Rev. Food Sci. Nutr.* **2017**, *57*, 3357–3372. [CrossRef] [PubMed]

33. Eyles, H.; Shields, E.; Webster, J.; Ni Mhurchu, C. Achieving the WHO sodium target: Estimation of reductions required in the sodium content of packaged foods and other sources of dietary sodium. *Am. J. Clin. Nutr.* **2016**, *104*, 470–479. [CrossRef] [PubMed]

34. Newson, R.S.; Elmadfa, I.; Biro, G.; Cheng, Y.; Prakash, V.; Rust, P.; Barna, M.; Lion, R.; Meijer, G.W.; Neufingerl, N.; et al. Barriers for progress in salt reduction in the general population. An international study. *Appetite* **2013**, *71*, 22–31. [CrossRef] [PubMed]

35. Okuda, N.; Stamler, J.; Brown, I.J.; Ueshima, H.; Miura, K.; Okayama, A.; Saitoh, S.; Nakagawa, H.; Sakata, K.; Yoshita, K.; et al. Individual efforts to reduce salt intake in China, Japan, UK, USA: What did people achieve? The INTERMAP Population Study. *J. Hypertens.* **2014**, *32*, 2385–2392. [CrossRef] [PubMed]

36. T.C. Sağlık Bakanlığı Türkiye Halk Sağlığı Kurumu. Türkiye Aşırı Tuz Tüketiminin Azaltılması Programı 2017–2021. Ankara, August 2016. Available online: http://beslenme.gov.tr/content/files/Tuz/t_rkiye_a_r_tuz_t_ketiminin_azalt_lmas_program_2017-2021.pdf (accessed on 9 June 2017).

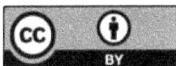

nutrients

MDPI

Article

Salt Use Behaviours of Ghanaians and South Africans: A Comparative Study of Knowledge, Attitudes and Practices

Elias Menyanu [1], Karen E. Charlton [1,2,*], Lisa J. Ware [3], Joanna Russell [4], Richard Biritwum [5] and Paul Kowal [6,7,8]

1   School of Medicine, Faculty of Science, Medicine and Health, University of Wollongong, Northfields Avenue, Wollongong, NSW 2522, Australia; ekm@uowmail.ed.au
2   Illawarra Health and Medical Research Institute, Wollongong, NSW 2522, Australia
3   Hypertension in Africa Research Team (HART), North-West University, Potchefstroom 2531, South Africa; lisa.jayne.ware@gmail.com
4   School of Health and Society, Faculty of Social Sciences, University of Wollongong, Northfields Avenue, Wollongong, NSW 2522, Australia; jrussell@uow.edu.au
5   Department of Community Health, University of Ghana, Accra, Ghana; biritwum@africaonline.com.gh
6   World Health Organization Study on global AGEing and adult health (SAGE), 1211 Geneva, Switzerland; kowalp@who.int
7   Research Centre for Generational Health and Ageing, University of Newcastle, Newcastle, NSW 2300, Australia
8   Department of Anthropology, University of Oregon, Eugene, OR 97403, USA
*   Correspondence: karenc@uow.edu.au; Tel.: +61-4221-4754

Received: 26 June 2017; Accepted: 23 August 2017; Published: 28 August 2017

Abstract: Salt consumption is high in Africa and the continent also shares the greatest burden of hypertension. This study examines salt-related knowledge, attitude and self-reported behaviours (KAB) amongst adults from two African countries—Ghana and South Africa—which have distributed different public health messages related to salt. KAB was assessed in the multinational longitudinal World Health Organisation (WHO) study on global AGEing and adult health (WHO-SAGE) Wave 2 (2014–2015). Respondents were randomly selected across both countries—Ghana ($n = 6746$; mean age 58 years old; SD 17; 41% men; 31% hypertensive) and South Africa ($n = 3776$, mean age 54 years old; SD 17; 32% men; 45% hypertensive). South Africans were more likely than Ghanaians to add salt to food at the table (OR 4.80, CI 4.071–5.611, $p < 0.001$) but less likely to add salt to food during cooking (OR 0.16, CI 0.130–0.197, $p < 0.001$). South Africans were also less likely to take action to control their salt intake (OR 0.436, CI 0.379–0.488, $p < 0.001$). Considering the various salt reduction initiatives of South Africa that have been largely absent in Ghana, this study supports additional efforts to raise consumer awareness on discretionary salt use and behaviour change in both countries.

Keywords: discretionary salt; dietary salt; sodium; health behaviour; blood pressure

1. Introduction

The Global Burden of Disease study has demonstrated that diet contributes significantly to risk of non-communicable diseases (NCDs) such as cancer, cardiovascular disease (CVD) and diabetes [1]. Dietary risk factors include diets low in fruits, vegetables, whole grains, nuts and seeds, fibre, omega-3 oils, and polyunsaturated fatty acids and diets that are high in sodium, red meat, processed meat, sweetened beverages, and trans fats [2–6]. The nutrition transition in many Sub-Saharan countries is resulting in a change in dietary patterns from traditional, plant-based diets to increasing intakes of processed foods that tend to be high in sugar and/or fat, known as energy dense, nutrient poor (EDNP) foods that are generally also high in salt [7]. Excess salt intake has been identified as one of the leading global health risks [8] and population level salt reduction is recognized as a cost-effective means of reducing blood pressure [9–12] and, in turn, reducing the risk of heart disease and stroke [13,14]. A 30% reduction in population level salt by 2020 is one of the voluntary global health targets identified by the World Health Organization [7].

On a global scale, it has been estimated that 1.7 million lives could be saved annually if salt consumption levels were decreased to recommended levels of less than 5g per day [15]. Across high and low-middle income countries, interventions to reduce population salt intake are considered cost effective (less than $1USD per person per year) [16,17].

Over 75% of cardiovascular deaths take place in low and middle-income countries [18] with the African region estimated to have around 20 million people with CVD [18]. As such, Africa shares the greatest burden of hypertension with almost half of adults aged 25 and older diagnosed and potentially more adults with undiagnosed, untreated and uncontrolled hypertension [19]. In Ghana, the prevalence of hypertension has continued to rise over the past 40 years [20–22]. South Africa (SA) equally shares a large burden of hypertension [23,24]. The direct healthcare costs attributable to non-optimal blood pressure in Sub-Saharan Africa (SSA) in 2001 were estimated to be two billion US dollars [25].

More than two-thirds of African populations attach low importance to dietary salt reduction as a significant approach to addressing hypertension [26,27]. In most African countries, salt is commonly added to food at the table and during cooking, and is a major ingredient found in commonly used sauces and seasonings [28,29]. Salted fish and meat are eaten frequently [30] while bread contains levels of salt that are generally higher than in countries in Europe and North America [31,32]. In SA, other sources of salt include cereals, meat and meat products, milk and dairy products, processed meats, meat pies and margarine. In that country, it is estimated that discretionary salt intake accounted for almost half of the total dietary intake in a sample of black urban dwelling people [33]. This represents a greater contribution as compared to many high income countries, where 75–85% of dietary salt intake is estimated to come from processed foods [34]. The Ghana Demographic and Health Survey indicated that 84% of women surveyed reported that someone in their household had consumed processed foods containing salt within the past 24 hours, while more than a third had consumed salted dried fish, 21% reported having had canned fish, meat and legumes and 24% reported the use of other processed foods containing salt [35]. The report identified a high use of salty foods in both rural and urban areas. Similarly, the South African Demographic and Health Survey 2003 indicated that more than 30% of survey respondents reported adding salt to food at the table and consuming salty snacks more than twice a week [36].

To reduce discretionary salt consumption in SA, there has been a concentrated focus on consumer education and awareness in recent years [37]. In addition, in June 2016, the SA government implemented mandatory legislation related to maximum levels of salt permitted in a wide range of processed food categories, including breads, meats, cereal products, fat spreads, snack foods and savoury products [38]. These foods have previously been shown to contribute significantly to overall non-discretionary salt intake in the South African population [33]. In contrast, in Ghana, there have been no concerted efforts by government or non-governmental organizations to implement salt reduction strategies. Instead, there has been a focus on the prevention of iodine deficiency through universal salt iodisation programmes [39–41] with the message to consume iodized salt widely disseminated through the mass media [39]. Public health concerns related to the association between increased salt intake and cardiovascular risk in Ghana have received comparatively little attention despite promising proof of concept studies [42]. Iodisation programmes and salt reduction strategies are not mutually exclusive, as has been demonstrated [43]. However, for both programmes to successfully coexist, different sectors of government (nutrition and NCDs) need to work together, to effectively monitor the iodine status of populations as salt content in the food supply decreases.

Given that the population in Ghana has been urged to consume iodised salt [39,40,44] combined with the generally increased accessibility of EDNP processed foods, it is timely to investigate knowledge, attitudes and behaviours (KAB) related to salt use in Ghana and to compare these against

SA, an African country in which salt reduction has been strongly emphasized. Ghana and SA share similar socio-demographic characteristics, as well as a high hypertension burden. The findings will be important—particularly for low and middle-income countries—for informing approaches to reducing the health risks through a better understanding of salt intake behaviours.

2. Materials and Methods

2.1. Study Design

Analysis for this study utilizes two nationally representative datasets collected in Ghan and South Africa (SA) during the World Health Organization's Study on global Ageing and dult health (SAGE-Wave 2) [45]. WHO SAGE is a multinational prospective cohort study that has been conducted in six low and middle-income countries since 2002. The purpose of the study is to examine the health and wellbeing of adults and the ageing process, with the aim of responding to health needs through policy, planning and research. SAGE Wave 2 was conducted in Ghana and SA in 2014/2015 with Wave 3 to be implemented in 2017–2018.

2.2. Participants

A total of 10,522 adults were recruited; n = 6746 in Ghana and n = 3776 in SA. Stratified sampling was conducted to respondents aged 50 years and older, with approximately 30% of adults aged 18–49 years as a comparative cohort. In selecting the sample, all SAGE Wave 1 households were included for SAGE Wave 2 data collection [45]. In SAGE SA, replacements for sample attrition used a systematic sampling approach to randomly select new households as previously described [46]. The sampling method used in SAGE Ghana followed a similar design, based on the 2003 World Health Survey/SAGE Wave 0 [47] with primary sampling units (PSUs) stratified by region and location (urban/rural). Selection of the PSUs was based on proportional allocation by size using the same follow-up and random systematic sampling method as South Africa.

2.3. Data Collection

Data collection in Ghana was completed by four field teams each comprising of 3–5 field workers who moved from region to region over an 11-month period (September 2014 to June 2015). In SA, twenty survey teams collected data from respondents across all provinces in the country over a 5-month period (August to December 2015). Surveys were administered in participants' home language. A computer assisted personal interview was used in collecting the data. All survey teams were trained with support from the WHO SAGE team, with survey teams using standardized training and survey materials [45]. Field teams visited respondents in their homes and workplaces to administer interviews.

2.4. Study Measures

The main outcome of the current analysis relates to reported salt KAB captured using a five-item questionnaire adapted from the WHO/PAHO protocol [48]. KAB is the usual term for such research and has been widely used, including in the context of salt behaviours [48–52]. One question investigated knowledge about salt and health—"Do you think that a high salt diet could cause a serious health problem?"—with answer options "yes" or "no". Another investigated attitudes about salt—"How much salt do you think you consume?"—with answer options of "far too much," "too much", "just the right amount", "too little", "far too little", "don't know", and "refused". The congruence between attitudes and perceptions has been explored [53], but for the purposes of comparison with other studies we prefer to retain the terminology of "attitudes". Three questions assessed salt use behaviours: (1) "Do you add salt to food at the table?"; (2) "In the food you eat at home, salt is added in cooking?"; and (3) "Do you do anything on a regular basis to control your salt or sodium intake?"—with answer options "always", "often", "sometimes", "rarely", and "never" for items 1 and 2, and "yes", "no", "don't know", and "refused" for item 3. Likert type response scales were provided, but for analysis of responses to the salt use behaviour questions categories of "always" and "often" were combined to represent "frequent" use, whilst "rarely" and "never" were combined to represent "infrequent" use.

"Currently working" was recorded as "having worked for at least 2 days during the last 7 days". "Recent use of alcohol" was recorded as "having consumed alcohol in the last 30 days", while "frequent alcohol intake" was recorded as "having consumed at least one alcoholic drink (on average) one or more days in a week" and "infrequent alcohol intake" was recorded as having consumed at least one alcoholic drink (on average) one to three days per month.

Age, sex, residential location (urban/rural), education, marital status, employment status, alcohol intake, smoking status, blood pressure (BP) and salt behaviour variables were recorded, as shown in Table 1. BP was measured using wrist worn validated Omron BP devices with positional sensors (Omron R6, Kyoto, Japan) [53]. Three BP readings were recorded on the left wrist (1-min between each measurement) while the participant sat with the wrist precisely at the level of the heart and legs uncrossed.

2.5. Ethics

Prior to data collection, the study measures were explained to the participants in their home language by the fieldworkers and written informed consent was obtained. The study complied with the ethical principles for medical research involving human subjects as stated in the Declaration of Helsinki [54]. The WHO Research Ethics Review Committee approved the study [RPC149]. Local ethical approval was obtained from the North-West University Human Research Ethics Committee (Potchefstroom, South Africa), the University of the Witwatersrand Human Research Ethics Committee (Johannesburg, South Africa), and the University of Ghana Medical School Ethics and Protocol Review Committee (Accra, Ghana).

2.6. Statistical Analysis

All data were collated and analysed using IBM SPSS Statistics for Windows, Version 20.0. (IBM Corp., Armonk, NY, USA). The normality of the data was checked by visual inspection and the Kolmogorov-Smirnov test. Descriptive statistics of frequencies, percentages and median (IQR) were used to describe respondents' characteristics and responses to survey items. Country differences were evaluated using Chi-square and Independent Samples Mann Whitney *U* tests. The significance level was set at $p < 0.05$. Logistic regression was applied to compare the probability of various salt behaviours between Ghana and SA and odds ratios and 95% confidence intervals (95% CI) were computed. The model was adjusted for potential confounders which included age, sex, residential location, educational level and hypertension prevalence as demonstrated in other studies [52,55–57]. BMI was not included in the final regression model as it was not statistically significant.

Table 1. Sociodemographic characteristics and selected health characteristics of the study samples in Ghana and South Africa, Study on Global Ageing and Adult Health (SAGE) Wave 2.

Characteristics	Age Categories—Countries Combined			Ghana *n* = 4753	South Africa *n* = 3392	*p* Value
	18–49 Years Old (*n* = 2279)	50+ Years Old (*n* = 5860)	*p* Value			
Age in years, median (IQR) 50 plus years, *n* (%)				*n* = 4743 58 (19.0) 3569 (75.2)	*n* = 3396 54 (24.0) 2291 (67.5)	<0.01 <0.01
Sex male, *n* (%)	*n* = 2277 871 (38.3)	*n* = 5857 2171 (37.0)	0.32	*n* = 4753 1954 (41.1)	*n* = 3392 1094 (32.3)	<0.01
Residence urban, *n* (%)	*n* = 2110 1176 (55.7)	*n* = 5560 2918 (52.5)	0.01	*n* = 4728 1970 (41.6)	*n* = 2924 2124 (72.8)	<0.01

Table 1. *Cont.*

| Characteristics | Age Categories—Countries Combined | | | Ghana $n = 4753$ | South Africa $n = 3392$ | p Value |
	18–49 Years Old $(n = 2279)$	50+ Years Old $(n = 5860)$	p Value			
Education			.			
Ever attended school, *n* (%)	$n = 2108$ 1839 (87.2)	$n = 5546$ 3327 (60.0)	<0.01	$n = 4734$ 2764 (58.4)	$n = 2920$ 2402 (82.3)	<0.01
Educational level high school or above, *n* (%)	$n = 2099$ 1164 (55.5)	$n = 5493$ 1646 (30)	<0.01	$n = 4706$ 678 (14.4)	$n = 2886$ 696 (24.1)	<0.01
Employment status: currently working, (%)	$n = 1473$ 1124 (76.3)	$n = 4832$ 2611 (54.0)	<0.01	$n = 4537$ 3169 (69.8)	$n = 1768$ 566 (32.0)	<0.01
Marital status: married/cohabiting, *n* (%)	$n = 937$ 231 (24.7)	$n = 1984$ 684 (34.5)	<0.01	$n = 4738$ 2692 (56.8)	$n = 2921$ 915 (31.3)	<0.01
Waist to height ratio <0.5, *n* (%)	$n = 1853$ 693 (37.4)	$n = 4807$ 1369 (28.5)	<0.01	$n = 4347$ 1553 (35.7)	$n = 2313$ 509 (22.0)	<0.01
Body Mass Index (BMI), median (IQR)	$n = 1904$ 25 (7.7)	$n = 4883$ 24.2 (8.4)	<0.01	$n = 4456$ 22.9 (6.2)	$n = 2331$ 28.6 (9.9)	<0.01
Alcohol intake						
Never *n* (%)	$n = 1597$ 397 (24.0)	$n = 1625$ 400 (24.6)	0.87	$n = 1168$ 786 (67.3)	$n = 2054$ 1639 (80.0)	<0.01
Recently yes, *n* (%)	$n = 515$ 351 (68.2)	$n = 1379$ 912 (66.1)	0.41	$n = 1379$ 916 (66.4)	$n = 515$ 347 (67.4)	0.69
Frequent, *n* (%)	$n = 508$ 203 (40.0)	$n = 1371$ 595 (43.4)	<0.01	$n = 1369$ 635 (46.4)	$n = 510$ 163 (32.0)	<0.01
Smoking status, current use of tobacco, *n* (%)	$n = 1616$ 137 (8.5)	$n = 1884$ 474 (25.2)	<0.01	$n = 1340$ 208 (15.5)	$n = 2160$ 403 (18.7)	0.06
Systolic blood pressure mmHg, median (IQR)	$n = 2030$ 119 (20.0)	$n = 5370$ 131 (28.0)	<0.01	$n = 4674$ 124.67 (28.0)	$n = 2726$ 130.7 (26.0)	<0.01
Diastolic blood pressure mmHg, median (IQR)	$n = 2030$ 75.7 (15.0)	$n = 5370$ 79.3 (17.0)	<0.01	$n = 4674$ 77 (16.0)	$n = 2726$ 80.67 (16.0)	<0.01
Hypertensive, *n* (%)	$n = 2079$ 401 (19.3)	$n = 5455$ 2320 (42.5)	<0.01	$n = 4675$ 1444 (30.9)	$n = 2859$ 1277 (44.7)	<0.01

Data recorded as median (inter quartile range) and frequencies (%). Smokers identified by self-report. Frequent alcohol use defined as the consumption of one or more alcoholic drinks a day/week. Hypertensive categorized as $BP \geq 140/90$ mmHg or previous diagnosis. Continuous variables were compared using the Independent Samples Mann Whitney U test; categorical variables were compared using the Chi-Square test.

3. Results

Approximately 30% of the recruited samples in both countries had data that could not be retrieved due to technical and data management issues during data collection and retrieval using the CAPI system. This loss of data was non-systematic and the sample size on which the current analysis is based is on a total samples size of $n = 8145$ (by sex). As such, in the sample for Ghana (41.1% ($n = 1954$) were male and 58.9% ($n = 2799$) were female, 75.2% ($n = 3569$) aged 50+ years old and 24.8% ($n = 1174$) aged 18–49 years old) and for SA (32.2% ($n = 1094$) were male and 67.8% ($n = 2298$) were female, 67.5% ($n = 2291$) aged 50+ years old and 32.5% ($n = 1105$) aged 18–49 years old). The characteristics of the population are presented in Table 1. Due to non-responses for some questionnaire items, the number of responses (n) for each variable is included in the tables. Significant differences were recorded between the two countries, with more older people (Ghana 75.2%; SA 67.5%; $p < 0.01$) and more men (Ghana 41.1%; SA 32.3%; $p < 0.01$) in Ghana than in SA, whereas SA had more urban residents (Ghana 41.6%; SA 72.8%), and more participants from SA had a higher educational status (Ghana 14.4%; SA 42.1%) and a higher level of hypertension prevalence (SA 44.7%; Ghana 30.9%; $p < 0.01$)

3.1. Knowledge

Approximately one-third (31.3%; $n = 2190$) of all respondents were not aware that a high salt diet could cause a serious health problem. This was consistently observed among older and younger adults, men and women and across both countries (Table 2). Significant associations were recorded between respondents' knowledge and their ethnicity within the South African cohort. Those with a "coloured" ethnic background recorded the highest knowledge (84%, $p < 0.01$).

Table 2. Association between salt knowledge, attitudes and behaviours (KAB) and demographic characteristics of Ghanaians ($n = 6746$) and South Africans ($n = 3776$); younger ($n = 2279$) and older ($n = 5860$); men ($n = 3048$) and women ($n = 5860$), SAGE Wave 2.

	Age Category—Countries Combined			Sex—Countries Combined			Ghana	SA	
	18–49 Years Old $n = 2279$	50+ Years Old $n = 5860$	*p* Value	Men $n = 3048$	Women $n = 5097$	*p* Value	$n = 4753$	$n = 3392$	*p* Value
Do you think that a high salt diet could cause a serious health problem? Yes *n* (%)	$n = 1940$ 1309 (67.5)	$n = 5061$ 3502 (69.2)	0.16	$n = 2602$ 1756 (67.5)	$n = 4399$ 3055 (69.4)	0.09	$n = 4328$ 2920 (67.5)	$n = 2673$ 1891 (70.7)	<0.01
How much salt do you think you consume? Just the right amount, *n* (%)	$n = 2047$ 1613 (78.8)	$n = 5392$ 3957 (73.4)	<0.01	$n = 2804$ 2176 (77.6)	$n = 4635$ 3394 (73.2)	<0.01	$n = 4622$ 3510 (75.9)	$n = 2817$ 2060 (73.1)	<0.01
Do you add salt to food at the table? "Always" and "Often" *n* (%)	$n = 1453$ 311 (21.4)	$n = 4026$ 673 (16.7)	<0.01	$n = 2024$ 393 (19.4)	$n = 3455$ 591 (17.1)	0.31	$n = 3552$ 350 (9.9)	$n = 1927$ 634 (32.9)	<0.01
In the food you eat at home, salt is added in cooking ... ? "Always" and "Often" *n* (%)	$n = 1822$ 1689 (92.7)	$n = 4771$ 4310 (90.3)	0.03	$n = 2552$ 2374 (93)	$n = 4041$ 3625 (89.7)	<0.01	$n = 4459$ 4294 (96.3)	$n = 2134$ 1705 (79.9)	<0.01
Do you do anything on a regular basis to control your salt or sodium intake? Yes *n* (%)	$n = 1990$ 688 (34.6)	$n = 5249$ 2034 (38.8)	0.01	$n = 2718$ 970 (35.7)	$n = 4521$ 1752 (38.8)	<0.01	$n = 4518$ 1939 (42.9)	$n = 2721$ 783 (28.8)	<0.01

Note: "All" represents respondents from both countries. Data was recorded in frequencies. Chi square tests were conducted.

3.2. Attitudes

Three quarters (74.9%; $n = 5570$) of all respondents perceived that they consumed just the right amount of salt. The perception of consuming "just the right amount of salt" was more frequently observed in younger adults, men, and in Ghanaians compared to South Africans

3.3. Salt Intake Behaviours

Among all respondents, 18% ($n = 984$) reported that they "always" and "often" (frequently) added salt to food at the table and the majority ($n = 5999$, 91%) reported that they frequently added salt to food at home during cooking. Almost two-thirds (62.4%) reported that they did not take any action to control their salt intake. The response to "taking actions to control salt intake on a regular basis" significantly differed according to knowledge about salt (knowledge and health, $p < 0.001$). For the two countries, fifty-two percent of respondents who did not think high salt could cause health problems reported that they never took actions on regular basis to reduce salt intake. Reported frequent alcohol intake was found to relate to less desirable salt intake behaviours. While 96.7% of respondents reporting frequent alcohol intake ($n = 1971$) also reported always or often adding salt to food while cooking, this behaviour was significantly lower (86.1%) in teetotalers ($n = 756$; $p < 0.01$). Additionally, significantly more teetotalers (51.0%) reported regularly attempting to control their salt intake when compared with frequent drinkers (33.7%; $p < 0.01$). Significant associations were ecorded between respondents who frequently added salt to food at the table and their ethnicity within the South African cohort. Those with African/black ethnic background reported adding more salt to food at the table than any other group (36.5%, $p < 0.01$).

Younger adults more frequently added salt to food at the table, added salt to food eaten at home during cooking and did less on a regular basis to control their salt intake than did older adults (Table 2). More South Africans than Ghanaians reported that they frequently added salt at the table (SA 32.9%; Ghana 9.9%; $p < 0.001$) and did not take actions to control their salt intake (SA 28.8%; Ghana 42.9%).

Significantly more Ghanaians than South Africans reported frequently adding salt to food during cooking (SA 79.9%; Ghana 96.3%; $p < 0.01$).

Multivariate analysis adjusted for sex, age, residence, educational level and hypertension prevalence showed that South Africans were more likely than Ghanaians to add salt to food at the table (OR 4.80, CI 4.071–5.611, $p < 0.001$) but less likely to add salt to food at home during cooking (OR 0.16, CI 0.130–0.197, $p < 0.001$) or to take action to control their salt intake regularly (OR 0.44, CI 0.379–0.488, $p < 0.01$); (Table 3). Men and younger adults were also significantly more likely to add salt to food and less likely to control salt intake. Those living in urban areas, educated to high school level or above, or those with hypertension were significantly more likely to regularly control their salt intake.

Table 3. Associations between sociodemographic variables and salt behaviours of adults in Ghana ($n = 6746$) and South Africa ($n = 3776$)—comparing the odds ratio for sub-optimal salt behaviours, SAGE Wave 2.

Variables	Salt Frequently Added to Food at the Table	Salt Frequently Added to Food during Cooking	Takes Regular Action to Control of Salt Intake
	OR (95% CI)	OR (95% CI)	OR (95% CI)
Ghana	Referent	Referent	Referent
SA	4.80 (4.071–5.611) *	0.16 (0.130–0.197) *	0.436 (0.379–0.488) *
Female	Referent	Referent	Referent
Male	1.40 (1.182–1.605) *	1.36 (1.118–1.654) *	0.78 (0.718–0.884) *
18–49 years old	Referent	Referent	Referent
50+ years old	0.78 (0.655–0.920)*	0.56 (0.450–0.711) *	1.23 (1.096–1.384) *
Rural	Referent	Referent	Referent
Urban	0.89 (0.762–1.041)	0.90 (0.744–1.099)	1.41 (1.271–1.565) *
Primary school and below	Referent	Referent	Referent
High school and above	0.87 (0.741–1.020)	0.86 (0.710–1.048)	1.12 (1.004–1.240) *
Normotensive	Referent	Referent	Referent
Hypertensives	1.11 (0.952–1.299)	0.88 (0.734–1.067)	1.48 (1.328–1.649) *

Note: Referent indicates reference category used for the comparison. Hypertension was categorized as BP $\geq 140/90$ mmHg or previous diagnosis, logistic regression was adjusted for sex, age category, residence, educational level and hypertension prevalence, * $p < 0.05$.

4. Discussion

The finding that 80% or more of adults in Ghana and SA frequently add salt to their food during cooking indicates that discretionary salt use remains high in both countries. Significant differences were observed between the two countries for various behaviours, such as a third of South Africans reported adding salt to food at the table as compared to only a tenth of Ghanaians. Significant differences were also observed between younger and older adults and between the genders. The most potentially detrimental behaviours were identified in men and younger adults. The contribution of discretionary salt intake to total salt intake cannot be under-emphasized even in societies where most salt comes from processed foods. Health promotion activities are needed to decrease individual level salt intake [7] in order to decrease salt preferences over time and thus decrease discretionary salt use [7,36,58].

Knowledge related to the adverse effects of salt on health was poor. Almost one third ($n = 2190$) of both Ghanaians and South Africans were not aware of the relationship between high salt intake and the possibility of a serious health problem. This could potentially explain practices of high discretionary salt use [55,59,60]. Conversely, individuals who know about the health effects of excess salt in the diet have been shown to be more likely to reduce their salt intake [49]. Knowledge of hypertension may influence both salt and self-care behaviours [61]. Our results show that responses to salt knowledge, attitudes and behaviours are significantly related as shown by other authors [56]

Our data indicates participants' high confidence in their perceived intake of the recommended levels of salt, since three-quarters of respondents reported that they consumed "just the right amount of salt." A limitation of this study relates to potential under-reporting of salt use, as shown in other studies [49,52,62,63] and responses to salt questions may not reflect actual intakes. Studies that measured 24 h urinary sodium excretion in addition to self-reported discretionary salt use in the same respondents revealed an underestimation in reported salt intake [33,64]. Hypertension levels were high in both samples but we did not investigate whether hypertensive individuals that were receiving treatment to control their blood pressure had also received advice on salt intake. There is a possibility of misreporting, as those who have received information on salt use may feel that they consume the recommended amount. Furthermore, there might be some lack of knowledge relative to the amount of salt recommended for daily consumption, as was the case in other studies [56]. This discrepancy between perceived and actual salt consumption has the potential to result in higher than anticipated salt intakes [65].

Our data indicates a need to intensify consumer education on salt intake awareness in both countries, including discretionary salt use. Previous research contributing to South African policy change [33] suggests that further investigation into particular food items that contribute high amounts of salt to the diet is needed in Ghana. Consistent with other studies [56], more attention should be directed towards the younger population (18–49 years old) and to men, who reported worse discretionary salt knowledge, attitudes and behaviours. Dietary salt education and awareness should also be integrated into school curricular and youth programmes, particularly as hypertension and associated morbidity and mortality typically occur at younger ages in Sub Saharan Africa (SSA) [66,67].

Our finding that Ghanaians add more salt to food at home during cooking compared with their South African counterparts may not be surprising given investment in campaigns to increase consumption of iodized salt [68–70]. Within Ghana, any action related to salt reduction for addressing NCDs appears to have been overshadowed by the strong focus on the prevention of iodine deficiencies [39–41,70]. This situation appears in contrast to WHO guidelines [14], which suggest compatibility of polices on salt reduction and salt iodisation. The guidelines advise that regular monitoring of sodium (salt) intake and iodine intake at country level is needed to adjust salt iodisation over time to ensure that individuals consume sufficient iodine while reducing overall intake of salt. If salt is sufficiently iodised, a reduction of salt intake to the recommended level of 5 g per day should still provide an adequate amount of iodine [43]. Ghana's strong emphasis on the reduction of iodine deficiencies provides a unique and untapped opportunity for addressing discretionary salt use and behaviour change. Salt used in food processing is not included in the mandatory Universal Salt Iodisation policies in either Ghana or South Africa, although there is some evidence from South Africa that indicates up to a third of margarines, bread, and savoury snack seasonings contain iodised salt [71].

We found that South Africans were almost 5 times more likely than Ghanaians to add salt to food at the table (controlling for sex, age, location, education level and hypertension prevalence). This finding was expected, as a greater proportion of the cohort in SA lived in urban areas compared with Ghana. Urbanization is one of the key drivers for excess salt consumption [15]. Further investigation regarding the effect of acculturation on addition of salt to food is of interest. The survey was conducted prior to salt legislation being introduced in SA, therefore it will be of importance to determine how the lowering of salt in processed foods impacts on both discretionary salt behaviours and actual salt intake levels in SA in the next wave of SAGE in 2017–2018.

The present study shows that almost two-thirds of the population were not taking any action to control their salt intake, and this may be explained by the finding that a third of respondents did not have any knowledge regarding the links between high salt intake and health problems. Among the key broad strategies for salt reduction is individual responsibility and action [7], for example, limiting the consumption of salty snacks and reducing the amount of salt used in cooking. The Health Belief Model explains that perceived seriousness, perceived susceptibility, perceived benefits and perceived barriers are critical evaluations an individual undertakes prior to engaging in a health behaviour [72]. Our data suggests that strategies are required to firstly increase awareness within the Health Belief Model of health promotion as a means of supporting behaviour change. The other broad strategy is at a systemic level—including measures like those adopted in South Africa to work with food manufacturers to lower salt levels in processed foods.

The findings of the present study were somewhat surprising because, despite the extensive public awareness campaign in SA to address population salt intake levels and influence salt related behaviour (Salt Watch) [37,73] and despite that population reporting greater salt knowledge, it was the Ghanaians who appeared to be more actively controlling their salt intake (Table 2). This highlights the point that knowledge alone is not sufficient to cause a change in behaviour. Consistent with the present study, research from Newson et al. (2013) [62] showed that almost half of survey respondents were not interested in reducing their salt intake and had no intention of making any changes to their salt consumption in the immediate future. With a large hypertension burden [24], it is likely that some South Africans may not feel empowered to make dietary changes. Additionally, cultural beliefs and practices that encourage salt consumption are also of concern. Salt use for spiritual and religious purposes is common place in SA [37] and this would need to be considered in health messages.

The finding that frequent alcohol intake was associated with less desirable salt intake behaviours has been reported by others [74]. Differences in reported alcohol intake between Ghanaian and South African study participants are similar to previous analyses of alcohol consumption from Wave 1 of SAGE which indicated that there were fewer "never" drinkers (lifetime abstainers) in Ghana than in SA, while the South African cohort had more "at risk" drinkers [75].

It is well established that reducing dietary salt to 3 g/day leads to a reduction in blood pressure in both in hypertensives and normotensives [76]. Given the current estimated prevalence of hypertension in the African region, it is imperative that salt reduction messages are included in public health campaigns alongside various strategies to support behaviour change while also modifying salt levels in commonly consumed foods. Provision of practical skills and strategies to encourage change in salt intake behaviours is key in this regard.

The present study had several strengths which included the use of large, nationally representative sample sizes in both SA and Ghana. A potential limitation relates to the oversampling of older people in keeping with the purpose of the SAGE, which may limit generalizability of the findings to the population younger than 50 in both countries. Regardless, these are relatively large representations of the 50+ population, with younger comparison groups in both countries.

5. Conclusions

This study provided important insights into salt knowledge, attitudes and behaviours (KAB) in SSA. High discretionary salt use remains common practice in the region and needs urgent attention in the face of high and rising hypertension levels. Significant differences in salt KAB were evident between the two countries which suggests the use of different strategies and approaches for combatting high discretionary salt intake may be appropriate, although strategies particularly targeting men and younger adults may be beneficial for both countries. The findings suggest that SA requires investment into public health campaigns to address the practice of adding salt to foods at the table, while in Ghana a focus on changing behaviours related to the use of salt in cooking is required. Campaigns and consumer education strategies—based on the Health Belief Model—may be useful to raise awareness for salt reduction in SSA.

Acknowledgments: This work is supported by an agreement with the CDC Foundation with financial support provided by Bloomberg Philanthropies, and a Partnerships & Research Development Fund (PRDF) grant from the Australia Africa Universities Network. SAGE is supported by WHO and the Division of Behavioral and Social Research (BSR) at the National Institute on Aging (NIA), US National Institutes of Health, through Interagency Agreements with WHO [OGHA 04034785; YA1323-08-CN-0020; Y1-AG-1005-01] and a Research Project Grant [R01AG034479]. Funding was provided through the grant for open access publication.

Author Contributions: K.E.C. and P.K. conceived and designed the research; E.M. and L.J.W. analyzed the data; E.M., K.E.C., L.J.W., J.R., R.B. and P.K. wrote the paper.

Conflicts of Interest: The authors declare no conflict of interest. The founding sponsors had no role in the design of the study; in the collection, analyses, or interpretation of data; in the writing of the manuscript, nor in the decision to publish the results.

References

1. Forouzanfar, M.H.; Afshin, A.; Alexander, L.T.; Forouzanfar, M.H.; Anderson, H.R.; Bachman, V.F.; Biryukov, S.; Brauer, M.; Burnett, R.; Casey, D.; et al. Global, regional, and national comparative risk assessment of 79 behavioural, environmental and occupational, and metabolic risks or clusters of risks in 188 countries, 1990–2013: A systematic analysis for the Global Burden of Disease Study 2013. *Lancet* **2016**, *388*, 2287–2323. [CrossRef]
2. Kromhout, D. Diet and cardiovascular diseases. *J. Nutr. Health Aging* **2001**, *5*, 144–149. [PubMed]
3. Grosso, G.; Mistretta, A.; Frigiola, A.; Gruttadauria, S.; Biondi, A.; Basile, F.; Vitaglione, P.; D'Orazio, N.; Galvano, F. Mediterranean Diet and Cardiovascular Risk Factors: A Systematic Review. *Crit. Rev. Food Sci. Nutr.* **2014**, *54*, 593–610. [CrossRef] [PubMed]
4. Siervo, M.; Lara, J.; Chowdhury, S.; Ashor, A.; Oggioni, C.; Mathers, J.C. Effects of the Dietary Approach to Stop Hypertension (DASH) diet on cardiovascular risk factors: A systematic review and meta-analysis. *Br. J. Nutr.* **2015**, *113*, 1–15. [CrossRef] [PubMed]
5. Donaldson, M.S. Nutrition and cancer: A review of the evidence for an anti-cancer diet. *Nutr. J.* **2004**, *3*. [CrossRef] [PubMed]
6. Psaltopoulou, T.I.; Alevizaki, M. The role of diet and lifestyle in primary, secondary, and tertiary diabetes prevention: A review of meta-analyses. *Rev. Diabet. Stud.* **2010**, *7*, 26–30. [CrossRef] [PubMed]
7. Salt Reduction. Available online: http://www.who.int/mediacentre/factsheets/fs393/en/ (accessed on 26 May 2017).
8. Sacks, F.M.; Svetkey, L.P.; Vollmer, W.M.; Appel, L.J.; Bray, G.A.; Harsha, D.; Obarzanek, E.; Conlin, P.R.; Miller, E.R.; Simons-Morton, D.G.; et al. Effects on blood pressure of reduced dietary sodium and the dietary approaches to stop hypertension (DASH) diet. *N. Engl. J. Med.* **2001**, *344*, 3–10. [CrossRef] [PubMed]
9. Campbell, N.R.C.; Neal, B.C.; MacGregor, G.A. Interested in developing a national programme to reduce dietary salt? *J. Hum. Hypertens.* **2011**, *25*, 705–710. [CrossRef] [PubMed]
10. World Health Organization. *Global Status Report on Noncommunicable Diseases 2010*; World Health Organisation: Geneva, Switzerland, 2011.
11. World Health Organisation. *WHO Global Strategy on Diet, Physical Activity and Health: The Americas Regional Consultation Meeting Report*; WHO: Geneva, Switzerland, 2003.
12. Yang, Q.H.; Liu, T.B.; Kuklina, E.V.; Flanders, W.D.; Hong, Y.L.; Gillespie, C.; Chang, M.H.; Gwinn, M.; Dowling, N.; Khoury, M.J.; et al. Sodium and Potassium Intake and Mortality Among US Adults Prospective Data From the Third National Health and Nutrition Examination Survey. *Arch. Intern. Med.* **2011**, *171*, 1183–1191. [CrossRef] [PubMed]
13. World Health Organisation. *Global Strategy on Diet, Physical Activity and Health*; WHO: Geneva, Switzerland, 2003.
14. Guideline: Sodium Intake for Adults and Children. Available online: http://www.who.int/nutrition/publications/guidelines/sodium_intake_printversion.pdf (accessed on 26 April 2017).
15. Healthy Diet. Available online: http://www.who.int/mediacentre/factsheets/fs394/en/ (accessed on 22 May 2017).
16. Asaria, P.; Chisholm, D.; Mathers, C.; Ezzati, M.; Beaglehole, R. Chronic disease prevention: Health effects and financial costs of strategies to reduce salt intake and control tobacco use. *Lancet* **2007**, *370*, 2004–2053. [CrossRef]
17. Beaglehole, R.; Bonita, R. Priority actions for the non-communicable disease crisis reply. *Lancet* **2011**, *378*, 565–566. [CrossRef]
18. Cardiovascular Diseases (CVDs). Available online: http://www.who.int/mediacentre/factsheets/fs317/en/ (accessed on 2 April 2017).
19. A Global Brief on Hypertension. Available online: http://apps.who.int/iris/bitstream/10665/79059/1/WHO_DCO_WHD_2013.2_eng.pdf?ua=1 (accessed on 7 January 2017).
20. Pobee, J.O.; Larbi, E.B.; Dodu, S.R.; Pisa, Z.; Strasse, T. Is systemic hypertension a problem in Ghana? *Trop. Dr.* **1997**, *9*, 89–92. [CrossRef] [PubMed]

21. Hyder, A.A.; Rotllont, G.; Morrow, R.H. Measuring the burden of disease: Healthy life-years. *Am. J. Public Health* **1998**, *88*, 196–202. [CrossRef] [PubMed]

22. Bosu, W.K. Epidemic of hypertension in Ghana: A systematic review. *BMC Public Health* **2010**, *10*. [CrossRef] [PubMed]

23. Seedat, Y.K. Control of hypertension in South Africa: Time for action. *SAMJ* **2012**, *102*, 25–26.

24. Ntuli, S.T.; Maimela, E.; Alberts, M.; Choma, S.; Dikotope, S. Prevalence and associated risk factors of hypertension amongst adults in a rural community of Limpopo Province, South Africa. *Afr. J. Prim. Health Care Fam. Med.* **2015**, *7*, 847. [CrossRef] [PubMed]

25. Gaziano, T.A.; Bitton, A.; Anand, S.; Weinstein, M.C. The global cost of nonoptimal blood pressure. *J. Hypertens.* **2009**, *27*, 1472–1477. [CrossRef] [PubMed]

26. Morris, R.C.; Sebastian, A.; Forman, A.; Tanaka, M.; Schmidlin, O. Normotensive salt sensitivity—Effects of race and dietary potassium. *Hypertension* **1999**, *33*, 18–23. [CrossRef] [PubMed]

27. Rayner, B.L.; Myers, J.E.; Opie, L.H.; Trinder, Y.A.; Davidson, J.S. Screening for primary aldosteronism—Normal ranges for aldosterone and renin in three South African population groups. *SAMJ* **2001**, *91*, 594–599. [PubMed]

28. World Health Organisation. *WHO Expert Consultation on Salt as a Vehicle for Fortification*; WHO: Geneva, Switzerland, 2007.

29. Webster, J.L.; Dunford, E.K.; Hawkes, C.; Neal, B.C. Salt reduction initiatives around the world. *J. Hypertens.* **2011**, *29*, 1043–1050. [CrossRef] [PubMed]

30. Kerry, S.M.; Emmett, L.; Micah, F.B.; Martin-Peprah, R.; Antwi, S.; Phillips, R.O.; Plange-Rhule, J.; Eastwood, J.B.; Cappuccio, F.P. Rural and semi-urban differences in salt intake, and its dietary sources, in Ashanti, West Africa. *Ethn. Dis.* **2005**, *15*, 33–39. [PubMed]

31. Wilson, N.; Nghiem, N.; Ryan, S.; Cleghorn, C.; Nair, N.; Blakey, T. Designing low-cost "heart healthy bread": Optimization using linear programing and 15-country comparison. *BMC Nutr.* **2016**, *2*. [CrossRef]

32. Nwanguma, B.C.; Okorie, C.H. Salt (sodium chloride) content of retail samples of Nigerian white bread: Implications for the daily salt intake of normotensive and hypertensive adults. *J. Hum. Nutr.* **2013**, *26*, 488–493. [CrossRef] [PubMed]

33. Charlton, K.E.; Steyn, K.; Levitt, N.S.; Zulu, J.V.; Jonathan, D.; Veldman, F.J.; Nel, J.H. Diet and blood pressure in South Africa: Intake of foods containing sodium, potassium, calcium, and magnesium in three ethnic groups. *Nutrition* **2005**, *21*, 39–50. [CrossRef] [PubMed]

34. Matlou, S.M.; Isles, C.G.; Higgs, A.; Milne, F.J.; Murray, G.D.; Schultz, E.; Starke, I.F. Potassium supplementation in blacks with mild to moderate essential-hypertension. *J. Hypertens.* **1986**, *4*, 61–64. [CrossRef] [PubMed]

35. Ghana Demographic and Health Survey, 2014. Available online: http://www.statsghana.gov.gh/docfiles/publications/2014%20GDHS%20%20Report.pdf (accessed on 9 December 2015).

36. Department of Health. *South Africa Demographic and Health Survey 2003*; Department of Heath: Pretoria, South Africa, 2007.

37. Eksteen, G.; Mungal-Singh, V. Salt intake in South Africa: A current perspective. *JEMDSA* **2015**, *20*, 9–13. [CrossRef]

38. Department of Health, South Africa. *Foodstuffs, Cosmetics and Disinfectants Act, 1972 (Act 54 of 1972): Regulations Relating to the Reduction in Certain Foodstuffs and Related Matters*; Government Gazette: Pretoria, South Africa, 2013.

39. Ghana: Stakeholder Campaign On the Use of Iodated Salt. Available online: http://allafrica.com/stories/201110060238.html (accessed on 7 May 2017).

40. Intensify Universal Salt Iodization Campaign—Official. Available online: http://www.ghananewsagency.org/print/36 (accessed on 10 May 2017).

41. ICCIDD. Progress of Household Consumption of Iodated Salt in Some African Countries. *Iodine Defic. Disord. Newsl.* **2008**, *31*, 71–78.

42. Cappuccio, F.P.; Kerry, S.M.; Micah, F.B.; Plange-Rhule, J.; Eastwood, J.B. A community programme to reduce salt intake and blood pressure in Ghana. *BMC Public Health* **2006**, *6*. [CrossRef] [PubMed]

43. Charlton, K.E.; Jooste, P.L.; Steyn, K.; Levitt, N.S.; Ghosh, A. A lowered salt intake does not compromise iodine status in Cape Town, South Africa, where salt iodization is mandatory. *Nutrition* **2013**, *29*, 630–634. [CrossRef] [PubMed]

44. Ghana Launches a New Advocacy Campaign on USI. Available online: http://www.ign.org/newsletter/idd_feb14_ghana.pdf (accessed on 9 May 2017).

45. Kowal, P.; Chatterji, S.; Naidoo, N.; Biritwum, R.; Fan, W.; Ridaura, R.L.; Maximova, T.; Arokiasamy, P.; Phaswana-Mafuya, N.; Williams, S.; et al. Data Resource Profile: The World Health Organization Study on global AGEing and adult health (SAGE). *Int. J. Epidemiol.* **2012**, *41*, 1639–1649. [CrossRef] [PubMed]

46. Charlton, K.; Ware, L.J.; Menyanu, E.; Biritwum, R.B.; Naidoo, N.; Pieterse, C.; Madurai, S.; Baumgartner, J.; Asare, G.A.; Thiele, E.; et al. Leveraging ongoing research to evaluate the health impacts of South Africa's salt reduction strategy: A prospective nested cohort within the WHO-SAGE multicountry, longitudinal study. *BMJ Open* **2016**, *6*, e013316. [CrossRef] [PubMed]

47. World Health Organisation. *National Report of the World Health Survey in Ghana, 2002–2004*; WHO: Geneva, Switzerland, 2006.

48. Prevention through Population-Wide Dietary Salt Reduction: Protocol for Population Level Sodium Determination in 24-h Urine Samples. Available online: http://www2.paho.org/hq/dmdocuments/2010/pahosaltprotocol.pdf (accessed on 12 June 2014).

49. Nasreddine, L.; Akl, C.; Al-Shaar, L.; Almedawar, M.M.; Isma'eel, H. Consumer Knowledge, Attitudes and Salt-Related Behavior in the Middle-East: The Case of Lebanon. *Nutrients* **2014**, *6*, 5079–5102. [CrossRef] [PubMed]

50. Land, M.A.; Webster, J.; Christoforou, A.; Johnson, C.; Trevena, H.; Hodgins, F.; Chalmers, J.; Woodward, M.; Barzi, F.; Smith, W.; et al. The association of knowledge, attitudes and behaviours related to salt with 24-h urinary sodium excretion. *Int. J. Behav. Nutr. Phys. Act.* **2014**, *11*. [CrossRef] [PubMed]

51. Magalhaes, P.; Sanhangala, E.J.R.; Dombele, I.M.; Ulundo, H.S.N.; Capingana, D.P.; Silva, A.B.T. Knowledge, attitude and behaviour regarding dietary salt intake among medical students in Angola. *Cardiovasc. J. Afr.* **2015**, *26*, 57–62. [CrossRef] [PubMed]

52. Claro, R.M.; Linders, H.; Ricardo, C.Z.; Legetic, B.; Campbell, N.R.C. Consumer attitudes, knowledge, and behavior related to salt consumption in sentinel countries of the Americas. *Rev. Panam. Salud Publica Pan Am. J. Public Health* **2012**, *32*, 265–273. [CrossRef]

53. Topouchian, J.A.; El Assaad, M.A.; Orobinskaia, L.V.; El Feghali, R.N.; Asmar, R.G. Validation of two automatic devices for self-measurement of blood pressure according to the International Protocol of the European Society of Hypertension: The Omron M6 (HEM-7001-E) and the Omron R7 (HEM 637-IT). *Blood Press. Monit.* **2006**, *11*, 165–171. [CrossRef] [PubMed]

54. WMA Declaration of HELSINKI—Ethical Principles for Medical Research Involving Human Subjects. Available online: https://www.wma.net/policies-post/wma-declaration-of-helsinki-ethical-principles-for-medical-research-involving-human-subjects/ (accessed on 12 May 2017).

55. Zhang, J.; Xu, A.Q.; Ma, J.X.; Shi, X.M.; Guo, X.L.; Engelgau, M.; Yan, L.X.; Li, Y.; Li, Y.C.; Wang, H.C.; et al. Dietary Sodium Intake: Knowledge, Attitudes and Practices in Shandong Province, China, 2011. *PLoS ONE* **2013**, *8*. [CrossRef] [PubMed]

56. Grimes, C.A.; Jane-Kelly, S.; Stanley, S.; Bolam, B.; Webster, J.; Khokhar, D.; Nowson, C. Knowledge, attitudes and behaviours related to dietary salt among adults in the state of Victoria, Australia 2015. *BMC Public Health* **2017**, *17*. [CrossRef] [PubMed]

57. Zhao, F.; Zhang, P.H.; Zhang, L.; Niu, W.Y.; Gao, J.M.; Lu, L.X.; Liu, C.X.; Gao, X. Consumption and Sources of Dietary Salt in Family Members in Beijing. *Nutrients* **2015**, *7*, 2719–2730. [CrossRef] [PubMed]

58. De Kock, H.L.; Zandstra, E.H.; Sayed, N.; Wentzel-Viljoen, E. Liking, salt taste perception and use of table salt when consuming reduced-salt chicken stews in light of South Africa's new salt regulations. *Appetite* **2016**, *96*, 383–390. [CrossRef] [PubMed]

59. Grimes, C.A.; Riddell, L.J.; Nowson, C.A. Consumer knowledge and attitudes to salt intake and labelled salt information. *Appetite* **2009**, *53*, 189–194. [CrossRef] [PubMed]

60. Kamran, A.A.; Azadbakht, L.; Sharifirad, G.; Mahaki, B.; Sharghi, A. Sodium intake, dietary knowledge, and illness perceptions of controlled and uncontrolled rural hypertensive patients. *Int. J. Hypertens.* **2014**, *2014*, 1–7. [CrossRef] [PubMed]

61. The Relationship between Patients' Knowledge on Primary Hypertension and Compliance with Sodium-Restricted Diet Therapy in the Kingdom of Swaziland, Southern Africa. Available online: https://stti.confex.com/stti/congrs07/techprogram/paper_33990.htm (accessed on 30 July 2017).

62. Newson, R.S.; Elmadfa, I.; Biro, G.; Cheng, Y.; Prakash, V.; Rust, P.; Barna, M.; Lion, R.; Meijer, G.W.; Neufingerl, N.; et al. Barriers for progress in salt reduction in the general population. An international study. *Appetite* **2013**, *71*, 22–31. [CrossRef] [PubMed]

63. Papadakis, S.; Pipe, A.L.; Moroz, I.A.; Reid, R.D.; Blanchard, C.M.; Cote, D.F.; Mark, A.E. Knowledge, attitudes and behaviours related to dietary sodium among 35- to 50-year-old Ontario residents. *Can. J. Cardiol.* **2010**, *26*, 164–169. [CrossRef]

64. Khaw, K.T.; Bingham, S.; Welch, A.; Luben, R.; O'Brien, E.; Wareham, N.; Day, N. Blood pressure and urinary sodium in men and women: The Norfolk Cohort of the European Prospective Investigation into cancer (EPIC-Norfolk)(1–3). *Am. J. Clin. Nutr.* **2004**, *80*, 1397–1403. [PubMed]

65. Cornelio, M.E.; Gallani, M.; Godin, G.; Rodrigues, R.C.M.; Nadruz, W.; Mendez, R.D.R. Behavioural determinants of salt consumption among hypertensive individuals. *J. Hum. Nutr. Diet.* **2012**, *25*, 334–344. [CrossRef] [PubMed]

66. Schutte, A.E.; Botha, S.; Fourie, C.M.T.; Gafane-Matemane, L.F.; Kruger, R.; Lammertyn, L.; Malan, L.; Mels, C.M.C.; Schutte, R.; Smith, W.; et al. Recent advances in understanding hypertension development in sub-Saharan Africa. *J. Hum. Hypertens.* **2017**, *31*, 491–500. [CrossRef] [PubMed]

67. Kayima, J.; Nankabirwa, J.; Sinabulya, I.; Nakibuuka, J.; Zhu, X.; Rahman, M.; Longenecker, C.T.; Katamba, A.; Mayanja-Kizza, H.; Kamya, M.R. Determinants of hypertension in a young adult Ugandan population in epidemiological transition—The MEPI-CVD survey. *BMC Public Health* **2015**, *15*. [CrossRef] [PubMed]

68. Campaign to Increase Iodine Intake Launched. Available online: http://ghanahospitals.org/news/details.php?id=625 (accessed on 2 June 2017).

69. At a Glance: Ghana. Available online: https://www.unicef.org/health/ghana_61446.html (accessed on 2 June 2017).

70. Combatting IDD in Ghana. Available online: http://www.ign.org/newsletter/idd_nl_may06_ghana.pdf (accessed on 10 June 2017).

71. Harris, M.J.; Jooste, P.L.; Charlton, K.E. The use of iodised salt in the manufacturing of processed foods in South Africa: Bread and bread premixes, margarine, and flavourants of salty snacks. *Int. J. Food Sci. Nutr.* **2003**, *54*, 13–19. [CrossRef] [PubMed]

72. Glanz, K.; Bishop, D.B. The Role of Behavioral Science Theory in Development and Implementation of Public Health Interventions. In *Annual Review of Public Health*; Fielding, J.E., Brownson, R.C., Green, L.W., Eds.; Annual Reviews: Palo Alto, CA, USA, 2010; Volume 31, pp. 399–418.

73. Webster, J.; Crickmore, C.; Charlton, K.; Steyn, K.; Wentzel-Viljoen, E.; Naidoo, P. South Africa's salt reduction strategy: Are we on track, and what lies ahead? *SAMJ* **2017**, *107*, 20–21. [CrossRef]

74. Chun, I.A.; Park, J.; Han, M.-A.; Choi, S.-W.; Ryu, S.-Y. The Association between smoking, alcohol intake, and low-salt diet: Results from the 2008 Community Health Survey. *J. Korean Diet. Assoc.* **2013**, *12*, 223–235. [CrossRef]

75. Martinez, P.; Landheim, A.; Clausen, T.; Lien, L. A comparison of alcohol use and correlates of drinking patterns among men and women aged 50 and above in Ghana and South Africa. *Afr. J. Drug Alcohol Stud.* **2011**, *10*, 75–87.

76. He, F.J.; Macgregor, G.A. How far should salt intake be reduced? *Hypertens* **2003**, *42*, 1093–1099. [CrossRef] [PubMed]

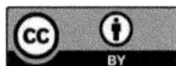

![nutrients logo] *nutrients*

MDPI

Article

Changes in Average Sodium Content of Prepacked Foods in Slovenia during 2011–2015

Igor Pravst [1],*, Živa Lavriša [1], Anita Kušar [1], Krista Miklavec [1] and Katja Žmitek [1,2]

[1] Nutrition Institute, Tržaška cesta 40, SI-1000 Ljubljana, Slovenia; ziva.lavrisa@nutris.org (Ž.L.);
   anita.kusar@nutris.org (A.K.); krista.miklavec@nutris.org (K.M.); katja.zmitek@vist.si (K.Ž.)
[2] VIST—Higher School of Applied Sciences, Gerbičeva cesta 51a, SI-1000 Ljubljana, Slovenia
* Correspondence: igor.pravst@nutris.org; Tel.: +386-590-68871; Fax: +386-1-300-79-81

Received: 5 July 2017; Accepted: 25 August 2017; Published: 29 August 2017

Abstract: A voluntary gradual reduction in the salt content of processed foods was proposed Slovenia in 2010. Our objective was to determine the sodium content of prepacked foods in 2015 and to compare these results with data from 2011. Labelled sodium content and 12-month sales data were collected for prepacked foods ($N = 5759$) from major food stores in Slovenia. The average and sales-weighted sodium content, as well as the share in total sodium sales (STSS) were calculated for different food category levels, particularly focusing on processed meat and derivatives (STSS: 13.1%; 904 mg Na/100 g), bread (9.1%; 546 mg), cheese (5.1%; 524 mg), and ready-to-eat meals (2.2%; 510 mg). Reduced sale-weighted sodium content was observed in cheese (57%), a neutral trend was observed in processed meat and derivatives (99%) and bread (100%), and an increase in sodium content was found in ready meals (112%). Similar trends were observed for average sodium levels, but the difference was significant only in the case of ready meals. No statistically significant changes were observed for the matched products, although about one-third of the matched products had been reformulated by lowering the sodium level by more than 3.8%. Additional efforts are needed to ensure salt reduction in processed foods in Slovenia. Such efforts should combine closer collaboration with the food industry, additional consumer education, and setting specific sodium content targets (limits) for key food categories.

Keywords: sodium; salt; processed foods; food composition; food labelling; food supply

1. Introduction

Excess dietary sodium intake is a well-recognised modifiable risk factor of high systolic blood pressure and a major cause of chronic non-communicable diseases [1,2]. Daily salt intake in most countries varies between 9–12 g [3], which is well above the World Health Organization (WHO) recommendations of a maximum of 5 g salt. It is estimated that globally reducing sodium intake to the recommended level would prevent about 2.5 million deaths annually, which has led to the WHO member states agreeing to cut the global population's sodium intake by 30% by 2025 [4]. Salt-reduction strategy programmes are now established in many countries. These programmes commonly include industry engagement (reformulation), setting sodium content targets for foods, consumer education, front-of-pack labelling schemes, and interventions in public institutions [5]. However, the efficacy of these programmes is not always systematically assessed. Decreasing the sodium intake in the population is considered the best verification of the efficacy of salt-reduction programmes. Major improvements by way of salt intake lowering are reported by a few countries where a long-term multifaceted approach was accompanied with strong political support. For example, a voluntary salt-reduction programme in the UK has led to a reduction in dietary sodium intake by 15% since 2003/2004 [6]. The programme involved collaboration with the food industry and media in addition to scientific and health professionals. Finland was also able to considerably reduce its population's sodium intake by applying similar voluntary codes of practice as part of the North Karelia project [7]. Several approaches were used, including greater education on a healthy diet and compulsory warning label use for high-salt products in many food categories, which resulted in the food industry reformulating numerous products in a bid to avoid such labels.

Although average sodium excretion in 24 h urine is recognised as the gold-standard marker for measuring salt intake in the population [8], this method cannot identify (changes in) food sources of sodium. Therefore, additional assessments of the efficacy of salt-reduction programmes also include monitoring sodium content in the food supply, especially in processed foods. This is very important in countries where salt-reduction programmes include the food industry voluntarily lowering salt content. Such studies have been more or less systematically performed in several countries, including in the USA [9,10], Australia [11,12], New Zealand [13], Canada [14] and the United Kingdom [15]. Studies mostly focus on monitoring the sodium content of processed prepacked foods and sometimes restaurant foods [16].

The sodium content of processed foods varies between different food categories. From a public health perspective, reformulation should be especially stimulated in food categories that present the largest contribution to sodium intake either due to their very high sodium content or their high consumption level by the population. Apart from plain salt (used as a condiment), the most important food sources of sodium include processed meat, bread and bakery products, cheese, as well as ready-to-eat prepared meals [15,17–19].

In Slovenia, the dietary salt intake is around 12 g daily [20], which is more than double the WHO recommendations. In 2010, a national Action Plan to Reduce Salt was accepted with the goal of cutting the population's salt intake to the recommended 5 g daily before 2020 [21]. Reduced salt intake is also a key objective of the recent National Programme on Nutrition and Physical Activity 2015–2025 [22]. In practice, the Action Plan entailed different activities, including increasing public awareness of the recommended salt intake and the risks of excess intake, as well as supporting food operators in gradually reducing the salt content of processed foods. a stepwise approach was taken to reduce salt in critical food categories contributing the most to people's salt intake. It was proposed that the industry should gradually cut processed foods' salt content in critical food categories by 3.8–5.8% each year. The first sodium content monitoring of prepacked foods occurred in 2011 using a sales-weighted approach [19]. This study showed that a robust and cost-effective approach to assessing prepacked foods' average sodium content could be achieved by employing a combination of 12-month food sales data, as provided by food retailers and covering most of the national market, and a comprehensive food composition database compiled using food labelling data. The study also revealed that in most investigated food categories, the market leaders had lower sodium levels than the average of that particular category [19].

The objective of this present study is to investigate sodium levels in prepacked foods in the Slovenian food supply in 2015 and to compare these results with the data available for 2011. We aim to particularly focus on processed meat and derivatives, plain bread, cheese, as well as ready-to-eat meals. The assessment relied on both the average sodium content of available prepacked foods and the sales-weighted average sodium content.

2. Materials and Methods

2.1. Collection of Data for 2015

Cross-sectional data on the nutritional composition of prepacked foods in the Slovenian food supply were collected during January–February 2015 in five shops (two mega markets, two supermarkets, and a discount market) of three major grocery chains with the largest nationwide shop networks (Spar, Mercator, and Hofer). Sampling was done in Ljubljana, Slovenia. In agreement with the retailers, all prepacked products with a unique European/International Article Number (EAN) barcode were systematically photographed and recorded in an online Composition and Labelling Information System (CLAS) database [23]. The database is supported by a specially developed computer application, which enables digital recognition of EAN codes to accelerate the database's formation and avoid duplicate entries. The information collected included a product's name, list of ingredients, nutritional values, packaging volume, price, and EAN barcode. For the purposes of this article, only sodium contents are reported. The CLAS database was further complemented with country-wide, 12-month sales data obtained from retailers. This data covered most of the national market and ensured proper data handling. These sales data refer to the national market and present food product sales for the 12 months prior to the data collection (January–December 2014). This was arranged on the condition that the results would not reveal any particular retailer's sales data. The sales data were given in universal form, including the EAN number, product description, number of products sold per year, and the quantity of food (kg or L) per packaging. The matching of foods was performed using EAN numbers. For the many products with the same EAN number that were available in different stores, the sales data from different retailers were combined to obtain the overall national yearly sales data for a product. According to the protocol developed within the Global Food Monitoring Initiative (GFMI) by Dunford et al. [24], we collected food data for the following categories: fruit and vegetable juices; soft drinks; cordials; coffee and tea; electrolyte drinks; waters; bread; biscuits; cakes; muffins and pastry; cereal bars; noodles; breakfast cereals; pasta; maize (corn); rice; couscous; unprocessed cereals; chocolate and sweets; jelly; chewing gum; pizza; soup; ready meals; pre-prepared salads and sandwiches; cheese; yoghurt products; milk; cream; desserts; ice cream and edible ices; butter and margarine; cooking oils; canned fish and seafood; chilled fish; frozen fish; baby foods; meal replacements; vegetables; fruit; jam and spreads; nuts and seeds; processed meat and derivatives; meat alternatives; crisps and snacks; sauces; mayonnaise/dressings; spreads; as well as honey and syrups. Alcoholic beverages and food supplements were not included. The samples included all foods available in the selected grocery stores at the time of sampling and for which sales data were available. In the next stage, food categories with less than 10 products with a nutritional declaration (sodium content) available were excluded from the analyses (maize; couscous; chewing gum; pre-prepared salads and sandwiches; chilled fish; meal replacements; as well as honey and syrups). The total food sample comprised 8323 products with available sales data, of which 5759 (69.2%) had their sodium content labelled and were therefore used for the calculations of the average sodium contents.

2.2. Use of Data for 2011

The comparison was performed with previously reported cross-sectional data for 2011 [19], which were collected in four shops (one mega market, two supermarkets, and a discount shop) of the same three major grocery chains as those collected in 2015. To enable easier comparison, all products in the 2011 database were re-categorised in line with the GFMI protocol [24]. Results are reported only for 22 (sub)categories for which the data collection included a complete food category as defined by GFMI: fruit and vegetable juices; soft drinks; electrolyte drinks; plain bread; biscuits; cakes, muffins and pastry; noodles; plain pasta; rice; pizza; ready meals; cheese; yoghurt products; milk; cream; butter and margarine; canned fish and seafood; processed meat and derivatives; pasta sauces; mayonnaise/dressings; meat spreads; vegetable spreads. Such dataset comprised 3745 products, of which 1374 (36.7%) were labelled with sodium content and used for the calculations of the average sodium contents.

2.3. Calculation of Average Sodium Content per (Sub)Category

The average sodium content of available prepacked foods (SCA; in mg of sodium per 100 g/mL) and average sodium content of sold prepacked foods (SCS; mg per 100 g/mL) were calculated for selected food (sub)categories for 2011 and 2015, according to the previously reported protocol [19]. SCa values present the average sodium content of all products within a specific (sub)category for which sodium/salt levels were labelled. SCS values present the average sodium content of all products sold within a specific category for which sodium levels were labelled. Ratios between SCa and SCS (SAR values) were also calculated.

2.4. Share in Total Sodium Sales (STSS)

Share in total sodium sales (STSS) was calculated using the data for 2015. Using the data related to the content of food per packaging, we calculated the amount (kg/L) of each product sold per year. In the next stage, the total sodium content of products sold within a specific food category (kg) was calculated using labelled sodium levels and 12-month sales data. STSS was calculated as the ratio between the total sodium in all sold foods in the (sub)category and the total sodium in all sold foods in the sample.

2.5. Data Processing and Statistical Analyses

The data were processed and evaluated using the computer programs Microsoft SQL Server Management Studio V13.0, Microsoft Analysis Services Client Tools 13.0, Microsoft Data Access Components (MDAC) 10.0, Microsoft Excel 2013 (Redmond, WA, USA), the program tool CLAS V1.0 (Composition and Labelling Information System; Nutrition Institute, Ljubljana, Slovenia), and the XLStat statistical software package V19.01 (Addinsoft, Barcelona, Spain). For SCA, the 95% confidence intervals (95% CI) were calculated. SCS was given as an exact value and, therefore, no confidence intervals are presented. Given that the samples consisted of all available foods in the food supply in the selected stores, a comparison between years was performed directly by calculating the SCa (2015/2011) and SCS (2015/2011) ratios. For statistical evaluation of differences in the average sodium content of available prepacked foods, a t-test or Mann-Whitney U test (for non-parametric variables) was used. For statistical comparison of the matched products in processed meat and derivatives, plain bread, cheese, and ready-to-eat meals between the years of 2011 and 2015, a paired t-test was used. $p < 0.05$ was considered to be statistically significant.

3. Results

SCa and SCS was calculated using the CLAS database with representative data on the availability of prepacked foods on the Slovenian market and 12-month, country-wide sales data for each product included in the database (see Table 1 for data on selected food categories, and Supplementary Table S1 for complete data). The food categories with the largest contribution to overall sodium sales (STSS >3%) were processed meat and derivatives (13.1%); vegetables (9.4%; particularly in canned vegetables: 9.1%); waters (9.4%); bread (9.1%); milk (8.6%); biscuits (6.6%); crisps and snacks (6.3%); cheese (5.1%); breakfast cereals (3.8%); and sauces (3.0%). The highest sodium average content (SCA) was observed in sauces (1131 mg/100 g; 95% CI: 877–1386 mg); processed meat and derivatives (984 mg/100 g; 95% CI: 910–1058 mg); crisps and snacks (787 mg/100 g; 95% CI: 742–833 mg); canned fish and seafood (659 mg/100 g; 95% CI: 478–840 mg); mayonnaise and dressings (580 mg/100 g; 95% CI: 512–648 mg); bread (546 mg/100 g; 95% CI: 512–580 mg); pizza (539 mg/100 g; 95% CI: 493–586 mg); cheese (524 mg/100 g; 95% CI: 480–567 mg); and ready-to-eat meals (510 mg/100 g; 95% CI: 469–551 mg). On the other hand, inclusion of sales data gave the highest SCS values for processed meat and derivatives (904 mg/100 g); crisps and snacks (804 mg/100 g); sauces (720 mg/100 g); pizza (519 mg/100 g); and bread (505 mg/100 g). The biggest differences between SCa and SCS values were observed in the categories of breakfast cereals (SAR: 7%); fruit and vegetable juices (14%); noodles (27%); as well as waters (321%).

The comparison of the determined average sodium levels in prepacked foods in the Slovenian food supply in 2015 was further assessed according to the data collected in 2011 [19]. The between-years SCA/SCS levels are presented in Table 1, Supplementary Table S1 and Figure 1 (SCS levels only; included (sub)categories with STSS > 0.5%, for which data for both 2011 and 2015 were available). In the food (sub)categories making a notable contribution to overall sodium intake, reduced sale-weighted sodium content was observed in biscuits (SCS 2015/2011 ratio: 80%); cheese (57%); and meat spreads (71%), while there was a neutral trend in sodium content in processed meat and derivatives (99%) and bread (100%). Interestingly, increased salt content was also observed in a considerable number of food categories with comparatively lower STSS ratios, including cakes, muffins, and pastry (105%); ready-to-eat meals (112%); mayonnaise/dressings (109%); and pasta sauces (111%). Similar trends were also found for the SCa values of most of the abovementioned categories. However, statistically significant changes between the years of 2011 and 2015 were observed only for the ready-to-eat meals and pasta sauces. In both cases, we determined an increase in SCa levels (SCa 2015/2011 ratio: 106% ($p = 0.013$) and 155% ($p = 0.002$), respectively). We noted a considerable increase in the proportion of products with labelled sodium content from 2011 to 2015 (from 34% to 66% for ready-to-eat meals; as well as from 21% to 65% for pasta sauces). Due to a lack of sodium content data, a considerable proportion of 2011 sample was not included into analyses, and this limited the comparison of both samples in food categories with the lowest penetration of nutrition declaration (meat spreads (Percentage of products with labelled sodium content (% LSC): 4%); canned fish and seafood (12%); cakes, muffins, and pastry (12%); cheese (13%); processed meat and derivatives (15%); cream (19%); pasta sauces (21%); plain bread (30%); noodles (31%); and ready meals (34%)).

Considering the national Action Plan to Reduce Salt [21], which had proposed voluntarily gradually reducing the salt content of processed foods in critical food categories by 3.8–5.8% per year, progress in cutting salt content was particularly expected in processed meat and derivatives, plain bread, cheese, and ready-to-eat meals. Therefore, we further focused on these (sub)categories and compared the composition of matching products (same brands) for which composition data were available in both 2011 and 2015 databases. a total of 98 such foods were identified. No statistically significant changes were observed for the matched products in the selected food categories ($p = 0.08$, 0.22, 0.25, and 0.76 for processed meat and derivatives; cheese; plain bread; and ready-to-eat meals, respectively), although about one-third of the matched products had been reformulated by lowering the sodium level by more than 3.8% (35%, 32%, 24%, and 21%, respectively).

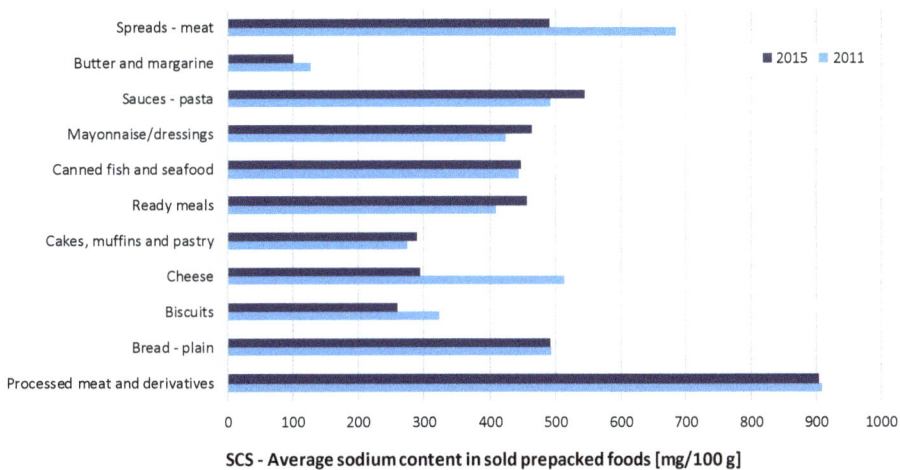

Figure 1. Comparison of the average sodium content of sold (SCS) prepacked foods for selected food (sub)categories (mg/100 g) in 2011 and 2015.

Table 1. Average sodium content of available (SCA) and sold (SCS) prepacked foods for selected food categories in 2011 and 2015.

Food Category	N	% LSC[1]	Year 2015 Average Sodium Content (mg per 100 g/mL) SCa (95% CI)[2]	SCS[3]	SAR: SCS/SCa Ratio[4]	STSS[5]	N	% LSC[1]	Year 2011 Average Sodium Content (mg per 100 g/mL) SCa (95% CI)[2]	SCS[3]	SCa Ratio 2015/2011	SCS Ratio 2015/2011
Waters	80	71%	15 (0–42)	47	321%	9.4%						
Bread	126	83%	546 (512–580)	505	92%	9.1%	155	30%	488 (449–527)	493	109%	100%
- plain	111	81%	530 (499–562)	492	93%	8.1%	485	45%	353 (312–394)	324	95%	80%
Biscuits	655	73%	335 (305–364)	259	78%	6.6%	73	12%	226 (169–283)	275	119%	105%
Cakes, muffins and pastry	285	71%	268 (246–289)	289	108%	2.5%	67	31%	94 (0–195)	20	109%	136%
Noodles	103	77%	103 (61–145)	27	27%	0.1%						
Breakfast cereals	212	94%	215 (182–248)	14	7%	3.8%						
Pasta	296	88%	128 (102–154)	75	58%	1.3%						
- plain	242	88%	61 (40–81)	55	91%	0.9%	281	53%	15 (7–23)	29	398% *	193%
- filled	54	87%	431 (380–482)	409	95%	0.4%						
Pizza	21	71%	539 (493–586)	519	96%	0.2%	23	70%	932 (649–1215)	799	58%	65%
Soups - concentrated	150	78%	425 (353–497)	387	91%	0.8%						
Ready meals	206	66%	510 (469–551)	457	90%	2.2%	152	34%	480 (367–579)	409	106% *	112%
Cheese	292	74%	524 (480–567)	294	56%	5.1%	381	13%	626 (429–823)	513	84%	57%
Butter and margarine	85	78%	144 (101–187)	101	71%	1.0%	74	62%	168 (100–236)	127	86%	80%
Canned fish and seafood	155	61%	659 (478–840)	447	68%	2.2%	180	12%	443 (375–511)	444	149%	101%
Vegetables	453	56%	395 (335–455)	319	81%	9.4%						
- canned	330	60%	484 (413–555)	382	79%	9.1%						
Processed meat and derivatives	362	47%	984 (910–1058)	904	92%	13.1%	363	15%	1116 (952–1258)	909	88%	99%
Meat alternatives	53	58%	453 (318–589)	220	48%	0.1%						
Crisps and snacks	206	86%	787 (742–833)	804	102%	6.3%						
Sauces	273	55%	1131 (877–1386)	720	64%	3.0%						
- pasta	108	65%	601 (528–673)	545	91%	1.1%	135	21%	386 (288–484)	492	155% *	111%
Mayonnaise/dressings	48	92%	580 (512–648)	464	80%	1.3%	36	47%	576 (481–671)	424	101%	109%
Spreads	234	57%	425 (359–490)	192	45%	1.0%						
- meat	131	45%	509 (469–548)	490	96%	0.6%	123	4%	626 (573–679)	686	81%	71%
- vegetable	48	71%	653 (454–853)	524	80%	0.1%	39	44%	578 (408–748)	459	113%	114%

Notes: Results for all food categories are presented in a Supplementary Table S1; [1] % LSC: Percentage of products with labelled sodium content; [2] SCA: Average sodium content of available prepacked foods (95% confidence interval); [3] SCS: Average sodium content of sold prepacked foods; [4] SAR: Ratio between SCa and SCS; [5] STSS: Share in total sodium sales; [6] Data from Korošec et al. 2014 [19], with foods categorised according to Dunford et al. 2012 [24]. * p-value < 0.05 (using t-test and Mann-Whitney test for comparison of Average sodium content of available prepacked foods (SCA) between both years).

4. Discussion

Using a combination of 12-month food sales data provided by food retailers covering most of the national market along with a comprehensive food composition database compiled using food labelling data, we showed that processed meat and derivatives (STSS: 13.1%), canned vegetables (9.1%), and plain bread (8.1%) were major sources of salt in prepacked foods in the Slovenian food supply in 2015 due to their high sodium levels and high level of consumption by the population.

Similar to the 2011 study [25], the highest sodium content was found in processed meats and derivatives (SCS: 904 mg/100 g) in 2015. The between-years comparison shows that although the average sodium content in the category was reduced (SCa 2015/2011: 82%), this change was not significant ($p = 0.13$) and there were also no important changes in the sales-weighted sodium content (SCS 2015/2011 ratio: 99%). Reduced sale-weighted sodium content was observed in cheese, butter and margarine, biscuits, as well as meat spreads (SCS 2015/2011: 57%, 80%, 80%, and 71%, respectively) (Table 1 and Supplementary Table S1). Differences in SCa levels showed similar but insignificant trends (SCa 2015/2011: 84%, 86%, 95%, and 81%, respectively).

Bread is considered a major source of sodium intake in the Slovenian population [26]. This was confirmed by our study as bread contributed 9.1% of total sodium sales. Unfortunately, we did not observe any shift towards lower sodium levels, even though this food category was a particular target of activities within the national Action Plan to Reduce Salt [21]. There was no statistical significant change in the SCa of plain bread between 2011 and 2015 (109%; $p = 0.12$). Furthermore, the sales-weighted sodium content in plain bread was the same as that in 2011 (SCS: 492 mg/100 g). For comparison, about 10% lower sales-weighted sodium levels in bread was reported in the UK study [15]. Considering that bread in Slovenia is chiefly sold as a non-prepacked product (not included in this study), this limits the generalisability of our results for this specific food category. It should be mentioned that a step towards cutting sodium content in bread was suggested by a very recent initiative for the self-regulation of foods produced in the bakery product sector, which is expected to be launched by the Slovenian Chamber of Commerce (SCC) in 2018. Changing sodium levels in bread will be particularly challenging since a very large number of food businesses operate in this sector, many of which are not SCC members. An interesting approach was taken in the Netherlands, where the bakery sector itself requested that mandatory maximum sodium levels be set for bread to ensure fair competition, while the levels for other categories are voluntary and do not attract formal sanctions [27].

Increased sodium content was observed in cakes, muffins, and pastry; ready-to-eat meals; mayonnaise/dressings; and pasta sauces (SCS 2015/2011: 105%, 112%, 109%, and 111%), which altogether contributed about 7% of the total sodium sales (STSS). Similar trends were observed with the SCa ratios where there was a statistically significant increase in sodium content of ready-to-eat meals and pasta sauces (SCa 2015/2011: 106% and 155% with $p < 0.05$ for both). Given that such "convenience" foods are gaining in importance for a large number of consumers [28], greater efforts should be targeted at these food groups. Several European Union (EU) member states already use such an approach [3,6,29]; however, harmonised activities on the EU level are essential, particularly in those food categories featuring a large proportion of internationally produced foods. An example of such an activity would be setting international minimum targets for salt reductions in key food categories. This can be done within the "EU platform for action on diet, physical activity and health" [30] with the support of "the high level group on nutrition and physical activity"—a group of European government representatives led by the European Commission (EC) [31]. Surprisingly, bottled water was also identified as a major contributor to total sodium sales among prepacked foods (STSS: 9.4%). To gain greater insight into this, we identified high sodium mineral waters as a major contributor to this large share. Among the 80 waters included in our analyses, sodium content levels were available for 56 of them. Ten mineral waters high in sodium (sodium $\geq$ over 200 mg/L) represented 99% of the abovementioned STSS value. It should be noted that in most natural mineral sodium waters, the predominant ion accompanying sodium is bicarbonate, which is considered to have a smaller effect on blood pressure than equivalent amounts of sodium chloride [32,33]. Water with the highest sodium level in our database contained 1700 mg of sodium (and only 58 g of chloride) per litre. This particular mineral water was labelled with a warning that the recommended intake is up to 0.3 L per day.

In line with observations made in 2011 [19], sales-weighted sodium levels were lower than average sodium levels for most food categories in Slovenia, which suggests lower than average sodium contents in market leaders (Table 1). However, this could be attributed to a mix of different factors, including brand trust, price, taste and texture expectations, as well as consumer experiences with a particular food product, rather than consumers' awareness of health risks created by a high sodium intake.

The first monitoring of sodium content in foods in the Slovenian food supply was performed just after the national Action Plan to Reduce Salt in 2011 was launched [21]. a limitation of the 2011 study [19] was that the food sample was originally collected to assess the penetration of different food labelling information, particularly nutrition and health claims [25]. Therefore, some food categories relevant to sodium intake were not included. However, a major strength of the 2011 data collection and of this present study is that all foods available in the selected food categories were included, while the varying importance (as dietary sources of sodium) of the different products was accounted for on a product-to-product basis by including sales data. Such an exact approach is rarely taken because researchers typically do not have access to sales data on a product-to-product basis. This approach was first taken in the UK by Mhurchu et al., who used a combination of commercial consumer panel food-purchasing data with nutrient data over 12 months for a more precise assessment of processed foods' sodium content and estimation of the population's exposure to sodium [15]. Since such a consumer panel does not exist in Slovenia, 12-month, nationwide sales data provided by retailers was used. The 2011 study protocol was revised for this present study to include all key prepacked food categories, resulting in a more extensive data collection. a strength of this present study is therefore the extent of the data collection and its employment of sales data to assess average sodium contents in various food categories. The database generated for such a study is useful for various purposes. Besides monitoring changes in the food supply, such a database can be also employed as a source of data in studies where food recalls or diaries are used. Considering that such a database should be regularly updated, this could present a considerable challenge in many countries. In addition, compiling such a comprehensive database is not always possible. Mutual trust must exist between academia and food retailers to successfully use our methodology (sales-weighted approach), which might not be feasible in all environments. In our case, such trust was gained with the national authorities' support for our efforts, an open discussion of issues related to data sharing, and by our strict commitment to protect the data. Another limitation of the study is that about 30% of the selected products were excluded from further analyses due to missing data on sodium levels. The mandatory labelling of salt content on processed prepacked foods in the EU, which was enforced since December 2016 [34], will enable an even larger proportion of foods to be used in such studies in the future. Furthermore, the study was not designed to investigate non-processed foods, which are a notable source of sodium intake.

5. Conclusions

The results of this study indicate that activities forming the national Action Plan to Reduce Salt had a limited effect on sodium levels in major prepacked food categories that are considered as major dietary sources of sodium. In this respect, extra efforts are needed to ensure further progress, which should entail even closer collaboration with the food industry and additional consumer education. Specific target sodium content values should be set for key food categories, rather than the expected annual lowering of sodium content in foods, as contained in the existing Action Plan. Further studies are needed to verify the efficacy of salt-reduction programmes, which should include both measuring the dietary intake of sodium and changes in sodium levels in foods in the future food supply.

Supplementary Materials: The following are available online at www.mdpi.com/2072-6643/9/9/952/s1. Table S1: Average sodium content of available (SCA) and sold (SCS) prepacked foods for selected food categories in 2011 and 2015.

Acknowledgments: The authors would like to thank the retailers for allowing access to their stores and sales data. We also acknowledge the help of collaborating students for their help in the data collection, and Murray Bales for providing assistance with the language. The work was financially supported by the Slovenian Research Agency (P3-0395: Nutrition and Public Health). The funding organisation had no role in the design, analysis, or writing of this article.

Author Contributions: I.P. was responsible for assuring the setup and funding of the study, he prepared the study design, collaborated in the data analyses, and contributed to writing the manuscript. Z.L. performed the data analyses, wrote the technical section, and prepared the first drafts of the tables and figures. K.M. coordinated the data collection and collaborated in data analyses. A.K. helped prepare the study design and critically reviewed the manuscript. K.Z. helped prepare the study design and data analyses, and wrote the manuscript.

Conflicts of Interest: The authors would like to acknowledge that I.P. has led/participated in various other research projects in the area of nutrition/public health/food technology, which were (co)funded by the Slovenian Research Agency, the Ministry of Health of the Republic of Slovenia, the Ministry of Agriculture, Forestry and Food of the Republic of Slovenia, and in case of specific applied research projects also by food businesses. The authors have no other conflicts of interest to disclose.

References

1. World Health Organization (WHO). *Reducing Salt Intake in Populations: Report of a WHO Forum and Technical Meeting*; World Health Organization: Geneva, Switzerland, 2007.
2. Forouzanfar, M.H.; Afshin, A.; Alexander, L.T.; Anderson, H.R.; Bhutta, Z.A.; Biryukov, S.; Brauer, M.; Burnett, R.; Cercy, K.; Charlson, F.J.; et al. Global, regional, and national comparative risk assessment of 79 behavioural, environmental and occupational, and metabolic risks or clusters of risks, 1990–2015: a systematic analysis for the Global Burden of Disease Study 2015. *Lancet* **2016**, *388*, 1659–1724. [CrossRef]
3. He, F.J.; MacGregor, G.A. a comprehensive review on salt and health and current experience of worldwide salt reduction programmes. *J. Hum. Hypertens.* **2009**, *23*, 363–384. [CrossRef] [PubMed]
4. WHO. Salt Reduction Faact Sheet. Available online: http://www.who.int/mediacentre/factsheets/fs393/en/ (accessed on 27 June 2017).
5. Trieu, K.; Neal, B.; Hawkes, C.; Dunford, E.; Campbell, N.; Rodriguez-Fernandez, R.; Legetic, B.; McLaren, L.; Barberio, A.; Webster, J. Salt Reduction Initiatives around the World—a Systematic Review of Progress towards the Global Target. *PLoS ONE* **2015**, *10*, e0130247. [CrossRef] [PubMed]
6. He, F.J.; Brinsden, H.C.; Macgregor, G.A. Salt reduction in the United Kingdom: a successful experiment in public health. *J. Hum. Hypertens.* **2013**, *28*, 345–352. [CrossRef] [PubMed]
7. Puska, P. Successful prevention of non-communicable diseases: 25 year experiences with North Karelia Project in Finland. *Public Health Med.* **2002**, *4*, 5–7.
8. Espeland, M.A.; Kumanyika, S.; Wilson, A.C.; Reboussin, D.M.; Easter, L.; Self, M.; Robertson, J.; Brown, W.M.; McFarlane, M. Statistical issues in analyzing 24-hour dietary recall and 24-hour urine collection data for sodium and potassium intakes. *Am. J. Epidemiol.* **2001**, *153*, 996–1006. [CrossRef] [PubMed]
9. Gillespie, C.; Maalouf, J.; Yuan, K.M.; Cogswell, M.E.; Gunn, J.P.; Levings, J.; Moshfegh, A.; Ahuja, J.K.C.; Merritt, R. Sodium content in major brands of US packaged foods, 2009. *Am. J. Clin. Nutr.* **2015**, *101*, 344–353. [CrossRef] [PubMed]
10. Ahuja, J.K.C.; Pehrsson, P.R.; Cogswell, M. a Comparison of Concentrations of Sodium and Related Nutrients (Potassium, Total Dietary Fiber, Total and Saturated Fat, and Total Sugar) in Private-Label and National Brands of Popular, Sodium-Contributing, Commercially Packaged Foods in the United States. *J. Acad. Nutr. Diet.* **2017**, *117*, 770–777. [CrossRef] [PubMed]
11. Trevena, H.; Neal, B.; Dunford, E.; Haskelberg, H.; Wu, J.H.Y. a Comparison of the Sodium Content of Supermarket Private-Label and Branded Foods in Australia. *Nutrients* **2015**, *7*, 7027–7041. [CrossRef] [PubMed]
12. Zganiacz, F.; Wills, R.B.H.; Mukhopadhyay, S.P.; Arcot, J.; Greenfield, H. Changes in the Sodium Content of Australian Processed Foods between 1980 and 2013 Using Analytical Data. *Nutrients* **2017**, *9*, 501. [CrossRef] [PubMed]
13. Monro, D.; Mhurchu, C.N.; Jiang, Y.N.; Gorton, D.; Eyles, H. Changes in the Sodium Content of New Zealand Processed Foods: 2003–2013. *Nutrients* **2015**, *7*, 4054–4067. [CrossRef] [PubMed]

14. Arcand, J.; Jefferson, K.; Schermel, A.; Shah, F.; Trang, S.; Kutlesa, D.; Lou, W.; L'Abbe, M.R. Examination of food industry progress in reducing the sodium content of packaged foods in Canada: 2010 to 2013. *Appl. Phys. Nutr. Metab.* **2016**, *41*, 684–690. [CrossRef] [PubMed]

15. Mhurchu, C.N.; Capelin, C.; Dunford, E.K.; Webster, J.L.; Neal, B.C.; Jebb, S.A. Sodium content of processed foods in the United Kingdom: Analysis of 44,000 foods purchased by 21,000 households. *Am. J. Clin. Nutr.* **2011**, *93*, 594–600. [CrossRef] [PubMed]

16. Ahuja, J.K.C.; Pehrsson, P.R.; Haytowitz, D.B.; Wasswa-Kintu, S.; Nickle, M.; Showell, B.; Thomas, R.; Roseland, J.; Williams, J.; Khan, M.; et al. Sodium monitoring in commercially processed and restaurant foods. *Am. J. Clin. Nutr.* **2015**, *101*, 622–631. [CrossRef] [PubMed]

17. Webster, J.L.; Dunford, E.K.; Neal, B.C. a systematic survey of the sodium contents of processed foods. *Am. J. Clin. Nutr.* **2010**, *91*, 413–420. [CrossRef] [PubMed]

18. Keogh, J.B.; Lange, K.; Hogarth, R.; Clifton, P.M. Foods contributing to sodium intake and urinary sodium excretion in a group of Australian women. *Public Health Nutr.* **2013**, *16*, 1837–1842. [CrossRef] [PubMed]

19. Korosec, Z.; Pravst, I. Assessing the average sodium content of prepacked foods with nutrition declarations: The importance of sales data. *Nutrients* **2014**, *6*, 3501–3515. [CrossRef] [PubMed]

20. Ribic, C.H.; Zakotnik, J.M.; Vertnik, L.; Vegnuti, M.; Cappuccio, F.P. Salt intake of the Slovene population assessed by 24 h urinary sodium excretion. *Public Health Nutr.* **2010**, *13*, 1803–1809. [CrossRef] [PubMed]

21. Ministry of Health of the Republic of Slovenia. National Action Plan for Reducing the Consumption of Salt in the Diet of the Population of Slovenia for the Period 2010–2020 (In Slovenian: Nacionalni Akcijski Načrt za Zmanjševanje Uživanja Soli v Prehrani Prebivalcev Slovenije za Obdobje 2010–2020). Available online: http://www.mz.gov.si/fileadmin/mz.gov.si/pageuploads/mz_dokumenti/delovna_podrocja/javno_zdravje/petric/Nacio_akcijski_nacrt_za_zmanj_uziv_soli_v_prehrani_preb_Slo_2010-2010.pdf (accessed on 27 June 2017).

22. Republic of Slovenia. Resolution on National Programme on Nutrition and Physical Activity 2015–2025 (In Slovenian: Resolucija o Nacionalnem Programu o Prehrani in Telesni Dejavnosti za Zdravje 2015–2025). Available online: http://www.mz.gov.si/fileadmin/mz.gov.si/pageuploads/javna_razprava_2015/Resolucija_o_nac_programu_prehrane_in_in_tel_dejavnosti_jan_2015.pdf (accessed on 27 June 2017).

23. Nutrition Institute. Podatkovna Baza CLAS Kot Orodje za Vrednotenje Sprememb na Področju Ponudbe Predpakiranih Živil v Sloveniji. Available online: http://www.nutris.org/clas/ (accessed on 16 August 2017).

24. Dunford, E.; Webster, J.; Metzler, A.B.; Czernichow, S.; Ni Mhurchu, C.; Wolmarans, P.; Snowdon, W.; L'Abbe, M.; Li, N.; Maulik, P.K.; et al. International collaborative project to compare and monitor the nutritional composition of processed foods. *Eur. J. Prev. Cardiol.* **2012**, *19*, 1326–1332. [CrossRef] [PubMed]

25. Pravst, I.; Kušar, A. Consumers' exposure to nutrition and health claims on prepacked foods: Use of sales weighting for assessing the food supply in Slovenia. *Nutrients* **2015**, *7*, 9353–9368. [CrossRef] [PubMed]

26. Hlastan Ribič, C.; Zakotnik, J.M.; Seljak, K.B.; Poličnik, R.; Blaznik, U.; Mis, F.N.; Eržen, I.; Ji, C.; Cappucio, F.P. Estimation of sodium availability in food in Slovenia: Results from household food purchase data from 2000 to 2009. *Slov. J. Public Health* **2014**, *53*, 209.

27. Centraal Bureau Levensmiddelhandel. National Agreement to Improve Product Composition 2014–2020. Available online: http://www.akkoordverbeteringproductsamenstelling.nl/en (accessed on 30 June 2017).

28. Sarmugam, R.; Worsley, A. Dietary Behaviours, Impulsivity and Food Involvement: Identification of Three Consumer Segments. *Nutrients* **2015**, *7*, 8036–8057. [CrossRef] [PubMed]

29. European Commission. Survey on Members States' Implementation of the EU Salt Reduction Framework. Available online: https://ec.europa.eu/health//sites/health/files/nutrition_physical_activity/docs/salt_report1_en.pdf (accessed on 16 August 2017).

30. European Commission. EU Platform for Action on Diet, Physical Activity and Health. Available online: https://ec.europa.eu/health/nutrition_physical_activity/platform_en (accessed on 16 August 2017).

31. European Commission. High Level Group: Salt Campaign. Available online: http://ec.europa.eu/health/nutrition_physical_activity/high_level_group/nutrition_salt_en.htm (accessed on 29 April 2014).

32. Casado, A.; Ramos, P.; Rodriguez, J.; Moreno, N.; Gil, P. Types and Characteristics of Drinking Water for Hydration in the Elderly. *Crit. Rev. Food Sci. Nutr.* **2015**, *55*, 1633–1641. [CrossRef] [PubMed]

33. Quattrini, S.; Pampaloni, B.; Brandi, M.L. Natural mineral waters: Chemical characteristics and health effects. *Clin. Cases Miner. Bone Metab.* **2016**, *13*, 173–180. [CrossRef] [PubMed]

34. European Comission. Regulation (EU) No 1169/2011 of the European Parliament and of the Council of 25 October 2011 on the Provision of Food Information to Consumers. Available online: http://eur-lex.europa.eu/legal-content/EN/TXT/PDF/?uri=CELEX:02011R1169-20140219 (accessed on 29 March 2017).

nutrients

MDPI

Article

Urinary Sodium-to-Potassium Ratio Tracks the Changes in Salt Intake during an Experimental Feeding Study Using Standardized Low-Salt and High-Salt Meals among Healthy Japanese Volunteers

Midori Sasaki Yatabe [1,2,3], Toshiyuki Iwahori [4,5], Ami Watanabe [1], Kozue Takano [1], Hironobu Sanada [2], Tsuyoshi Watanabe [2], Atsuhiro Ichihara [3], Robin A. Felder [6], Katsuyuki Miura [5,7], Hirotsugu Ueshima [5,7], Junko Kimura [1] and Junichi Yatabe [1,2,3,*]

[1] Department of Pharmacology, Fukushima Medical University School of Medicine, Fukushima 960-1295, Japan; midorisy@endm.twmu.ac.jp (M.S.Y.); amichacha3@gmail.com (A.W.); takak1209@gmail.com (K.T.)
[2] Department of Nephrology, Hypertension, Diabetology, Endocrinology and Metabolism, Fukushima Medical University School of Medicine, Fukushima 960-1295, Japan; sndmak2006@yahoo.co.jp (H.S.); twat0423@fmu.ac.jp (T.W.)
[3] Department of Medicine II, Endocrinology and Hypertension, Tokyo Women's Medical University, Tokyo 162-8666, Japan; atzichi@endm.twmu.ac.jp
[4] Research and Development Department, Omron Healthcare Co., Ltd., Muko 617-0002, Japan; iwahori@belle.shiga-med.ac.jp
[5] Department of Public Health, Shiga University of Medical Science, Shiga 520-2192, Japan; miura@belle.shiga-med.ac.jp (K.M.); hueshima@belle.shiga-med.ac.jp (H.U.)
[6] Department of Pathology, University of Virginia Health System, Charlottesville, VA 22908, USA; raf7k@virginia.edu
[7] Center for Epidemiologic Research in Asia, Shiga University of Medical Science, Shiga 520-2192, Japan
*   Correspondence: jyatabe@endm.twmu.ac.jp; Tel.: +81-333-538-111

Received: 6 June 2017; Accepted: 25 August 2017; Published: 29 August 2017

Abstract: The Na/K ratio is considered to be a useful index, the monitoring of which allows an effective Na reduction and K increase, because practical methods (self-monitoring devices and reliable individual estimates from spot urine) are available for assessing these levels in individuals. An intervention trial for lowering the Na/K ratio has demonstrated that a reduction of the Na/K ratio mainly involved Na reduction, with only a small change in K. The present study aimed to clarify the relationship between dietary Na intake and the urinary Na/K molar ratio, using standardized low- and high-salt diets, with an equal dietary K intake, to determine the corresponding Na/K ratio. Fourteen healthy young adult volunteers ingested low-salt (3 g salt per day) and high-salt (20 g salt per day) meals for seven days each. Using a portable urinary Na/K meter, participants measured their spot urine at each voiding, and 24-h urine was collected on the last day of each diet period. On the last day of the unrestricted, low-salt, and high-salt diet periods, the group averages of the 24-h urine Na/K ratio were 4.2, 1.0, and 6.9, while the group averages of the daily mean spot urine Na/K ratio were 4.2, 1.1, and 6.6, respectively. The urinary Na/K ratio tracked changes in dietary salt intake, and reached a plateau approximately three days after each change in diet. Frequent monitoring of the spot urine Na/K ratio may help individuals adhere to an appropriate dietary Na intake.

Keywords: dietary sodium intake; experimental feeding study; salt restriction; standardized diet; urinary sodium-to-potassium ratio

1. Introduction

It has previously been demonstrated that excess dietary sodium (Na) and insufficient dietary potassium (K) cause blood pressure (BP) elevation [1]. Additionally, epidemiological studies have demonstrated that high dietary Na and low dietary K intakes are also associated with increased cardiovascular disease (CVD) risks [2–5]. Despite rigorous campaigns to reduce Na and increase K intake, there remains a large discrepancy between the recommended and actual intakes of both Na and K [6–8]. Therefore, exact measurement methods are required to facilitate more accurate association studies between dietary salt intake and CVD risk, and avoid discrepant findings arising from technical issues [9,10]. However, the reliable measurement of individual Na and K intake values depends on high-quality, repeated 24-h urine collection (over a period of several days), which is inconvenient and expensive [10–14]. Methods using single spot urine sampling, which are considerably easier than repeated 24-h urine collection, to estimate urinary Na excretion over a single 24-h period have been proposed for the evaluation of population means [15–17], but these techniques have inherent problems in terms of accuracy [10,18,19].

The Na/K ratio is considered to be a useful index for use in achieving effective Na reduction and K increase [20]. Epidemiological studies have suggested that the urinary Na/K ratio is a better measurement of dietary Na reduction and K increase in relation to BP and CVD risk assessments than separate Na or K levels [21–27]. Additionally, the former is easier to measure than the latter, due to its independence from urine collection and creatinine measurement; indeed, repeated Na/K ratio measurements from spot urine samples provide more reliable estimates than those from 24-h urine samples [28–30]. Previous studies have demonstrated that single spot urine samples can be used to estimate the population mean values of the 24-h urine Na/K ratio [28], and that four to seven repeated measurements of the Na/K ratio in spot urine samples can be used to estimate the 24-h urine Na/K ratio in individuals [29,30]. Moreover, a recent report on the self-monitoring of the Na/K ratio for both Na reduction and K increase has emphasized that an individual approach can be used; reduction of the Na/K ratio mainly involved Na reduction, while K only changed a little in healthy volunteers recruited from the general population [31].

Although there are separate dietary recommendations for Na and K, currently, no generally accepted target urinary Na/K ratio level has been established [20]. A recent report speculated that a rough estimate of the mean salt intake (g/day) of a population may be derived by calculating approximately two to four times the population mean 24-h urinary Na/K molar ratio in different populations [20]. However, the urinary Na/K ratio levels that correspond to particular Na or K excretion or dietary intake levels have not yet been determined. Additionally, Na and K are excreted through different pathways [13], and the time lapse observed between Na and K intake and their excretion, reflected as the Na/K ratio, remains unknown. Once this is known, the urinary Na/K ratio may be a useful index to monitor when targeting effective Na reduction and K increase [20].

Therefore, we performed this experimental dietary study with the aim of determining a recommended cutoff value for the Na/K ratio for practical salt reduction by monitoring daily Na/K ratios. To this end, we sought to clarify the urinary Na/K ratio corresponding to dietary Na and K intake, and to examine the daily changes in the urinary Na/K ratio after an abrupt change in Na intake, using standardized meals.

2. Materials and Methods

2.1. Participants

The participants were healthy volunteers without hypertension (defined as an office blood pressure exceeding 140/90 mmHg, at baseline), diabetes, or other known diseases, and who were not taking regular medication. Sixteen individuals were recruited for the study. The study was conducted in accordance with the Declaration of Helsinki, and the Ethics Committee of Fukushima Medical

University (Approval No. 1555; Approval Date, 22 Nov. 2012) approved the protocol. All participants provided written informed consent, and no adverse events associated with the study were recorded.

2.2. Dietary Protocol

The participants consumed a low-salt (LS) diet (3 g/day sodium chloride (NaCl) = 51 mmol/day) for seven days, which was immediately followed by a high-salt (HS) diet (20 g NaCl/day = 342 mmol/day) for another seven days. The menu plan was designed by three registered dietitians. The mean dietary K intake reported among the Japanese population ranged from approximately 2.2 to 2.8 g/day [32,33]. Thus, we set the K amount to 2.5 g/day (64 mmol/day) throughout the LS and HS diet periods. The K and protein intake amounts were standardized between the LS and HS diets, but the total energy intake was adjusted for each individual. The participants were allowed to consume low-Na, low-K snacks provided to them, but were instructed not to consume food outside of that provided by the study. The meals were cooked from scratch in the test kitchen in accordance with the menu plan. Moreover, all participants gathered in a dining hall for three meals a day during the entire period (both the LS and HS diet periods). Before the LS diet period, and again after the HS diet period, the participants followed their own regular, unrestricted (NS) diet under free-living conditions, without any restrictions on Na or K intake.

2.3. Urinary Na/K Ratio and Blood Pressure Measurements

The spot urinary Na/K ratio was measured using a portable personal device throughout the study period (HEU-001-F; Omron Healthcare Co., Muko, Japan; Figure S1a,b) [31], which weighed about 50 g. The device has flat iron electrodes that measure the urinary Na/K ratio, and it displays the result within 1 min. The participants were asked to measure and record their urinary Na/K ratio at every voiding.

2.4. Biochemical Analyses of Urine and Blood

On the last day of each diet period, including the NS diet period before commencing the LS diet period, 24-h urine collections were conducted, in addition to spot urine Na/K ratio measurements. Participants were instructed to collect all urine samples using a measuring cup, with all urine saved in 2 L bottles, unless urine collection was unsuccessful or contaminated with feces. To avoid under- and overcollection, the start and end times of the 24-h urine collection were supervised by clinic staff. The 24-h urine collection began with the participants voiding urine to empty their bladder during the first visit and finished during the visit on the following day when the participants collected their urine in the bottles on-site and returned with their 24-h urine collection bottles. Urine was collected for 24 h and kept cold during the collection period. The samples were handled by certified staff. The Na, K, creatinine, and plasma aldosterone concentrations and plasma renin activity were determined in these samples, as described previously [34].

2.5. Statistical Analysis

2.5.1. Dietary Intake vs. Urinary Excretion

Participants obtained a fixed amount of dietary Na and K from the controlled meals provided during the study, and the Na/K ratio, and Na and K excretions measured from the urine were compared in order to clarify the relationship between dietary Na intake and the urinary Na/K molar ratio. All p values were two-sided, and p values < 0.05 were considered to indicate statistically significant differences. Statistical analyses were performed using IBM SPSS Statistics (IBM Japan, Tokyo, Japan). The differences between the groups were analyzed using one-way repeated-measure analysis of variance with Bonferroni correction or the Friedman test, where applicable. Data are presented as mean $\pm$ standard deviation (SD), unless otherwise noted.

2.5.2. Daily Na/K ratio Assessment from Multiple Spot Urine Samples for Estimating the 24-h Urine Na/K Ratio

Since participants were consuming a controlled diet in this study, the day-to-day variability of Na and K were expected to be minimized. Thus, we used a single 24-h urine sample and daily repetitive measurements of the spot urine Na/K ratio to evaluate the dietary levels of Na and K for each individual in this study. Iwahori et al. previously proposed repetitive measurements of the spot urine Na/K ratio sampling from different days to estimate the seven-day 24-h Na/K ratio [29,30]; however, daily repetitive spot urine Na/K ratio sampling from the same day has not yet been established for estimating a single-day 24-h urine Na/K ratio under controlled dietary conditions. Thus, this estimation method was additionally evaluated in this study. Spearman's rho values for Na/K ratios were calculated to examine the correlation between the daily mean values of the spot urine Na/K ratio and the corresponding values for 24-h urine specimens. Agreement between the daily mean values of the spot urine Na/K ratio and the 24-h urine Na/K ratio was examined using the Bland-Altman method [35]. Bland-Altman plots showing the daily means of the spot urine Na/K ratio and the 24-h urine Na/K ratio values versus the difference between these two values, were used to assess the mean difference (bias). The upper and lower agreement limits (mean difference $\pm$ 1.96 $\times$ SD of difference) between the daily means of the spot urine Na/K ratio and the 24-h urine Na/K ratio were calculated, as was the difference between the upper and lower agreement limits (defined as 95% limit of the difference).

3. Results

3.1. Baseline Parameters of the Participants

Table 1 shows the baseline parameters of the participants on an unrestricted diet. We performed the study from January to February 2014. Excluding two participants who dropped out for personal reasons, 14 eligible individuals, comprising five men and nine women, aged 21 to 26 years, completed the study and their data were included in the final analysis.

Table 1. Baseline parameters of the participants on an unrestricted diet.

Parameter	Unit	Mean $\pm$ SD (Range)
Men/women		5:9 = 35.7%
Age	Years	22.5 $\pm$ 0.3 (21–26)
Weight	kg	53.3 $\pm$ 5.1 (44.9–63.1)
BMI	kg/m^2	20.4 $\pm$ 2.0 (17.2–25.6)
Fasting serum glucose	mg/dL	83 $\pm$ 7
Insulin	μIU/mL	7.2 $\pm$ 2.6
Morning pulse rate	Beats per min	66 $\pm$ 12
Evening pulse rate	Beats per min	65 $\pm$ 10

BMI, body mass index; SD, standard deviation.

3.2. Changes in 24-h Urinary Na/K Ratio and Basic Parameters During the Study

Data from urine samples with a low creatinine content (<0.8 g/day or <70% of maximal urinary creatinine excretion) were excluded from the analysis. The average urinary Na/K molar ratios of the 14 participants, which was calculated from 24-h urine collection, were 4.2 $\pm$ 1.9, 1.0 $\pm$ 0.3, and 6.9 $\pm$ 1.5, (mean $\pm$ SD) on the last day of the NS, LS (3 g/day), and HS (20 g/day) diet periods, respectively. Their average dietary NaCl levels, based on urinary excretions calculated from 24-h urine collection, were 7.3, 1.7, and 17.1 g/day for the NS, LS, and HS diet periods, respectively. Additionally, the urinary K excretion level was 1.16 g/day for the NS diet period. The NaCl excretion percentages, calculated based on Na excretion from 24-h urine for the LS and HS diet periods, were 57% and 86%, respectively, of the designed dietary NaCl content of each respective diet. The urinary K excretion level increased by 33% during the HS diet period, even though a constant dietary K intake was maintained. Furthermore, the urinary K excretion percentages were 48% and 66% of the designed dietary K content for the LS and HS diets, respectively, under the assumption that 90% and 70% of dietary Na and K, respectively, would be excreted in the urine.

No significant differences in blood pressure between the three diet periods were observed (Table 2). Hematocrit was significantly reduced during the HS diet period. Additionally, the urine volume increased by 1.5-fold, but the plasma renin activity significantly decreased during the HS diet period as compared to the LS diet period.

Table 2. Parameters measured at the end of each diet period.

Parameter	Unit	Unrestricted	Low Salt	High Salt	*p* Value
Morning SBP	mmHg	104 ± 9	103 ± 7	102 ± 11	0.769
Morning DBP	mmHg	69 ± 7	65 ± 8	70 ± 7	0.102
Morning MBP	mmHg	76 ± 15	78 ± 7	81 ± 7	0.341
Morning pulse rate	/min	66 ± 12	67 ± 13	64 ± 9	0.652
Hematocrit	%	44.3 ± 3.3	44.4 ± 3.9	42.7 ± 3.0 *	0.045
PAC	pg/mL	208 ± 97	391 ± 204 $	133 ± 63 *,#	0.001
PRA	ng/mL/h	1.3 ± 1.1	2.9 ± 1.5 $	1.0 ± 1.4 *	0.006
Creatinine	mg/dL	0.69 ± 0.13	0.71 ± 0.14	0.65 ± 0.11 *,#	0.000
Serum Na	mEq/L	141 ± 2	141 ± 1	141 ± 2	0.220
Serum K	mEq/L	4.0 ± 0.2	4.0 ± 0.2	4.1 ± 0.3	0.940
Urine volume	mL/day	926 ± 369	978 ± 336	1416 ± 495 *,#	0.016
Urine Na	mmol/day	128 ± 47	30 ± 7 $	281 ± 42 *,#	0.001
Urine K	mmol/day	32.3 ± 9.4	29.5 ± 6.0	39.2 ± 7.6 *	0.032
Urine creatinine	g/day	1.20 ± 0.25	1.14 ± 0.20	1.23 ± 0.29	0.093
Morning SBP	mmHg	104 ± 9	103 ± 7	102 ± 11	0.769
Morning DBP	mmHg	69 ± 7	65 ± 8	70 ± 7	0.102

SBP, systolic blood pressure; DBP, diastolic blood pressure; MBP, mean blood pressure; PAC, plasma aldosterone; PRA, plasma renin activity. Mean ± SD. For urinary data, those with urinary creatinine excretion of <0.8 g/day or <70% of the maximal urinary creatinine excretion were excluded from the analysis (*n* = 11–12). $ *p* < 0.05 for unrestricted versus low-salt diet. * *p* < 0.05 for low-salt versus high-salt diet. # *p* < 0.05 for unrestricted versus high-salt diet.

3.3. Changes in Self-Measured Urinary Na/K Ratio During the Study

In this study, the group means of the urinary Na/K ratio obtained from the daily mean of repetitive spot urine Na/K ratio determinations were 4.2 ± 2.1, 1.1 ± 0.8, and 6.6 ± 2.1 (mean ± SD) on the last day of the NS, LS (3 g/day), and HS (20 g/day) diet periods, respectively. The individual spot urine Na/K ratio fluctuated under the controlled diets, with the variation being large during the HS diet period, but small during the LS diet period (Figure 1a). Diurnal variation was readily observed in most participants during the HS diet period. The group average urinary Na/K ratio clearly showed a plateau approximately three days after the change in the dietary Na level (Figure 1b). In individual traces, the time to reaching the plateau varied between three and four days (Figure 1a).

The daily mean range of the device-measured individual urinary Na/K molar ratio was narrow during the LS diet period (0.23–2.80), but wide during the HS diet period (3.16–10.14). In fact, 74% and 94% of the 207 individual-based urinary Na/K molar ratio measurements taken during days four to seven of the LS diet were ≤1.0 and ≤2.0, respectively. During the last four days of the HS diet, 7.6%, 42.6%, 31.4%, 29.4%, and 15.2% of the 278 individual-based urinary Na/K molar ratio measurements were ≤4.0, 4.1–6.0, 6.1–8.0, 8.1–10.0, and >10, respectively.

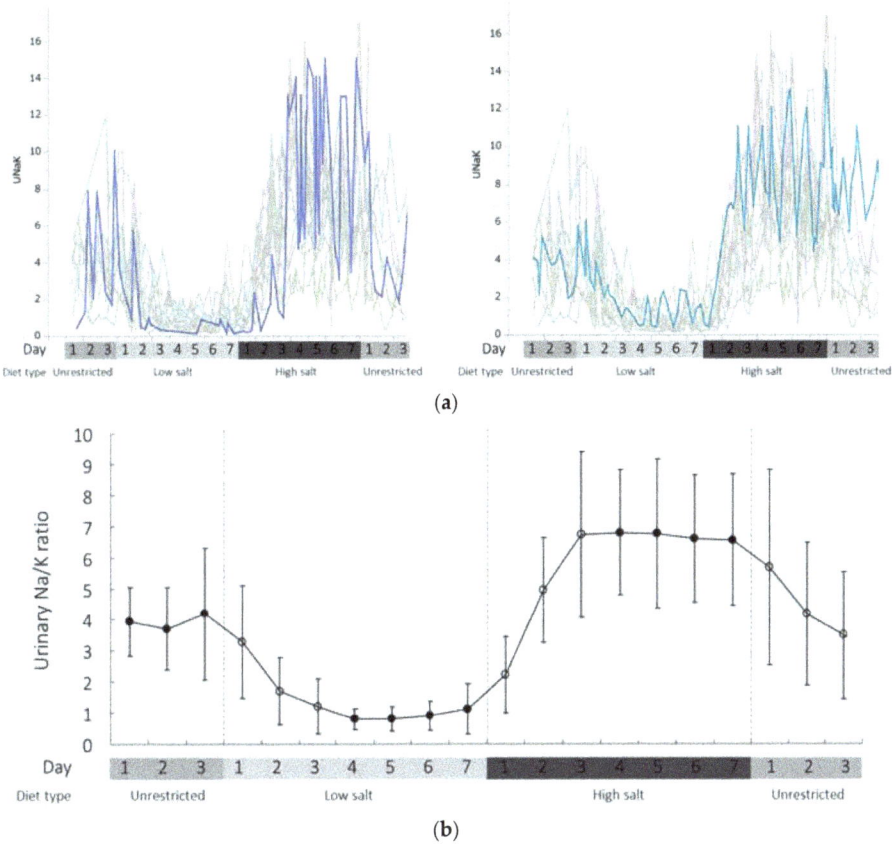

Figure 1. Time-dependent changes in urinary Na/K ratio (UNaK) during unrestricted, low-salt (3 g NaCl/day), and high-salt (20 g NaCl/day) diet periods measured by the device. (**a**) Individual trends and (**b**) group average throughout the study.

3.4. Validation of Daily Mean Spot Urine Na/K Ratio for Estimating 24-h Urine Na/K Ratio

The individual daily means of the spot urine Na/K ratio for the last three days of each diet period correlated well with the 24-h urine Na/K ratio of the last day of each diet period (Figure 2). For the daily mean spot urine Na/K ratio determined on the last day of each diet period, the bias estimate, defined as the difference between the Na/K ratios of the 24-h and spot urine collections, was 0.13, whereas the 95% limit of the difference ranged from −2.96 to 3.21, according to the Bland–Altman method (Figure 2). The voiding frequency ranged from three to eight times per day (mean: 4.0 and 5.0 times per day during the LS and HS diet periods, respectively) in this study. Figure S2 shows the correlations between the 24-h urine Na/K ratio on the last day and the means of different numbers of randomly selected spot urine Na/K ratios during the last three days of each diet period. The correlation coefficient ranged from 0.74 to 0.88, the bias ranged from 0.16 to 0.39, and the 95% lower and upper limits of difference ranged from −0.45 to −0.19 and 0.72 to 1.1, respectively, among these combinations. The correlation between the mean Na/K ratio of three to seven spot urine samples and the 24-h urine collection remained high, and their agreement was good (Figure S2).

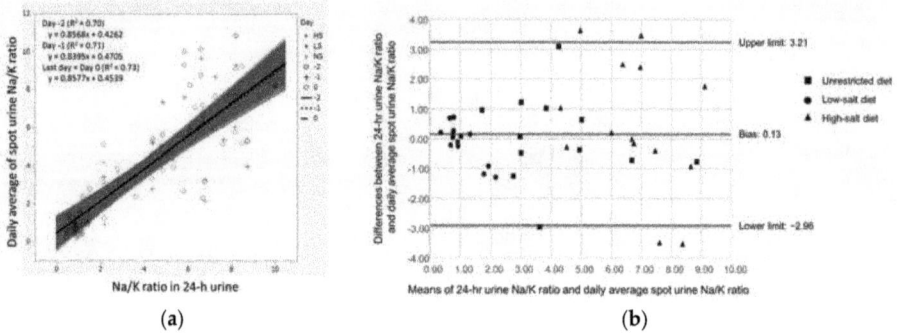

(a)   (b)

Figure 2. Correlation and agreement analyses between individual daily means of the spot urine Na/K ratio and 24-h urine Na/K ratio: (**a**) Spearman's correlation between the 24-h urine Na/K ratio during the last day of each diet period and individual daily means of the spot urine Na/K ratio of the last three days of each diet period. Data points from unrestricted (NS), low-salt (LS), and high-salt (HS) diet periods are shown in green, blue, and red, respectively. The regression lines calculated for the last day (0), the day before (−1), and two days before the last day (−2) are shown with 95% confidence interval in gray areas. (**b**) Bland-Altman plot of the 24-h urine Na/K ratio and daily means of the spot urine Na/K ratio on the last day of each diet period.

4. Discussion

The relationship between the urinary Na/K ratio and dietary Na/K ratio, Na, and K levels has been unclear. Frequent monitoring of the urinary Na/K ratio during acute changes in salt intake has not been reported previously. This nonparallel, experimental dietary study demonstrated the relationship between standardized dietary Na and K intake levels and the corresponding urinary Na/K ratio among healthy volunteers. Association studies have demonstrated the benefits of monitoring the Na/K ratio to assess Na reduction and K increase in relation to BP and CVD risks, as compared with monitoring Na and K levels separately. However, the urinary and dietary Na/K ratio levels used for assessing risk scores differed among these previous studies due to the percentage of diet reflected in the urine [25–27,36,37]. In the present study, the urinary Na/K ratio tracked the changes in dietary Na intake; changes were reflected in the urinary Na/K ratio within approximately three days under standardized dietary conditions. Furthermore, the daily means of the urinary Na/K ratio correlated well with those of the dietary Na/K ratio, and the former was approximately 1.3 times the value of the latter.

Use of formulas to estimate 24-h urinary Na excretion from a single spot urine sample depends on other parameters, such as body weight and creatinine clearance [15–17], and may be biased [18,19], whereas the Na/K ratio is independent of both creatinine excretion and body weight, and is also unbiased [26]. Repeated spot urine Na/K ratios may therefore be a useful and practical means for obtaining individual values of the urinary Na/K ratio [29,30]. The spot urine Na/K ratio showed higher correlations and better agreements with 24-h urine values than the Na or K level alone [28–30], especially when using repeated spot urine measurements [29,30]. The results of the agreement and correlation analyses of four to seven repeated measurements of the spot urine Na/K ratio were similar to those of one to two-day 24-h urine Na/K ratios, when compared with the gold standard seven-day 24-h urine Na/K ratio [29,30].

In this study, we primarily used the daily mean of the spot urine Na/K ratio, but we also examined the use of different repetitions of spot urine sampling to determine their agreement with the 24-h urine Na/K ratio under standardized and unrestricted dietary conditions. Increasing the number of random spot urine Na/K ratio samples is known to improve the correlation with the seven-day 24-h urine Na/K ratio [29,30], as confirmed by our findings, although the level of agreement in our study was slightly less than that reported previously. This may be because only a single 24-h urine sample collection was performed for each dietary condition in the present study. However, the correlation data indicated that the mean of multiple spot urine Na/K ratios reflected the 24-h Na/K ratio well. The daily mean of the spot urine Na/K ratio was roughly equivalent to the mean of five random spot urine Na/K ratio measurements. This may be explained by voiding frequency. For relatively short-term studies, the daily mean spot urine Na/K ratio measured at least four days after a change in diet may serve as a simple substitute for a 24-h urine Na/K ratio.

In this regard, a self-monitoring device for the urinary Na/K ratio measurement, which provides prompt on-site feedback, has been evaluated with a view to supporting an individual approach for Na reduction and K increase [31]. Repeated measurement of the spot urine Na/K ratio may be a low-burden method for monitoring adherence to World Health Organization (WHO) guidelines on Na and K intake. However, interpretation of the individual estimate obtained through the repeated spot urine Na/K ratio measurement is difficult, because the urinary Na/K ratio corresponding to the dietary Na and K intake has not yet been reported. Moreover, a formally recommended cutoff value for this ratio has not been established to date. Our findings provide a basis for Na/K monitoring, which is a prerequisite for setting such goals.

Rakova et al. have demonstrated that individual urinary Na excretion fluctuated under controlled dietary conditions, which was similar to the results of our study [14]. However, the amount of dietary salt intake correlated well with the group mean 24-h urinary Na/K ratio, based on a 24-h sample collected during the last day of each period, and the urinary Na/K ratio obtained by determining the daily mean of repetitive spot urine Na/K ratio measurements at least three days after changing the standardized diet. Thus, the single-day 24-h urine collection on the last day of LS and HS diet periods reasonably represented the group estimate of Na intake during these periods, as the day-to-day variation in Na excretion was minimized by means of the standardized diets. Additionally, the urinary Na/K ratio is known to show diurnal variation [38]. Thus, daily repetitive spot urine Na/K ratio sampling may have corrected the effect of diurnal variation and therefore show a good association with dietary salt intake and the 24-h urine Na/K ratio under controlled dietary conditions.

We determined the urinary Na/K molar ratio corresponding to the Na and K intake using our standardized diets. The dietary Na/K molar ratios in this study were designed to be 0.80 and 5.3 on the LS (NaCl, 3 g/day; K, 2.5 g/day; Na/K molar ratio = 51.3/64.1 mmol/mmol) and HS (NaCl, 20 g/day; K, 2.5 g/day; Na/K molar ratio = 341.9/64.1 mmol/mmol) diets. Previous reports have indicated that 80–95% of dietary Na [13,39–42] and 63–77% of dietary K [13,40,41] is excreted in the urine. Thus, if 90% and 70% of dietary Na and K, respectively, are excreted in the urine, the urinary Na/K ratio would be 1.3 times the dietary Na/K ratio, which indicates that the theoretical urinary Na/K molar ratio should be 1.0 and 6.8 on the LS and HS diets, respectively, in the present study. The actual group averages of the 24-h urine Na/K molar ratio were 1.0 and 6.9 on the LS and HS diets, respectively; the urinary Na/K molar ratio obtained as the daily mean of spot urine Na/K ratios were 1.1 and 6.6, which were close to these theoretical values. However, the 24-h urine Na and K excretions were 58–81% and 48–66%, respectively, of the designed dietary content during the LS and HS diet periods.

As shown in Table 2, the component of the urinary Na/K ratio that showed the predominant change was the amount of Na excreted, which reflected NaCl consumption. Although there was a significant increase in urinary K excretion during the HS diet period, which may have resulted from increased Na delivery to the distal tubules of the kidney [43,44], the change in K was much smaller than that in Na, and K excretion did not differ between the HS and the NS diet periods. Moreover, a recent self-monitoring intervention study on lowering the urinary Na/K ratio mainly resulted in Na reduction, with little change observed in K [31]. These findings suggest that the change in urinary Na/K ratio in real world conditions (with Na and K intake levels close to the average of the general population) would be mainly due to changes in Na, and would be relatively independent of K. However, these assumptions may not be applicable to individuals with an extreme K intake or to patients with kidney diseases. Furthermore, a decrease in urinary Na excretion during the LS diet period may have been due to sustained extra-renal Na loss, and the lower-than-expected Na and K excretion seen throughout the study may have been due to the loss of Na in sweat, as some participants participated in sports during the study, in addition to possible incomplete urine collection. Considering that 24-h urine Na and K measurements may result in Na and K intake underestimations due to incomplete collections [10], the use of the Na/K ratio is more advantageous than separate Na or K excretion assessments, because it is resistant to systematic errors related to urine volume. The finding that the rate of K excretion was lower than that of Na excretion in our study may also be explained by a relative K deficiency in our study participants and due to racial differences in the K balance [40].

Changes associated with salt intake were appropriately observed in this study, such as those in urine volume, voiding frequency, serum creatinine levels, hematocrit, plasma aldosterone concentrations, and plasma renin activity. No significant changes in blood pressure were observed in our study, which may be due to the inclusion of young normotensive participants and a short salt-loading duration. The normotensive population has been reported to display a lower percentage of blood pressure salt-sensitivity than the hypertensive population [45].

Dietary NaCl intake may be roughly estimated from the urinary Na/K ratio by examining the population mean 24-h urine Na/K molar ratio and the population mean 24-h urine salt (NaCl) (g/day) concentration [30]. In this study, the ratio of dietary NaCl (g/day) to urinary Na/K molar ratio was approximately 3, in different dietary conditions; the group mean 24-h urine Na/K molar ratio during LS and HS diet periods were 1.0 and 6.9, when the group mean salt intake was 3 (g/day) and 20 (g/day), respectively. Findings from the INTERMAP (International study of macro- and micro-nutrients and blood pressure) study showed that the population mean dietary salt intake of 11.8 (g/day) corresponded to a population mean 24-h urine Na/K molar ratio of 4.3, in four Japanese cohort centers [32]. Thus, a rough estimate of the group mean salt intake (g/day) may be taken as being approximately three times the group mean 24-h urinary Na/K molar ratio. Thus, considering that the group mean urinary Na/K molar ratio during the NS diet period was 4.2, the group mean salt intake may have ranged from 12 to 13 g/day.

WHO reports suggest that guideline-targeted Na and K intake levels would yield a Na/K ratio of approximately 1.0 [46,47]. Extrapolating from the present study, an average urinary Na/K molar ratio of approximately 1 would correspond to a dietary salt intake of 3 g per day, rather than 5 g per day. However, given that the K intake level during the LS period in our study was lower than that recommended by the WHO guideline, the dietary salt intake level needed to satisfy the Na/K ratio of 1 should be lower than the Na level recommended by the WHO guideline. This phenomenon may occur in a real-world setting. During the LS diet period, more than 70% and 90% of spot urine Na/K molar ratio measurements were ≤1.0 and ≤2.0, respectively. Considering that Cook et al. reported that a Na/K molar ratio of between 1 and 2 resulted in the lowest CVD risk [25], a urinary Na/K ratio of <2 might be a reasonable current goal for most individuals, in terms of lowering BP and reducing CVD risk. Further investigations are needed to explore the possibility that a lower target than that currently aspired to might be optimal.

This study has several limitations. First, the participants were young Japanese individuals, and the sample size was relatively small. Second, it is not known whether the urinary Na/K ratio acclimatizes over a longer period after an acute change in diet. Another limitation of the study is that the actual food intake and data collection were dependent on the participants, although we attempted to achieve high-quality 24-h urine collection in this study by monitoring the start and end of the collection period [10,48]. However, the urinary excretion-to-dietary intake ratio of electrolytes were somewhat lower than those previously reported [13,14,39–42]. The relatively low NaCl and K excretion values and the low urine volume may be partly due to incomplete urine collection, as well as to excess Na loss in sweat during sports participation.

Nutrients **2017**, *9*, 951

5. Conclusions

In conclusion, we determined that the group average of the individual daily means of the spot urine Na/K ratio tracked the changes in dietary levels of Na. Frequent urinary Na/K ratio monitoring may be a useful index of individuals' dietary Na and K levels, which may help individuals to adhere to appropriate Na intake amounts, and thereby may contribute to the reduction of cardiovascular complications.

Supplementary Materials: The following are available online at www.mdpi.com/2072-6643/9/9/951/s1. Figure S1: (a) Urinary Na/K ratio monitor (HEU-001F, Omron Healthcare Co., Ltd., Kyoto, Japan); (b) Pearson's correlation coefficient for the urinary Na/K ratios measured by the portable urinary Na/K ratio monitor (HEU-001F, Omron Healthcare Co., Ltd., Kyoto, Japan) and by a biochemical inspection center (BML Inc., Tokyo, Japan). Figure S2: Correlation between one random spot urine Na/K ratio as well as the average of three, five, or seven random spot urine Na/K ratios obtained during the last three days of each diet period and the 24-h urine Na/K ratio obtained on the last day of each diet period.

Acknowledgments: This study was conducted at Fukushima Medical University in cooperation with the Department of Public Health of Shiga University of Medical Science and Omron Healthcare Co., Ltd. We gratefully acknowledge the excellent technical assistance of Ayumi Haneda. We also thank the dieticians, Fumie Taguchi, Emi Ohashi, and Izumi Ishida, for designing the menus. Satsuki Kurosawa, Yuri Ikeda, Mizuho Yonemoto, and Momoko Nochi participated in the data collection and analysis. This work was supported by a step-up project grant from Fukushima Medical University (MSY), JPS KAKENHI Grant Number 15K21263 (MSY) and NIH grants, HL074940 (RAF) and DK039308 (RAF).

Author Contributions: M.S.Y., T.I., and J.Y. contributed to the design of the study. M.S.Y. and J.Y. participated in the data collection and analysis. M.S.Y., T.I., K.M., H.U., and J.Y. contributed to the drafting of the manuscript. All authors participated in the critical revision of the manuscript and approved the final version of the manuscript for submission.

Conflicts of Interest: Toshiyuki Iwahori is an employee of Omron Healthcare Co., Ltd. Hirotsugu Ueshima serves as a consultant for Omron Healthcare Co., Ltd. Katsuyuki Miura received a research fund from Omron Healthcare Co. Ltd.

References

1. Adrogué, H.J.; Madias, N.E. Sodium and potassium in the pathogenesis of hypertension. *N. Engl. J. Med.* **2007**, *356*, 1966–1978. [CrossRef] [PubMed]
2. Gay, H.C.; Rao, S.G.; Vaccarino, V.; Ali, M.K. Effects of different dietary interventions on blood pressure: Systematic review and meta-analysis of randomized controlled trials. *Hypertension* **2016**, *67*, 733–739. [CrossRef] [PubMed]
3. He, F.J.; Li, J.; MacGregor, G.A. Effect of longer term modest salt reduction on blood pressure: Cochrane systematic review and meta-analysis of randomized trials. *BMJ* **2013**, *346*, f1325. [CrossRef] [PubMed]
4. Aburto, N.J.; Ziolkovska, A.; Hooper, L.; Elliott, P.; Cappuccio, F.P.; Meerpohl, J.J. Effect of lower sodium intake on health: Systematic review and meta-analyses. *BMJ* **2013**, *346*, f1326. [CrossRef] [PubMed]
5. Aburto, N.J.; Hanson, S.; Gutierrez, H.; Hooper, L.; Elliott, P.; Cappuccio, F.P. Effect of increased potassium on cardiovascular risk factors and disease: Systematic review and meta-analyses. *BMJ* **2013**, *346*, f1378. [CrossRef] [PubMed]
6. Brown, I.J.; Tzoulaki, I.; Candeias, V.; Elliott, P. Salt intakes around the world: Implications for public health. *Int. J. Epidemiol.* **2009**, *38*, 791–813. [CrossRef] [PubMed]
7. Cogswell, M.E.; Zhang, Z.; Carriquiry, A.L.; Gunn, J.P.; Kuklina, E.V.; Saydah, S.H.; Yang, Q.; Moshfegh, A.J. Sodium and potassium intakes among US adults: NHANES 2003–2008. *Am. J. Clin. Nutr.* **2012**, *96*, 647–657. [CrossRef] [PubMed]
8. Bernstein, A.M.; Willett, W.C. Trends in 24-h urinary sodium excretion in the United States, 1957–2003: A systematic review. *Am. J. Clin. Nutr.* **2010**, *92*, 1172–1180. [CrossRef] [PubMed]
9. Cogswell, M.E.; Mugavero, K.; Bowman, B.A.; Frieden, T.R. Dietary sodium and cardiovascular disease risk-measurement matters. *N. Engl. J. Med.* **2016**, *375*, 580–586. [CrossRef] [PubMed]
10. Cobb, L.K.; Anderson, C.A.; Elliott, P.; Hu, F.B.; Liu, K.; Neaton, J.D.; Whelton, P.K.; Woodward, M.; Appel, L.J. American Heart Association Council on Lifestyle and Metabolic Health. Methodological issues in cohort studies that relate sodium intake to cardiovascular disease outcomes: A science advisory from the American Heart Association. *Circulation* **2014**, *129*, 1173–1186. [CrossRef] [PubMed]

11.   Liu, K.; Stamler, J. Assessment of sodium intake in epidemiological studies on blood pressure. *Ann. Clin. Res.* **1984**, *16* (Suppl. 43), 49–54. [PubMed]

12.   Lerchl, K.; Rakova, N.; Dahlmann, A.; Rauh, M.; Goller, U.; Basner, M.; Dinges, D.F.; Beck, L.; Agureev, A.; Larina, I.; et al. Agreement between 24-hour salt ingestion and sodium excretion in a controlled environment. *Hypertension* **2015**, *66*, 850–857. [CrossRef] [PubMed]

13.   Kawasaki, T.; Itoh, K.; Uezono, K.; Sasaki, H. A simple method for estimating 24 h urinary sodium and potassium excretion from second morning voiding urine specimen in adults. *Clin. Exp. Pharmacol. Physiol.* **1993**, *20*, 7–14. [CrossRef] [PubMed]

14.   Tanaka, T.; Okamura, T.; Miura, K.; Kadowaki, T.; Ueshima, H.; Nakagawa, H.; Hashimoto, T. A simple method to estimate populational 24-h urinary sodium and potassium excretion using a casual urine specimen. *J. Hum. Hypertens.* **2002**, *16*, 97–103. [CrossRef] [PubMed]

15.   Brown, I.J.; Dyer, A.R.; Chan, Q.; Cogswell, M.E.; Ueshima, H.; Stamler, J.; Elliott, P.; INTERSALT Co-Operative Research Group. Estimating 24-hour urinary sodium excretion from casual urinary sodium concentrations in Western populations: The INTERSALT study. *Am. J. Epidemiol.* **2013**, *177*, 1180–1192. [CrossRef] [PubMed]

16.   Polonia, J.; Lobo, M.F.; Martins, L.; Pinto, F.; Nazare, J. Estimation of populational 24-h urinary sodium and potassium excretion from spot urine samples: Evaluation of four formulas in a large national representative population. *J. Hypertens.* **2017**, *35*, 477–486. [CrossRef] [PubMed]

17.   Huang, L.; Crino, M.; Wu, J.H.; Woodward, M.; Barzi, F.; Land, M.A.; McLean, R.; Webster, J.; Enkhtungalag, B.; Neal, B. Mean population salt intake estimated from 24-h urine samples and spot urine samples: A systematic review and meta-analysis. *Int. J. Epidemiol.* **2016**, *45*, 239–250. [CrossRef] [PubMed]

18.   Iwahori, T.; Miura, K.; Ueshima, H. Time to consider use of the sodium-to-potassium ratio for practical sodium reduction and potassium increase. *Nutrients* **2017**, in press. [CrossRef] [PubMed]

19.   INTERSALT Co-operative Research Group. INTERSALT: An international study of electrolyte excretion and blood pressure. Results for 24-hr urinary sodium and potassium excretion. *BMJ* **1988**, *297*, 319–328.

20.   Stamler, J.; Rose, G.; Stamler, R.; Elliott, P.; Dyer, A.; Marmot, M. INTERSALT study findings. Public health and medical care implications. *Hypertension* **1989**, *14*, 570–577. [CrossRef] [PubMed]

21.   Tzoulaki, I.; Patel, C.J.; Okamura, T.; Chan, Q.; Brown, I.J.; Miura, K.; Ueshima, H.; Zhao, L.; Van Horn, L.; Daviglus, M.L.; et al. A nutrient-wide association study on blood pressure. *Circulation* **2012**, *126*, 2456–2464. [CrossRef] [PubMed]

22.   Perez, V.; Chang, E.T. Sodium-to-potassium ratio and blood pressure, hypertension, and related factors. *Adv. Nutr.* **2014**, *5*, 712–741. [CrossRef] [PubMed]

23.   Cook, N.R.; Obarzanek, E.; Cutler, J.A.; Buring, J.E.; Rexrode, K.M.; Kumanyika, S.K.; Appel, L.J.; Whelton, P.K. Trials of Hypertension Prevention Collaborative Research Group. Joint effects of sodium and potassium intake on subsequent cardiovascular disease: The Trials of Hypertension Prevention follow-up study. *Arch. Intern. Med.* **2009**, *169*, 32–40. [CrossRef] [PubMed]

24.   Cook, N.R.; Appel, L.J.; Whelton, P.K. Sodium intake and all-cause mortality over 20 years in the Trials of Hypertension Prevention. *J. Am. Coll. Cardiol.* **2016**, *68*, 1609–1617. [CrossRef] [PubMed]

25.   Cook, N.R.; Cutler, J.A.; Obarzanek, E.; Buring, J.E.; Rexrode, K.M.; Kumanyika, S.K.; Appel, L.J.; Whelton, P.K. Long term effects of dietary sodium reduction on cardiovascular disease outcomes: Observational follow-up of the Trials of Hypertension Prevention (TOHP). *BMJ* **2007**, *334*, 885–888. [CrossRef] [PubMed]

26.   Iwahori, T.; Miura, K.; Ueshima, H.; Chan, Q.; Dyer, A.R.; Elliott, P.; Stamler, J.; INTERSALT Research Group. Estimating 24-hour urinary sodium/potassium ratio from casual ("spot") urinary sodium/potassium ratio: The INTERSALT Study. *Int. J. Epidemiol.* **2016**, in press. [CrossRef] [PubMed]

27.   Iwahori, T.; Ueshima, H.; Miyagawa, N.; Ohgami, N.; Yamashita, H.; Ohkubo, T.; Murakami, Y.; Shiga, T.; Miura, K. Six random samples of casual urine on different days are sufficient to estimate daily sodium/potassium ratio as compared to 7-day 24-h urine collections. *Hypertens. Res.* **2014**, *37*, 765–771. [CrossRef] [PubMed]

28.   Iwahori, T.; Ueshima, H.; Torii, S.; Saito, Y.; Fujiyoshi, A.; Ohkubo, T.; Miura, K. Four to seven random casual urine specimens are sufficient to estimate 24-h urinary sodium/potassium ratio in individuals with high blood pressure. *J. Hum. Hypertens.* **2016**, *30*, 328–334. [CrossRef] [PubMed]

29. Iwahori, T.; Ueshima, H.; Ohgami, N.; Yamashita, H.; Miyagawa, N.; Kondo, K.; Torii, S.; Yoshita, K.; Shiga, T.; Ohkubo, T.; et al. Effectiveness of a self-monitoring device for urinary sodium/potassium ratio on dietary improvement in free-living adults: A randomized controlled trial. *J. Epidemiol.* **2017**, in press.

30. Hunter, D. Biochemical indicators of dietary intake. In *Nutritional Epidemiology*, 2nd ed.; Willet, W., Ed.; Oxford University Press: New York, NY, USA, 1998; pp. 174–243.

31. Stamler, J.; Chan, Q.; INTERSALT Co-operative Research Group. INTERMAP appendix tables. *J. Hum. Hypertens.* **2003**, *17*, 665–758. [CrossRef]

32. Ministry of Health, Labour and Welfare. *National Nutrition and Health Survey, 2010*; Daiichi Shuppan: Tokyo, Japan, 2012.

33. Yatabe, M.S.; Yatabe, J.; Yoneda, M.; Watanabe, T.; Otsuki, M.; Felder, R.A.; Jose, P.A.; Sanada, H. Salt sensitivity is associated with insulin resistance, sympathetic overactivity, and decreased suppression of circulating renin activity in lean patients with essential hypertension. *Am. J. Clin. Nutr.* **2010**, *92*, 77–82. [CrossRef] [PubMed]

34. Bland, J.; Altman, D.G. Statistical methods for assessing agreement between two methods of clinical measurement. *Lancet* **1986**, *1*, 307–310. [CrossRef]

35. Yang, Q.; Liu, T.; Kuklina, E.V.; Flanders, W.D.; Hong, Y.; Gillespie, C.; Chang, M.H.; Gwinn, M.; Dowling, N.; Khoury, M.J.; et al. Sodium and potassium intake and mortality among US adults: Prospective data from the Third National Health and Nutrition Examination Survey. *Arch. Intern. Med.* **2011**, *171*, 1183–1191. [CrossRef] [PubMed]

36. Okayama, A.; Okuda, N.; Miura, K.; Okamura, T.; Hayakawa, T.; Akasaka, H.; Ohnishi, H.; Saitoh, S.; Arai, Y.; Kiyohara, Y.; et al. Dietary sodium-to-potassium ratio as a risk factor for stroke, cardiovascular disease and all-cause mortality in Japan: The NIPPON DATA80 cohort study. *BMJ Open.* **2016**, *6*, e011632. [CrossRef] [PubMed]

37. Rakova, N.; Jüttner, K.; Dahlmann, A.; Schröder, A.; Linz, P.; Kopp, C.; Rauh, M.; Goller, U.; Beck, L.; Agureev, A.; et al. Long-term space flight simulation reveals infradian rhythmicity in human Na$^+$ balance. *Cell. Metab.* **2013**, *17*, 125–131. [CrossRef] [PubMed]

38. Iwahori, T.; Ueshima, H.; Torii, S.; Yoshino, S.; Kondo, K.; Tanaka-Mizuno, S.; Arima, H.; Miura, K. Diurnal variation of urinary sodium-to-potassium ratio in free-living Japanese individuals. *Hypertens. Res.* **2017**. [CrossRef] [PubMed]

39. Pietinen, P.I.; Findley, T.W.; Clausen, J.D.; Finnerty, F.A.; Altschul, A.M. Studies in community nutrition: Estimation of sodium output. *Prev. Med.* **1976**, *5*, 400–407. [CrossRef]

40. Voors, A.W.; Dalferes, E.R., Jr.; Frank, G.C.; Aristimuno, G.G.; Berenson, G.S. Relation between ingested potassium and sodium balance in young blacks and whites. *Am. J. Clin. Nutr.* **1983**, *37*, 583–594. [PubMed]

41. Clark, A.J.; Mossholder, S. Sodium and potassium intake measurements: Dietary methodology problems. *Am. J. Clin. Nutr.* **1986**, *43*, 470–476. [PubMed]

42. Holbrook, J.T.; Patterson, K.Y.; Bodner, J.E.; Douglas, L.W.; Veillon, C.; Kelsay, J.L.; Mertz, W.; Smith, J.C., Jr. Sodium and potassium intake and balance in adults consuming self-selected diets. *Am. J. Clin. Nutr.* **1984**, *40*, 786–793. [PubMed]

43. Palmer, B.F.; Clegg, D.J. Physiology and pathophysiology of potassium homeostasis. *Adv. Physiol. Educ.* **2016**, *40*, 480–490. [CrossRef] [PubMed]

44. Palmer, B.F. Regulation of potassium homeostasis. *Clin. J. Am. Soc. Nephrol.* **2015**, *10*, 1050–1060. [CrossRef] [PubMed]

45. Armando, I.; Villar, V.A.; Jose, P.A. Genomics and pharmacogenomics of salt-sensitive hypertension. *Curr. Hypertens. Rev.* **2015**, *11*, 49–56. [CrossRef] [PubMed]

46. World Health Organization. WHO Guideline: Sodium intake for adults and children. In *Geneva: World Health Organization (WHO)*; WHO: Genève, Switzerland, 2012.

47.   World Health Organization. WHO Guideline: Potassium intake for adults and children. In *Geneva: World Health Organization (WHO)*; WHO: Genève, Switzerland, 2012.
48.   The INTERSALT Co-operative Research Group. INTERSALT study: An international co-operative study on the relation of blood pressure to electrolyte excretion in populations, I: Design and methods. *J. Hypertens.* **1986**, *4*, 781–787.

nutrients

MDPI

Article

Collecting Evidence to Inform Salt Reduction Policies in Argentina: Identifying Sources of Sodium Intake in Adults from a Population-Based Sample

Natalia Elorriaga [1,2,*], Laura Gutierrez [1], Iris B. Romero [2], Daniela L. Moyano [1], Rosana Poggio [1], Matías Calandrelli [3], Nora Mores [4], Adolfo Rubinstein [5] and Vilma Irazola [1]

[1] Centro de Excelencia en Salud Cardiovascular para el Cono Sur (CESCAS), C1414CPV Ciudad Autónoma de Buenos Aires, Argentina; lgutierrez@iecs.org.ar (L.G.); dmoyano@iecs.org.ar (D.L.M.); rpoggio@iecs.org.ar (R.P.); virazola@iecs.org.ar (V.I.)

[2] Escuela de Nutrición, Universidad de Buenos Aires, C1122AAD Ciudad Autónoma de Buenos Aires, Argentina; irisbromero@yahoo.com.ar

[3] Sanatorio San Carlos, Pcia de Río Negro, 8400 Bariloche, Argentina; matiascalandrelli@yahoo.com.ar

[4] Municipalidad de Marcos Paz, Pcia de Buenos Aires, 1727 Marcos Paz, Argentina; oliveramores@gmail.com

[5] Ministerio de Salud de la Nación, C1073ABA Ciudad Autónoma de Buenos Aires, Argentina; adolfo.rubinstein@gmail.com

* Correspondence: nelorriaga@iecs.org.ar; Tel.: +54-011-4777-8767

Received: 25 July 2017; Accepted: 23 August 2017; Published: 31 August 2017

Abstract: The maximum content of sodium in selected processed foods (PF) in Argentina was limited by a law enacted in 2013. Data about intake of these and other foods are necessary for policy planning, implementation, evaluation, and monitoring. We examined data from the CESCAS I population-based cohort study to assess the main dietary sources among PF and frequency of discretionary salt use by sex, age, and education attainment, before full implementation of the regulations in 2015. We used a validated 34-item FFQ (Food Frequency Questionnaire) to assess PF intake and discretional salt use. Among 2127 adults in two Argentinean cities, aged 35–76 years, mean salt intake from selected PFs was 4.7 g/day, higher among male and low education subgroups. Categories of foods with regulated maximum limits provided near half of the sodium intake from PFs. Use of salt (always/often) at the table and during cooking was reported by 9% and 73% of the population, respectively, with higher proportions among young people. Reducing salt consumption to the target of 5 g/day may require adjustments to the current regulation (reducing targets, including other food categories), as well as reinforcing strategies such as education campaigns, labeling, and voluntary agreement with bakeries.

Keywords: salt; sodium intake; food sources; processed foods; Argentina; adults; food frequency questionnaire; food policy

1. Introduction

Noncommunicable diseases (NCDs) are the main contributor to mortality and morbidity globally [1,2] and interventions to reduce the burden of NCDs are highly cost-effective [3]. Elevated sodium intake has been associated with a number of NCDs (including hypertension, cardiovascular disease, and stroke), and decreasing sodium intake may reduce blood pressure and the risk of associated NCDs [4]. In Argentina, cardiovascular disease (CVD) is the first cause of death in the general population [5] and 37% of all cardiovascular deaths in Argentina are attributable to hypertension [6]. Hypertension is more frequent among those with the lowest educational level and lowest income subgroups [7]. Although no studies have measured total sodium consumption in a population-based sample of Argentina, consensus among experts suggests that current sodium intake is at least double of the WHO 2000 mg/day recommendation [8].

Population-based interventions to reduce sodium intake are being successfully implemented in various countries worldwide, and have the potential to reduce the prevalence of high blood pressure and the burden of cardiovascular diseases [9]. The Argentinean government has shown leadership in developing strategies to reduce sodium consumption. In 2009, the national program called Menos Sal Más Vida ("Less Salt More Life") was launched, promoting the reduction of salt consumption by the Argentinean population [10]. It has included actions like a voluntary agreement with the Argentinean Federation of Bakeries (FAIPA, by its Spanish acronym) to reduce salt levels in breads [8]. In 2011, the initiative was consolidated through the signing of agreements for Voluntary and Progressive Reduction of the Sodium content of the Processed Foods celebrated between the Ministry of Health (MoH), the Ministry of Agriculture, Livestock and Fisheries and large food industries of the country [4]. The initiative required food companies to reduce 5% to 15% of the sodium content of four groups of food: (1) processed meats; (2) cheese and dairy products; (3) soups and dressings; and (4) cereals, cookies, pizza, and pasta (farinaceous). In 2013, National Act 26905 [11] was passed, establishing different lines of action in order to strengthen public health policies to promote the reduction of the consumption of sodium. One of the strategies was the definition of mandatory maximum levels of sodium in selected processed foods included in the former voluntary agreement, with the MoH being the implementation authority to set new progressive and gradual reduction targets and to include new food categories. In 2017, according to the Joint Resolution 1-E/2017 [12], these maximum limits were included in the Argentinean Food Code (CAA, by its Spanish acronym).

A key component of any sodium reduction intervention must be monitoring sodium consumption at the population level [9]. It should provide essential information to policymakers and all interested stakeholders on the population levels of sodium consumption; the main dietary sources of sodium; the goals and objectives to be reached and the progress, and limitations and results of the implementation of the intervention [2]. As was previously mentioned, measurements of total sodium intake through 24 h urinary excretion at the national level in Argentina have not been undertaken yet, but using the spot urines from a pilot study conducted in the province of La Pampa, a mean sodium consumption of 4832 mg/day for men, 3983 mg/day for women, and 4407 mg/day on average, was estimated, equivalent to 12.1, 10, and 11 grams/day of salt, respectively [13]. Although urinary sodium excretion can indicate the magnitude of the problem within a population, neither the sources of sodium intakes nor the means to reduce it can be identified through this measure. A complete determination of sodium sources involves assessment of several separate elements including dietary intake, sodium content of food consumed, and discretionary salt use in cooking or at table [9]. Frequency of discretionary salt use at the table has been assessed at the three waves of the National Risk Factor Surveys (NRFS) [7,14,15], showing that population that have reported adding always or almost always salt at the table represented 23.1%, 25.3%, and 17.3% in 2005, 2009, and 2013. Discretionary salt use in cooking has been less studied and, according to qualitative studies, it may be an important source of sodium in Latin America [16,17]. Updated information on diet sources of sodium from studies with individual data at the national level is scarce, but based on data from National Health and Nutrition Survey (ENNyS, by its Spanish acronym) conducted in 2004–2005 among children and women less than 50 years, the MoH estimated that between 65% and 70% of dietary sodium intakes come from processed foods [8]. A recent work analyzing sodium content in processed foods based on nutritional panels has indicated that in 2014, before the national law had entered into force, most of the regulated products were below or at the upper-levels defined by the regulation [18]. However, full interpretation of the achieved reduction of sodium content in these foods required dietary intake data of these food products. Henceforth, some knowledge gaps should be filled to effectively guide policy development and monitoring; mainly: (a) which are the main food products that are currently providing most of the sodium at the population level; (b) how much sodium are they contributing? (c) how often is the consumption of low-salt food alternatives? (d) do the main sources differ across subgroups of age, sex, and level of education? (e) are the implemented strategies covering the main sources of sodium at different population groups? Although the national level is the target for a national policy, and a second wave of the ENNyS is planned to be conducted in the short-term, before those results are ready, analysis of dietary population-based information at sub-national levels will be useful to feed the policy implementation process by supporting interventions tending to achieve the goal of consuming less than 5 g of salt per day.

Thus, the purpose of this study is to contribute to the implementation, monitoring, and evaluation of salt reduction policies and the design of new courses of action by providing policy makers and stakeholders with valuable information about the main diet sources of sodium among adults in Argentina and their variation across subgroups of sex, age, and level of education. With this aim, we used Argentinean data from a Southern Cone multicentric population-based cohort study, to examine estimated sodium intakes from selected food products, the consumption of main available low-salt alternatives, the frequency of discretionary salt use in cooking and at the table among adults in 2014, before the full implementation of the national law.

2. Materials and Methods

2.1. Design and Population

We conducted a cross-sectional study in a random subset of participants of the CESCAS I (Centro de Excelencia en Salud Cardiovascular para América del Sur) Study [19]. Details of the study design and sampling methods of the CESCAS I study have been published elsewhere [20]. Briefly, a random multiple-stage stratified sampling was used to select representative samples of the general population, aged 35–74 years old from four cities in Latin America: Bariloche and Marcos Paz in Argentina, Temuco in Chile and Canelones in Uruguay. The sampling design included four stages: In the first stage, census enumeration areas were randomly selected in each location using probability proportional to size, with stratification by socioeconomic level of the enumeration area. In the second stage, blocks per census enumeration area were also randomly selected. In the third stage, households from each block were selected through systematic random sampling methods. In the fourth stage, one household member between 35–74 years old was selected for the study.

In the present study, we assessed the frequency of consumption of cooking/table salt among the participants of the CESCAS cohort living in Bariloche and Marcos Paz (n = 3026). In addition, we administered a food frequency questionnaire to a random subsample of 2127 participants from these Argentinean cities. Data was collected from September 2013 to June 2014.

2.2. Ethical Statement

All subjects gave their informed consent for inclusion before they participated in the study. The study was conducted in accordance with the Declaration of Helsinki, and the protocol was approved by the *Comité de Protocolos de Investigación del the Hospital Italiano de Buenos Aires* (Project 1489).

2.3. Dietary Assessment

Frequency of consumption and average portions of selected foods sources of sodium as well as their low-sodium alternatives were estimated by a short Food Frequency Questionnaire (FFQ) recently developed and validated in Argentina [21] for monitoring nutrition policies of reduction of sodium and trans fat recently implemented at the country. Items were selected based on categories of foods potentially affected by the new legislation, and local food composition and consumption data. The questionnaire was evaluated by expert nutritionists to assess face-validity, and then it was compared with three 24-h recalls. The short FFQ showed good inter-method reliability to estimate sodium intake from processed foods (paired *t*-test, $p > 0.05$; percent difference <10%; Spearman correlations > 0.5; cross-classification in opposite quartile < 10%), with no proportional bias (Bland–Altman correlation, $p > 0.05$) [21]. The short FFQ queries the frequency of intake of 34 food items during the last 12 months and asks the portion size for most of them (Table S1). Three food items represent low-sodium products that are currently available in the country (cheese, bread, and crackers without added salt), which are alternatives to frequently consumed foods with high sodium content. Average consumption of each food item per day was calculated based on frequency of consumption and portion size [22,23]. Sodium provided by each food item was calculated considering the average consumption of each food item per day and data of sodium content in food products [8,18,24,25] (Table S2).

Frequency of use of cooking/table salt was also assessed through two questions with 5 response options each (never, rarely, sometimes, often, and always).

The questionnaire was administered at home by trained interviewers.

2.4. Covariables

Age, sex, and highest level of education data were collected. Marital status, health insurance coverage (yes/no), prevalence of hypertension (defined as systolic blood pressure $\geq$140 mm Hg and/or diastolic blood pressure $\geq$90 mm Hg, and/or use of antihypertensive medication), overweight and obesity (defined as body mass index >25 to $\leq$30 kg/m^2 and >30 kg/m^2), central obesity (defined as waist circumference $\geq$102 for men and $\geq$88 cm for women), smoking, and low physical activity (<600 MET-minutes/per week) were obtained from CESCAS I baseline database [19]. Blood pressure, height, weight, and waist circumference were measured by trained nurses at the baseline stage of the study.

2.5. Data Analysis

We estimated daily intake of sodium from selected foods overall and by subgroups of sex (male and female), age (35 to 54, 55 to 74 years old) and level of education (less than <8 years, 8–12 years, >12 years). We also estimated frequency of consumption, average intake/day, and average contribution of sodium from the selected food items and frequency of discretionary salt use. For descriptive purposes and to assess associations between discretionary salt use and demographic characteristics, response options were contracted into two categories: Never, rarely, or sometimes; and often or always. To assess associations, education level options were also contracted in two categories. Assessment of the association of demographic variables with sodium intake from processed foods was adjusted using multivariable linear regression. We derived odds ratios using multivariable logistic regression to assess associations of demographic variables with discretionary salt use.

Data were analyzed using Stata/SE 12 (StataCorp, College Station, TX, USA) and all analyses were weighted considering the survey's complex design.

3. Results

3.1. Characteristics of the Sample

Socio-demographic, lifestyle, and clinical characteristics of the participants are presented in Table 1.

Table 1. General characteristics of the study population.

Characteristics	Discretionary Salt Data (*n* = 3026) (%)	Short FFQ (*n* = 2129) (%)
Female	62.0	61.5
Age		
35–54 years	50.4	53.1
$\geq$55 years	49.5	46.9
Education		
$\leq$7 years	56.0	54.0
8–12 years	30.8	31.8
>12 years	13.2	14.2
Marital Status [1]		
Married	67.7	68.6
Single, divorced or widowed	32.3	31.4

Table 1. *Cont.*

Characteristics	Discretionary Salt Data (n = 3026) (%)	Short FFQ (n = 2129) (%)
Health Insurance coverage	56.0	49.0
City		
Bariloche	46.2	42.8
Marcos Paz	53.8	57.2
Lifestyle and clinical characteristics [1,2]		
Low physical activity (<600 MET-minutes/week)	22.7	23.4
Current smoker	27.2	28.4
Overweight (BMI $\geq$ 25 and < 30 kg/m^2)	37.5	36.7
Obesity (BMI $\geq$ 30 kg/m^2)	36.6	37.4
Central Obesity [3]	49.6	48.5
Hypertension [4]	43.9	41.4

BMI: Body mass index, FFQ: Food frequency questionnaire; [1] Data from baseline (2011–2012); [2] Weighted data; [3] Waist circumference $\geq$102 for men and $\geq$88 cm for women; [4] Systolic blood pressure $\geq$140 mm Hg and/or diastolic blood pressure $\geq$90 mm Hg and/or use of antihypertensive medication.

3.2. Sodium Intake from Processed Foods

Table 2 shows the average daily sodium intake from the selected processed foods by sex, age, and level of education. The average intake of sodium from these foods was 1861 mg/day (4.7 g of salt), 1651 mg/day (4.1 g of salt) and 2098 mg/day (5.3 g of salt) overall, among women and men, respectively. Sex and level of education were independent predictors of sodium consumption ($p < 0.001$ and $p = 0.006$, Supplementary Table S3). Sodium intake from processed foods among men were 439 mg/day (95% CI: 304–574 mg/day) higher than women, and those with more than 8 years of formal education reported a mean consumption 192 mg/day (95% CI: 328–56 mg/day) lower.

Table 2. Weighted mean, standard error (SE), and 95% confidence interval (95% CI) of estimates of daily intakes of sodium (mg) from food items included in the short FFQ by sex, age, and level of education.

	Overall (n = 2129)			Female (n = 1310)			Male (n = 819)		
	Mean (mg/day) [1]	SE	(95% CI)	Mean (mg/day)	SE	(95% CI)	Mean (mg/day)	SE	(95% CI)
All	1861	33.7	(1795–1928)	1651	37.6	(1578–1725)	2098	56.9	(1987–2210)
				Age					
<55 y	1875	45	(1788–1963)	1675	50	(1577–1772)	2104	76	(1956–2252)
$\geq$55 y	1831	46	(1741–1921)	1604	52	(1503–1705)	2085	77	(1933–2237)
				Education					
$\leq$7 y	1966	48	(1871–2061)	1792	57	(1681–1903)	2147	79	(1991–2302)
8–12 y	1825	61	(1706–1944)	1575	64	(1449–1701)	2139	107	(1930–2349)
>12 y	1691	72	(1550–1831)	1492	77	(1341–1643)	1912	122	(1670–2151)

SE: Standard error; y: Years; [1] Values are expressed in mg of sodium; to calculate grams of salt, multiply mg of sodium by 0.0025.

3.3. Main Sources of Sodium Among Processed Food Groups and Food Categories Affected by the Current Legislation (National Act 26.905)

The frequency of consumption of each food item is described in Supplementary Table S4. Briefly, farinaceous such as breads and crackers were the food products more frequently consumed. Bread sold at bakeries was the product with the highest frequency of consumption. More than 70% of the participants reported they had consumed this type of bread at least once a week during the past 12 months and 26% had done so every day. Also, crackers were consumed by 21% of the population daily. Regarding alternatives with less sodium, almost 30% of participants reported consuming crackers without added salt at least once a week. Mean consumptions of without-added-salt crackers, breads, and cheeses were 6.8 (SE: 0.3), 8.3 (SE: 0.6), and 19 (SE: 0.8) g/day, and provided less than 1% of sodium from processed foods. Other processed foods such as cheeses and bouillon cubes/powders were consumed more than once a week by at least 25% of the population, and meat products such as cold cuts, and other convenient foods such as pizzas, empanadas/pies puff were consumed by near 45% of participants at least once a week. By contrast, less than 10% of the population reported consuming salted snacks every week.

Mean daily intakes and sodium provided from each product as well as their relative importance out of the total sodium from all processed foods in the questionnaire are summarized in Table 3 and Figure 1. In the same table, products were classified as regulated with maximum limits of sodium content by Act 26.905 or not regulated. The main food groups providing sodium were: "Soups and other convenience foods", "Bread, crackers and cookies", "Meat products", and "Cheeses". It was estimated that they accounted for 36.1%, 24.9%, 18.7%, and 15.0% of the sodium provided by processed foods, respectively. In particular, some food products were estimated to represent the major sources of sodium from processed foods in this population, including meat products (18.7%), bread from bakeries (18.1%), bouillon cubes/powder and instant soups (17.5%), cheeses (15%), and puff pastry for pies/empanadas (9.2%), as well as pizza (4.6%). Nearly half of the sodium (47.6%) was provided by products regulated by the law. Among those products not included in the law, French bread and other packaged foods products not yet regulated provided the rest of the salt. Figure 2 presents the main sources of sodium among food products and potential interventions to reduce the intakes at the population level.

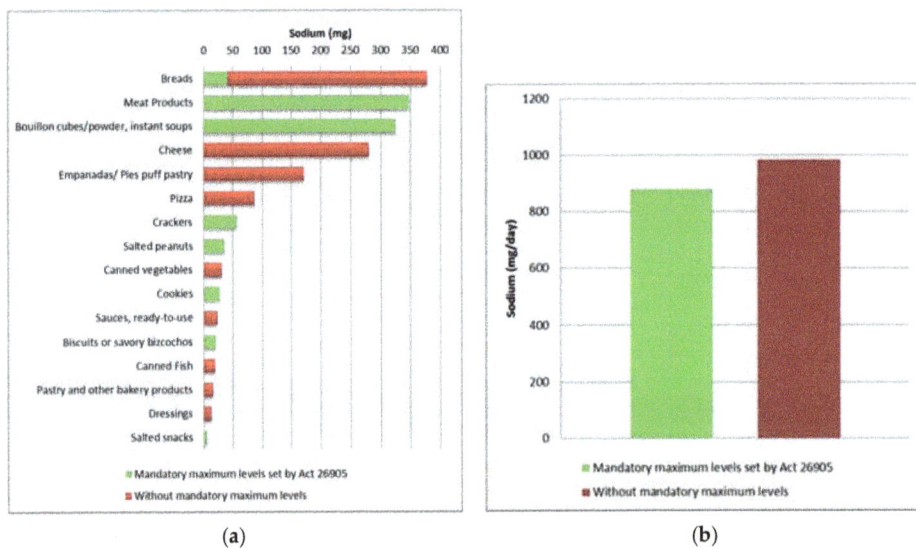

(a)   (b)

Figure 1. Dietary food categories sources of sodium and National Act 26.905: (**a**) Ranking of main dietary sources of sodium and food groups regulated by Act 26.905; (**b**) Sodium intakes from food categories with and without mandatory maximum levels.

Ranking of food sources among processed foods by age, sex, and educational level are presented in Supplementary Tables S5.1–S5.4. Bread, meat products, bouillon cubes/powder or instant soups, and chesses were the most important sources. In general, the first two food sources of sodium among men were bread from bakeries and meat products. Among women, bouillon cubes/powder or soups and meat products were the principal sources, but there were some differences of relative importance of food sources according to the educational attainment (e.g., bread intake was lower and cheese intake was higher at higher educational level). Food sources of sodium among women and low level of education were more frequently categories of foods with maximum limits included in the current national law. (Supplementary Material Figure S1).

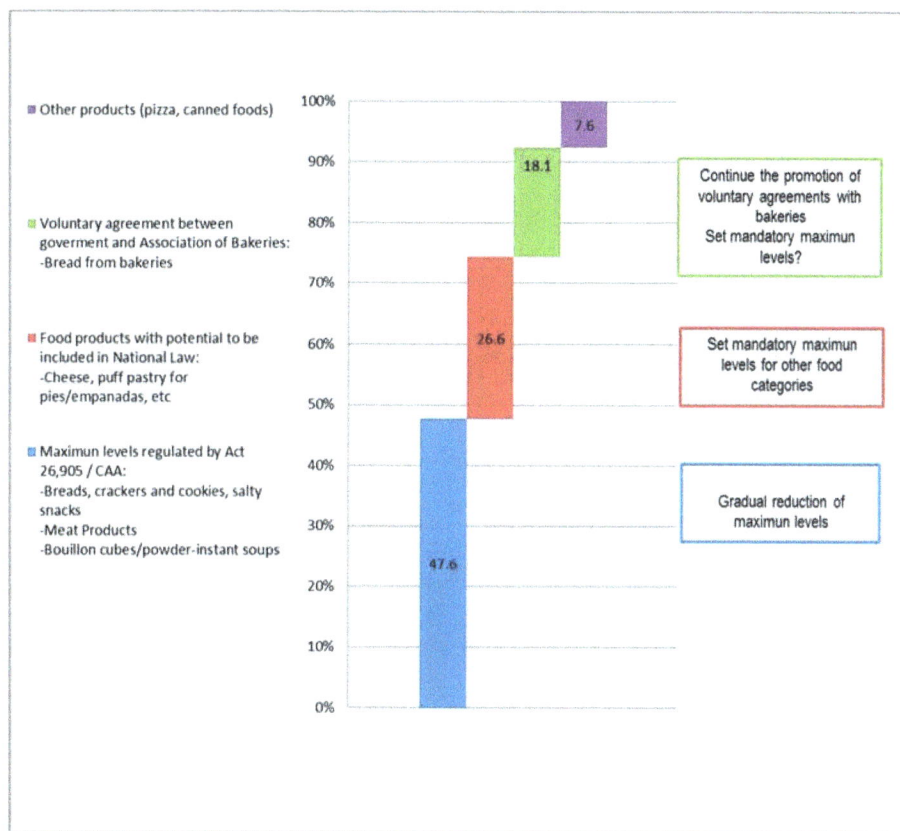

Figure 2. Main sources of sodium among food products and potential interventions to reduce the intakes at the population level.

Table 3. Mean intakes of food products and sodium by food categories with or without mandatory maximum limits regulated by National Act 26.905.

Food Groups	Food Intake/Person (g/Day or ml/Day) * Mean (SE)	Estimated Sodium Consumed per Person (mg/Day) Mean (SE)	Percentage of Sodium Provided by Food Category [1]	Maximum Limit Set by Act 26.905
Soups, dressings, canned foods, and other convenience foods			36.1	
Bouillon cubes or powder	60 (1.9) *	213 (6.9)	11.5	Yes
Instant soups	47 (2.1) *	112 (5)	6.0	Yes
Puff pastry for pies/quiches	17 (0.5)	106 (3.3)	5.7	No
Puff pastry for *empanadas* [2]	10.5 (0.3)	65 (1.6)	3.5	No
Pizza	17.1 (0.4)	86 (2.2)	4.6	No
Canned vegetables/legumes	15 (0.5)	32 (1.1)	1.7	No
Canned Fish	5.8 (0.2)	20 (0.6)	1.1	No
Sauces, ready-to-use	6.1 (0.2)	24 (0.8)	1.3	No
Dressings: Mayonnaise, mustard, ketchup, etc.	1.4 (0.1)	13 (0.6)	0.7	

Table 3. *Cont.*

Food Groups	Food Intake/Person (g/Day or ml/Day) * Mean (SE)	Estimated Sodium Consumed per Person (mg/Day) Mean (SE)	Percentage of Sodium Provided by Food Category [1]	Maximum Limit Set by Act 26.905
Breads, crackers, cookies			24.9	
Bread, French or whole wheat (from bakeries)	42 (1.5)	336 (11.7)	18.1	No
Bread, Sliced or sandwich (packaged)	5.8 (0.4)	29 (1.8)	1.5	Yes
Bread, Vienna, hot dog/hamburger bun (packaged)	2.9 (0.2)	14 (1)	0.7	Yes
Crackers, white or whole wheat (packaged)	9.1 (0.4)	57 (2.5)	3.1	Yes
Cookies (packaged)	4.1 (0.2)	12 (0.6)	0.6	Yes
Filled/sandwich cookies such as Oreo	6.4 (0.3)	16 (0.8)	0.9	Yes
Meat Products			18.7	
Vienna sausage	5 (0.2)	49 (2.1)	2.6	Yes
Chorizo/Chorizo sausage/Argentinean sausage	8.5 (0.3)	89 (3.1)	4.8	Yes
Other cold cuts (such as ham, salami, bologna, etc.)	7.5 (0.2)	62 (2)	3.3	Yes
Pre-processed hamburgers	11.3 (0.5)	81 (3.6)	4.4	Yes
Frozen pre-cooked breaded chicken, nuggets or fish	12.8 (0.5)	66 (2.8)	3.5	Yes
Cheeses			15.0	
Soft cheeses	29.1 (1)	129 (4.4)	6.9	No
Semi-hard cheeses	21 (0.7)	131 (4.5)	7.0	No
Hard cheese	2.5 (0.1)	20 (0.5)	1.1	No
Pastry, other bakery products, sweets			2.0	
Biscuits or savory bizcochos	2.8 (0.1)	21 (0.9)	1.1	Yes [3]
Cakes, pies, muffins, etc.	2.9 (0.1)	8 (0.4)	0.4	Yes
Danish/croissants and other Argentine facturas [4]	9.2 (0.3)	5 (0.2)	0.3	No
Alfajores [5]	2.9 (0.2)	3 (0.2)	0.2	No
Other			2.7	
Salted snacks	0.8 (0)	6 (0.3)	0.3	Yes
Salted peanuts	2.5 (0.1)	37 (1.6)	2.0	Yes
Butter/Margarine	2.1 (0.1)	3.8 (0.2)	0.2	No

SE: Standard error. * All values are g/day, except bouillon cubes and instant soup, which are expressed as ml/day of reconstituted product. [1] Percentage out of 1861 mg/day from the sum of these foods and alternative low-salt foods. [2] Small pie. [3] Partially, only packaged products. [4] Traditional pastry. [5] Sweet biscuit with filling.

3.4. Use of Discretionary Salt

The reported frequencies of use of salt at the table often or always, and in cooking were 9.9% and 73.3%, respectively (Table 4). In multivariable analysis (Supplementary Table S6), older adults were more likely to report avoiding salt use in cooking and at the table (OR of often/always adding salt in cooking: 0.66, 95% CI: 0.59–0.73; at the table: 0.67, 95% CI: 0.53–0.85). Men were more likely than women to report salt use at the table (OR: 1.38; 95% CI 1.09–1.73). There was no association of level of education with reported salt use in cooking or at the table.

Table 4. Weighted frequency, standard error (SE), and 95% confidence interval (95% CI) of discretional use of salt in cooking and at the table by sex, age, and level of education.

Characteristics	Overall (n = 3026)			Female (n = 1879)			Male (n = 1147)		
	%	SE	(95% CI)	%	SE	(95% CI)	%	SE	(95% CI)
			Use of salt in cooking (often or always)						
All	73.3	0.9	(71.5–75.1)	72.7	1.1	(70.5–74.9)	74	1.5	(71.1–76.9)
				Age					
≤55 y	79.4	1.2	(77.2–81.7)	78.6	1.4	(75.8–81.4)	80.3	1.9	(76.7–84)
>55 y	61.7	1.4	(59–64.4)	61.7	1.8	(58.2–65.2)	61.7	2.2	(57.5–66)
				Education					
≤7 y	70.8	1.2	(68.3–73.2)	68.9	1.6	(65.8–72.0)	72.9	1.9	(69–76.7)
8–12 y	77.6	1.5	(74.6–80.6)	77.7	1.9	(74.0–81.03)	77.5	2.4	(72.7–82.3)
>12 y	71.5	2.5	(66.5–76.5)	72.5	3	(66.6–78.4)	70.3	4.2	(62.1–78.6)
			Use of salt at the table (often or always)						
All	9.9	0.7	(8.5–11.3)	9.2	0.9	(7.5–10.9)	10.8	1.2	(8.5–13.1)
				Age					
≤55 y	11.0	1.0	(9.0–12.9)	10.4	1.2	(8.1–12.8)	11.6	1.6	(8.4–14.7)
>55 y	8.0	0.8	(6.3–9.6)	6.8	1.0	(4.8–8.9)	9.3	1.4	(6.5–12.0)
				Education					
≤7 y	8.6	0.9	(6.8–10.4)	8	1.1	(5.8–10.2)	9.3	1.5	(6.4–12.2)
8–12 y	10.5	1.2	(8.1–13)	10.1	1.6	(7–13.2)	11	2	(7.1–14.8)
>12 y	12.5	2	(8.5–16.5)	10.5	2.2	(6.1–14.9)	14.8	3.5	(7.9–21.6)

SE: Standard Error; y: years.

4. Discussion

This study identified sodium intake from selected food products and the top contributors to dietary sodium intake as well as frequency of discretional salt use in adults older than 35 years old in two Argentinean cities. Separate estimates for groups of age, sex, and level of education are also described.

While bread from bakeries is known to be the major source of sodium in Argentina, our study set forth identifying other food sources of sodium to monitor and develop strategies to reduce sodium intake in our population. Once identified, we sought to study if these other sources had been included in the 2013 National Law. The food categories included in the law provided 2.1 g/day of salt (875 mg/day of sodium), with meat products and bouillon cubes/powders as top contributors (near 1.7 g/day of salt or 675 mg/day of sodium). As Allemandi et al. [18] have previously reported, based on sodium content declared in food labels, all the evaluated bouillon cubes and soups (n = 27) and almost all (51 out of 55) meat products were below the mandatory targets before the act was full implemented. Some snacks and packaged bakery products were also above the target in 2013–2014 [25]. In our study, if mean content of sodium in meat products, snacks, and packaged baked products that were above the target (Table S1) were reduced to mandatory maximum levels, the sodium intake would be reduced in less than 30 mg/day of sodium. In this scenario, food categories included in the National Law would provide 849 mg/day of sodium instead of 875 mg/day. Thus, reaching further reduction of sodium intake would require monitoring and also adjusting the maximum limits of these products.

In addition to the foods currently included in the law, we also identified other products that are contributors of sodium intake and could be incorporated into the regulation in the future. For instance, cheeses were important contributors to the overall sodium intake (0.7 g/day of salt or 280 mg of sodium), and therefore would be good candidates to be included in further regulations, mainly because there were previous experiences of voluntary agreement of progressive reduction of salt in these products [26]. Other food products categorized as convenience foods, such as puff pastry for "empanadas" (small filled pies) and pies/quiches, which are quite frequently consumed in Argentina, were moderate but consistent contributors of sodium (170 mg/day of sodium and 0.4 g/day of salt) and could be considered for salt reduction and setting of maximum levels of sodium content.

As expected, artisanal bread, like French bread sold at bakeries, was frequently consumed and resulted an important contributor of sodium (336 mg/day sodium and 0.8 g/day of salt). These results were somewhat lower but still consistent with those estimated by the National Nutrition and Health Survey (ENNyS) conducted in 2004–2005 among women aged 10–49 [27] in Argentina, but represented nearly a fourth of the estimated national per capita consumption of 190 g/day in 2010 [28], based on the production and sales. Besides those differences, which could be explained by the different methodologies to measure salt intake such as food production/sales against food consumption, the national "Less Salt More Life" Program reported that between 2009 and 2015 more than 9000 traditional bakeries and hypermarkets had voluntarily adhered to 25% sodium reduction in breads [26]. We used in our work an estimation of 2% of salt in bread [8], however the current contribution of sodium may be lower since we are not considering the last Less Salt More Life actions. More efforts should be made to reach most of the bakeries at local levels. If the content of salt in bread from all bakeries was 1.5%, the reduction in sodium intake in this population would be of 84 mg/day or 0.21 g/day of salt. The baseline level of sodium in breads in Argentina was similar to other South American countries like Paraguay and Chile. Mandatory and voluntary reduction policies have been implemented in other Latin American countries. Initial reduction of salt in bread in those countries was similar to that implemented in Argentina (25%), but further reductions seem to be feasible, like the experience of Chile [29], and countries in other regions (e.g., UK, Ireland, and Australia) [30]. Most of the reduction of sodium in bread in Argentina was voluntary. If these reformulation efforts were mandatory in Argentina and maximum limits were the same as that for the packaged breads without bran (maximum limit of 501 mg/100 g), the reduction in sodium intake in this population would be of 126 mg/d or 0.31 g/d of salt. Based on previous estimations, both scenarios, as well as further reductions, would have a significant impact on the mortality and morbidity of the population [31].

In our work, discretionary salt use at the table proved to be in good agreement with results of the National Risk Factors Survey conducted in 2013 [7], including the gradient across age groups and gender. Moreover, the most remarkable result about discretionary salt use that emerged from our data was that almost 3/4 of the population reported they often/always use salt in cooking, with higher frequencies among younger adults. In our study, the percentage of people that have reported table salt usage often or very often was near the proportion reported in USA [32] and slightly lower than in Australia [33] and the UK [34]. However, adding salt "often or very often" during cooking was very much more frequent than reported in those countries. Nowson et al. [35] have reported a relationship between the discretionary salt used sometimes or often/always and higher salt excretion. Thus, implemented strategies to reduce the use of salt at the table should be maintained (e.g., education, interventions reducing salt shakers at the table in restaurants) though changing discretional use of salt in cooking may require other actions. The Argentinean Food Guidelines [36,37] explicitly recommend reducing salt use while cooking along with replacement with herbs and condiments. However, recent qualitative studies have reported that people trying to reduce the amount of salt may use strategies like using seasonings such as mayonnaise, balsamic vinegar, lemon, or consommés [17], some of them with high sodium-content such as bouillon cubes/powders, which were not recognized as sources of salt [16]. Additionally, other studies conducted in Argentina have reported that reducing consumption of salt tended to be a reactive event when personal/family health events took place, rather than a proactive behavior [16,38], and that people tended to perceive to have a high intake of salt based only on table salt [38].

In our study, sodium intake from processed foods almost reached the maximum recommended intake of salt, and also a high percentage of the population reported adding salt during cooking. While in developed regions, such as European and Northern American countries, sodium intake is dominated by sodium added in manufactured foods ($\geq$75% of intake) [39], in Latin American countries both discretionary salt and processed foods can be identified as important sources of sodium [17]. For example, more than 70% of dietary sodium in Brazil is provided by salt and salt-based condiments added to foods [40]. However, consumption of processed foods and ready meals is rapidly growing [41] in Brazil and other countries of the region [42].

This study has several strengths. First, the sample is representative of the general population in those cities, and since it has been conducted immediately before the law entered into force, it can provide useful baseline data to allow monitoring of future progress. To our knowledge, this is the first study in our country to analyze sources of sodium in subgroups of adults of both sexes according to age and education level in a population-based sample. This information is very useful to adapt policies to facilitate and promote a healthy food environment to specific vulnerable subgroups of the population. Also, in this work, we have estimated sodium consumption provided by a list of foods from a short FFQ, which have shown good inter-method reliability to obtain population estimations compared with three 24-h recalls. There are also some limitations. Data about sodium content in food products were estimated mainly for indirect sources. However, this approach allows including information representative of sodium content of main available food products at one time point and could be then updated to perform comparisons. Also, these results need to be interpreted with caution because they might not be generalized to the national level or people younger than 35 years old. Regarding the questionnaire, reported sodium intake here represents only estimated sodium from processed foods, which is likely to be lower than the total sodium intake because of the exclusion of salt added in cooking, at the table, fresh foods, and from fresh foods, supplements, and medicines. Besides that, it has been the first application of this tool in a large-population study and the FFQ seems to be feasible to implement in other settings, or to repeat its application in the future in the same population to assess changes in consumption of processed food sources of sodium. Because the original questionnaire aims to assess sodium and trans fatty acids, some foods (e.g., margarine and butter) providing very low dietary sodium could be avoided in future applications.

Identified food sources could be targets for interventions by reducing sodium content in these foods and/or reducing the intake of these products. Since salt in foods has many functions [43] and several actors are involved in reformulation processes, selection of new food categories to be included in the legislation and/or further reduction of sodium content in products already included should be made based on feasibility, opportunity, technology, and implementation issues [8,44,45]. It is a primary responsibility of the government to guide and facilitate these processes as it is its duty to provide relevant information and education that allow the population to make informed food choices, like the diffusion and updating of the national food guidelines and devising a more clear food labeling strategy [17,46].

5. Conclusions

In summary, the results of our study have helped to identify the main sources of sodium intake among adults in two Argentinean cities. The identification of these foods will be important for monitoring and developing strategies to reduce sodium intake in this population. It is concluded that in these Argentine cities, selected processed foods such as bread, meat products, bouillon cubes/powders, soups, cheeses, other convenience foods, and bakery products are important contributors of sodium to the adult's diet in these Argentine cities, with some differences among sex and level of education. In addition, discretional salt use is very frequent, particularly in cooking among both sexes. Nearly half of the sodium from processed foods is estimated to have been provided by products with maximum limits set in 2013 by National Act 26.905. Based on our findings, government strategies to reduce salt consumption at the national population level are well directed, but further interventions are necessary to offer a healthy food environment and promote healthy food choices. Among them, the government should consider: (a) progressive reductions of already defined targets, which could positively influence sodium consumption of all the population, and particularly women and people with less educational level; (b) inclusion of maximum limits for other food products that represent important contributions of sodium such as cheese and bread rom bakeries; (c) development of new and clearer labeling strategies to allow the population to better identify food sources of salt as well as regulation of publicity of foods; (d) the launch of campaigns targeting salt use and other high-sodium ingredients in cooking such as bouillon cubes that are not recognized as food high in salt. Continuing the implementation of salt reduction policies in Argentina will contribute to the progress in preventing and controlling cardiovascular diseases and their associated risk factors and will also help accomplish global targets of reducing premature deaths from NCDs by 2025.

Supplementary Materials: The following are available online at www.mdpi.com/2072-6643/9/9/964/s1, Table S1: Food items included in the short questionnaire, household measuring units to estimate quantities per time, sodium content per 100 g of food and maximum values set by National Act 26905; Table S2: Sodium content in food products/100 g of food: Source of data; Table S3: Weighted linear regression models of sodium intake from food products; Table S4: Reported weighted frequency of consumption of separated food items included in the short questionnaire during the last 12 months; Table S5.1: Main dietary sources of sodium among women by age group; Table S5.2: Main dietary sources of sodium among men by age group; Table S5.3: Main dietary sources of sodium among women by level of education; Table S5.4: Main dietary sources of sodium among men by level of education; Table S6: Multiple-adjusted odds ratios of adding salt associated with demographic characteristics in adults aged 35–74 years, Bariloche and Marcos Paz, Argentina, *n* = 3026; Figure S1: Sources of sodium from food products considering the inclusion in the National Act 26905, by sex and level of education.

Acknowledgments: This work was supported by the National Heart, Lung, and Blood Institute of the National Institutes of Health under contract No. 268200900029C and the International Development Research Center, Ottawa, ON, Canada. IDRC Project 106881-001.

Author Contributions: N.E., V.I. and A.R. conceived and designed the study; N.E., R.P., N.M. and M.C. coordinated and conducted the field work; N.E., L.G., I.B.R. and D.L.M. analyzed the data; N.E. and I.R wrote the first draft of the paper; all authors read and approved the last version of the paper.

Conflicts of Interest: The authors declare no conflict of interest. The founding sponsors had no role in the design of the study; in the collection, analyses, or interpretation of data; in the writing of the manuscript, and in the decision to publish the results.

References

1. WHO. *Preventing Chronic Disease: A Vital Investment*; World Health Organization: Geneva, Switzerland, 2005.
2. WHO. *Global Status Report on Noncommunicable Diseases 2010*; World Health Organization: Geneva, Switzerland, 2011.
3. Murray, C.J.; Lauer, J.A.; Hutubessy, R.C.; Niessen, L.; Tomijima, N.; Rodgers, A.; Lawes, C.M.; Evans, D.B. Effectiveness and costs of interventions to lower systolic blood pressure and cholesterol: A global and regional analysis on reduction of cardiovascular-disease risk. *Lancet* **2003**, *361*, 717–725. [CrossRef]
4. Bibbins-Domingo, K.; Chertow, G.M.; Coxson, P.G.; Moran, A.; Lightwood, J.M.; Pletcher, M.J.; Goldman, L. Projected effect of dietary salt reductions on future cardiovascular disease. *N. Engl. J. Med.* **2010**, *362*, 590–599. [CrossRef] [PubMed]
5. Natalidad y Mortalidad 2014. Síntesis Estadística 1. Available online: http://www.deis.msal.gov.ar/wp-content/uploads/2016/05/Sintesis-estadistica-Nro1.pdf (accessed on 10 February 2017).
6. Rubinstein, A.; Colantonio, L.; Bardach, A.; Caporale, J.; Marti, S.G.; Kopitowski, K.; Alcaraz, A.; Gibbons, L.; Augustovski, F.; Pichon-Riviere, A. Estimation of the burden of cardiovascular disease attributable to modifiable risk factors and cost-effectiveness analysis of preventative interventions to reduce this burden in Argentina. *BMC Public Health* **2010**, *10*, 627. [CrossRef] [PubMed]
7. Ministerio de Salud de la Nación. *Tercera Encuesta Nacional de Factores de Riesgo Para Enfermedades No Transmisibles*, 1st ed.; Ministerio de Salud de la Nación, Instituto Nacional de Estadísticas y Censos: Buenos Aires, Argentina, 2015.
8. Ferrante, D.; Apro, N.; Ferreira, V.; Virgolini, M.; Aguilar, V.; Sosa, M.; Perel, P.; Casas, J. Feasibility of salt reduction in processed foods in Argentina. *Rev. Panam. Salud Publ.* **2011**, *29*, 69–75. [CrossRef]
9. WHO. *Strategies to Monitor and Evaluate Population Sodium Consumption and Sources of Sodium in the Diet: Report of a Joint Technical Meeting Convened by Who and the Government of Canada*; World Health Organization (WHO): Geneva, Switzerland, 2011.
10. Ministry of Health. Menos sal más Vida (Less Salt More Life). Available online: http://www.msal.gob.ar/ent/index.php/informacion-para-ciudadanos/menos-sal--vida (accessed on 10 March 2016).
11. National Act 26.905. *Consumo de Sodio. Valores Máximos*; El Senado y Cámara de Diputados de la Nación Argentina reunidos en Congreso: Buenos Aires, Argentina, 2013.
12. *Resolución Conjunta 137/10 y 941/10*; Secretaría de Políticas Regulación e Institutos; Secretaría de Agricultura Ganadería y Pesca: Buenos Aires, Argentina, 2010.
13. Ministerio de Salud de la Nación. *Estrategia Piloto Para Reducir el Consumo de Sal en la Provincia de la Pampa*; Ministerio de Salud: Buenos Aires, Argentina, 2013.
14. Ferrante, D.; Virgolini, M. Encuesta nacional de factores de riesgo 2005: Resultados principales: Prevalencia de factores de riesgo de enfermedades cardiovasculares en la Argentina. *Rev. Argent Cardiol.* **2007**, *75*, 20–29.

15. Daniels, S.R.; Linetzky, B.; Konfino, J.; King, A.; Virgolini, M.; Laspiur, S. Encuesta nacional de factores de riesgo 2009: Evolución de la epidemia de enfermedades crónicas no transmisibles en argentina. Estudio de corte transversal. *Rev. Argent Salud Públ.* **2011**, *2*, 34–41.

16. Peña, L.; Bergesio, L.; Discacciati, V.; Majdalani, M.P.; Elorriaga, N.; Mejía, R. Actitudes y comportamientos acerca del consumo de sodio y grasas trans en Argentina. *Rev. Argent Salud Públ.* **2015**, *6*, 7–13.

17. Sanchez, G.; Peña, L.; Varea, S.; Mogrovejo, P.; Goetschel, M.L.; Montero-Campos Mde, L.; Mejia, R.; Blanco-Metzler, A. Knowledge, perceptions, and behavior related to salt consumption, health, and nutritional labeling in Argentina, Costa Rica, and Ecuador. *Rev. Panam. Salud Publ.* **2012**, *32*, 259–264.

18. Allemandi, L.; Tiscornia, M.V.; Ponce, M.; Castronuovo, L.; Dunford, E.; Schoj, V. Sodium content in processed foods in Argentina: Compliance with the national law. *Cardiovasc. Diagn. Ther.* **2015**, *5*, 197–206. [PubMed]

19. Rubinstein, A.L.; Irazola, V.E.; Calandrelli, M.; Elorriaga, N.; Gutierrez, L.; Lanas, F.; Manfredi, J.A.; Mores, N.; Olivera, H.; Poggio, R.; et al. Multiple cardiometabolic risk factors in the southern cone of Latin America: A population-based study in Argentina, Chile, and Uruguay. *Int. J. Cardiol.* **2015**, *183C*, 82–88. [CrossRef] [PubMed]

20. Rubinstein, A.L.; Irazola, V.E.; Poggio, R.; Bazzano, L.; Calandrelli, M.; Lanas Zanetti, F.T.; Manfredi, J.A.; Olivera, H.; Seron, P.; Ponzo, J.; et al. Detection and follow-up of cardiovascular disease and risk factors in the southern cone of Latin America: The CESCAS I study. *BMJ Open* **2011**, *1*, 1–6. [CrossRef] [PubMed]

21. Mejia, R. *Assesing the Impact of Current National Policies to Reduce Salt and Ans-Fatty Acids in Argentina. IDRC Project Final Technical Report*; CEDES: Buenos Aires, Argentina, 2015.

22. Suarez, M.M.; Lopez, L.B. *Alimentacion Saludable. Guia Practica Para su Realizacion*; Libreria Editorial Akadia: Buenos Aires, Argentina, 2005.

23. Vázquez, M.; Witriw, A. Modelos Visuales de Alimentos & Tablas de Relación Peso/Volumen. Buenos Aires, Argentina, 1997.

24. Allemandi, L.; Garipe, L.; Schoj, V.; Pizarro, M.; Tambussi, A. Análisis del contenido de sodio y grasas trans de los alimentos industrializados en Argentina. *Rev. Argent Salud Públ.* **2013**, *4*, 14–19.

25. Elorriaga, N.; Bardach, A.E.; Defago, M.D.; Levi, L.; Nessier, M.C.; Irazola, V. Development, implementation and evaluation of tools for decision-making on healthy eating policies in Argentina. In *Anuario Becas de Investigación "Carrillo Oñativia" 2012*; Ministerio de Salud: Buenos Aires, Argentina, 2016; pp. 250–251.

26. Ministerio de Salud. Programa Menos sal más vida 2015. Available online: http://www.msal.gob.ar/ent/images/stories/programas/pdf/2015-11_menos-sal-mas-vida_ppt.pdf (accessed on 25 November 2016).

27. Mangialavori, G.; Guidet, A.B.; Abeyá-Gilardon, E.; Durán, P.; Kogan, L. *Alimentos Consumidos en Argentina. Resultados de la Encuesta Nacional de Nutrición y Salud-ENNyS 2004/5*; Ministerio de Salud: Buenos Aires, Argentina, 2012.

28. Lezcano, E.P. Analisis de producto: Productos panificados. In *Alimentos Argentinos*; Ministerio de Agroindustria: Buenos Aires, Argentina, 2011.

29. Valenzuela, L.K.; Quitral, R.V.; Villanueva, A.B.; Zavala, M.F.; Atalah, S.E. Evaluación del programa piloto de reducción de sal/sodio en el pan en santiago de Chile. *Rev. Chil. Nutr.* **2013**, *40*, 119–122. [CrossRef]

30. Valverde Guillén, M.; Picado Pérez, J. World strategies in salt/sodium reduction in bread. *Rev. Costarric. Salud Públ.* **2013**, *22*, 61–67.

31. Konfino, J.; Mekonnen, T.A.; Coxson, P.G.; Ferrante, D.; Bibbins-Domingo, K. Projected impact of a sodium consumption reduction initiative in Argentina: An analysis from the CVD policy model—Argentina. *PLoS ONE* **2013**, *8*, e73824. [CrossRef] [PubMed]

32. Quader, Z.S.; Patel, S.; Gillespie, C.; Cogswell, M.E.; Gunn, J.P.; Perrine, C.G.; Mattes, R.D.; Moshfegh, A. Trends and determinants of discretionary salt use: National health and nutrition examination survey 2003–2012. *Public Health Nutr.* **2016**, *19*, 2195–2203. [CrossRef] [PubMed]

33. Grimes, C.A.; Riddell, L.J.; Nowson, C.A. The use of table and cooking salt in a sample of Australian adults. *Asia Pac. J. Clin. Nutr.* **2010**, *19*, 256–260. [PubMed]

34. Sutherland, J.; Edwards, P.; Shankar, B.; Dangour, A.D. Fewer adults add salt at the table after initiation of a national salt campaign in the UK: A repeated cross-sectional analysis. *Br. J. Nutr.* **2013**, *110*, 552–558. [CrossRef] [PubMed]

35. Nowson, C.; Lim, K.; Grimes, C.; O'Halloran, S.; Land, M.A.; Webster, J.; Shaw, J.; Chalmers, J.; Smith, W.; Flood, V.; et al. Dietary salt intake and discretionary salt use in two general population samples in Australia: 2011 and 2014. *Nutrients* **2015**, *7*, 10501–10512. [CrossRef] [PubMed]

36. AADYND. *Guías Alimentarias Para la Población Argentina*, 1st ed.; Asociación Argentina de Dietistas y Nutricionistas; Federación Argentina de Graduados en Nutrición: Buenos Aires, Argentina, 2000.

37. Ministerio de Salud de la Nación. *Guías Alimentarias Para la Población Argentina*; Ministerio de Salud: Buenos Aires, Argentina, 2016.

38. Vázquez, S.M.B.; Lema, R.S.N.; Contarini, C.A.; Kenten, C.C. Sal y salud, el punto de vista del consumidor argentino obtenido por la técnica de grupos focales. *Rev. Chil. Nutr.* **2012**, *39*, 182–190. [CrossRef]

39. Brown, I.J.; Tzoulaki, I.; Candeias, V.; Elliott, P. Salt intakes around the world: Implications for public health. *Int. J. Epidemiol.* **2009**, *38*, 791–813. [CrossRef] [PubMed]

40. Sarno, F.; Claro, R.M.; Levy, R.B.; Bandoni, D.H.; Monteiro, C.A. Estimativa de consumo de sódio pela população brasileira, 2008–2009. *Rev. Saúde Públ.* **2013**, *47*, 571–578. [CrossRef]

41. Louzada, M.L.D.C.; Martins, A.P.B.; Canella, D.S.; Baraldi, L.G.; Levy, R.B.; Claro, R.M.; Moubarac, J.-C.; Cannon, G.; Monteiro, C.A. Ultra-processed foods and the nutritional dietary profile in Brazil. *Rev. Saúde Públ.* **2015**, *49*. [CrossRef] [PubMed]

42. Pan American Health Organization. *Ultra-Processed Food and Drink Products in Latin America: Trends, Impact on Obesity, Policy Implications*; PAHO: Washington, DC, USA, 2015.

43. Doyle, M.E.; Glass, K.A. Sodium reduction and its effect on food safety, food quality, and human health. *Compr. Rev. Food Sci. Food Saf.* **2010**, *9*, 44–56. [CrossRef]

44. Speroni, F.; Szerman, N.; Vaudagna, S.R. High hydrostatic pressure processing of beef patties: Effects of pressure level and sodium tripolyphosphate and sodium chloride concentrations on thermal and aggregative properties of proteins. *Innov. Food Sci. Emerg. Technol.* **2014**, *23*, 10–17. [CrossRef]

45. Dominguez, M.; Kleiman, E.; Vaudagna, S.; Vitale-Gutierrez, J.A.; Masana, M. *Escenarios Sobre Exigencias de Calidad e Inocuidad en el Sector Productor de Materias Primas y Alimentos Elaborados en Argentina (2030)*; Ministerio de Ciencia, Tecnología e Innovación Productiva: Buenos Aires, Argentina, 2017.

46. *The Right to Adequate Food*; Fact Sheet No. 34; Office of the United Nations High Commissioner for Human Rights, United Nations Office: Geneva, Switzerland, 2010.

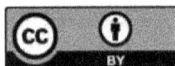

nutrients

MDPI

Review

Infants' and Children's Salt Taste Perception and Liking: A Review

Djin G. Liem

Centre for Advanced Sensory Science, School of Exercise and Nutrition Sciences, Deakin University,
221 Burwood Highway, Burwood, VIC 3125, Australia; gie.liem@deakin.edu.au; Tel.: +61-03-9244-6039

Received: 17 August 2017; Accepted: 8 September 2017; Published: 13 September 2017

Abstract: Sodium is an essential nutrient for the human body. It is widely used as sodium chloride (table salt) in (processed) foods and overconsumed by both children and adults, placing them at risk for adverse health effects such as high blood pressure and cardiovascular diseases. The current review focusses on the development of salt taste sensitivity and preferences, and its association with food intake. Three -to- four month old infants are able to detect and prefer sodium chloride solutions over plain water, which is thought to be a biological unlearned response. Liking for water with sodium chloride mostly decreases when infants enter early childhood, but liking for sodium chloride in appropriate food contexts such as soup and snack foods remains high. The increased acceptance and preference of sodium chloride rich foods coincides with infants' exposure to salty foods, and is therefore thought to be mostly a learned response. Children prefer higher salt concentrations than adults, but seem to be equally sensitive to salt taste. The addition of salt to foods increases children's consumption of those foods. However, children's liking for salt taste as such does not seem to correlate with children's consumption of salty foods. Decreasing the exposure to salty tasting foods during early infancy is recommended. Salt plays an important role in children's liking for a variety of foods. It is, however, questionable if children's liking for salt per se influences the intake of salty foods.

Keywords: taste; smell; salt; foods; nutrition; children; sensory; intake; development

1. Introduction

Sodium is essential for the regulation of the osmotic pressure and extracellular fluids in the human body. It has been estimated that humans need about 180 to 230 mg of sodium per day for normal bodily functioning [1]. Sodium cannot be produced by the human body and therefore needs to be ingested, which, in modern society, is done so mostly in the form of sodium chloride (i.e., table salt). Despite the biological need for sodium, excessive sodium consumption has been related to a range of adverse health outcomes, such as hypertension, gastric cancer and obesity [2–4]. Therefore, the WHO has recommended for adults to consume no more than 2 g of sodium per day. For children (2–16 years) this limit is adjusted downwards, based on energy requirements [5]. In Australia the National Health and Research Council recommends an increasing upper limit with age starting with 1 g of sodium/day as the upper limit for 2–3 years old, which should not exceed 2.3 g sodium/day when children enter the adolescence years (14–18 years) [6]. This is similar to upper limits published by the Center for Disease Control in the United States of America (US) [7].

Sodium chloride is a relatively cheap and widely used ingredient in processed foods [8] and serves a variety of functions. The addition of salt limits microbial growth by lowering the water activity [9]. Texture and juiciness of foods are enhanced by the interaction of salt with protein, and by the enhancement of the hydration and water holding capacity of foods [10]. In bakery products, salt strengthens the gluten network, which improves the elasticity of the dough [11,12]. Moreover, salt is added to foods to improve the flavour profile. The addition of salt not only increases saltiness, but also suppresses bitterness. When bitterness is decreased the sweet taste of food is more noticed, resulting in a generally liked flavour profile [13]. As a result of the wide spread use of sodium chloride in processed foods and the reliance of modern consumers on processed foods, the majority of sodium (75%) in the Western diet comes from processed foods and restaurant foods [14,15]. Only a small proportion of total sodium intake comes from natural sources and from what consumers add to their food during preparation and consumption (i.e., 10 to 15%) [9].

The biological need for sodium, combined with a scarcity of sodium in the diet of the primate ancestors of humans, likely resulted in an evolutionary human drive to consume sodium [16]. Nowadays, the wide spread use of sodium chloride in processed foods has made sodium extremely accessible. This, not surprisingly, leads to an overconsumption of sodium. Yet, it is important to note that well before the existence of modern processed foods, sodium consumption has been well above (i.e., 3–5 g of sodium/day) the human physiological requirements [15]. The consistency in intake over time and across different ethnic populations suggest that the modern food industry is not the only factor involved in humans' high sodium consumption and that unknown physiological or nutritional factors might be involved.

The excessive consumption of sodium by adults and children is, nowadays, mostly derived from sodium chloride. In a large study including 187 countries it was found that 99.2% of the adult population consumed more sodium than the WHO's recommended upper limit of 2 g of sodium per day. The vast majority (88.3%) of the adult population consumed more than 3 g of sodium per day [3]. An Australian study found that sodium intake rapidly doubled in the first 2 years of life, to an estimated 1 g of sodium per day by the age of 17 months [17]. By the age of 4 years the average sodium intake has been estimated at almost 1.5 g of sodium per day [18]. Data from the US [19] suggested that children's sodium intake further increases with age (6–13 years: 3.1 g/day, 14–18 years: 3.6 g/day). Such an increase can partly be explained by an increased total food consumption with age, but can also be a consequence of an increased sodium density of children's diets [19]. It has been estimated that about half of the sodium children in the US consume comes from only 10 food categories that include pizza, Mexican-mixed dishes, sandwiches, breads, cold cuts, soups, savoury snacks, cheese, plain milk, and poultry [19]. This is in line with 9- to 13-year-old children in Australia (mean sodium intake = 2.7 g/day), who consumed most of their sodium from cereal based products, and meat and poultry products [20]. The problem with these high levels of sodium consumption at a young age is two-fold. Firstly, it sets children up for developing high blood pressure during childhood and adulthood [21,22]. Secondly, children might get used to eating high levels of salt, and expect a certain level of saltiness in their foods. This potentially leads to unhealthy food choices during child-and adulthood.

This signifies the need to understand why infants and children consume such high amounts of sodium, which far exceeds their biological need. In this quest it is worth investigating how the ability to sense sodium and a liking for salty foods develops, given that food-liking plays a key role in children's [23] and infants' [24] food choice and consumption. This review aims to provide an overview of the current knowledge about the development of salt taste perception and salt taste liking during infancy and childhood and its relationship to food consumption and health outcomes. This review focusses on human research in non-clinical populations and will not provide an extensive review of neurological processes and brain structures involved in salt appetite in severely sodium deficient populations or animals.

2. Literature Search

A systematic literature search was conducted as of 6 June 2017 using Medline Complete, PsycINFO, Social Sciences Citation Index, Scopus, Psychology and Behavioural Science Collection, Cochrane Database of Systematic Reviews and Emerald Insight. The following search terms were used: (taste OR preference OR sensory) AND (salt OR sodium) AND (infants OR baby OR newborn OR neonate). This resulted in 330 references. A complete manual search of the reference lists of original studies was also conducted. Studies which did not have salty taste preferences or perception as either a dependent variable or independent variable, or were conducted in only adults or animals were excluded. After excluding duplicates, and irrelevant titles, 54 references were considered relevant for the present review.

3. Taste Perception

When salty foods or beverages are tasted, both physiological and cognitive related processes take place. Salt taste perception is derived from the interaction of sodium with amiloride-sensitive epithelial sodium channels (ENaC) in the human taste buds on the tongue [9]. In addition ENaCs have been located in the distal nephron, distal colon and airway epithelia, where they play an important role in Na^+ reabsorption [25]. This suggests a potential link between salt taste perception and other (e.g., renal) functions in the body [26]. Furthermore, it has been suggested that salt taste perception through the interaction of sodium with ENaCs is not the only mechanism involved in human salt taste perception. Additional cellular and molecular mechanisms are not yet understood fully [15].

Neurological signals which result from the interaction between sodium and sodium sensing channels are transmitted to the brain and interpreted in specific parts of the brain. A strong enough signal results in the perception of a variety of taste related aspects such as detection, intensity, taste quality (e.g., sweet, sour, bitter, salty, umami), and hedonics [27].

Humans' ability to detect sodium, which is part of taste sensitivity, mainly represents the physiological process of taste perception, whereas hedonics (e.g., liking, preference, acceptance) is a result of the cognitive interpretation of the physiological taste signals. Although both are part of taste functioning, the underlying principles and methods on how to assess these are different. It is generally found that taste sensitivity and taste hedonics do not correlate well [28], emphasising that both represent different pathways. This makes it important to investigate both taste sensitivity and hedonics, in order to understand the relationship between taste functioning and health outcomes.

Many animals, including humans, are able to sense sodium in the food supply by taste [29], however not all sodium in foods can easily be tasted [30]. For example, sodium in bread can be reduced to some extent without children [31] nor adults [32] noticing the difference. Sodium chloride is the only food grade chemical which elicits a pure salt taste [26]. More precisely, it is the positively charged sodium ion, rather than the chloride anion, which is mainly responsible for salty taste [33]. Other salts such as potassium chloride elicit a salty taste, but often taste bitter when used in high quantity. Lithium chloride does elicit a pure salt taste, but cannot be used in foods because of its toxicity (for review see [34]). In the absence of effective salt replacers, sodium chloride (hereafter referred to as "salt") is the only chemical which in practice can be used to make food taste saltier.

Humans have a high liking for salty tasting foods, which, from an evolutionary point of view, would result in humans preferring foods with sodium, which is needed for survival. The addition of salt to food changes the complete sensory profile, beyond making a food taste saltier. In both children [35] and adults [13,36], it has been shown that the addition of salt to food can make the food taste less bitter. Such suppression of bitter taste can increase perceived sweetness of particular foods [36]. Salt is mostly consumed in the contexts of specific foods, rather than pure salt itself. Therefore, the measurement of salt taste sensitivity is usually carried out with salted water, whereas the measurement of children's hedonic response to salt in foods is usually carried out with stimuli in which salt is deemed appropriate such as soups, broth, and crackers.

4. Salt Taste Detection and Acceptance in Infants

Infants' ability to detect salt taste is mainly measured by the quantity the infant ingests, sucking patterns and facial expression in response to ingestion of water solutions with different concentrations of salt [37,38]. Because of the nature of these measurements it is hard to distinguish between infants' ability to detect sodium and infants' preference for, or liking of, sodium.

With these limitations in mind, it has been found that infants go through different developmental stages of acceptance of salted water and salted foods. When newborns (1–4 days old) are presented with 4.3 g of salt/100 mL of water, facial expressions suggest an indifference to salty taste [37,38]. This is unlikely to be due to the newborns' inability to respond to taste per se. Facial and ingestive responses to bitter, sweet and to some extent sour taste, suggest that newborns can discriminate between different taste stimuli [37–40]. Animal studies suggest that the specific central and/or peripheral mechanisms, underlying salt taste perception, mature postnatally [41]. In other words, newborns might not be able to detect salt taste until further maturation of the salt taste system. It needs, however, to be mentioned that one study observed that newborns decrease their sucking burst frequency in response to mild salt tasting solutions (0.58 g of salt/100 mL of water) [42]. It has been hypothesised that such signs of lower acceptance (compared to water) is caused by the interaction of sodium with taste fibres which are not specific to sodium and might therefore elicit other taste responses such as slight bitterness, which infants reject [43].

Newborns have a biological need for sodium, which brings up the question of why newborns are not able to show a preferential response to salty taste, like they show for sweet taste [38]. The lack of a salt taste response might have an evolutionary reason. Although there is a need for sodium at birth, the first food the infant naturally encounters is breastmilk, which is dominated by sweet taste [44] and contains a sufficient concentration of sodium for the baby to thrive [45]. Children have an inborn preference for sweet taste, which would lead to a natural acceptance and consumption of breastmilk. This makes an inborn acceptance of salt taste, from an evolutionary point of view, not needed per se.

By the age of approximately 4 to 6 months, when sodium channels have further matured, infants show a preference for salty water over plain water [38,46], and salted baby cereal over plain baby cereal [47], as measured by ingestion. This shift from indifference to preference of salted water is thought to reflect an unlearned biological response to salty taste, rather than a learned response [48]. This does not mean, however, that the addition of salt to any baby food would ensure an increase in consumption. When salt was added to baby formula, 6- to 7-months-old infants found it less palatable, as measured by frequency of sucks, than baby formula without added salt [43]. Presumably because the addition of salt made the baby formula less sweet, which was confirmed by a trained adult sensory panel [43]. Alternatively, but not mutually exclusively, the addition of salt created an unknown flavour combination, which infants rejected because of its novelty.

In summary, infants' ability to detect salt taste develops postnatally such that infants younger than about 3 months of age are most likely not able to detect salt taste. Once infants can detect salt taste they show a preference for salt taste in water. There is no prior exposure to salt taste needed for infants to prefer salted water, which suggests an unlearned biological response to salt taste.

The changes in salt preferences in the first year of life are expressed in Figure 1.

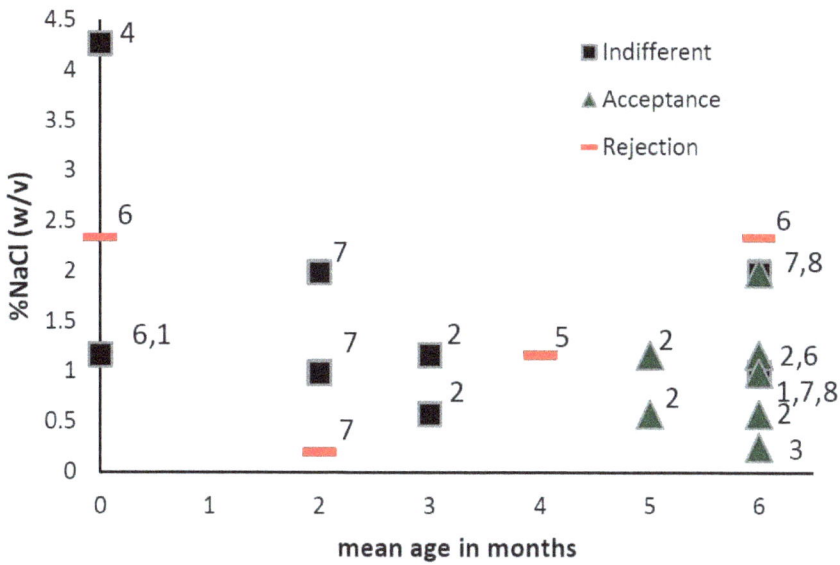

Figure 1. Infants' (0–6 months) Indifference, acceptance and rejection responses to different concentrations of NaCl water (%NaCl *w/v*). Age on the y-axis represent mean age in months. 1 Maller & Desor 1973, measure: intake, stimuli: salt water [40]; 2 Beauchamp,Cowart &Moran 1986, measure: intake, stimuli: salt water [49]; 3 Harris & Booth 1987, measure: intake, stimuli: cereals [50]; 4 Rossenstein &Oster, 1988, measure facial expression and sucking, stimuli: water [37]; 5 Crystal & Bernstein, 1998, measure: facial expression, intake, stimuli: salt water [51]; 6 Beauchamp, Cowart, Mennella, Marsh 1994, measure: sucks and intake, stimuli: salt water [43]; 7 Stein, Cowart & Beauchamp, 2006. measure: intake, stimuli: salt water [52]; 8 Stein, Cowart & Beauchamp, 2012, measure: intake, stimuli: salt water [53].

5. Variation in Salt Preference of Infants

5.1. Prenatally

Infants' preference for salty taste varies depending on a variety of factors such as physiological triggers before birth. Studies in rats suggest that extracellular dehydration and electrolyte imbalance of the mother rat can increase the salt appetite in the offspring [54]. Extracellular dehydration (as well as a fall in NaCl concentration) causes the kidneys to release renin into the circulation where it acts as an enzyme to activate angiotensin into angiotensin I, which is converted by angiotensin converting enzyme, produced mainly by the lungs, into angiotensin II. Angiotensin II plays a key role in maintaining body fluid balance and is the main stimulus for the secretion of the hormone aldosterone [55]. Angiotensin II and aldosterone are known to induce salt appetite. Both can cross the placenta and hypothetically influence the salt appetite of the off spring [54].

Extracellular dehydration and electrolyte imbalance can be caused by severe fluid loss, such as repeated severe vomiting. Relating this to humans, infants born from mothers with severe morning sickness are shown to be more likely to prefer high salt solutions, than infants from mothers who did not, or to a lesser extent, suffered from morning sickness during pregnancy [51]. This seems to have long lasting effects, as adult offspring from mothers who experienced severe morning sickness had a higher preference for salty foods, had a higher salt use, and ate more salty snack foods, than peers whose mothers did not experience such extreme morning sickness [56]. Furthermore, severe morning sickness of the mother has been associated with low birth weight of the offspring [57]. Infants with a low birth weight are more likely to prefer high salt solutions (as measured by consumption), than infants born with a normal birth weight [52].

Physiological triggers induced by severe morning sickness, as described above, are supposedly rare. It has been suggested that although around 50% of pregnant women experience morning sickness, only 0.3 to 1% of pregnant women experience severe vomiting which could lead to dehydration [58]. So although salt taste preferences seem to be influenced by physiological triggers before birth on an individual level, the impact on a population level is likely to be minimal.

5.2. Postnatally

Postnatally either a severe shortage of sodium as well as an over consumption of sodium might result in an enhanced preference for salty taste. Sodium deficiency during infancy and childhood is rare, except in clinical populations [59]. However, the repeated consumption of certain chloride-deficient baby formulas during infancy is suggested to result in a hormonal state (e.g., elevated plasma aldosterone levels and renin activity), which is similar to that of sodium deficiency. The long term consumption of these formulas during infancy has been positively correlated with dietary behaviours which suggest a high preference for salty foods [60]. Along the same lines, adolescents who went through severe episodes of vomiting and/or diarrhoea as an infant, causing electrolyte imbalance, show a high preference for salty foods [61].

On the other hand, the introduction of a diet high in sodium might lead to a preference for salty foods as well. Generally, by the age of 3 to 4 months infants are introduced to solid foods, including foods high in sodium such as cereals. An Australian longitudinal study shows that when infants grow from 9 to 18 months, their sodium intake doubles, with bread and rolls being the largest contributor to total sodium intake [17]. Such increased exposure to salty foods during infancy is thought to be correlated with the infants' increased preference for salt tasting foods [50]. Potentially delaying the introduction of salty foods to infants can lower their preference for salty taste [53]. These studies have, however, a number of short comings. Harris and Booth (1987) did a very rough measurement of infants' consumption of sodium rich foods from which it is not possible to determine the salty taste of foods and which foods were consumed [50]. Stein and colleagues (2012) focused on specific sodium rich foods (e.g., starchy foods, salted water) [53]. None of the studies investigated the specificity of sodium exposure. That is, it remains unclear if a high preference for salty foods is related to a general liking of more intense tasting foods, or if such high salt preference specifically alters the intake of salty foods. It is also not clear if preference for salty taste as measured in one medium or food relates to the intake of a wide range of salty foods. Moreover, both studies were observational and causality can not be concluded. One of the rare, but well designed, studies to investigate the causal relationship between salt consumption and salt preferences in infants was conducted in the 1980s. In a controlled study, researchers fed infants (3–8 months) either a low (2 mmol Na/100 kcal) or high (9 mmol Na/100 kcal) sodium dense diet for 5 months, and assessed their liking for salty taste and consumption of salty foods at the age of 8 years. The results show no evidence to support the hypothesis that a high salt intake during infancy resulted in either a high salt consumption or high salt preference in childhood [62]. However, the number of infants and children tested in this study was fairly small ($n = 27$).

To summarise, there is some suggestion that infants' preference for salty taste is influenced by physiological disturbances which are initiated by severe fluid loss by either the pregnant mother or during early infancy. In addition, feeding regimes which either trigger similar hormonal systems as sodium deficiency, as well as the introduction of salty foods, potentially increase infants' preference for salty foods. However, it remains questionable whether the consumption of high amounts of salty foods during infancy impacts liking for salty foods beyond infancy.

6. Salt Taste Perception of Children

Over the past 40 years, children's taste perception and liking have been reasonably well investigated [63]. Below we provide a review of studies focused on children's salt taste sensitivity and liking and how these relate to health outcomes such as weight status and blood pressure. Studies investigating children's sensitivity to salt taste might provide us with insight into the physiological development of salt taste perception, whereas children's hedonic response to salt taste might provide us with insights into children's food choice behaviour with respect to salty foods. Therefore, both salt taste sensitivity and liking will be reviewed below.

Children Salt Taste Sensitivity

Unlike the difficulties of measuring salt taste sensitivity with infants, salt taste sensitivity in children can be measured rather precisely. Salt taste sensitivity can be expressed as, the detection threshold (i.e., the lowest detectable concentration of NaCl), recognition threshold (i.e., the lowest NaCl concentration at which a subject can identify salty taste), or supra-threshold (i.e., the lowest difference in concentration in NaCl—in the detectable range—that is clearly perceived by a subject) [64]. To our knowledge, studies investigating salt taste sensitivity of children only focused on detection and recognition thresholds.

In order to measure detection thresholds, different methodologies have been used. Some researchers used a range of salt solutions and paired all solutions with distilled water in a 2-Alternative-Forced-Choice test (e.g., taste two samples, of which one contains salt) [65], or a 3-Alternative- Forced-Choice test (e.g., taste three samples, of which one contains salt) [66]. During the execution of this method children received all pairs of salted and distilled water, independent of the accuracy of the answers. Other researchers used a range of salt solutions and presented them in a staircase method. In this method, an inaccurate answer leads to the presentation of a higher salt concentration and an accurate answer leads to the presentation of a lower salt concentration. The presentation mode in the staircase method has either been a 2-Alternative-Forced-Choice [67–69], or an alternative like "taste four samples of which one contains salt" [70] or "taste 8 samples of which 4 contain salt" [71]. Most studies found detection thresholds of around 0.02% (w/v) NaCl, with one exception which found a threshold of 0.006% (w/v) NaCl. However, the latter study was conducted with a specific clinical population [71].

As suggested by Table 1, in general the staircase method seems to find lower salt taste detection thresholds than any of the other methods. In comparison, salt threshold in adults varies widely with some studies finding a threshold of 0.01% (w/v) NaCl [72], and others a three times higher threshold at 0.03% (w/v) NaCl [73]. Only two studies compared the salt detection threshold of children to those of adults in one study design. One study found higher salt detection threshold in 10- to 19-year-olds, compared with 20- to 29-year-olds [70]. Another study only found such difference when comparing boys with women [65]. None of the studies listed in Table 1 could confirm any associations between salt taste detection threshold and salt intake. One study found a higher salt taste detection threshold for those who liked soup/stews [66], whereas others failed to see such an association [67]. In adults it is generally found that salt detection threshold as measured using water solutions are not related to liking or intake [73].

Salt taste recognition thresholds are commonly conducted with a range of salt solutions and presented one at a time. Children simply reported whether they could identify the taste [74–77]. Children's recognition thresholds of salty taste fall about 9 times above children's salt detection threshold and vary from 0.17 to 0.18% (w/v) NaCl. Two studies found higher thresholds, but technically speaking they did not measure thresholds because of the limited number of solutions which were offered [76,77]. In adults, salt recognition thresholds vary, as is the case with children. For example, Wise and colleagues found a salt recognition threshold of 0.08% NaCl [72], whereas Lucas and colleagues found a recognition threshold of 0.11% [73]. See Table 1 for an overview.

Table 1. Children's salt taste detection and recognition threshold.

Population N, Age Range, Country	Type of Threshold (Design)	Solution Range %NaCl in Water	Threshold	Remarks	Reference
N = 251, 10–12 years, Japan	Detection (filter paper, paired comparison)	0.6–1.6	0.6%	0.6%NaCl was lowest concentration presented.	Thresholds not related to liking or salt intake	Matsuzuki et al., 2008 [67]
N = 24 10–19 years, UK	Detection (staircase, one in 4)	0.004–0.58	0.04%	Mean based on interpretation of figure	Threshold 10–19 years old is higher than 20–29 years old	Baker et al., 1983 [70]
N = 70, 12–13 years, Korea	Detection (triangle test)	0.005–0.15	0.03%		Higher thresholds for those liking soup/stew	Kim and Lee, 2009 [66]
N = 97, 8–14 years, USA	Detection (staircase, paired comparison)	0.0003–5.8	0.021%	52% overweight children	Threshold not related to salt intake	Bobowski & Mennella, 2015 [68]
N = 68, 8–9 years, Australia	Detection (paired comparison)	0.0009–0.029	0.016–0.036%	Boys were less sensitive than adults	Boys had higher threshold than women	James, Laing, & Oram, 1997, [65]
N = 72, Age unknown, Spain	Detection (staircase paired comparison)	0.0012–0.08	0.027%			Arguelles et al., 2006 [69]
N = 22, 9–19 years, USA	Detection (staircase 4 in 8)	0.00006–5.8	0.006%	Clinical population		Hertz et al., 1975 [71]
N = 421, 14–19 years, Brazil	Recognition	0.02–5.8	0.17%		Threshold not related to body composition	Kirsten & Wagner, 2014, [74]
N = 237, 6–15 years, Japan	Recognition (one solution)	-	0.4%	0.4% was the only solution presented	Sensitivity lowest in 4–6 graders	Ohnuki et al., 2014 [77]
N = 40, 5–12 years, Italy	Recognition (two solutions)	0.18, 1.8	1.8%	Only two solutions tested		Majorana et al., 2012 [76]
N = 319, 9–17 years, Nigeria	Recognition threshold (range)	0.18–1	0.18%		Higher threshold in boys than girls	Okoro et al., 1998 [75]

Salt taste thresholds might reflect biological processes in the body. Sodium sensitive channels (ENaC) have been found throughout the body, including the kidneys where they play an important role in Na^+ regulation [25]. Furthermore, animal studies suggest that salt taste sensitivity, salt uptake by the gut and salt excretion by the kidney share similar physiological pathways [78]. Differences in salt taste sensitivity might therefore be linked to high blood pressure. In adults, it has been suggested that there is a potential link between salt taste sensitivity and high blood pressure [79–82], however such a link is not uniformly shown [83–85].

Several studies looked into the potential link between children's salt taste sensitivity and high blood pressure. Bobowski et al. found that systolic blood pressure was positively associated with salt taste detection thresholds in normal weight, but not overweight/obese, children [68]. This is in line with earlier findings in a group of Spanish children [69]. Kirsten and colleagues [74] investigated 14- to 19-year-olds' ability to detect NaCl in a water solutions (e.g., 4 mmol/L, 8 mmol/L, 15 mmol/L, 30 mmol/L, 60 mmol/L, 120 mmol/L, 250 mmol/L, 500 mmol/L, 1000 mmol/L). The median concentration at which salt taste was detected was 30 mmol/L. About one third (i.e., 36%) had a detection threshold of higher than 30 mmol/L. The mean diastolic blood pressure was higher amongst those 36% than amongst the remaining sample. The mechanism behind the association between children's salt taste perception and high blood pressure remains unknown. Potentially, salt taste perception and high blood pressure share similar physiological mechanisms.

In summary, from the limited data available there is, to our knowledge, no strong evidence to suggest that children and adults differ in their sensitivity to salt taste. However, it needs to be noted that differences in methodologies make it difficult to compare studies. There is no evidence that children's salt taste sensitivity is related to food consumption and some evidence that lower salt sensitivity is related to higher blood pressure in some, but not all children.

7. Children's Liking of Salty Taste

Unlike young infants, children as young as 3 years of age show an adult-like rejection of salted water, but show a high liking for salted soup [46]. This suggests that in general children this age might only like salt in a food context they are familiar with. The shift from acceptance to rejection of salt in water might, therefore, be influenced by the experience children have with salt tasting foods. However, it needs to be said that some researchers have found that a small proportion of children might accept salt in water [86]. Such preference might reflect a biological driver, rather than a learned preference for salty taste.

Similar to sweet taste preferences [87], there is some evidence that children prefer higher salt concentrations than adults do. Already back in 1975 Desor and colleagues showed that 9- to 15-year-old children were more likely to prefer 2.3 g NaCl/100 mL in water than adults did [86]. Such a difference in salt preference has also been demonstrated in soups [88], popocorn [89] and broth [90].

Interestingly, similar to previous findings in adults [91], children's liking for salt is suggested to be positively related to children's liking for sweet [90]. This suggests that liking for high levels of salt does not exclude liking for high levels of sweetness. At least two explanations for this finding can be put forward. Firstly, the increased need for energy and minerals in stages of rapid growth might simultaneously drive salt and sweet preferences in children [90]. Secondly, repeated dietary salt consumption might drive the consumption of sugar sweetened beverages [92,93] and subsequently increase liking for salt and sweet simultaneously. Both these hypotheses need further investigation.

It is not clear why children prefer higher levels of salt in foods than adults do. As shown earlier, there is no clear evidence that children and adults differ in their sensitivity to salty taste. Moreover, it is generally found that salt taste sensitivity and salt liking are not related [73]. Because exposure to, and liking of specific foods are generally found to be positively correlated in children [94], it could be hypothesised that children are more exposed to salty foods than adults, resulting in children's higher preference for salt taste than adults. However, large population data suggest that the sodium density of children's and adults' diets are similar [19]. This, however does not give a clear indication of how salty the diets of children and adults taste. Lastly, it has been suggested that children's preference for high salty foods reflects their biological need for minerals at certain stages of growth [90]. In clinical populations it has been shown that salt preferences can be increased when there is a high loss of sodium, for example in the case of congenital adrenal hyperplasia (CAH) [95]. In this disease, a genetic mutation results in adrenal insufficiency which can lead, in its severest form, to a persistent urinary loss of sodium, known as salt-wasting. Children suffering from the severe form of CAH showed an increased salt appetite, meaning they liked salt more and used salt more often. Salt wasters added 130% to 160% more NaCl (as measured with a questionnaire) to their foods than controls. In addition, Salt wasters were more likely to lick or eat pure salt. Subsequent qualitative interviews revealed that Salt Wasters developed, from a young age, strategies to deliberately consume more salt [95,96]. However a disease like CAH is extremely rare and only occurs in about 0.007% of children [96]. There is also no evidence that children have a higher need for sodium than adults do [6].

Figure 2 provides an overview of the different salt concentrations children like/prefer/accept in different foods.

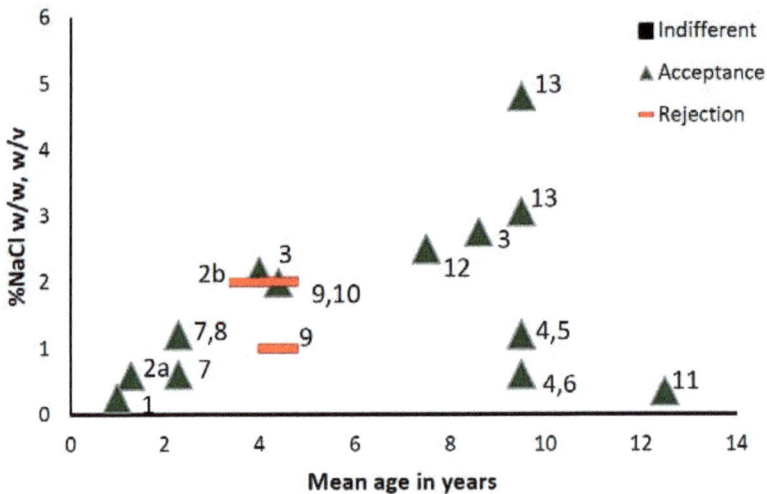

Figure 2. Children's (1–13 years) indifference, acceptance and rejection responses to different concentrations of NaCl in foods (%NaCl *w/w*) and liquids (%NaCl *w/v*). 1 Harris & Booth 1987, higher consumption compared to unsalted version, mashed potatoes [50]; 2 Beauchamp & Moran 1986, higher (2a) or lower (2b) consumption compared to unsalted version, water [49]; 3 Beauchamp, Cowart & Moran 1990, most preferred, soup [88]; 4 Bouhlal, Chabanet, Issanchou & Nicklaus 2013, more liked than unsalted version, Pasta and green beans [97]; 5 Bouhlal, Chabanet, Issanchou & Nicklaus 2013, higher consumption compared to unsalted version, pasta [97]; 6 Bouhlal, Chabanet, Issanchou & Nicklaus 2013, higher consumption compared to unsalted version, green beans [97]; 7 Bouhlal, Issanchou & Nicklaus 2011, higher consumption compared to unsalted version, green beans [98]; 8 Bouhlal, Issanchou & Nicklaus 2011, higher consumption compared to unsalted version, pasta [98]; 9 Cowart & Beauchamp 1986, lower consumption compared to unsalted version, water [48]; 10 Cowart & Beauchamp 1986, higher consumption compared to unsalted version, soup [48]; 11 Kim & Lee 2009, most preferred, soup [66]; 12 Mennella, Finkbeiner, Lipchock, Hwang & Reed 2014, most preferred, broth [90]; 13 Verma, Mittal, Ghildiyal, Chaudhary & Mahajan 2007, more liked than unsalted version, popcorn (unclear statistics) [89].

8. Children's Salt Liking and Intake of Sodium

It is generally thought that food liking plays a key role in children's food consumption [23]. Some studies, but not all, have been able to find a positive correlation between the liking for salt taste in adults, as tested in a controlled setting, and the consumption of sodium in everyday life [99,100]. The research into a potential association between salt taste liking and salt consumption encounters a number of challenges. Firstly, some of the sodium in the food supply cannot be tasted as being salty [30] and is mainly added to processed foods for preservation and food structural reasons [101]. Secondly, the addition of salt to foods, as mentioned earlier, influences the complete sensory profile of foods, which goes beyond making foods taste saltier [13,36]. It is therefore likely that children's liking of added salt in one food does not necessarily translate to children's liking of added salt in another food. Related to that, studies in adults suggest that liking for salt is food specific. That is, some foods such as salty snacks are liked when they are salty, whereas the reverse is true for foods in which salt taste deemed less appropriate [99]. Thirdly, insensitive methodology to measure children's salt taste liking and/or salt consumption can result in a lack of correlation between salt taste liking and salt consumption. Lastly, tasting a small amount of food might not be a good predictor of consuming large amounts of the liked food [102], due to, for example, sensory specific satiety [103] or boredom [104].

The majority of studies show that the addition of salt to a variety of foods, such as soup [48,90], green beans, pasta [97,98], ricotta cheese [105], carrots [106], and popcorn [89], increases children's liking and—if measured—consumption of that food. A large cross cultural study in 8 countries including close to two thousand children, showed that the majority of children preferred a cracker with added salt (1.6 g/100 g food) compared to a cracker with a lower concentration of salt (0.7 g/100 g food) [107]. However despite the fact that salt seems to be able to increase food liking and consumption, it does not mean that an increase in liking will always result in an increase in consumption. For example Cowart and Beauchamp (1986) showed that for half of the 3- to 6-year old children they tested, the most liked soup did not correspond to the soup they drank the most of [48]. In a study with 8- to 11-year-old it was found that small additions of salt would increase liking, but not consumption of pasta [108]. Furthermore, it is important to notice that the addition of salt does not influence children's liking, nor intake equally across different foods [105,108]. Hypothetically, children like the changed flavour profile of the foods, as a result of the addition of salt, rather than salt taste itself.

Potentially, liking of salty foods is related to small increases in salt consumption which cannot be measured in single foods, but can be measured when focusing on daily sodium consumption. A study which measured 5- to 10-year-old children's liking for salt (0.92–6.14 g NaCl/100 g of broth) in broth, found that liking for salt in broth was positively related to daily sodium intake (r = 0.24). It was, however, not reported which foods contributed most to the daily sodium consumption [90]. The latter is important because the sodium content of food does not necessarily mean they taste salty. So it is likely that children's salt preference is correlated with some foods, but not others. Kim et al. suggested that salt preference as measured in soup was positively associated with the frequent consumption of certain salty foods (i.e., pork cutlets and hamburgers), but not with other foods (e.g., pizza, fried chicken) [66]. If one assumes that there is some positive relationship between children's salt taste liking and intake of salty foods, one might also expect an association between children's salt taste liking and health outcomes such as weight status and high blood pressure. However, to our knowledge such associations have not been found [107,109]. This supports the view that children's salt taste preferences are unlikely to have a generic effect on children's diet.

All these studies are, however, observational studies, and causality cannot be concluded. How modifiable are children's salt preferences? Repeated exposure to a salted food has been shown to increase children's liking for that particular salted food, but not for a salted food to which the child was not exposed [105]. Another study confirmed that repeated exposure to salted foods increases intake of that food, but it is not clear if such exposure leads to a high liking for salt taste [108]. These studies suggest that liking for a particular salted food can be changed by repeated exposure. However, it does not support the hypothesis that repeated exposure to salty foods increase children's generic liking for salty taste.

In adults, salt taste liking can be shifted downwards by exposing individuals to low sodium diets. Such shifts have been observed in randomized controlled studies in which adults were placed on a low sodium diet for 2 weeks to several months (see [110] for review). Not only liking for salt taste can be adjusted downwards, but salt taste intensity can be increased as a result of a low sodium diets which is maintained for at least 2 months [111]. For an extensive review on this topic see [15]. It is important to note that all these intervention studies applied an overall reduction of sodium in the diet, rather than a sodium reduction in one single food. To date it remains unclear if a reduction in one single food would result in an overall liking of reduced levels of sodium in a variety of foods.

One can speculate that by repeated exposure, children become familiar with foods. This familiarisation can drive liking [94]. However, to our knowledge, there are no experimental studies carried out with children to verify if a repeated exposure to either low salty or high salty food can modify children's generic liking for salt.

In summary, there is some evidence that children, compared to adults, prefer higher concentrations of salt in soups and crackers. However, there seem to be no studies that investigated if children, compared to adults, prefer higher concentrations of salt in a variety of foods, such as salt-fat foods, meats, and vegetables, than adults. Most studies suggest that the addition of salt to foods increases children's liking for the salted food, however it is unlikely that such liking represents a generic liking for salty taste. The evidence for a positive association between the liking of a salty taste and ingestion of salty foods in general is not convincing. It is also worth noting that although children seem to have a liking for higher concentrations of salt than adults, such a difference does not manifest itself in a difference in the sodium density of children's and adults' diets [19].

9. Conclusions

The high consumption of sodium by children is worrisome and a better understanding of what might contribute to this high consumption might aid to the development of strategies to decrease this high sodium consumption. The present review highlights the role of taste in infants' and children's consumption of high sodium foods.

The current review suggests that both biology and learned experiences influence infants' and children's liking for salty foods. Although the liking of salty taste starts as an unlearned response in early infancy, this liking soon develops as a result of repeated exposure to salty foods. The available studies seem to suggest that infancy is a potentially sensitive period in which salt taste preferences could be modified. Generally speaking, a low exposure to salty foods is associated with a low preference for salty foods. Randomised controlled trials, however, are needed to provide clarity about the causality of such relationship. No study, to our knowledge, suggested that decreasing the exposure to salty foods during infancy is associated with an increased liking or desire for salty foods. Therefore, limiting infants' consumption of salty foods to decrease sodium consumption and potentially decrease liking for salty foods seems to be a sensible approach. At the same time it is not recommended to try to eliminate sodium from the infants' diet all together, because severe sodium deficiency has been linked to an increased liking of salty taste amongst other medical complications. The role of repeated exposure to salty foods during infancy and subsequent liking of salty taste and consumption of salty foods during childhood, adolescence and adulthood requires, however, more systematic research. Randomised controlled trials are needed to provide insight into whether avoiding high sodium foods during infancy can have a long-lasting effect on the development of salt taste liking and the consumption of salty foods.

Several studies showed that children have a preference for a higher level of saltiness than adults. Such heightened preference does not seem to result in a general diet higher in sodium density. However, studies in which salt is added to a variety of foods have consistently shown that children's food consumption can be increased when salt is added. The amount of salt which needs to be added to significantly increase consumption is, however, food dependent. This seems to suggest that it is not salt taste per se which drives consumption, but the effect salt has on the complete sensory profile of foods which drives consumption. To date there is a lack of research investigating mechanisms by which a change of salt content can modify children's liking, desire and intake of a variety of foods.

Hypothetically, by slowly decreasing the amount of salt in specific foods children consume, one might be able to decrease children's liking for these specific salty foods as has been suggested in adults. However, such strategy should include the whole diet rather than single foods and needs to be informed by randomised controlled trials. A similar strategy has been suggested for adults [15].

In conclusion, decreasing exposure to salty tasting foods during early infancy is recommended. Salt plays an important role in children's liking for a variety of foods. It is questionable whether children's liking for salt per se influences their intake of salty foods.

Acknowledgments: The author would like to acknowledge Julie Mennella and Russell Keast for their excellent comments on earlier drafts of the manuscript.

Conflicts of Interest: The author declares no conflict of interest.

References

1. World Health Organization (WHO). *Reducing Salt Intake in Populations*; World Health Organization: Geneva, Switzerland, 2007.
2. He, F.J.; MacGregor, H.E. A comprehensive review on salt and health and current experience of worldwide salt reduction program. *J. Hum. Hypertens.* **2009**, *23*, 363–384. [CrossRef] [PubMed]
3. Mozaffarian, D.; Fahimi, S.; Singh, G.M.; Micha, R.; Khatibzadeh, S.; Engell, R.E.; Lim, S.; Danaei, G.; Ezzati, M.; Powles, J. Global sodium consumption and death from cardiovascular causes. *N. Engl. J. Med.* **2014**, *371*, 624–634. [CrossRef] [PubMed]
4. Ma, Y.H.; He, F.J.; MacGregor, G.A. High salt intake: Independet risk factor for obesity. *Hypertension* **2015**, *66*, 843–849. [CrossRef] [PubMed]
5. World Health Organization (WHO). *Guideline: Sodium Intake for Adults and Children*; WHO: Geneva, Switzerland, 2012.
6. NHMRC. Nutrient Reference Values for Australia and New Zealand, Sodium. Available online: https://www.nrv.gov.au/sites/default/files/content/n35-sodium_0.pdf (accessed on 6 July 2017).
7. CDC. Sodium and Potassium Intakes among US Infants and Preschool Children, 2003–2010. Available online: https://www.cdc.gov/salt/pdfs/mmwr_journal_highlights.pdf (accessed on 1 September 2017).
8. Webster, J.L.; Dunford, E.K.; Neal, B. A systematic survey of the sodium contents of processed foods. *Am. J. Clin. Nutr.* **2009**, *91*, 413–420. [CrossRef] [PubMed]
9. Dötsch, M.; Busch, J.; Batenburg, M.; Liem, G.; Tareilus, E.; Mueller, R.; Meijer, G. Strategies to reduce sodium consumption: A food industry perspective. *Crit. Rev. Food Sci. Nutr.* **2009**, *49*, 841–851. [CrossRef] [PubMed]
10. Inguglia, E.S.; Zhang, Z.; Tiwari, B.K.; Kerry, J.P.; Burgess, C.M. Salt reduction strategies in processed meat products—A review. *Trends Food Sci. Technol.* **2017**, *59*, 70–78. [CrossRef]
11. Silow, C.; Axel, C.; Zannini, E.; Arendt, E.K. Current status of salt reduction in bread and bakery products—A review. *J. Cereal Sci.* **2016**, *72*, 135–145. [CrossRef]
12. Beck, M.; Jekle, M.; Becker, T. Impact of sodium chloride on wheat flour dough for yeast-leavened products. I. Rheological attributes. *J. Sci. Food Agric.* **2012**, *92*, 585–592. [CrossRef] [PubMed]
13. Breslin, P.A.; Beauchamp, G.K. Salt enhances flavour by suppressing bitterness. *Nature* **1997**, *387*, 563. [CrossRef] [PubMed]
14. Mattes, R.D.; Donnelly, D. Relative contributions of dietary sodium sources. *J. Am. Coll. Nutr.* **1991**, *10*, 383–393. [CrossRef] [PubMed]
15. Institute of Medicine (IOM). Taste and flavor roles of sodium in foods: A unique challenge to reducing sodium intake. In *Strategies to Reduce Sodium Intake in The United States*; Henney, J.E., Taylor, C.L., Boon, C.S., Eds.; National Academies Press: Washington, DC, USA, 2010.
16. Beauchamp, G.K. The human preference for excess salt. *Am. Sci.* **1987**, *75*, 27–33.

Nutrients **2017**, *9*, 1011

17. Campbell, K.J.; Hendrie, G.; Nowson, C.; Grimes, C.A.; Riley, M.; Lioret, S.; McNaughton, S.A. Sources and correlates of sodium consumption in the first 2 years of life. *J. Acad. Nutr. Diet.* **2014**, *114*, 1525–1532. [CrossRef] [PubMed]

18. O'Halloran, S.A.; Grimes, C.; Lacy, K.E.; Nowson, C.; Campbell, K. Dietary sources and sodium intake in a sample of australian preschool children. *BMJ Open* **2015**, *6*, e008698. [CrossRef] [PubMed]

19. Quader, Z.S.; Gillespie, C.; Sliwa, S.A.; Ahuja, J.K.C.; Burdg, J.P.; Moshfegh, A.; Pehrsson, P.R.; Gunn, J.P.; Mugavero, K.; Cogswell, M.E. Sodium intake among US school-aged children: National health and nutrition examination survey, 2011–2012. *J. Acad. Nutr. Diet.* **2017**, *117*, 39–47.e5. [CrossRef] [PubMed]

20. Grimes, C.A.C.; Campbell, K.J.; Riddell, L.J.; Nowson, C.A. Sources of sodium in australian children's diets and the effect of the application of sodium targets to food products to reduce sodium intake. *Br. J. Nutr.* **2011**, *105*, 468–477. [CrossRef] [PubMed]

21. Yang, Q.; Zhang, Z.; Kuklina, E.V.; Fang, J.; Ayala, C.; Hong, Y.; Loustalot, F.; Dai, S.; Gunn, J.P.; Tian, N.; et al. Sodium intake and blood pressure among US children and adolescents. *Pediatrics* **2012**, *130*, 611–619. [CrossRef] [PubMed]

22. Lawlor, D.A.; Smith, G.D. Early life determinants of adult blood pressure. *Curr. Opin. Nephrol. Hypertens.* **2005**, *14*, 259–264. [CrossRef] [PubMed]

23. Birch, L.L. Influences on the development of children's eating behaviours: From infancy to adolescence. *Can. J. Diet. Pract. Res.* **2007**, *68*, s1–s56. [PubMed]

24. Mennella, J.A. Ontogeny of taste preferences: Basic biology and implications for health. *Am. J. Clin. Nutr.* **2014**, *99*, 704S–711S. [CrossRef] [PubMed]

25. Boscardin, E.; Alijevic, O.; Hummler, E.; Frateschi, S.; Kellenberger, S. The function and regulation of acid-sensing ion channels (asics) and the epithelial Na(+) channel (ENAC): Iuphar review 19. *Br. J. Pharmacol.* **2016**, *173*, 2671–2701. [CrossRef] [PubMed]

26. Roper, S.D. The taste of table salt. *Pflüg. Arch.* **2015**, *467*, 457–463. [CrossRef] [PubMed]

27. Bachmanov, A.A.; Beauchamp, G.K. Taste receptor genes. *Annu. Rev. Nutr.* **2007**, *27*, 389–414. [CrossRef] [PubMed]

28. Webb, J.; Bolhuis, D.P.; Cicerale, S.; Hayes, J.E.; Keast, R. The relationships between common measurements of taste function. *Chemosens. Percept.* **2015**, *8*, 11–18. [CrossRef] [PubMed]

29. Beauchamp, G.K.; Dulbecco, R. Salt preference in humans. In *Encyclopedia of Human Biology*; Academic Press: San Diego, CA, USA, 1997; pp. 669–675.

30. Henney, J.E.; Taylor, C.L.; Boon, C.S. Taste and flavor roles of sodium in foods: A unique challenge to reducing sodium intake. In *Strategies to Reduce Sodium Intake in The United States*; National Academies Press: Washington, DC, USA, 2010.

31. Kovac, B.; Knific, M. The perception of low-salt bread among preschool children and the role of educational personnel in creating a positive attitude towards reformulated food. *Zdr. Varst.* **2016**, *56*, 39–46. [CrossRef] [PubMed]

32. Girgis, S.; Neal, B.; Prescott, J.; Prendergast, J.; Dumbrell, S.; Turner, C.; Woodward, M. A one-quarter reduction in the salt content of bread can be made without detection. *Eur. J. Clin. Nutr.* **2003**, *57*, 616–620. [CrossRef] [PubMed]

33. Barthosuk, L.M. Sensory analyses of taste. In *Biological and Behavioral Aspects of Salt Intake*; Kare, M.R., Fregly, M.J., Bernard, R.A., Eds.; Academic Press: New York, NY, USA, 1980; pp. 83–98.

34. Liem, D.G.; Miremadi, F.; Keast, R.S.J. Reducing sodium in foods: The effect of flavor. *Nutrients* **2011**, *3*, 694–711. [CrossRef] [PubMed]

35. Mennella, J.A.; Pepino, M.Y.; Beauchamp, G.K. Modification of bitter taste in children. *Dev. Psychobiol.* **2003**, *43*, 120–127. [CrossRef] [PubMed]

36. Keast, R.S.; Breslin, P.A. An overview of taste-taste interactions. *Food Qual. Pref.* **2003**, *14*, 111–124. [CrossRef]

37. Rossenstein, D.; Oster, H. Differential facial responses to four basic tastes in newborns. *Child Dev.* **1988**, *59*, 1555–1568. [CrossRef]

38. Steiner, J.E.; Weiffenbach, J.M. Facial expressions of the neonate infant indication the hedonics of food-related chemical stimuli. In *Taste and Development: The Genesis of Sweet Preference*; U.S. Government Printing Office: Washington, DC, USA, 1977; pp. 173–188.

39. Desor, J.A.; Maller, O.; Andrews, K. Ingestive responses of human newborns to salty, sour, and bitter stimuli. *J. Comp. Physiol. Psychol.* **1975**, *89*, 966–970. [CrossRef] [PubMed]

40. Maller, O.; Desor, J.A. *Effect of Taste on Ingestion by Human Newborns*; NIH 73-546; Government Printing Office: Washington, DC, USA, 1973; pp. 279–291.

41. Hill, D.L.; Mistretta, C.M. Developmental neurobiology of salt taste sensation. *Trends Neurosci.* **1990**, *13*, 188–195. [CrossRef]

42. Cowart, B.J.; Beauchamp, G.K.; McBride, R.L.; MacFie, H.J.H. Early development of taste perception. In *Psychological Basis of Sensory Evaluation*; Elsevier Applied Science: New York, NY, USA, 1990; pp. 1–16.

43. Beauchamp, G.K.; Cowart, B.J.; Mennella, J.A.; Marsh, R.R. Infant salt taste: Developmental, methodological, and contextual factors. *Dev. Psychobiol.* **1994**, *27*, 353–365. [CrossRef] [PubMed]

44. McDaniel, M.R.; Barker, E.; Lederer, C.L. Sensory characterization of human milk. *J. Dairy Sci.* **1989**, *72*, 1149–1158. [CrossRef]

45. Manganaro, R.; Marseglia, L.; Mamı, C.; Palmara, A.; Paolata, A.; Loddo, S.; Gargano, R.; Mondello, M.; Gemelli, M. Breast milk sodium concentration, sodium intake and weight loss in breast-feeding newborn infants. *Br. J. Nutr.* **2007**, *97*, 344–348. [CrossRef] [PubMed]

46. Beauchamp, G.K.; Cowart, B.J. Congenital and experiential factors in the development of human flavor preferences. *Appetite* **1985**, *6*, 357–372. [CrossRef]

47. Harris, G.; Thomas, A.; Booth, D.A. Development of salt taste in infancy. *Dev. Psychobiol.* **1990**, *26*, 534–538. [CrossRef]

48. Cowart, B.J.; Beauchamp, G.K. The importance of sensory context in young children's acceptance of salty tastes. *Child Dev.* **1986**, *57*, 1034–1039. [CrossRef] [PubMed]

49. Beauchamp, G.K.; Cowart, B.J.; Moran, M. Developmental changes in salt acceptability in human infants. *Dev. Psychobiol.* **1986**, *19*, 17–25. [CrossRef] [PubMed]

50. Harris, G.; Booth, D.A. Infants' preference for salt in food: Its dependence upon recent dietary experience. *J. Reprod. Infant Psychol.* **1987**, *5*, 97–104. [CrossRef]

51. Crystal, S.R.; Bernstein, I.L. Infant salt preference and mother's morning sickness. *Appetite* **1998**, *30*, 297–307. [CrossRef] [PubMed]

52. Stein, L.; Cowart, B.; Beauchamp, G. Salty taste acceptance by infants and young children is related to birth weight: Longitudinal analysis of infants within the normal birth weight range. *Eur. J. Clin. Nutr.* **2006**, *60*, 272–279. [CrossRef] [PubMed]

53. Stein, L.J.; Cowart, B.J.; Beauchamp, G.K. The development of salty taste acceptance is related to dietary experience in human infants: A prospective study. *Am. J. Clin. Nutr.* **2012**, *94*, 123–129. [CrossRef] [PubMed]

54. Nicolaidis, S.; Galaverna, O.; Metzler, C.H. Extracellular dehydration during pregnancy increases salt appetite of offspring. *Am. J. Physiol.* **1990**, *258*, R281–R283. [PubMed]

55. Hurley, S.W.; Johnson, A.K. The biopsychology of salt hunger and sodium deficiency. *Pflüg. Arch.* **2015**, *467*, 445–456. [CrossRef] [PubMed]

56. Crystal, S.R.; Bernstein, I.L. Morning sickness: Impact on offspring salt preference. *Appetite* **1995**, *25*, 231–240. [CrossRef] [PubMed]

57. Zhou, Q.; O'brien, B.; Relyea, J. Severity of nausea and vomiting during pregnancy: What does it predict? *Birth* **2001**, *26*, 108–114. [CrossRef]

58. Niebyl, J.R. Nausea and vomitting in pregnancy. *N. Engl. J. Med.* **2010**, *361*, 1544–1550. [CrossRef] [PubMed]

59. Mansour, F.; Petersen, D.; De Coppi, P.; Eaton, S. Effect of sodium deficiency on growth of surgical infants: A retrospective observational study. *Pediatr. Surg. Int.* **2014**, *30*, 1279–1284. [CrossRef] [PubMed]

60. Stein, L.J.; Cowart, B.J.; Epstein, A.N.; Pilot, L.J.; Laskin, C.R.; Beauchamp, G.K. Increased liking for salty foods in adolescents exposed during infancy to a chloride-deficient feeding formula. *Appetite* **1996**, *27*, 65–77. [CrossRef] [PubMed]

61. Leshem, M. Salt preference in adolescence is predicted by common prenatal and infantile mineralofluid loss. *Physiol. Behav.* **1998**, *63*, 699–704. [CrossRef]

62. Whitten, C.; Stewart, R. The effect of dietary sodium in infancy on blood pressure and related factors. Studies of infants fed salted and unsalted diets for five months at eight months and eight years of age. *Acta Paediatr. Scand. Suppl.* **1980**, *2791*, 1–17. [CrossRef]

63. Mennella, J.A.; Bobowski, N.K.; Reed, D.R. The development of sweet taste: From biology to hedonics. *Rev. Endocr. Metab. Disord.* **2016**, *17*, 171–178. [CrossRef] [PubMed]

64. Meilgaard, M.; Civille, G.V.; Carr, B.T. *Sensory Evaluation Techniques*; CRC Press: London, UK, 1999.

65. James, C.E.; Laing, D.G.; Oram, N. A comparison of the ability of 8–9-year-old children and adults to detect taste stimuli. *Physiol. Behav.* **1997**, *62*, 193–197. [CrossRef]
66. Kim, G.H.; Lee, H.M. Frequent consumption of certain fast foods may be associated with an enhanced preference for salt taste. *J. Hum. Nutr. Diet.* **2009**, *22*, 475–480. [CrossRef] [PubMed]
67. Matsuzuki, H.; Muto, T.; Haruyama, Y. School children's salt intake is correlated with salty taste preference assessed by their mothers. *Tohoku J. Exp. Med.* **2008**, *215*, 71–77. [CrossRef]
68. Bobowski, N.K.; Mennella, J.A. Disruption in the relationship between blood pressure and salty taste thresholds among overweight and obese children. *J. Acad. Nutr. Diet.* **2015**, *115*, 1272–1282. [CrossRef] [PubMed]
69. Arguelles, J.; Diaz, J.J.; Malaga, I.; Perillan, C.; Costales, M.; Vijande, M. Sodium taste threshold in children and its relationship to blood pressure. *Braz. J. Med. Biol. Res* **2006**, *40*, 721–726. [CrossRef]
70. Baker, K.A.; Didcock, E.A.; Kemm, J.R.; Patrick, J.M. Effect of age, sex and illness on salt taste detection thresholds. *Age Ageing* **1983**, *12*, 159–165. [CrossRef] [PubMed]
71. Hertz, J.; Cain, W.S.; Bartoshuk, L.M.; Dolan, J.T.F. Olfactory and taste sensitivity in children with cystic fibrosis. *Physiol. Behav.* **1975**, *14*, 89–94. [CrossRef]
72. Wise, P.M.; Breslin, P.A.S. Individual differences in sour and salt sensitivity: Detection and quality recognition thresholds for citric acid and sodium chloride. *Chem. Senses* **2013**, *38*, 333–342. [CrossRef] [PubMed]
73. Lucas, L.; Riddell, L.; Liem, G.; Whitelock, S.; Keast, R. The influence of sodium on liking and consumption of salty food. *J. Food Sci.* **2011**, *76*, S72–S76. [CrossRef] [PubMed]
74. Kirsten, V.R.; Wagner, M.B. Salt taste sensitivity thresholds in adolescents: Are there any relationships with body composition and blood pressure levels? *Appetite* **2014**, *81*, 89–92. [CrossRef] [PubMed]
75. Okoro, O.E.; Uroghide, G.E.; Jolayemi, T.E.; George, O.O.; Enobakhare, C.O. Studies on taste thresholds in a group of adolescent children in rural Nigeria. *Food Qual. Pref.* **1998**, *9*, 205–210. [CrossRef]
76. Majorana, A.; Campus, G.; Anedda, G.; Piana, G.; Bossu, M.; Cagetti, M.G.; Conto, G.; D'Alessandro, G.; Strohmneger, L.; Polimeni, A. Development and validation of a taste sensitivity test in a group of healthy children. *Eur. J. Paediatr. Dent.* **2012**, *13*, 147–150. [PubMed]
77. Ohnuki, M.; Ueno, M.; Zaitsu, T.; Kawaguchi, Y. Taste hyposensitivity in japanese schoolchildren. *BMC Oral Health* **2014**, *14*, 36. [CrossRef] [PubMed]
78. Evans, L.C.; Ivy, J.R.; Wyrwoll, C.; McNairn, J.A.; Menzies, R.I.; Christensen, T.H.; Al-Dujaili, E.A.S.; Kenyon, C.J.; Mullins, J.J.; Seckl, J.R.; et al. Conditional deletion of hsd11b2 in the brain causes salt appetite and hypertension. *Circulation* **2016**, *133*, 1360–1370. [CrossRef] [PubMed]
79. Zumkley, H.; Vetter, H.; Mandelkow, T.; Spieker, C. Taste sensitivity for sodium chloride in hypotensive, normotensive and hypertensive subjects. *Nephron* **1987**, *47*, 132–134. [CrossRef] [PubMed]
80. Nikam, L.H. Salt taste threshold and its relation to blood pressure in normotensive offspring of hypertensive parents amongst indian adolescents. *Indian J. Physiol. Pharmacol.* **2015**, *59*, 34–40. [PubMed]
81. Wotman, S.; Mandel, I.D.; Thompson, R.H.; Laragh, J.H. Salivary electrolytes and salt taste thresholds in hypertension. *J. Chron. Dis.* **1967**, *20*, 833–840. [CrossRef]
82. Fallis, N.; Lasagna, L.; Tetreault, L. Gustatory thresholds in patients with hypertension. *Nature* **1962**, *196*, 74–75. [CrossRef]
83. Mattes, R.D. Salt taste and hypertension: A critical review of the literature. *J. Chronic Dis.* **1984**, *37*, 195–208. [CrossRef]
84. Azinge, E.C.; Sofola, O.A.; Silva, B.O. Relationship between salt intake, salt-taste threshold and blood pressure in nigerians. *West Afr. J. Med.* **2011**, *30*, 373–376. [PubMed]
85. Henkin, R.I. Salt taste in patients with essential hypertension and with hypertension due to primary hyperaldosteronism. *J. Chronic Dis.* **1974**, *27*, 235–244. [CrossRef]
86. Desor, J.A.; Greene, L.S.; Maller, O. Preferences for sweet and salty in 9- to 15-year-old and adult humans. *Science* **1975**, *190*, 686–687. [CrossRef] [PubMed]
87. Beauchamp, G.K.; Cowart, B.J.; Dobbing, J. Development of sweet taste. In *Sweetness*; Springer: Berlin, Germany, 1987; pp. 127–138.
88. Beauchamp, G.K.C.; Moran, M. Preference for high salt concentrations among children. *Dev. Psychobiol.* **1990**, *26*, 539–545. [CrossRef]
89. Verma, P.; Mittal, S.; Ghildiyal, A.; Chaudhary, L.; Mahajan, K.K. Salt preference: Age and sex related variability. *Indian J. Physiol. Pharmacol.* **2007**, *51*, 91–95. [PubMed]

90. Mennella, J.A.; Finkbeiner, S.; Lipchock, S.V.; Hwang, L.-D.; Reed, D.R. Preferences for salty and sweet tastes are elevated and related to each other during childhood. *PLoS ONE* **2014**, e92201. [CrossRef] [PubMed]

91. Stone, L.; Pangborn, R. Preferences and intake measures of salt and sugar, and their relation to personality traits. *Appetite* **1990**, *15*, 63–79. [CrossRef]

92. He, F.J.; Marrero, N.M.; MacGregor, G.A. Salt intake is related to soft drink consumption in children and adolescents: A link to obesity? *Hypertension* **2008**, *51*, 629–634. [CrossRef] [PubMed]

93. Grimes, C.A.; Riddell, L.J.; Campbell, K.J.; Nowson, C.A. Dietary salt intake, sugar-sweetened beverage consumption, and obesity risk. *Pediatrics* **2013**, *131*, 14–21. [CrossRef] [PubMed]

94. Cooke, L. The importance of exposure for healthy eating in childhood: A review. *J. Hum. Nutr. Diet.* **2007**, *20*, 294–301. [CrossRef] [PubMed]

95. Kochli, A.; Tenenbaum-Rakover, Y.; Leshem, M. Increased salt appetite in patients with congenital adrenal hyperplasia 21-hydroxylase deficiency. *Am. J. Physiol. Regul. Integr. Comp. Physiol.* **2005**, *288*, R1673–R1681. [CrossRef] [PubMed]

96. Trapp, C.M.; Speiser, P.W.; Oberfield, S.E. Congenital adrenal hyperplasia: An update in children. *Curr. Opin. Endocrinol. Diabetes Obes.* **2011**, *18*, 166–170. [CrossRef] [PubMed]

97. Bouhlal, S.; Chabanet, C.; Issanchou, S.; Nicklaus, S. Salt content impacts food preferences and intake among children. *PLoS ONE* **2013**, *8*, e53971. [CrossRef] [PubMed]

98. Bouhlal, S.; Issanchou, S.; Nicklaus, S. The impact of salt, fat and sugar levels on toddler food intake. *Br. J. Nutr.* **2011**, *105*, 645–653. [CrossRef] [PubMed]

99. Hayes, J.; Sullivan, B.; Duffy, V. Explaining variability in sodium intake through oral sensory phenotype, salt sensation and liking. *Physiol. Behav.* **2010**, *100*, 369–380. [CrossRef] [PubMed]

100. Mattes, R.D. The taste for salt in humans. *Am. J. Clin. Nutr.* **1997**, *65*, 692S–697S. [PubMed]

101. Albarracı, W.; Sanchez, I.C.; Grau, R.I.; Barat, J.M. Salt in processsing; usage and reduction: A review. *Food Sci. Technol.* **2011**, *46*, 1329–1336.

102. Zandstra, E.H.; De Graaf, C.; van Trijp, H.C.; van Staveren, W.A. Laboratory hedonic ratings as predictors of consumption. *Food Qual. Pref.* **1999**, *10*, 411–418. [CrossRef]

103. Rolls, B.J.; Rolls, E.T.; Rowe, E.A.; Sweeney, K. Sensory specific satiety in man. *Physiol. Behav.* **1981**, *27*, 137–142. [CrossRef]

104. Liem, D.; Zandstra, E.H. Children's liking and wanting of snack products: Influence of shape and flavour. *Int. J. Behav. Nutr. Phys. Act.* **2009**, *6*, 38. [CrossRef] [PubMed]

105. Sullivan, S.A.; Birch, L.L. Pass the sugar, pass, the salt: Experience dictates preference. *Dev. Psychol.* **1990**, *26*, 546–551. [CrossRef]

106. Beauchamp, G.K.; Moran, M. Acceptance of sweet and salty tastes in 2-year-old children. *Appetite* **1984**, *5*, 291–305. [CrossRef]

107. Ahrens, W. Sensory taste preferences and taste sensitivity and the association of unhealthy food patterns with overweight and obesity in primary school children in Europe—A synthesis of data from the idefics study. *Flavour* **2015**, *4*, 8. [CrossRef]

108. Bouhlal, S.; Issanchou, S.; Chabanet, C.; Nicklaus, S. 'Just a pinch of salt'. An experimental comparison of the effect of repeated exposure and flavor-flavor learning with salt or spice on vegetable acceptance in toddlers. *Appetite* **2014**, *83*, 209–217. [CrossRef] [PubMed]

109. Alexy, U.; Schaefer, A.; Sailer, O.; Busch-Stockfisch, M.; Huthmacher, S.; Kunert, J.; Kersting, M. Sensory preferences and discrimination ability of children in relation to their body weight status. *J. Sens. Stud.* **2011**, *26*, 409–412. [CrossRef]

110. Bobowski, N. Shifting human salty taste preference: Potential opportunities and challenges in reducing dietary salt intake of americans. *Chemosens. Percept.* **2015**, *8*, 112–116. [CrossRef] [PubMed]

111. Bertino, M.; Beauchamp, G.K.; Engelman, K. Long-term reduction in dietary sodium alters the taste of salt. *Am. J. Clin. Nutr.* **1982**, *36*, 1134–1144. [PubMed]

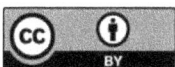

nutrients

Article

Baseline and Estimated Trends of Sodium Availability and Food Sources in the Costa Rican Population during 2004–2005 and 2012–2013

Adriana Blanco-Metzler [1,*], Rafael Moreira Claro [2], Katrina Heredia-Blonval [3], Ivannia Caravaca Rodríguez [4], María de los A. Montero-Campos [1], Branka Legetic [5] and Mary R. L'Abbe [6,*]

[1] Costa Rican Institute of Research and Training in Nutrition and Health, Tres Rios 4-2250, Costa Rica; mmontero@inciensa.sa.cr

[2] Nutrition Department (NUT), Federal University of Minas Gerais (UFMG), Belo Horizonte MG 30.130-100, Brazil; Rafael.claro@gmail.com

[3] Independent Nutritionist, San José 10203-1000, Costa Rica; katrihe@gmail.com

[4] Ministry of Health, San José 10123-1000, Costa Rica; ivannia.caravaca@misalud.go.cr

[5] Independent Consultant, Novi Sad 21000, Serbia; legeticb@gmail.com

[6] Department of Nutritional Sciences, University of Toronto, Toronto, ON M5S 3E2, Canada

* Correspondence: ablanco@inciensa.sa.cr (A.B.-M.); mary.labbe@utoronto.ca (M.R.L.); Tel.: +506-2279-9911 (A.B.-M.)

Received: 16 June 2017; Accepted: 11 September 2017; Published: 15 September 2017

Abstract: In 2012, Costa Rica launched a program to reduce salt and sodium consumption to prevent cardiovascular disease and associated risk factors, but little was known about the level of sodium consumption or its sources. Our aim was to estimate the magnitude and time trends of sodium consumption (based on food and beverage acquisitions) in Costa Rica. Data from the National Household Income and Expenditure Surveys carried out in 2004–2005 (n = 4231) and 2012–2013 (n = 5705) were used. Records of food purchases for household consumption were converted into sodium and energy using food composition tables. Mean sodium availability (per person/per day and adjusted for a 2000-kcal energy intake) and the contribution of food groups to this availability were estimated for each year. Sodium availability increased in the period from 3.9 to 4.6 g/person/day ($p < 0.001$). The income level was inversely related to sodium availability. The main sources of sodium in the diet were domestic salt (60%) in addition to processed foods and condiments (with added sodium) (27.4%). Dietary sources of sodium varied within surveys ($p < 0.05$). Sodium available for consumption in Costa Rican households largely exceeds the World Health Organization-recommended intake levels (<2 g sodium/person/day). These results are essential for the design and implementation of effective policies and interventions.

Keywords: salt; sodium; population intervention; policy; food consumption; socioeconomic factors; Costa Rica; Latin America

1. Introduction

Recent data on sodium intake show that populations around the world are consuming an amount of sodium that is excessive to what is physiologically necessary. In many cases, intake also exceeds the current World Health Organization (WHO) recommendations on sodium consumption for adults, which is 2 g sodium/day (equivalent to 5 g salt/day) [1,2]. A direct relationship between excessive sodium intake and the development of hypertension exists, which is responsible for 30% of the hypertension burden worldwide [3].

Globally, high blood pressure (hypertension) is the main risk factor for and the leading cause of death as well as being the second risk for disability related to cardiovascular disease (CVD) [4,5]. An estimated 17.9 million people died from CVD in 2015, representing 31% of all deaths. Over three quarters of CVD deaths take place in low- and middle-income countries [6].

In Costa Rica, a middle-income country, CVDs represent the leading cause of death since 1970 [7,8]. Two surveys of cardiovascular risk factors based on the Stepwise methodology of the Pan American Health Organization/World Health Organization (PAHO/WHO) have been recently carried out in the country [7,9], showing similar results for hypertension. The national prevalence of hypertension in adults over 19 years of age has remained constant at 37.8% in 2010 and 36.2% in 2014 (no significant difference) [9].

Reducing sodium intake is recognized as the most cost-effective intervention in preventing hypertension, CVD, and several other related conditions [10,11]. This is the main reason for the PAHO/WHO launching the "Cardiovascular Disease Prevention Initiative by Reducing Salt Consumption in the Americas" in 2009. This policy statement established a gradual reduction of sodium intake to reach a target of 2 g per person per day by 2020 (or 5 g of salt/person/day) [10].

Sodium intake can be estimated by a wide range of methods. According to PAHO, the Household Budget Survey (HBS) methodology represents a viable option to estimate sodium consumption by household members in countries with limited economic resources [10]. Brazil [12,13], Poland [14], and Slovenia [15] have used this method to measure salt intakes and identify the main dietary sources.

The objective of this study was to estimate the magnitude, distribution, and time trends in the availability of sodium in households of Costa Rica as well as the main food sources by analyzing the HBS conducted in Costa Rica during the years of 2004–2005 and 2012–2013. This scientific evidence is essential for the development of the sodium reduction national program and to achieve the salt goal of the WHO Global Action Plan for the Prevention and Control of Non-Communicable Diseases 2013–2020 [16].

2. Materials and Methods

The design of the study is ecological. The data analyzed were collected during the National Household Income and Expenditure Surveys (ENIGH) performed during 2004–2005 (ENIGH 2004–2005) and 2012–2013 (ENIGH 2012–2013). ENIGH is the specific name given to the HBS in Costa Rica. These surveys were carried out by the National Institute of Statistics and Censuses of Costa Rica (INEC). These surveys provide information on the composition of the budget in the country's households through knowledge of their income and expenditures on goods and services.

A probabilistic sampling design was employed, resulting in data that is representative of all households in Costa Rica and in the two zones of the country (urban and rural households). The sampling was based on a complex strategy that applies the previous definition of the socioeconomic strata and integrates the 348 (ENIGH 2004–2005) and 468 (ENIGH 2012–2013) sectors in the same territorial domain (zone and region) in strata that are economically homogeneous. Following this, sectors were selected in each stratum and households were selected within each sector. Finally, in order to standardize the data collection in the four quarters of the year, interviews were conducted in each sector throughout the 12 months of the study. A detailed description of the ENIGH sampling strategy is available in previous studies [17,18].

The records of all food and beverage purchases by the household for a period of seven consecutive days were analyzed (in ENIGH, the weekly records are converted to a month for the end registers). More details about ENIGH methodology can be found in previous studies [17,18]. A total of 96,336 purchases (by 4231 households) were recorded in ENIGH 2004–2005 and 186,308 (by 5705 households) in ENIGH 2012–2013. Information regarding the acquisition of foods outside the home was not available in ENIGH 2004–2005 and in 2012–2013, although the acquisition of snacks outside the home were registered. Foods outside the home corresponds to food items purchased and consumed outside the home, with snacks corresponding to one type of these food items. The criterion adopted for the recording of expenditure in ENIGH is "acquired", as the information available for each household is a proxy measure and not "actual intake".

The income per household used in both HBSs is the total net income of the household and includes the income that the household members receive in an average month for the last 12 months. This includes income from wages; self-employment with deductions from law; financial assets and rental of properties; transfers in cash or in kind; imputed rent (non-monetary income of the value of the imputed rental of own housing); as well as financial or capital transactions [17,18].

The methodology developed by Monteiro [12,13] consists of converting the food and beverage acquisition records of the family budget survey into nutrients by means of food composition tables. A national food composition table was constructed by collecting the sodium and energy contents of approximately 980 foods and typical recipes. Due to the lack of sodium content data in the national food composition tables, the United States Department of Agriculture's (USDA) nutrient database [19] was used as the main data source. In the case of fortified foods and native foods, the tables of food composition published by the Costa Rican Institute for Research and Teaching in Nutrition and Health [20,21] were used. To determine the sodium content in typical Costa Rican recipes, the database of the Nutrition School of the University of Costa Rica ValorNut [22] was used. The nutritional content of food recipes or preparations was calculated based on the methodology established by the Food and Agriculture Organization of the United Nations [23]. A comprehensive review of the built table was performed and food was classified into the five food groups established by the research team.

The availability of sodium/person/day and the contribution for each food group was calculated. The results of ENIGH 2012–2013 were compared with those of ENIGH 2004–2005 before trends were established.

Items were grouped based on the categories established by Monteiro [12,24], which consisted of separating common salt from salt-based condiments. The final classification was defined by five categories: common salt; condiments with added sodium; processed foods without added sodium; prepared dishes; "natura" (foods in their natural state, without any processing), and processed foods with added sodium (excluding condiments).

Food and beverage acquisition records (containing the amount acquired in kilograms or liters) from ENIGH 2004–2005 and 2012–2013 were initially linked to sodium and energy content. The net quantity of each product was estimated by removing the non-edible fraction from the total acquired quantity (gross quantity) and used in the determination of the sodium amount of each acquisition. Following this, the availability of sodium was estimated (per capita/day, by dividing the total acquired quantity by the number of people in the household and by 30.33 (average number of days per month) for the entire set of foods and beverages, according to food groups. This was estimated for the total population and according to zone (rural and urban) and income level (using t-test).

As this survey is not designed for nutritional purposes, and in order to mitigate errors in the analysis and allow for comparisons between surveys, the results were standardized to 2000 kcal, which is the average energy consumption of a healthy adult [25].

Consumption trends were identified and compared between both surveys. The surveys are methodologically comparable except that in ENIGH 2004–2005, the sample does not allow stratification at the regional level (due to inconsistencies in some regional information, INEC decided not to recommend this stratification). This comparison was conducted for the entire population of each survey and according to income levels. For this, the per capita income was first estimated in each household (by dividing total income by the number of individuals in each household using information available at ENIGH) and used to divide the population into five income levels (based on the quintiles of per capita income distribution). Student's t-tests were used to compare each income level between the surveys, while a regression model (Generalized Linear Model was used to investigate trends between the income levels within each survey.

Analyzes were performed with the statistical program SPSS version 20 (IBM Corp, New York, NY, USA). In each unit of analysis, the expansion factor was considered. This factor is obtained as the inverse of the probability of selecting each house at the time of selecting the sample. We tested the hypothesis at the significance level of 5% by the Student's *t*-test [26].

3. Results

Household energy and sodium availability in Costa Rica, unadjusted and adjusted to 2000 kcal, is shown in Table 1 according to the zone and year of survey. The amount of sodium available for consumption in 2004–2005 and 2012–2013 was 3.9 and 4.6 g/person/day, respectively. A statistically significant increasing trend was found ($p < 0.0001$). In both surveys, a significant difference ($p < 0.0001$) was found between the availability of sodium in rural compared to urban areas. In all areas, the available sodium was always greater than 3.6 g/person/day. Adjusting the sodium availability to a 2000-kcal diet did not substantially alter the scenario. The available sodium analysis of ENIGH 2012–2013 showed no significant differences between regions ($p > 0.05$).

Table 1. Household energy and sodium availability according to region and zone of residence in Costa Rica with comparisons of the data from 2004–2005 and 2012–2013.

Zone	*n*		Energy (kcal/Person/Day)		Sodium (g/Person/Day)		Sodium (g/Person/Day/2000 kcal)	
	2004–2005	2012–2013	2004–2005	2012–2013	2004–2005	2012–2013	2004–2005	2012–2013
Costa Rica	1,134,433	1,396,747	2315	2390	3.9	4.6 [a]	3.4	3.8 [a]
Urban	705,111	1,023,061	2263	2344	3.6	4.4 [a,b]	3.2	3.8 [a,b]
Rural	429,322	373,686	2400	2531	4.5	5.2 [a,b]	3.8	4.1 [a,b]

[a] Statistically significant differences between 2004–2005 and 2012–2013 ($p < 0.0001$); and [b] rural vs. urban ($p < 0.0001$).

The energy and sodium available in households according to income levels (quintiles) is shown in Table 2. In both surveys, all income quintiles exceeded the maximum recommended intake of sodium (2 g/person/day) with a minimum of 3.8 g/person/day in 2012–2013, which had no linear relation with income level in the unadjusted data. However, the analysis of energy values showed that the sodium intake had an inversely proportional relationship with the income (Figure 1). On the other hand, when comparing sodium availability (g/person/day) surveys conducted during 2004–2005 and 2012–2013, we found differences in sodium available between quintiles II, IV, and V ($p < 0.05$), with none found between quintiles I and III ($p > 0.05$).

Table 2. Household energy and sodium availability based on food purchases according to increasing quintiles of income distribution in Costa Rica with comparisons of the data from 2004–2005 and 2012–2013.

Quintile	*n*		Energy (kcal/Person/Day)		Sodium (g/Person/Day)		Sodium (g/Person/Day/2000kcal)	
	2004–2005	2012–2013	2004–2005	2012–2013	2004–2005	2012–2013	2004–2005	2012–2013
Costa Rica	1,134,433	1,396,747	2315	2390	3.9	4,6 [a]	3.4	3.9 [a]
I	225,773	279,044	1896	1724	3.9	3,8 [b]	4.1	4.4 [b]
II	226,647	279,642	2065	2195	3.5	4.7 [a]	3.4	4.3 [a]
III	228,332	279,437	2276	2494	4.0	4.7	3.5	3.8
IV	226,503	279,409	2626	2679	4.4	4.9 [a]	3.4	3.7 [a]
V	227,178	279,215	2712	2669	3.9	4.7 [a]	2.9	3.5 [a]

[a] Statistically significant differences between 2004–2005 and 2012–2013 ($p < 0.0001$); and [b] between quintiles of income ($p < 0.05$).

Sodium g/person/2000 kcal

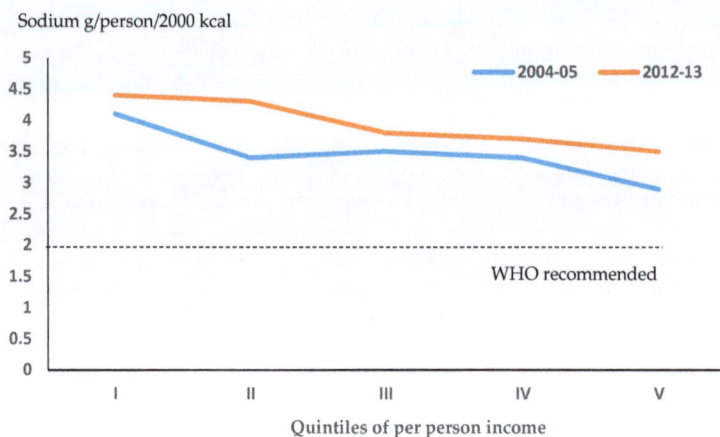

Figure 1. Trends in household availability of sodium * according to increasing quintiles of per person family income in Costa Rica with a comparison of the data from 2004–2005 and 2012–2013. * Adjusted to a 2000-kcal diet. For more information, see Section 2.

Table 3 shows the sources of sodium in the diet of the population of Costa Rica by household per person income. Common salt (table or kitchen salt) was the main source, with an estimated intake of 2.4 and 2.8 g/person/day in the ENIGH 2004–2005 and 2012–2013, respectively. In both surveys, common salt contributes 60% of total sodium available in the households, followed by processed foods and condiments. The dietary source that contributed least to dietary sodium was natural and processed foods with no added sodium, which accounted for only 5% of sodium availability. Statistical differences ($p < 0.05$) were found between the food sources of sodium in both surveys. A significant trend over time ($p < 0.05$) was found due to an increase in the sodium intake per person from processed foods and condiments with sodium added. In comparison, in ready-to-eat meals and natural foods, the sodium availability tended to decrease or remain constant between surveys. Socioeconomic income was inversely associated with common salt availability, as well as being directly associated with a greater acquisition of processed foods, natural foods, and prepared dishes ($p < 0.05$). No association was found between socioeconomic income and acquisition of condiments.

Table 3. Dietary sources of sodium acquired for household consumption (g/person/day) according to increasing quintiles of income distribution based on food purchases in Costa Rica with the comparison of the data from 2004–2005 and 2012–2013.

2012–2013

Food Group	n	Costa Rica		Quintiles of Per Capita Income Distribution				
		g/Person/Day	%	I	II	III	IV	V
Common salt (table or kitchen)	1,396,747	2.78	60.2	72.4 [b]	66.3 [b]	61.6 [b]	58.2 [b]	45.2 [b]
Processed foods	1,396,747	0.65 [a]	14.2 [a]	10.1 [b]	10.9 [b]	14.1 [b]	15.8 [b]	19.4 [b]
Sodium-based condiments	1,396,747	0.61 [a]	13.2 [a]	11.8 [b]	15.0 [b]	13.1 [b]	11.8 [b]	14.0 [b]
Ready to eat meals	1,396,747	0.33 [a]	7.2 [a]	2.4 [b]	3.8 [b]	6.1 [b]	8.7 [b]	14.3 [b]
In natura foods	1,396,747	0.24	5.1	3.4 [b]	4.0 [b]	5.2 [b]	5.5 [b]	7.3 [b]
Total	1,396,747	4.61	100	100	100	100	100	100

Table 3. *Cont.*

2004–2005								
Food Group	*n*	Costa Rica		Quintiles of Per Capita Income Distribution				
		g/person/day	%	I	II	III	IV	V
Common salt (table or kitchen)	1,134,433	2.37	60.2	77.2	66.3	62.4	54.7	41.2
Processed foods	1,134,433	0.61	15.4	8.1	13.9	15.3	17.1	22.5
Sodium-based condiments	1,134,433	0.36	9.3	6.4	7.7	9.3	11.7	10.8
Ready to eat meals	1,134,433	0.38	9.8	5.1	7.6	8.0	10.7	17.2
In natura foods	1,134,433	0.21	5.4	3.2	4.6	4.9	5.8	8.3
Total	1,134,433	3.94	100	100	100	100	100	100

[a] Statistically significant differences between food groups in 2012–2013 and 2004–2005 ($p < 0.05$); and [b] between food groups in 2012–2013 and 2004–2005 of quintiles of income ($p < 0.05$).

4. Discussion

The household availability of sodium in Costa Rica is within the internationally reported range (3.6 to 4.8 g/person/day) [10], but exceeds the WHO maximum intake recommendation [2]. The higher amount of sodium available in the rural areas can be explained by the greater availability of energy and, therefore, of foods that provide sodium. Other authors have reported that the consumption of salt is directly proportional to energy [12].

We found that there was a trend of increased sodium acquisition in households over time, with a 15% increase in per person household acquisition in less than a decade. This result is extremely relevant for public health, as it indicates the urgent need for effective actions capable of stopping this expansion and methods aiming to reduce sodium consumption in the country. The results of the present study also indicate that Costa Rica, up to 2013, was failing to meet the goal set out in the "National Strategy for Comprehensive Management of Chronic Non-Communicable Diseases and Obesity 2014–2021", which was an average relative reduction of "15% in daily salt/sodium intake" [27]. This goal was based on the sodium available in the homes estimated in the ENIGH 2004–2005 [18] and, until the publication of this study, no results from ENIGH 2012–2013 were available.

This study is the first one that estimates sodium availability in Costa Rican households at a national level. Previously, the consumption of sodium in Costa Rica has only been estimated in the metropolitan areas. Using the method of seven-day food diaries, the mean consumption of sodium was estimated as 3.6 g/person/day in the metropolitan city of Cartago [28]. Using the technique of 24-h urine in a sample of 30 adult men with hypertension in San Jose, the capital of the country, sodium intake was found to be 3.8 g/person/day [29]. These studies estimated 0.8 and 1.0 g/person/day less sodium than what we estimated in the HBS 2012–2013. Differences may be due to the methodology used, the size of the populations, and their representativeness, as more sodium is consumed in the rural population [12,13]. The amount of domestic salt estimated in the present study is within the range reported in previous studies conducted in the country [28–30].

Despite differences in the methodology used to estimate sodium consumption [28,29], all studies show that the consumption of sodium and of common salt (kitchen or table) in Costa Rica considerably exceeds the international recommendation [2].

An inverse relationship was found between sodium availability in households (energy-adjusted) and income, which is similar to that reported in studies conducted in developing [12,13] and developed countries [31]. Although a poorer diet quality among low-income families may be one of the reasons for high sodium intake [31], this result might also relate to the main source of sodium consumption in Costa Rica, namely common salt (table or kitchen).

Regarding the main sources of dietary sodium, income level is known to play a major influence. In developed countries, the main sources of sodium are processed foods and meals outside the home. In addition, a smaller contribution of common salt and condiments has been reported [32], since cooking in the home is less common in developed countries [33]. In Costa Rica and Brazil, food is still prepared in home, with common salt and condiments representing the main sources of sodium in the diet [13]. However, in both countries, there is has been increasing availability of ultra-processed foods seen in recent years [24,34].

Contrary to expectations, the contribution of prepared dishes on the household availability of sodium decreased between surveys (from 9.8% to 7.2%). These differences are due to changes in food collection and classification between two surveys in a way that resulted in the comparison for this food group not being recommended. Natural and processed foods without added sodium represented the groups that provide less sodium to the diet. This behavior is similar in both surveys and shows that, unfortunately, the acquisition of natural foods did not increase in this period. The reduced household availability of natural foods is directly associated with a better economic income in Costa Rica.

Condiments, mainly consommés and cubes, was the food group whose sodium contribution to diet increased most over the course of nine years, with their availability in households having almost doubled. In the late 1990s, the Costa Rican Ministry of Health found an important substitution of domestic salt for condiments in household daily food preparations. For this reason, as a part of the salt fortification policy, the government established that salt used in the manufacture of consommés and cubes must contain iodine and fluorine at the levels stipulated for domestic salt since 2001 [35]. This policy was designed to prevent an iodine deficiency in the population and it may have contributed to the increase in the acquisition of commercial condiments high in salt. However, as we demonstrate in this study, there has been an increase not only in the intake of condiments but also in domestic salt.

The results of the present study serve as an important driver for the inclusion of condiments in the preparation of the PAHO regional targets on sodium reduction [36]. They also have been used in the establishment of the national goal of salt reduction; the preparation of the action plan of the national strategy for the management of chronic non-communicable diseases in Costa Rica [27]; and the establishment of national sodium reduction targets in key processed foods.

The HBS method has its limitations, because the survey was designed for economic reasons and not for nutritional purposes. Due to this ecological type of study, there are several main limitations. Firstly, our method overestimates the consumption of sodium because it is assumed that every food and beverage item purchased is for human consumption. Secondly, it is impossible to estimate the consumption of sodium away from home, since only food and beverages acquired for household consumption are recorded with enough information. Thirdly, the use of food composition tables does not always precisely estimate the sodium content of the foods consumed by participants. Furthermore, most of the data for the sodium content of foods was determined from the food composition table of the USDA, with a lack of updated local food data. There needs to be further confirmation with more precise studies, especially considering that a homogenous distribution is assumed in this present study. However, the advantage of this ecological method is economical, because the data already exists and results are quickly generated. Although the HBS methodology is not as accurate as 24-h urine excretion or national nutritional surveys, it allows for an approximate estimation and permits monitoring changes in the consumption of sodium in the population [32].

5. Conclusions

In Costa Rica, in urban and rural zones and across income stratum, the sodium available for consumption at the household level (based on households' food and beverage acquisitions) considerably exceeds the maximum WHO recommendation. Rural areas and individuals with lower income are those with the greater risk of having high sodium consumption. It is imperative to promote public health interventions in Costa Rica to reduce excessive consumption of sodium in the population, both at home and in the processed foods supply. This must be conducted in order to contribute to the reduction of hypertension and associated chronic diseases and to meet public health interventions [27,28,32,37]. The pattern of sodium consumption by the population of Costa

Rica is typical of a developing country. Continued nutritional analysis of the ENIGH database is recommended in order to evaluate and monitor actions to reduce salt/sodium intake in the population. Results need to be confirmed by 24-h urine excretion. In addition, it is desirable that the salt reduction program works in conjunction with the National Salt Fortification Program, as both health policies should strive to work in a synchronized way so that each one achieves its purpose without being to the detriment of the other.

Acknowledgments: External financial support was from the International Development Research Center, Canada (IDRC Project # 106 888). The Instituto Nacional de Estadística y Censos (INEC) of Costa Rica supplied the ENIGH databases for free. David Lopez Marin was the national consultant in statistics that was hired by the project.

Author Contributions: A.B., M.L., B.L. and M.M. conceived the study and designed the research protocol of the complete project. A.B., K.H., I.C. and R.C. outlined the plan for the analysis and effectively conducted the data organization and analysis. A.B. and R.C. wrote the initial version of the manuscript. All authors reviewed and approved the final version of the manuscript.

Conflicts of Interest: The authors declare no conflicts of interest. The founding sponsor had no role in the design of the study; in the collection, analyses, or interpretation of data; in the writing of the manuscript, and in the decision to publish the results.

References

1. Global Burden of Disease 2015 Risk Factors Collaborators. Global, regional, and national comparative risk assessment of 79 behavioural, environmental and occupational, and metabolic risks or clusters of risks, 1990–2015: A systematic analysis for the Global Burden of Disease Study 2015. *Lancet* **2016**, *388*, 1659–1724. Available online: https://www.ncbi.nlm.nih.gov/pubmed/27733284 (accessed on 28 July 2017).
2. World Health Organization (WHO). *Guideline: Sodium Intake for Adults and Children*; WHO: Geneva, Switzerland, 2012. Available online: http://www.who.int/nutrition/publications/guidelines/sodium_intake_printversion.pdf (accessed on 28 July 2017).
3. He, F.J.; MacGregor, G.A. A comprehensive review on salt and health and current experience of worldwide salt reduction programmes. *J. Hum. Hypertens.* **2009**, *23*, 363–384. Available online: https://www.ncbi.nlm.nih.gov/pubmed/19110538 (accessed on 15 June 2017). [PubMed]
4. Lawes, C.M.; Vander Hoorn, S.; Rodgers, A.; International Society of Hypertension. Global burden of blood-pressure-related disease, 2001. *Lancet* **2008**, *371*, 1513–1518. Available online: https://www.ncbi.nlm.nih.gov/pubmed/18456100 (accessed on 28 August 2017). [PubMed]
5. World Health Organization (WHO). *Reducing Sodium Intake to Reduce Blood Pressure and Risk of Cardiovascular Diseases in Adults*; e-Library of Evidence for Nutrition Actions (eLENA), WHO: Geneva, Switzerland, 2017. Available online: http://www.who.int/mediacentre/factsheets/fs317/en/ (accessed on 3 May 2017).
6. GBD 2015 Mortality and Causes of Death Collaborators. Global, regional, and national life expectancy, all-cause mortality, and cause-specific mortality for 249 causes of death, 1980–2015: A systematic analysis for the Global Burden of Disease Study 2015. *Lancet* **2016**, *388*, 1459–1544. Available online: https://www.researchgate.net/publication/308904659_Global_regional_and_national_life_expectancy_all-cause_mortality_and_cause-specific_mortality_for_249_causes_of_death_1980-2015_a_systematic_analysis_for_the_Global_Burden_of_Disease_Study_2015 (accessed on 29 July 2017).
7. Caja Costarricense del Seguro Social. *Vigilancia de los Factores de Riesgo Cardiovascular*; Servicios Gráficos: San José, Costa Rica, 2011; p. 41. Available online: http://www.binasss.sa.cr/informesdegestion/vigilancia.pdf (accessed on 3 May 2017).
8. Costa Rica. Ministerio de Salud, Instituto Costarricense de Investigación y Enseñanza en Nutrición y Salud, Caja Costarricense del Seguro Social y Organización Panamericana de la Salud. *Encuesta Multinacional de Diabetes Mellitus, Hipertensión Arterial y Factores de Riesgo Asociados, Área Metropolitana, San José, 2004*; El Ministerio: San José, Costa Rica, 2009; pp. 12–15. Available online: http://www2.paho.org/hq/index.php?option=com_docman&task=doc_view&gid=16262&Itemid=270 (accessed on 3 May 2017).
9. Caja Costarricense del Seguro Social. *Vigilancia de los Factores de Riesgo Cardiovascular. Segunda Encuesta, 2014*; Editorial Nacional de Salud y Seguridad Social: San José, Costa Rica, 2016; pp. 34–92. Available online: http://www.binasss.sa.cr/informesdegestion/encuesta2014.pdf (accessed on 4 June 2017).

10. World Health Organization. Salt Reduction. Available online: http://www.who.int/mediacentre/factsheets/fs393/en/ (accessed on 1 August 2017).

11. He, F.J.; Campbell, N.R.; MacGregor, G.A. Reducing salt intake to prevent hypertension and cardiovascular disease. *Rev. Panam. Salud Pública* **2012**, *32*, 293–300. Available online: https://www.ncbi.nlm.nih.gov/pubmed/23299291 (accessed on 3 May 2017). [CrossRef] [PubMed]

12. Sarno, F.; Moreira, R.; Bertazzi, R.; Henrique, D.; Gouvea, S.; Monteiro, C.A. Estimated sodium intake by the Brazilian population, 2002–2003. *Rev. Saúde Pública* **2009**, *43*, 1–6. Available online: https://www.ncbi.nlm.nih.gov/pubmed/19225699 (accessed on 6 May 2017).

13. Sarno, F.; Claro, R.M.; Levy, R.B.; Bandoni, D.H.; Monteiro, C.A. Estimated sodium intake for the Brazilian population, 2008–2009. *Rev. Saude Publica* **2013**, *47*, 571–578. Available online: https://www.ncbi.nlm.nih.gov/pubmed/24346570 (accessed on 6 May 2017). [CrossRef] [PubMed]

14. European Commission. *Survey on Members States Implementation of the EU Salt Reduction Framework*; Publications Office of the European Union: Luxemberg, Belgium, 2012; p. 14. Available online: http://ec.europa.eu/health/sites/health/files/nutrition_physical_activity/docs/salt_report1_en.pdf (accessed on 6 May 2017).

15. Hlastan, R.; Zakotnik, J.M.; Seljak, B.K.; Polinick, R.; Blaznik, U.; Mis, N.F.; Erzen, I.; Ji, C.; Cappuccio, F.C. Estimation of sodium availability in food in Slovenia: Results from household food purchase data from 2000 to 2009. *Slov. J. Public Health* **2014**, *53*, 209–219. Available online: https://www.degruyter.com/view/j/sjph.ahead-of-print/sjph-2014-0021/sjph-2014-0021.xml (accessed on 6 May 2017).

16. World Health Organization. *Global Action Plan for the Prevention and Control of Noncommunicable Diseases 2013–2020*; WHO document Production Services: Geneva, Switzerland, 2013; pp. 1–91. Available online: http://apps.who.int/iris/bitstream/10665/94384/1/9789241506236_eng.pdf?ua=1 (accessed on 6 May 2017).

17. Instituto Nacional de Estadistica y Censos. *Encuesta Nacional de Ingresos y Gastos de los Hogares 2013: Principales Resultados*; INEC: San José, Costa Rica, 2014. Available online: http://www.inec.go.cr/sites/default/files/documentos/pobreza_y_presupuesto_de_hogares/gastos_de_los_hogares/metodologias/documentos_metodologicos/mepobrezaenig2013-2014-01_1.pdf (accessed on 6 May 2017).

18. Instituto Nacional de Estadística y Censos. *Encuesta Nacional de Ingresos y Gastos 2004: Principales Resultados*; INEC: San José, Costa Rica, 2006; p. 302.

19. USDA Food Composition Databases 2015. Available online: https://ndb.nal.usda.gov/ndb/search/list (accessed on 6 May 2017).

20. Alfaro, T.; Salas, M.T.; Ascencio, M. *Tabla de Composición de Alimentos de Costa Rica: Alimentos Fortificados*; Instituto Costarricense de Investigación y Enseñanza en Nutrición y Salud: Tres Ríos, Costa Rica, 2006; p. 20. Available online: https://www.inciensa.sa.cr/vigilancia_epidemiologica/informes_vigilancia/tablas%20composicion/Alimentos%20fortificados.pdf (accessed on 6 May 2017).

21. Blanco-Metzler, A.; Montero-Campos, M.A.; Fernández-Piedra, M. *Tabla de Composición de Alimentos de Costa Rica. Macronutrientes y Fibra Dietética*; Instituto Costarricense de Investigación y Enseñanza en Nutrición y Salud: Tres Ríos, Costa Rica, 2006; pp. 22–39. Available online: http://www.inciensa.sa.cr/vigilancia_epidemiologica/informes_vigilancia/tablas%20composicion/Macronutrientes%20y%20fibra.pdf (accessed on 6 May 2017).

22. ValorNut (1) (Software). Available online: http://nutricion2.ucr.ac.cr/valornut/ (accessed on 6 May 2017).

23. Greenfield, H.; Southgate, D.A.T. *Food Composition Data. Production, Management and Use*, 2nd ed.; FAO: Rome, Italy, 2003; p. 225. Available online: http://www.fao.org/docrep/008/y4705e/y4705e00.htm (accessed on 17 May 2017).

24. Monteiro, C.A.; Bertazzi, R.; Claro, R.M.; de Castro, I.R.; Cannon, G. Increasing consumption of ultra-processed foods and likely impact on human health: evidence from Brazil. *Public Health Nutr.* **2010**, *14*, 5–13. Available online: https://www.cambridge.org/core/services/aop-cambridge-core/content/view/C36BB4F83B90629DA15CB0A3CBEBF6FA/S1368980010003241a.pdf/increasing_consumption_of_ultraprocessed_foods_and_likely_impact_on_human_health_evidence_from_brazil.pdf (accessed on 6 May 2017).

25. COMIECO. Reglamento Técnico Centroamericano. In *RTCA 67.01.60:10 Etiquetado Nutricional de Productos Alimenticios Preenvasados Para Consumo Humano Para la Poblacion a Partir de 3 Años de Edad*; Diario Oficial La Gaceta N°71; Imprenta Nacional: San José, Costa Rica, 2011. Available online: https://extranet.who.int/nutrition/gina/sites/default/files/COMIECO%202011%20Etiquetado%20Nutricional%20de%20Productos%20Alimenticios%20Preenvasados%20para%20Consumo%20Humano.pdf (accessed on 13 June 2017).

26. Downey, N.M.; Heath, R.W. *Métodos Estadísticos Aplicados*, 3rd ed.; Harla S.A. de C.V.: México City, Mexico, 1973.

27. Costa Rica. Ministerio de Salud. *Estrategia Nacional Abordaje Integral de las Enfermedades Crónicas No Transmisibles y Obesidad 2014–2021*; El Ministerio: San José, Costa Rica, 2014; 100p. Available online: http://www.iccpportal.org/sites/default/files/plans/CRI_B3_COR_Libro_Estrategia_ECNT.pdf (accessed on 7 May 2017).

28. Costa Rica. Ministerio de Salud. *Encuesta Basal de Factores de Riesgo Para Enfermedades no Transmisibles. Cartago 2001. Módulo 1: Factores Alimentarios*; Ministerio de Salud: San José, Costa Rica, 2003.

29. Brenes, M.; Villalobos, D. Evaluación del Estado Nutricional de un Grupo de Funcionarios con Hipertensión Arterial Atendidos en la Oficina de Bienestar y Salud, Sede Universitaria Rodrigo Facio de la Universidad de Costa Rica, 2012. Bachelor's Thesis, Universidad de Costa Rica, San Pedro, Costa Rica, 2013.

30. Instituto Nacional de Estadistica y Censos. Costo de la Canasta Basica Alimentaria, enero 2011. In *Boletín Mensual Nueva Canasta Basica Alimentaria*; INEC: San Jose, Costa Rica, 2011; p. 9. Available online: www.inec.go.cr/sites/default/files/documentos/economia/costo_canasta_basica_alimentaria/publicaciones/reeconomcba012011-01.pdf (accessed on 20 May 2017).

31. De Mestral, C.; Mayén, A.L.; Petrovic, D.; Marques-Vidal, P.; Bochud, M.; Stringhini, S. Socioeconomic Determinants of Sodium Intake in Adult Populations of High-Income Countries: A Systematic Review and Meta-Analysis. *Am. J. Public Health* **2017**, *107*, 563. Available online: https://www.ncbi.nlm.nih.gov/pubmed/28272962 (accessed on 15 June 2017). [PubMed]

32. Pan American Health Organization (PAHO). *Salt Smart Americas: Guide for Country-Level Action*; PAHO: Washington DC, USA, 2013; pp. 91–104. Available online: http://www2.paho.org/hq/index.php?option=com_content&view=article&id=8677%3A2013-technical-document-salt-smart-americas&catid=5387%3Asalt-reduction-media-center&Itemid=40601 (accessed on 3 May 2017).

33. Holden, J.M.; Pehrsson, P.R.; Nickle, M.; Haytowitz, D.B.; Exler, J.; Showell, B.; Williams, J.; Thomas, R.G.; Ahuja, J.K.C.; Patterson, K.Y.; et al. USDA monitors levels of added sodium in commercial packaged and restaurant foods. *Procedia Food Sci.* **2013**, *2*, 60–67. Available online: http://ac.els-cdn.com/S2211601X13000114/1-s2.0-S2211601X13000114-main.pdf?_tid=57a8dd34-520d-11e7-ba88-00000aacb35d&acdnat=1497560471_7749e969b438c7a977b5ebad16c598c4 (accessed on 15 June 2017).

34. Pan American Health Organization. *Ultra-Processed Food and Drink Products in Latin America: Trends, Impact on Obesity, Policy Implications*; PAHO: Washington DC, USA, 2015. Available online: http://iris.paho.org/xmlui/bitstream/handle/123456789/7699/9789275118641_eng.pdf?sequence=5&isAllowed=y (accessed on 14 May 2017).

35. Reforma Norma Oficial para la Sal de Calidad Alimentaria, N° 30032-S. Diario Oficial La Gaceta N° 247. Alcance N 88-A a. Imprenta Nacional, San José, Costa Rica. 2001. Available online: http://www.pgrweb.go.cr/scij/Busqueda/Normativa/Normas/nrm_texto_completo.aspx?param1=NRTC&nValor1=1&nValor2=47668&nValor3=88169&param2=1&strTipM=TC&lResultado=2&strSim=simp (accessed on 14 May 2017).

36. Pan American Health Organization (PAHO). SaltSmart Consortiumn Consensus Statement to Advance Target Harmonization by Agreeing on Regional Targets for the Salt/Sodium Content of Key Food Categories. 2015. 11p. Available online: http://www2.paho.org/hq/index.php?option=com_docman&task=doc_download&gid=28929&Itemid=270&lang=en (accessed on 14 May 2017).

37. Costa Rica. Ministerio de Salud. *Plan Nacional Para la Reducción del Consumo de Sal/Sodio en la Población de Costa Rica, 2011–2021*; El Ministerio: San José, Costa Rica, 2011; pp. 3–20. Available online: https://www.ministeriodesalud.go.cr/index.php/biblioteca-de-archivos/sobre-el-ministerio/politcas-y-planes-en-salud/planes-en-salud/1103-plan-nacional-para-la-reduccion-del-consumo-de-sal-sodio-en-la-poblacion-de-costa-rica-2011-2021/file (accessed on 14 May 2017).

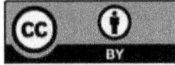

nutrients

MDPI

Article

Evaluation of a Mass-Media Campaign to Increase the Awareness of the Need to Reduce Discretionary Salt Use in the South African Population

Edelweiss Wentzel-Viljoen [1,*]**, Krisela Steyn** [2]**, Carl Lombard** [3]**, Anniza De Villiers** [4]**,**
Karen Charlton [5,6] **, Sabine Frielinghaus** [7]**, Christelle Crickmore** [8] **and Vash Mungal-Singh** [8]

[1] Centre for Excellence in Nutrition (CEN), Faculty of Health Sciences, North-West University,
    Potchefstroom 2520, South Africa
[2] Chronic Disease Initiative for Africa, University of Cape Town, Private Bag X3 Observatory,
    Cape Town 7925, South Africa; krisela.steyn@uct.ac.za
[3] Biostatistics Unit, South African Medical Research Council, Tygerberg, Cape Town 7505, South Africa;
    carl.lombard@mrc.ac.za
[4] Non-Communicable Diseases Research Unit, South African Medical Research Council, Tygerberg,
    Cape Town 7505, South Africa; Anniza.deVilliers@mrc.ac.za
[5] School of Medicine, Faculty of Science, Medicine and Health, University of Wollongong, Wollongong,
    NSW 2522, Australia; karenc@uow.edu.au
[6] Illawarra Health and Medical Research Institute, Wollongong, NSW 2522, Australia
[7] MQ Market Intelligence, 5 Windward Turn, Atlantic Beach, Cape Town 7441, South Africa; sabine@mqmi.net
[8] Heart and Stroke Foundation South Africa, Unit 5B, 5th Floor, Graphic Centre, 5 Buiten Street, Cape Town
    8001, South Africa; christelle@heartfoundation.co.za (C.C.); vash@heartfoundation.co.za (V.M.-S.)
*   Correspondence: edelweiss.wentzel-viljoen@nwu.ac.za; Tel.: +27-82-379-0023

Received: 11 October 2017; Accepted: 7 November 2017; Published: 12 November 2017

Abstract: The South African strategic plan to reduce cardiovascular disease (CVD) includes reducing population salt intake to less than 5 g/day. A mass media campaign was undertaken to increase public awareness of the association between high salt intake, blood pressure and CVD, and focused on the reduction of discretionary salt intake. Community based surveys, before and after the campaign, were conducted in a cohort of black women aged 18–55 years. Questions on knowledge, attitudes and beliefs regarding salt use were asked. Current interest in engaging with salt reduction behaviors was assessed using the "stage of change" model. Five hundred fifty women participated in the baseline study and 477 in the follow-up survey. Most of the indicators of knowledge, attitudes and behavior change show a significant move towards considering and initiating reduced salt consumption. Post intervention, significantly more participants reported that they were taking steps to control salt intake (38% increased to 59.5%, $p < 0.0001$). In particular, adding salt while cooking and at the table occurred significantly less frequently. The findings suggest that mass media campaigns may be an effective tool to use as part of a strategy to reduce discretionary consumption of salt among the population along with other methods.

Keywords: salt reduction; mass-media public health campaign; salt strategy

1. Introduction

Reducing mean population salt intake by 30% by 2025 is one of the World Health Organization's (WHO) [1] global targets to reduce and control hypertension and non-communicable diseases (NCDs). In rural South Africans, stroke, the second most common cause of death and the leading cause of disability [2], is associated with high blood pressure and excess weight [3]. In their strategic plan for the prevention and control of non-communicable diseases (2013–2017), the South African National

Department of Health includes the target to reduce the mean population intake of salt to less than 5 g per day [4]. Current salt intake by the South African population is well above this amount [5,6] with about 30% taking in more than 10 g of salt/day [6], as confirmed by a recent systematic review of the sub-Saharan Africa region [7].

To achieve these targets, two essential complementary strategies are needed. The first relates to changes to the food supply. It is estimated that approximately 60% of total salt intake is provided from processed foods, while the remaining 40% comes from discretionary use of salt in domestic food preparation and salt added to food during meals [8]. The South African government has adopted a legislative approach (implemented June 2016) that requires the food industry to comply with maximum targets for salt levels in a wide range of food categories, with a further reduction required by 2019 [9]. From the time that the Minister of Health initiated the national salt reduction strategy for South Africa, there have been a number of activities undertaken by the Department of Health and non-governmental organizations which have received wide coverage in the media. Examples include newspaper and magazine articles and TV airing that reported about the excessive salt intake of the population, promulgation of the salt reduction regulations and high level meetings held in the country on NCDs including the WHO/United Nations United Nations High-level meeting on NCD Prevention and control to shape the international agenda from 19 to 20 September 2011 in New York, USA.

The second strategy relates to efforts to change consumer behavior related to salt use. An advocacy group, Salt Watch (www.heartfoundation.co.za), that was formed in 2014 and funded, in part, by the National Department of Health through the Heart and Stroke Foundation South Africa (HSFSA), was mandated to run a mass-media campaign to increase public awareness related to the association between a high salt intake, blood pressure and cardiovascular disease, and to highlight the need to reduce discretionary salt intake. In addition, it also provided some information on which foods contain less salt. The campaign was based on sound behavior change principles [10,11] and the evaluation of the intended impact of the campaign was central to its initial planning. The progression through the different stages of change [12,13] was used as an outcome measure. The campaign supports the revised South African Food-Based Dietary Guidelines that state, as part of a healthy eating pattern, the population should "Use salt and foods high in salt sparingly" [5]. It consisted of television and radio advertisements as well as various supporting activities aimed at strengthening the advertisement message and providing additional information and education materials regarding salt reduction. The primary target audience were adult black women as the persons primarily responsible for food purchases and preparation in the household.

In this paper, we report on the baseline and follow-up survey after the intervention to assess the impact of a public awareness campaign by recording shifts after the intervention period, such as reach and participation, as well as changes in the knowledge, attitudes, beliefs and intended behaviors of the target audience.

2. Materials and Methods

2.1. Development and Implementation of the Public Awareness Campaign

A multi-sectorial group of salt reduction stakeholders formed an advocacy group called Salt Watch, which was launched during the Salt Summit meeting held in Johannesburg, South Africa on 13 March 2014. Salt Watch is led by the HSFSA and endorsed by the South African National Department of Health and was responsible for implementing the Public Awareness Campaign (for more information visit www.heartfoundation.co.za).

The campaign aimed to impact on several of the key processes described in the Theory of Reasoned Action (TRA) [10] to be instrumental in an individual deciding to change their behavior, namely: knowledge, attitudes, beliefs and intentions. In keeping with this theory, a successful salt awareness campaign will therefore require in the first instance an increase in knowledge about the dangers of high salt intake and then show improvements in the population's attitudes to, and beliefs about the need to reduce high salt intake. Changes in these intermediary factors can be reasonably expected to increase the likelihood of an increase in the appropriate behaviors to reduce salt intake in the future.

The public awareness campaign consisted of two aspects. The main activity involved the development of one 30 s television advertisement and two 30 s radio advertisements for the most popular television channels and radio stations that are utilized by the target population. The two radio advertisements were translated into three commonly spoken languages in South Africa (English, isiXhosa and isiZulu) (six in total). The television advertisement was in English with isiXhosa subtitles and in isiZulu with English subtitles (two in total). These were accompanied by sign language in the case of the television advertisements. Thus a total of eight advertisements were developed (six radio and two TV). The advertisements featured a well-known South African medical doctor and media personality who emphasized the message that South Africans are consuming too much salt and that too much salt leads to hypertension, which can cause heart attacks and strokes. The doctor further urged South Africans to reduce their discretionary salt intake and ask their local clinic or doctor for more information. After extensive piloting of the content of the advertisement in the target population, the advertisements ran for a total of six months from 14 August 2014 to 24 May 2015 with an average of 44 television airings and 131 radio airings per month. The advertisements were not aired from beginning of December 2014 to end of February 2015 since this is the summer holiday period in South Africa and fewer listeners and viewers were anticipated.

The second aspect of the public awareness campaign included various supporting activities aimed at strengthening the advertisement message and providing additional information and education materials regarding salt reduction. The Salt Watch website (www.heartfoundation.co.za/), housed a mobile site function that utilized unstructured supplementary service data (USSD) technology that enabled the public to engage with Salt Watch in order to obtain more information and lower-salt recipes. Salt Watch brochures were developed and translated into five different languages for distribution, free of charge, and could be downloaded from the Salt Watch website. Distribution was implemented through various platforms, scientific congresses, symposiums, and brochures were provided upon request from the public or health care practitioners, as well as at free HSFSA public health screenings and HSFSA wellness days. Further awareness activities made use of the HSFSA infrastructure and existing media relationships to engage mass media to carry content provided through media releases ($n = 8$) at regular intervals throughout the campaign. These activities generated broadcast clips ($n = 162$), and yielded print and online articles ($n = 195$). The HSFSA further dedicated their social media platforms to salt reduction messaging and awareness during relevant periods of the campaign, including Facebook, twitter and their monthly newsletter titled Heart Zone. Through a partnership with a local pharmaceutical company, the HSFSA launched a second edition of their recipe book "Cooking from the Heart" which contained 36 reduced-salt recipes, in addition to general healthy eating information. The recipe book ($n = 58,000$ printed), which was only available in English, featured dedicated salt reduction messaging on six of its pages and was mainly distributed free of charge via health care professionals.

Health care professionals (dietitians, nutritionists, general practitioners, physicians, nurses and community health workers) were engaged during the campaign as they were identified as being highly influential stakeholders to provide salt reduction messages during health care interactions with individuals. Information regarding the Salt Watch campaign as well as educational tools and resources (e.g., patient brochures, a "Salt and Health" educational presentation with speaker notes, and a salt information manual) were shared with the identified healthcare professionals through various platforms. These included presentations and/or exhibitions at relevant congresses and meetings, a medical journal editorial [14], continued professional development articles ($n = 2$) for health care professionals and informative e-mails sent by professional associations/societies to their members. Table 1 provides detailed information on the number of individual health care professionals reached.

Table 1. Information regarding the Salt Watch campaign shared with health care professionals.

Type of Information	General Medical Practitioners	Nurses	Dietitians/Nutritionists	Community Health Workers	Totals
Talks	30	30	1250	95	1405
Stand Interactions (Questions filled in)			92		92
Brochures	450		952	50,000	51,402
Emails			1717		1717
Editorials	2180	160,315	400		162,895
CPD			400		400
Total	**2660**	**160,345**	**4811**	**50,095**	**217,911**

CPD: Continuous professional development.

2.2. The Setting and Study Population

Community based surveys were conducted in a cohort of a convenience stratified sample of black women aged 18–55 years. A research agency, MQ (Market Intelligence) Market Intelligence of Cape Town was commissioned to undertake participant recruitment, obtain consent and administer the questionnaire within the participants' homes using experienced fieldworkers. The surveys were conducted in urban areas of three South African provinces: Gauteng (14 suburbs); Eastern Cape (14 suburbs); and KwaZulu-Natal (19 suburbs). The selection of the provinces was informed by the campaign's prime target market. In these provinces, consumers speak mainly isiXhosa or isiZulu. Within each suburb, there were predetermined quotas to ensure optimal representation of the women in the study areas. The number of participants per province was calculated based prorata on the number of people living in that province. Once this was known, the agency used a map to choose the specific towns and suburbs ensuring a wide geographical coverage of the province. The fieldworkers then looked for households that were willing to conduct an interview with them for the baseline as well as the after study. The fieldworkers also ensured that the interviewee has not been interviewed for at least three months and that she fits other recruitment criteria. In order to get a good spread of each of the three provinces the number of interviews was distributed over different areas. For example, not more than 5 households were interviewed in a specific area. The woman selected to be interviewed in each household were black women aged 18–55 years who self-identified as the main purchaser and decision maker of household food and groceries and were classified as meeting the South African Living Standards Measurement (LSM) category of 3–7 [15]. In addition, we also selected English, isiXhosa or isiZulu speaking women. LSM is a marketing segmentation tool developed by the South African Audience Research Foundation that divides the South African population into relatively homogeneous groups according to their ownership of major household appliances and their degree of urbanization using 29 variables as indicators [15]. South Africans 16 years and older are categorized into 10 LSM categories with LSM 10 indicating a high standard of living and wealth and LSM 1 reflecting extreme poverty. The sample was stratified according to Province, age, LSM group, gender, race, language and purchasing and decision making power. We did not control for education, family size, family stage or blood pressure status.

2.3. Data Collection

The data collection was coordinated by the HSFSA. The original English baseline and follow-up survey questionnaires were developed by the research team and translated into the vernacular language of each region. The interview was conducted by a trained interviewer in the home in a one-on-one situation. The data were captured in an English paper version of the questionnaire. The baseline survey included questions on the socio-demographic characteristics of the participants, their knowledge, attitudes, and beliefs as well as past and current behavior in relation to salt intake and its relationship to health. Both open ended and closed questions were included in the survey instrument. Questions were either prompted or unprompted.

A "stages of change" questionnaire based on the theoretical framework of Proshaska and DiClemente [12] was included. Questions related to participants' current interest in engaging with salt reduction behaviors and included the following: "I am not interested in lowering salt in my diet" (pre-contemplation); "I have the intention of doing that within the next six months" (contemplation); "I have the intention of doing that within the next months"(preparation); "I have started lowering my salt intake during the last six months"(action); "I have already lowered my salt intake for longer than six months" (maintenance). The follow-up questionnaire used the same baseline questions and added questions related to the recall of the participant's exposure to the television and radio advertisements, as well as specific questions related to aspects of the intervention program.

Baseline interviews were conducted between the 6 and 12 August 2014 and follow-up interviews between 11 May and the 4 June 2015 by teams of experienced multilingual trained interviewers who lived locally. Interviews were conducted in the language preferred by the respondent, which was predominantly either IsiZulu or IsiXhosa. Back checks were performed for a minimum of 25% of the respondents to verify the interviewing process, as well as the quota requirements for each suburb.

2.4. The Analyses of Data

Quantitative data sets of the baseline and follow-up surveys were computerized and merged. The marginal frequency distributions of the responses in each period were tabulated and compared, using logistic and multinomial regression models and taking into account the dependency of the within participant pre-post responses through a cluster variance specification at this level. Through this setup, all 550 women were included in all the inferential analysis. A logistic regression model for dropout was used to investigate the association of baseline demographic factors for this outcome. For one of the key outcomes, stage of change, the mediation of region, level of education, age group and LSM group was investigated. Region specific results for stage of change are reported as result of this analysis. A p value of ≤ 0.05 is considered a significant change in the categories studied.

A coding frame for the open ended questions was developed after data from 15% of the sample was extracted. The responses were categorized to identify main and sub-categories. These categories were all maintained in 2015. In 2015, we added a number of new codes of answers that were not mentioned in the 2014 study. Some of the open ended questions that related to correct knowledge about the impact of a high salt intake, and questions about the content of the advertisements were pre-coded. The open ended questions were analyzed by hand by trained coders according to the developed coding frame.

3. Results

3.1. Demographics

Five hundred fifty black females participated in the baseline study and 477 of those who participated in the baseline survey were included in the follow-up survey. Seventy-one of the baseline participants (43 from Gauteng province) could not be found or refused to participate and two women's data was excluded as they reported different names to those provided at the baseline survey. The participants from Gauteng province (a highly urbanized area) indicated that they do not have time to complete the questionnaire again or the cell phone number provided was not in operation. This provided a response rate of 86.7%. The majority of the participants were IsiZulu speaking, lived in Gauteng, had 7–12 years of schooling, were in the LSM 5–7 category, and had children younger than six years of age. Nearly 40% of the women reported that they knew their blood pressure status (Table 2).

Table 2. Characteristics of participants in the baseline survey (*n* = 550).

Characteristics	Characteristics	Participants (*n*)	Participants (%)
Age group	18–35 years	276	50.2
	>35–55 years	274	49.8
Province	Gauteng	212	38.6
	KwaZuluNatal	208	37.8
	Eastern Cape	130	23.6
LSM group	LSM 3–4	155	28.2
	LSM 5–7	395	71.8
Education	Less than 7 years schooling	20	3.6
	Seven to 12 years schooling	375	68.2
	Any tertiary education	151	27.5
Family stage	No children	78	14.2
	With children under 6 years	231	42.0
	With children 7–12 years	139	25.3
	With children 13–18 years	71	12.9
	With children older than 18 years	28	5.1
Language	English	2	0.4
	IsiXhosa	138	25.1
	IsiZulu	392	71.3
Blood pressure (BP) status	Person knows their BP value	210	38.2
	Has been informed by a doctor or nurse? that they had high BP	112	20.4
	Currently taking BP medication	62	11.3

3.2. Exposure to the Intervention

During the follow-up survey, over 40% of the participants (*n* = 202) reported having heard, read, or seen any food and/or health related advertisement campaign in the last few months, compared to less than 20% at baseline (*p* < 0.0001), across all age and LSM groups. At baseline, 60.8% of the participants reported that they had seen/heard some sort of salt-related health information. However, the question did not identify specific media activities. In the follow-up survey more than three-quarter (77.8%) of the participants (*n* = 202) reported that they had seen the specific Salt Watch media campaign that included salt-related health information on TV or heard the messages on the radio. Table 3 shows the unprompted recall of the content of the campaign advertisements by those participants who had seen or heard the advertisements (*n* = 202). The most frequently recalled messages were that "too much salt is bad for your health" followed by "you should eat less salt".

Table 3. Unprompted recalls by participants who reported having seen or heard the advertisements of the content of the advertisements during the follow-up survey (*n* = 202).

Open Ended Question Answers	Participants (%) *n* = 202
The food you buy already contains salt	9
Salt was poured on the table (TV image shown) and information given about how much salt we should use each day	15
You should use less salt	17
South Africans eat too much salt every day	24
High blood pressure can cause heart attacks and strokes	25
Too much salt can lead to high blood pressure	28
Too much salt is bad for your health	64

Besides the television and radio advertisements, participants (*n* = 143) also recalled health information on posters at clinics/hospitals (20%), in magazines (7%), by word of mouth (5%), general practitioner/dietitian (2%), and newspaper (1%).

3.3. Changes in the Knowledge, Attitude or Beliefs and Intended Behaviors

The changes in knowledge, attitudes, beliefs and self-reported behaviors are shown in Table 4. Most of the indicators of knowledge, attitudes and behavior change show a significant move towards considering and initiating reduced salt consumption.

Significant increases were found for knowledge items that were related to high salt intake and its health outcomes. All these items mentioned were presented in both the radio and television advertisements. Many of the target population knew before the intervention that high salt intake is a risk for developing hypertension.

In terms of salt behavior, most participants thought that they consumed the right amount of salt both before and after the intervention. However, in general terms, after the intervention, the participants thought that it was important to reduce the amount of salt consumed.

Post intervention, significantly more participants reported that they were taking steps to control their salt intake. In particular, adding salt while cooking and at the table occurred significantly less frequently after the campaign than before.

Table 4. Knowledge, attitude, beliefs and self-reported behavior of participants regarding salt use before and after the campaign.

Questions	Baseline 2014 (n = 550) Participants (%)	Follow-Up 2015 (n = 477) Participants (%)	p
Knowledge			
High salt intake is bad for your health (when directly prompted)	75.5	89.4	≤0.0001
High salt intake is related to suffering strokes (unprompted)	8	50	Not available
Salt intake is related to heart disease (unprompted)	28	59	Not available
High salt intake is related to developing hypertension (unprompted)	75	77	Not available
Attitudes and beliefs			
Consume just the right amount of salt	74.4	71.2	0.609
It is very important to lower the salt in your diet	66.6	74.5	<0.001
Behavior			
Confirmed that they are controlling their salt intake	38.0	59.5	<0.0001
Add salt at the table			
Rarely	22.9	27.1	
Sometimes	22.6	30.3	
Often	11.5	9.6	0.0015 [1]
Always	20.6	15.0	
Add salt when cooking			
Rarely	6.2	11.3	
Sometimes	10.4	25.3	
Often	17.5	20.0	<0.0001 [2]
Always	63.3	40.3	

Not available: Multinomial regression analyses were not done on this unprompted data. [1] A significant change overall, p = 0.0015. A significant shift to lower usage of salt at the table as reflected in increased reporting of "rarely" and "sometimes" in 2015 compared to 2014. [2] A significant change overall, p < 0.0001. A significant shift in using salt in cooking to "rarely", "sometimes" and "often" relative to "always".

Reported salt practices after the campaign indicated significant reductions in the amount of salt used in cooking and at the table, accompanied by a significantly higher use of herbs and spices. No significant changes were found in any of the other prompted salt reduction behaviors (see Table 5).

Table 5. Percentage of respondents before and after the intervention who reported changing their salt consumption behavior on direct questioning.

Salt Consumption Behavior	Baseline 2014 (%) n = 209	Follow-Up 2015 (%) n = 285	p
Avoid/minimize consumption of processed foods	64.2	64.2	0.992
Look at the salt or sodium labels on food	54.2	56.1	0.571
Avoid adding salt at table	14.2	20.1	0.049
Buy low **salt** alternatives	61.0	59.6	0.708
Buy low **sodium** alternatives	52.9	54.7	0.594
Do not add salt when cooking	45.2	59.1	<0.0001
Use herbs or spices other than salt when cooking	70.0	77.8	0.023
Avoid eating out	45.2	45.8	0.594

Figure 1 illustrates the shift in the stages of change in salt consumption for the study. The multinomial logistic regression analyses identified a differential intervention effect (p < 0.0001) between the three regions with Gauteng showing no intervention effect ($p = 0.2405$) in contrast to the other two regions, KwaZulu-Natal and Eastern Cape, where a significant ($p < 0.0001$) shift towards initiation of salt reduction was observed ($p < 0.0001$).

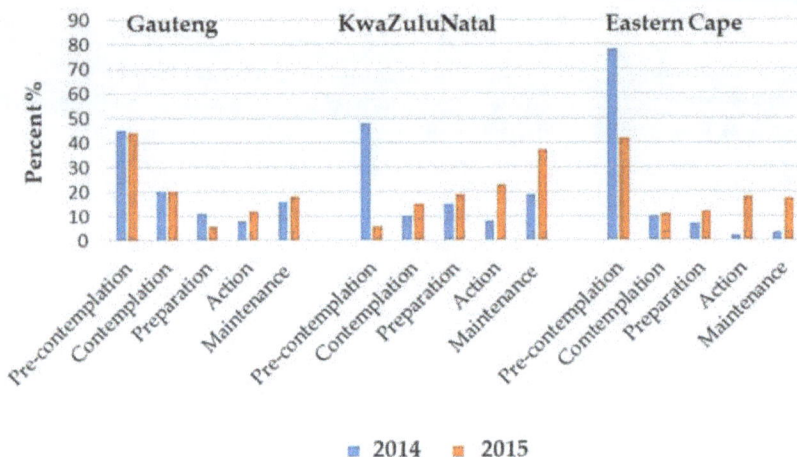

Figure 1. Percentage of participants in the various stages of change of salt consumption before and after the intervention in each region. The stages of change in salt consumption categories: pre-contemplation: no intention to reduce salt intake; contemplation: plans to reduce salt intake in the next 6 months; preparation: plans to reduce salt intake in the next month; action: reduction in salt intake has been initiated; maintenance: reduced salt intake has been maintained for 6 months.

4. Discussion

The evaluation demonstrated the effectiveness of a public health awareness campaign to increase knowledge and awareness of the health consequences of a high salt diet in South African black women of low-middle socioeconomic status. Our data also suggested shifts in salt behaviors in some of the target population. This positive change among black women to considering a reduction in their discretionary salt intake has not previously been achieved in other low and middle income countries through the use of a mass media public health awareness campaign. This is particularly important in this setting as South Africans consume about 40% of their salt from discretionary sources [8]. One of the staple foods in South Africa is homemade maize meal and consumers tend to add soup powder, stock cubes and/or a monosodium glutamate-based flavoring (all are high in salt) for a change in taste. Furthermore, South Africans, being from a low income country, probably eat less processed foods than consumers in high-income countries. This is, however, likely to change. From 1999 to 2012, there has been an increase in the consumption of processed foods and beverages (soft drinks, sauces, dressings and condiments, and sweet and savory snacks), which is typical of an upwardly mobile consumer population [16]. This contrasts with the situation in the United Kingdom where discretionary salt intake provides a minor contribution to overall salt intake (15%) [17].

We showed a significant shift to lower reported usage of salt at the table as reflected in increased reporting of "rarely" and "sometimes" in 2015 compared to 2014. This could be explained by our finding of significant improvement in the salt knowledge of the participants from 2014 to 2015. The improved knowledge reflected the content of the television and radio advertisements. Nearly a third of the participants reportedly had been diagnosed with hypertension, which may explain why there was a relatively high knowledge at baseline that "a high salt intake is bad for your health" (75.5%) and "a high salt intake is related to developing hypertension" (75%).

In this study, 59% of participants at follow-up, on direct questioning, reported not adding salt while cooking. This is much higher than reported in an Australian cross-sectional study where 35.1% of the participants reported this behavior [18] which was similar to reported behavior at baseline in our cohort. In addition, we found a significant shift to lower usage of salt at the table as reflected in increased reporting of "rarely" and "sometimes" in 2015 compared to 2014. This again suggests the positive impact of our awareness campaign. In the United Kingdom, one of the contributing factors to the success of efforts to reduce population-level salt intake [19] through their national salt reduction campaign, is a reduction in the practice of adding salt at the table [20]. The difficulty in showing an association between reported salt-related behavior change and biological outcomes is illustrated by a recent Australian study, which found no evidence of an association between any measure of knowledge, attitudes or behaviors and a single 24-h urinary salt excretion (before or after adjustment for age, gender, body mass index and highest level of education) [21]. In our study, we did not investigate the association between actual salt intake using biomarkers and the categorization of individual stages of change. However, the High-Risk and Population Strategy for Occupational Health Promotion (HIPOP-OHP) Study [22] demonstrated a significant association between stage of change for reported dietary salt intake behavior and spot urinary sodium excretion for both males and non-obese females. In that study, those with in the pre-contemplation stage had a higher salt intake than those classified as being at a later stage of change. The unprompted reporting of the participants of the actual content of the advertisements also strongly suggests that the discretionary salt reduction campaign resulted in a reduced discretionary salt use by the target population. The finding that there was a significant positive shift in participants reporting increasing use of herbs and spices, rather than salt in food preparation, is also very encouraging. These actions to reduce salt intake were not included in the content of the television and radio adverts but only in the additional materials that was made available by Salt Watch. This reflects the increased impact of the use of multimedia in conveying health messages to a study population and suggests that such an approach should be used whenever feasible in population-based health campaigns.

It is encouraging that there were positive shifts in the stages of change categories towards reducing salt intake, at least in two of the three provinces sampled, as this holds promise that the campaign achieved its goals (Figure 1). Possible reasons why Gauteng participants did not demonstrate a significant shift in their stage of change may be related to a greater degree of urbanization compared to the other two provinces, or that these residents may have been more exposed to general salt reduction messages before the beginning of the mass media campaign. A combined analysis using the multinomial logistic regression identified this shift towards initiation of salt reduction to be significant (<0.001) (data not shown).

Furthermore, these increased desirable actions were also confirmed by the significant reported shifts towards less discretionary salt use. The data also illustrates that changes in the initial steps described in the Theory of Reasoned Action of behavior change occurred in our study population; knowledge improved and beliefs and attitudes shifted towards the desired steps that may lead to less salt use in future [10]. In addition, a previous multi-country survey on the stages of change regarding salt reduction in high LSM groups (internet access and email address were inclusion criteria) reported that about 55% of the studied group (in South Africa) of men and women were in the first three stages combined [23]. It thus seems as if the lower LSM groups moved to a similar pattern of the stages of change in 2015 (first three stages combined) as compared to the higher LSM groups in the multi-country study published in 2013. Participants were from Brazil, India, China, Germany/Austria, Hungary and United States of America.

The World Health Organization has clearly identified a 30% salt reduction as one of the essential targets to control NCDs. It has also been identified of one of the "Best Buys" that countries can undertake to achieve reduced NCD burden [24]. The South African government has initiated its salt policy activities by formulating salt reduction regulations [9] and by supporting the Salt Watch led salt awareness campaign. This evaluation of a media campaign and additional supported activities of

Nutrients **2017**, *9*, 1238

Salt Watch indicates that the strategy holds promise to reduce discretionary salt intake in South Africa, particularly if the health promotion components become incorporated as part of an ongoing health promotion campaign for the country.

4.1. Limitations

There are limitations to our study. The study has limited generalizability as the study population included only black women from urban settings from low to middle living standards measures. The follow-up survey was conducted soon after the end of the airing of the advertisements and it cannot be assumed that the impact of the salt reduction messages would be maintained over the longer term. It would have been useful to re-evaluate the participants some months after the population-based intervention was completed to assess how frequently such campaigns would need to be repeated to ensure long term maintenance of the messages. In addition, the same individuals were included in the baseline and follow-up surveys. They could have been prompted to investigate the facts surrounding salt consumption as a direct result of taking part in the study, hence influencing your findings during the follow-up survey.

The respondents in the study were selected as a convenience sample in 47 suburbs of the selected three provinces. Thus although the study has some regional representativeness it is not based on any formal sampling frame. The statistical inference conducted therefore assumes a random sample from the target population. The significance of the results reported is therefore only illustrative under this required assumption.

The same people were interviewed in 2014 and 2015 thus resulting in potential reporter bias because of social desirability as reported in the literature [25]. The lack of a control group is a major limitation to the study design but could not be included because of the population level intervention strategy which necessitated a pre-post quasi experimental study design. It was not possible to use, for example, a neighboring country as a control group since no information is available on the usual eating habits, salt intake or existing salt reduction strategies of neighboring southern African countries.

Theory of Reasoned Action (TRA) [10] suggests that a person's behavior is determined by his/her intention to perform the behavior. This intention is predicted by their knowledge, beliefs and attitudes regarding a specific behavior, and by their beliefs about whether individuals who are important to them approve or do not approve of the behavior (subjective norm). In this paper, we did not interrogate the last aspect of the TRA.

Blood pressure status was not ascertained during the study and the possible association with baseline knowledge could not be adjusted for the analysis.

4.2. Possible Additional Research

Additional research is needed on the stages of salt change. Since the Australian study [21] did not investigate the association between stages of salt change and salt intake as measured by 24-h urine excretion (gold standard method), it would be worthwhile to do so. Collection of 24-h urinary samples in order to measure salt intake is expensive and logistically complex to conduct on a population level. If an association between salt intake (using 24-h urinary samples) and stages of behavior change could be demonstrated, the use of the stages of behavior change could be a less invasive method of evaluating salt intake of a population.

5. Conclusions

The success of a public health campaign that aimed to improve population-level knowledge and attitudes related to discretionary salt use has been demonstrated in black South African women from low income settings. However, the findings should be extrapolated to other groups with care. Significantly more participants reported that they were taking steps to control salt intake following the intervention. In particular, reported behaviors of adding salt to food while cooking, and at the table occurred significantly less frequently. The findings suggest that mass media campaigns may be an effective tool that can make an important contribution to strategies to reduce the consumption of discretionary salt intake among the South African population. Trieu and colleagues [25] in a recent review concluded that education or awareness campaigns alone are unlikely to be adequate to achieve the WHO target of a 30% reduction in average salt intake. We agree that multi-pronged strategies using multiple channels of communication need to accompany the salt reduction regulations of certain foods stuffs.

Acknowledgments: Funding for the development and implementation of the public awareness campaign and the research were received from the Heart and Stroke Foundation South Africa, the South African National Department of Health, Directorate: Non-communicable diseases and the Centre of Nutrition for Excellence, North-West University, South Africa. No funds were received for covering the costs to publish in open access journal.

Author Contributions: E.W.-V. and K.S. substantially contributed to the conception and design, analysis and interpretation of the data and wrote the manuscript. K.C., A.D.V. and C.C. contributed to the design, analysis and interpretation of the data and critically revised the manuscript for important intellectual content. C.L. was responsible for the statistical analysis of the data. S.F. contributed to the design of the questionnaires, was responsible for the collection of the data, analysis of the data and critically revised the manuscript for important intellectual content. V.M.-S. and C.C. was responsible for the development and implementation of the intervention and critically revised the manuscript for important intellectual content.

Conflicts of Interest: The authors declare no conflict of interest. South African National Department of Health, Directorate: Non-communicable diseases had no role in the design of the study; in the collection, analyses, or interpretation of data; in the writing of the manuscript, and in the decision to publish the results.

References

1. World Health Organization. *Global Action Plan for the Prevention and Control of Noncommunicable Diseases 2013–2020*; WHO: Geneva, Switzerland, 2013. Available online: http://www.who.int/nmh/publications/ncd-action-plan/en/ (accessed on 1 August 2014).

2. Pillay-van Wyk, V.; Msemburi, W.; Laubscher, R.; Dorrington, R.E.; Groenewald, P.; Matzopoulos, R. Second national burden of disease study South Africa: national and subnational mortality trends, 1997–2009. *Lancet* **2013**, *381*. [CrossRef]

3. Maredza, M.; Bertram, M.Y.; Gómez-Olivé, X.F.; Tollman, S.M. Burden of stroke attributable to selected lifestyle risk factors in rural South Africa. *BMC Public Health* **2016**, *16*, 1–11. [CrossRef] [PubMed]

4. South African National Department of Health. *Strategic Plan for the Prevention and Control of Non-Communicable Diseases 2013–2017*; Department of Health: Pretoria, South Africa, 2013.

5. Wentzel-Viljoen, E.; Steyn, K.; Ketterer, E.; Charlton, K. Use salt and foods high in salt sparingly: A food-based dietary guideline for South Africa. *SA J. Clin. Nutr.* **2013**, *26*, S105–S113.

6. Swanepoel, B.; Schutte, A.E.; Cockeran, M.; Steyn, K.; Wentzel-Viljoen, E. Sodium and potassium intake in South Africa: An evaluation of 24-hour urine collections in a white, black, and Indian population. *J. Am. Soc. Hypertens.* **2016**, *10*, 829–837. [CrossRef] [PubMed]

7. Oyebode, O.; Oti, S.; Chen, Y.-F.; Lilford, R.J. Salt intakes in sub-Saharan Africa: A systematic review and meta-regression. *Popul. Health Metr.* **2016**, *14*, 1. [CrossRef] [PubMed]

8. Charlton, K.E.; Steyn, K.; Levitt, N.S.; Zulu, J.V.; Jonathan, D.; Veldman, F.J.; Nel, J.H. Diet and blood pressure in South Africa: Intake of foods containing sodium, potassium, calcium, and magnesium in three ethnic groups. *Nutrition* **2005**, *21*, 39–50. [CrossRef] [PubMed]

9. South African Department of Health. Foodstuffs, Cosmetics and Disinfectants ACT, 1972 (ACT No. 54 of 1972). Regulations Relating to the Reduction of Sodium in Certain Foodstuffs and Related Matters. Republic of South Africa. Government Gazette, 20 March 2013. Available online: http://www.heartfoundation.co.za/sites/default/files/articles/South%20Africa%20salt%20legislation.pdf (accessed on 16 April 2015).

10. Fishbein, M.; Yzer, M.C. Using theory to design effective health behavior interventions. *Commun. Theory* **2003**, *13*, 164–183. [CrossRef]

11. Painter, J.E.; Borba, C.P.; Hynes, M.; Mays, D.; Glanz, K. The use of theory in health behavior research from 2000 to 2005: A systematic review. *Ann. Behav. Med.* **2008**, *35*, 358–362. [CrossRef] [PubMed]

12. Prochaska, J.O.; DiClemente, C.C. Transtheoretical therapy: Toward a more integrative model of change. *Psychother. Theory Res. Pract.* **1982**, *19*, 276. [CrossRef]

13. Prochaska, J.O.; Velicer, W.F. The transtheoretical model of health behavior change. *Am. J. Health Promot.* **1997**, *12*, 38–48. [CrossRef] [PubMed]

14. Eksteen, G.; Mungal-Singh, V. Salt intake in South Africa: A current perspective. *J. Endocrinol. Metab. Diabetes S. Afr.* **2015**, *20*, 9–14. [CrossRef]

15. Haupt, P. The SAARF Universal Living Standards Measure (SU-LSM™) 12 Years of Continuous Development. Available online: http://www.saarf.co.za/LSM/lsm-article.asp (accessed on 3 March 2014).

16. Ronquest-Ross, L.-C.; Vink, N.; Sigge, G.O. Food consumption changes in South Africa since 1994. *S. Afr. J. Sci.* **2015**, *111*, 1–12. [CrossRef]

17. He, F.; MacGregor, G. A comprehensive review on salt and health and current experience of worldwide salt reduction programmes. *J. Hum. Hypertens.* **2009**, *23*, 363–384. [CrossRef] [PubMed]

18. Sarmugam, R.; Worsley, A.; Wang, W. An examination of the mediating role of salt knowledge and beliefs on the relationship between socio-demographic factors and discretionary salt use: A cross-sectional study. *Int. J. Behav. Nutr. Phys. Act.* **2013**, *10*, 25–33. [CrossRef] [PubMed]

19. Sadler, K.; Nicholson, S.; Steer, T.; Gill, V.; Bates, B.; Tipping, S.; Cox, L.; Lennox, A.; Prentice, A. *National Diet and Nutrition Survey: Assessment of Dietary Sodium in Adults (Aged 19 to 64 Years) in England, 2011*; Public Health England: London, UK, 2012.

20. Sutherland, J.; Edwards, P.; Shankar, B.; Dangour, A.D. Fewer adults add salt at the table after initiation of a national salt campaign in the UK: A repeated cross-sectional analysis. *Br. J. Nutr.* **2013**, *110*, 552–558. [CrossRef] [PubMed]

21. Land, M.; Webster, J.; Christoforou, A.; Johnson, C.; Trevena, H.; Hodgins, F.; Chalmers, J.; Woodward, M.; Barzi, F.; Smith, W. The Association of Knowledge, Attitudes and Behaviours Related to Salt with 24-hour Urinary Sodium Excretion. *Int. J. Behav. Nutr. Phys. Act.* **2014**, *11*, 47–55. [CrossRef] [PubMed]

22. Tamaki, J.; Kikuchi, Y.; Yoshita, K.; Takebayashi, T.; Chiba, N.; Tanaka, T.; Okamura, T.; Kasagi, F.; Minai, J.; Ueshima, H. Stages of change for salt intake and urinary salt excretion: Baseline results from the High-Risk and Population Strategy for Occupational Health Promotion (HIPOP-OHP) study. *Hypertens. Res.* **2004**, *27*, 157–166. [CrossRef]

23. Newson, R.; Elmadfa, I.; Biro, G.; Cheng, Y.; Prakash, V.; Rust, P.; Barna, M.; Lion, R.; Meijer, G.; Neufingerl, N. Barriers for progress in salt reduction in the general population. An international study. *Appetite* **2013**, *71*, 22–31. [CrossRef] [PubMed]

24. World Health Organization. *Scaling Up Action against Noncommunicable Diseases: How Much Will It Cost?*; WHO: Geneva, Switzerland, 2011. Available online: http://www.who.int/nmh/publications/cost_of_inaction/en/ (accessed on 12 April 2016).

25. Trieu, K.; McMahon, E.; Santos, J.A.; Bauman, A.; Jolly, K.-A.; Bolam, B.; Webster, J. Review of behaviour change interventions to reduce population salt intake. *Int. J. Behav. Nutr. Phys. Act.* **2017**, *14*, 17. [CrossRef] [PubMed]

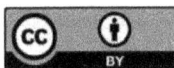

nutrients

MDPI

Article

Assessment of a Salt Reduction Intervention on Adult Population Salt Intake in Fiji

Arti Pillay [1], Kathy Trieu [2,7], Joseph Alvin Santos [2,7], Arleen Sukhu [1], Jimaima Schultz [3], Jillian Wate [1], Colin Bell [4], Marj Moodie [4,5], Wendy Snowdon [4], Gary Ma [6], Kris Rogers [2] and Jacqui Webster [2,7,*]

[1] Pacific Research Centre for the Prevention of Obesity and Noncommunicable Diseases (C-POND), Fiji National University, Nasinu, Suva, Fiji; arti.pillay@fnu.ac.fj (A.P.); arleen.sukhu@fnu.ac.fj (A.S.); jillian.wate@fnu.ac.fj (J.W.)
[2] The George Institute for Global Health, University of New South Wales, Sydney NSW 2052, Australia; ktrieu@georgeinstitute.org.au (K.T.); jsantos@georgeinstitute.org.au (J.A.S.); krogers@georgeinstitute.org (K.R.)
[3] Independent Nutrition Consultant, Suva, Fiji; jimaima63@gmail.com
[4] Global Obesity Centre, Deakin University, Geelong VIC 3220, Australia; colin.bell@deakin.edu.au (C.B.); marj.moodie@deakin.edu.au (M.M.); wendy.snowdon@deakin.edu.au (W.S.)
[5] Deakin Health Economics, Centre for Population Health Research, Faculty of Health, Deakin University, Burwood VIC 3125, Australia
[6] School of Medicine, University of Western Sydney, Campbell town, Sydney 2560, Australia; G.Ma@westernsydney.edu.au
[7] School of Public Health, University of Sydney, Sydney 2006, Australia
* Correspondence: jwebster@georgeinstitute.org.au; Tel.: +61-2-8052-4520

Received: 6 October 2017; Accepted: 7 December 2017; Published: 12 December 2017

Abstract: Reducing population salt intake is a global public health priority due to the potential to save lives and reduce the burden on the healthcare system through decreased blood pressure. This implementation science research project set out to measure salt consumption patterns and to assess the impact of a complex, multi-faceted intervention to reduce population salt intake in Fiji between 2012 and 2016. The intervention combined initiatives to engage food businesses to reduce salt in foods and meals with targeted consumer behavior change programs. There were 169 participants at baseline (response rate 28.2%) and 272 at 20 months (response rate 22.4%). The mean salt intake from 24-h urine samples was estimated to be 11.7 grams per day (g/d) at baseline and 10.3 g/d after 20 months (difference: -1.4 g/day, 95% CI -3.1 to 0.3, $p = 0.115$). Sub-analysis showed a statistically significant reduction in female salt intake in the Central Division but no differential impact in relation to age or ethnicity. Whilst the low response rate means it is not possible to draw firm conclusions about these changes, the population salt intake in Fiji, at 10.3 g/day, is still twice the World Health Organization's (WHO) recommended maximum intake. This project also assessed iodine intake levels in women of child-bearing age and found that they were within recommended guidelines. Existing policies and programs to reduce salt intake and prevent iodine deficiency need to be maintained or strengthened. Monitoring to assess changes in salt intake and to ensure that iodine levels remain adequate should be built into future surveys.

Keywords: population sodium intake; salt reduction; nutrition intervention; Pacific Islands; behavior change; health policy; salt targets; blood pressure; hypertension

1. Introduction

Increased blood pressure (BP) is associated with increased risk of heart diseases and stroke. Increased dietary salt intake is associated with increased BP [1]. The World Health Organization

(WHO) recommends a salt intake of less than 5 grams per day [2]. Reducing salt intake to less than 5 grams per day in adults has shown to reduce systolic blood pressure by 3.47 mmHg (0.76 to 6.20) and diastolic blood pressure by 1.81 mmHg (0.54 to 3.08) [3].

In Fiji, noncommunicable diseases (NCD) were the top ten causes of mortality in 2015 [4], with ischaemic heart diseases and hypertensive diseases accounting for 16.6% and 4.6% of proportionate mortality, respectively [4]. The 2011 WHO STEPwise approach to surveillance of noncommunicable disease risk factors (STEPS) survey showed an increase from 2002 in the prevalence of high blood pressure (systolic blood pressure (SBP) $\geq$ 140 and/or diastolic blood pressure (DBP) $\geq$ 90 mmHg or currently on medication for raised BP) from 24.2% to 31% [5]. While there are other contributors to high blood pressure, a shift in diet patterns has also been observed over time, showing more reliance on processed and imported food products [6], which tend to be higher in salt [7].

Monitoring and lowering population salt intake have been identified as important steps towards reducing the burden of NCDs [8]. In Fiji, available information for salt intake was based on 24-h recall data from the 2004 National Nutrition Survey (NNS). The estimated overall mean salt intake was 3.86 grams, which was widely understood to be an underestimation [9]. Mean data on salt intake based on 24-h urine samples was previously unavailable, which meant that targeting interventions towards specific groups and monitoring salt intakes over time was difficult. Major sources of salt in the Fijian diet, identified by the 2004 NNS 24-h recall data, were iodized table salt (27.1%), bread (17.4%), roti (14.5%), fish and seafood, including canned fish (12.1%), and meat, including canned meat (7.0%) [9]. The use of salt and salty condiments is also common in households for food preparation.

The aim of this study was to evaluate the impact of an intervention to reduce population salt intake in Fiji based on changes in mean salt intake measured through 24-h urine samples. Salt has been used as a vehicle for fortification of iodine in Fiji since 1996, in order to address iodine deficiency amongst pregnant women and school children [10]. Thus, iodine levels were also measured in this study to ensure that interventions on salt reduction did not affect iodine interventions.

The project was part of the Global Alliance for Chronic Diseases Hypertension research program.

2. Materials and Methods

The study took place between 2012 and 2016 in Fiji, an upper-middle income Melanesian island country in the South Pacific Ocean, north of New Zealand. Fiji has a total population of 837,271 [11], and is divided into four major jurisdictions: Central, Eastern, Western and Northern. Currently, 87% of the population live on the two major islands—with just under half of the population living in urban areas and just over half in rural areas, but with more rapid rates of population increase in urban areas. The Fiji population is categorized as iTaukei (natives of the country), Fijians of Indian descent (FID) and Fijians of Other descent (FOD) (Chinese, Pacific Islanders, Europeans, and all other nationalities) [11]. For the purposes of this study, we compared iTaukei with all other Fijians.

The study comprised three phases: (1) a nationally representative survey to measure baseline population salt consumption patterns, (2) the implementation of a multi-faceted salt reduction intervention and; (3) a survey after 20 months, to assess any changes in salt intake resulting from the intervention to date. A detailed methodology was published in the protocol [12]. Ethical Approval for the survey was granted by the University of Sydney, Human Research Ethics Council (15,359), Deakin University (2013-020), and the Fiji National Research Ethics and Review Committee (FNRERC 201307).

2.1. The Intervention

Between the baseline and 20-month surveys, a multi-sectorial and multi-faceted intervention targeted towards (i) food manufacturers and retailers (ii) caterers and bakers, and (iii) consumers through health workers, media and community leaders, was undertaken by the study team at the Pacific Research Centre for the Prevention of Obesity and Noncommunicable Diseases (C-POND), in collaboration with the Ministry of Health and Medical Services (MoHMS) and the National Food and Nutrition Centre (NFNC). Based on similar programs in other countries [13], and informed by the baseline monitoring of salt consumption and behaviors, the intervention aimed to increase awareness of the link between salt and health, to reduce the use of discretionary salt, and to reduce salt in the food supply through product reformulations (See Table 1). Prior to this study, salt intervention activities were implemented by the MoHMS, and voluntary salt targets for a range of food categories had been agreed by the food industry [14].

Table 1. Intervention activities.

Strategy and Goal	Actions
Strategic health communication Goal: To increase consumer awareness on salt and health	Train and engage health educators including health workers, government workers, faith-based and voluntary organizations to disseminate messages on salt and health Distribution of information materials to consumers through nurses and dietitians in 21 districts Public awareness campaign on television, radio, websites, billboards "Kick the salt, lower you blood pressure". Dissemination of communication materials: pamphlets, posters, booklets and salt message DVDs.
Industry engagement Goal: To reduce sodium content in processed foods through reformulation and improve the food environment	Engage food manufacturers to lower the salt content of foods towards the Fiji salt targets for different food categories. Engage food retailers to import reduced salt products and lower salt alternatives for similar brands of products. Engage restaurants, bakeries and catering facilities through training Environmental Health Officers, caterers and canteen managers on salt reduction and providing Information Education Communication (IEC) materials for dissemination. Incorporate the removal of salt shakers from tables as part of the Ministry of Health and Medical Services (MoHMS) restaurant grading scheme.
Salt reduction in the main Fiji hospital Goal: To educate and improve the food supply for hospital patients and staff	Educate hospital staff on salt and health. Educate food service staff in the preparation of low salt meals Improve the food environment in hospitals through removing the salt shakers from tables and lowering the sodium content of hospital meals Educate patients and their relatives on salt and health

2.2. Participant Recruitment

Both surveys used a multi-stage cluster sampling approach to select samples representative of the adult population in Fiji. The baseline survey used the sampling frame from the WHO STEPS survey conducted in 2011. The 20-month survey used the 2014 National Nutrition Survey as the sampling frame. In both surveys, Enumeration areas (EAs) were selected through probability proportional to sampling size. Households were then randomly selected from each EA and within each household; one individual was randomly selected without replacement using the KISH method [15]. At baseline, a subsample of 600 individuals aged 25–64 years, from the total sample of 2515, was selected to participate in the salt sub-study. Based on the 40% response rate during the baseline survey, a sample of 1215 was estimated for the 20-month survey. This was to provide 80% power with an alpha of 0.05, to detect a 10% difference in salt intake from the baseline.

2.3. Data Collection

The objective of the surveys was to collect information on demographics and salt intake through urine samples. Data collection took place from August 2012 to the end of December 2013 at baseline, and from November 2015 to end of August 2016 at 20 months. Data collection was carried out by 60 trained Public Health nurses from their respective divisions during baseline and 8 trained research assistants carried out the survey at 20 months. The training covered recruitment, data collection, data storage and record keeping procedures. A refresher training post-cyclone Winston was conducted for the 20-month survey.

Participants were contacted via telephone and through home visits. Once the participants were recruited, and their written informed consent was obtained, they were provided with a 2.5-litre container for a 24-h urine collection, with verbal and written instructions for the collection. Participants were instructed to start the 24-h urine collection on a new day, to exclude the first urine of the day and to start the collection from the second urine till the first urine of the second day. The date, start and finish times were recorded on the bottles.

Demographic data and physical measurements (height to the nearest 0.1 cm and weight to the nearest 0.01 kg for calculating body mass index (BMI), and BP from three readings for determining blood pressure) were collected according to the WHO STEPS surveillance protocol [15], as part of the first visit. Appointments for a second visit were made to collect the 24-h urine samples. When all of the information had been collected, participants were presented with a $FJ20.00 supermarket voucher in appreciation for their participation. Urine sample volumes were measured, aliquots of 100 mL were extracted, labeled and sent to the Vanua Medical Lab where they were stored at less than 20 °C until they could be analyzed.

At 20 months, an additional spot urine aliquot for all non-pregnant females of child-bearing age between 25–45 years was sent to Westmead Hospital in Sydney for an analysis of iodine concentration.

2.4. Data Analysis

Analysis of the sodium and creatinine concentrations was undertaken at baseline and 20 months, with additional analysis for iodine and potassium at 20 months. Creatinine per day (mmol) was used as a marker for completion of the 24-h collection. For both baseline and the 20-month surveys, incomplete collections less than 500 mL total urine volume for both sexes, and creatinine of less than 4.0 mmol/day for women and less than 6.0 mmol/day for men were excluded [16].

Baseline and 20-month survey data were weighted by age, sex, and ethnicity (a total of 8 groups for each time point) based on the distribution of the 2007 Fiji Census. All analyses were done using the *svy command* in STATA/IC 13.1 for Windows (StataCorp LP, College Station, TX, 77845, USA), taking into account the survey design, cluster effect (EA), strata effect (division), and finite population correction factor (395,464), using the Taylor linearization approach for variance estimation [17].

3. Results

3.1. Response Rate

At baseline, of the 600 invited participants, 241 (40%) urine samples were obtained and at 20 months, of the 1215 invited participants, 497 (41%) urine samples were obtained. At baseline, 14 participants were excluded due to missing urine volumes and seven for missing demographic information. At 20 months, 58 participants were excluded for missing urine volumes and one for missing sex information. Furthermore, 51 and 166 were excluded from the analysis for suspected incomplete 24-h urine collection, leaving a total of 169 at baseline, and 272 participants at 20 months (28.2% and 22.4% participation rates).

3.2. Population Characteristics

Participant characteristics for both baseline and 20-month survey participants are summarized in Table 2. The mean age of the sample was 42 years for both surveys, with an almost even distribution of sex and ethnicity. For both baseline and 20-month surveys, the majority of the participants (about 80%) were from the Central and Western Divisions. About 40% were educated to primary and secondary level, while only a small proportion had no formal schooling. Aside from DBP, there were no significant differences in characteristics between baseline and 20-month survey participants ($p > 0.05$).

Table 2. Characteristics of participants surveyed at baseline and after 20 months.

Characteristics	Unweighted			Weighted (Age, Sex, Ethnicity)			2007 Fiji Census Data ($n = 395,464$)
	Baseline ($n = 169$)	20 months ($n = 272$)	*p*-value	Baseline	20 months	*p*-value	
Age, years (mean, SE)	46.7 (0.8)	44.1 (0.6)	0.013	42.6 (0.9)	42.4 (0.6)	0.890	
Age group (%)							
25–44 years	42.0	53.7	0.017	63.2	63.2	1.000	63.2
45–64 years	58.0	46.3		36.8	36.8		36.8
Female (%)	55.6	53.7	0.690	49.1	49.1	1.000	49.1
Ethnicity (%)							
iTaukei	50.3	57.0	0.170	52.5	52.5	1.000	52.5
FID and FOD	49.7	43.0		47.5	47.5		47.5
Division (%)							
Central	42.0	40.8	0.142	42.6	40.6	0.846	40.4
Eastern [a]	1.8	6.6		1.7	5.7		4.2
Northern	20.9	17.3		17.2	20.2		15.9
Western	37.3	35.3		38.6	35.4		39.5
Education (%)							
No formal schooling	0.0	3.0	0.014	0.0	2.4	0.299	
Primary school level	52.7	40.3		46.1	38.7		
Secondary school level	35.3	39.9		39.8	41.1		
Tertiary school level and post-graduate	12.0	16.8		14.1	17.9		
Height, cm (mean, SE)	166.4 (0.7)	167.4 (0.6)	0.310	167.9 (1.1)	167.8 (0.9)	0.924	
Weight, kg (mean, SE)	78.9 (1.5)	82.8 (1.2)	0.046	79.8 (2.1)	82.4 (1.4)	0.321	
Body Mass Index, kg/m² (mean, SE)	28.4 (0.5)	29.5 (0.4)	0.072	28.2 (0.6)	29.2 (0.4)	0.199	
SBP, mmHg (mean, SE)	132.9 (1.7)	133.1 (1.2)	0.906	129.1 (1.5)	131.5 (1.3)	0.203	
DBP, mmHg (mean, SE)	82.1 (0.9)	83.4 (0.8)	0.281	80.3 (0.8)	82.8 (0.9)	0.037	
History of hypertension (%)	28.1	27.9	0.976	21.7	25.2	0.497	
Urinary volume, mL (mean, SE)	1764.3 (52.6)	1639.7 (46.0)	0.082	1788.2 (63.2)	1650.9 (61.3)	0.130	
Creatinine, mmol (mean, SE)	9.9 (0.4)	10.6 (0.3)	0.165	10.0 (0.5)	10.6 (0.3)	0.352	

FID: Fijians of Indian descent; FOD: Fijians of Other descent. [a] Sample size from the Eastern Division was small at both surveys ($n = 3$ at baseline; $n = 18$ at 20 months).

3.3. Changes in Salt Intake

The weighted mean population salt intake was 11.7 g/day (standard error (SE) 0.7) at baseline and 10.3 g/day (SE 0.5) after 20 months, but the difference was not statistically significant (-1.4 g/day, 95% confidence interval (CI) -3.1 to 0.3, $p = 0.115$). The proportion with salt intake above the WHO maximum target of 5 g/day was 86.4% and 78.2% at baseline and 20 months respectively (Table 3).

Table 3. Changes in estimated mean Fiji population salt intake (after weighting age, sex, and ethnicity).

Salt intake, g/day (mean, SE)	Baseline ($n = 169$)	20 Months ($n = 272$)	Change (95% CI)
Overall	11.7 (0.7)	10.3 (0.5)	-1.4 (-3.1 to 0.3); $p = 0.115$
Males	13.6 (1.2)	11.3 (0.7)	-2.3 (-5.0 to 0.4); $p = 0.099$
Females	9.7 (0.7)	9.2 (0.6)	-0.5 (-2.3 to 1.3); $p = 0.611$
Salt intake above the WHO 5 g target (%)	86.4	78.2	-8.2; $p = 0.083$

3.4. Subgroup Analysis Disaggregated by Gender

There was a significant reduction in salt intake among females in the Central Division from baseline to follow-up (-3.34 g/day, 95% CI -6.07 to -0.61; $p = 0.017$). In the other divisions combined, female salt intake increased although this was not statistically significant (1.23 g/day). Further analysis (i.e., difference-in-differences) showed that there was a differential effect between females in the Central Division compared to other divisions (-4.57 g/day, 95% CI -7.92 to -1.21; $p = 0.008$). There was no differential effect by division for males (0.71 g/day, 95% CI -4.64 to 6.06; $p = 0.792$). There was also no differential effect by ethnicity or age for both sexes (Table 4).

Table 4. Changes in salt intake disaggregated by gender (mean, SE) by division, ethnicity and age.

		Baseline (n = 169)	20 Months (n = 272)	Difference (95% CI, p-value)
By division				
Central	Male	13.20 (1.27)	11.28 (0.96)	−1.92 (−5.08 to 1.23); $p = 0.230$
	Female	12.41 (0.83)	9.07 (1.10)	−3.34 (−6.07 to −0.61); $p = 0.017$
Other division	Male	13.92 (2.02)	11.29 (0.92)	−2.63 (−6.95 to 1.69); $p = 0.229$
	Female	8.15 (0.71)	9.38 (0.71)	1.23 (−0.72 to 3.18); $p = 0.213$
By ethnicity				
iTaukei	Male	12.62 (1.13)	11.04 (0.96)	−1.58 (−4.51 to 1.34); $p = 0.286$
	Female	9.49 (1.00)	8.15 (0.58)	−1.34 (−3.61 to 0.91); $p = 0.240$
FID and FOD	Male	14.61 (2.05)	11.56 (0.84)	−3.05 (−7.43 to 1.32); $p = 0.169$
	Female	9.96 (0.75)	10.49 (1.06)	0.53 (−2.05 to 3.11); $p = 0.683$
By age Group				
25–44 years	Male	14.01 (1.63)	10.68 (0.87)	−3.32 (−6.97 to 0.33); $p = 0.074$
	Female	9.81 (0.81)	8.90 (0.66)	−0.91 (−2.93 to 1.11); $p = 0.375$
45–64 years	Male	12.82 (1.14)	12.33 (0.96)	−0.50 (−3.44 to 2.45); $p = 0.739$
	Female	9.55 (0.86)	9.84 (0.94)	0.29 (−2.22 to 2.81); $p = 0.817$

FID: Fijians of Indian descent; FOD: Fijian of Others descent.

3.5. Comparison of Results of Those Affected and Not Affected by the Cyclone for Participants at 20 Months

Data collection in Central Division participants was completed prior to Tropical Cyclone Winston. In the regions that were affected by the cyclone, data collection was delayed for 3 months which allowed diets to return to normal. In total, 105 of the 272 participants with usable urine samples at 20 months were recruited from the affected regions, and their mean salt intake was considerably higher compared to those surveyed prior to the cyclone (Table 5).

Table 5. Differences in salt intakes of people surveyed before and after the cyclone.

	Total (n = 272)	Affected by Cyclone (n = 105)	Not Affected by Cyclone (n = 167)	Difference (95% CI)
Salt intake, g/d (mean, SE)	10.3 (0.5)	12.0 (0.7)	9.2 (0.6)	2.8 (1.0–4.6)

3.6. Potassium and Iodine Intakes

At 20 months, mean potassium intake was 79.9 mmol/day (SE 5.0) (sodium-to-potassium ratio was 2.6 (0.1)) which is below the WHO guideline of at least 90 mmol/day for adults.

A total of 131 useable spot urine samples were collected from non-pregnant women of child-bearing age surveyed at 20 months (11% of original sample). Mean urinary iodine (UI) concentration was found to be 207 µg/L which meets the recommendations for women. However, the proportion of the sample with UI concentration less than 50 µg/L was 4.6% and the proportion of the sample with UI concentration less than 100 µg/L was 19.1%.

4. Discussion

This study aimed to assess the impact of a national population-wide salt reduction intervention in Fiji and highlights the need for strengthened interventions. We found that population salt intakes were high, using a 24-h urine analysis. However, we were unable to demonstrate any statistically significant reduction in population salt intake, as a result of the intervention to date. The lack of a significant effect was potentially due to the low response rate, as the sample sizes were possibly too small to detect any changes. The low response rate could also have resulted in a sampling bias which could also affect the results. The limited intervention dose, based on trying to target the whole population spread out over different islands in a relatively short timescale, might also explain the lack of impact. Whilst it is not possible to draw firm conclusions in relation to the impact on salt intake, we observed some improvements in knowledge and salt-related behaviors, suggesting that the communication campaign was starting to have an impact. These findings are being explored further in a subsequent paper.

The data does show a statistically significant reduction in salt intake for females in the Central Division, which is interesting to consider. However, the small sample sizes again mean that it is difficult to draw firm conclusions. Female salt intake was much higher at baseline in the Central Division (12.41g/day (0.83)) than in the other divisions (8.15g/day (0.71)). This could potentially be explained by the fact that there are more urban areas in the Central Division, so females are more likely to be working and have access to a greater range of processed foods and places to eat out. The higher baseline for female salt intake would make it easier to achieve a reduction. The intervention may also have been more intense in the Central Division due to its proximity to the capital city Suva, which is where the project staff and government organizations involved in the interventions are based. This data highlights the importance of disaggregating results in relation to sex, in view of the fact that females tend to have a different salt intake to males, and in order to understand any differential impact of the interventions.

The potential impact of Cyclone Winston in relation to any differential impact on the regions also needs to be considered. In contrast to other regions, the monitoring in the Central Division took place before Cyclone Winston which struck Fiji in February 2016. This means that the Central Division was the only area where people had not been provided with food rations for any period prior to the survey. Rations distributed after Cyclone Winston comprised of rice and milk, plus canned fish, canned meat, instant noodles and biscuits, most of which are contributors to dietary salt [18]. Despite the research team allowing several months after the cyclone before resuming the survey, so that people could resume their normal routines, mean salt intake amongst those surveyed after the cyclone was found to be significantly higher, 12 g/day (SE 0.7), than those surveyed before the cyclone, 9.2 g/day (SE 0.6) $p = 0.003$. Whilst it is not possible to be certain due to the small sample size, an examination of differences between the regions at baseline showed that there were no similar disparities, while the regional sub-analysis of changes in salt intake showed that there was a significant reduction in the Central Division which was not observed in the other divisions, suggesting that the cyclone may have impacted diets.

Population salt intake, measured at baseline and at 20 months, was similar to global mean estimates of population salt intake [19]. The high salt intake in Fiji could be attributed to the shift in diet patterns that has been observed over time with more reliance on processed and imported food products [6]. The link between increased salt intake and increased blood pressure, leading to cardiovascular diseases [20,21] strokes [22], and kidney diseases [23], is well established. The 2011 WHO STEPS survey showed that there had already been an increase in the prevalence of high blood pressure (SBP $\geq$ 140 and/or DBP $\geq$ 90 mmHg or people currently on medication for raised BP) from 24.2% in 2002 to 31% in 2011 [5]. There is strong evidence that reducing salt intake will reduce blood pressure, which in turn is associated with reduced risk of stroke and fatal coronary disease in adults [3].

The multi-sector, complex population-wide intervention, combining voluntary government agreements with the food industry with community mobilization and awareness in Fiji was challenging to implement effectively in the short timescale. It is unlikely that the voluntary agreements with industry were translated into significant changes in the levels of salt in the overall food supply during the intervention period. Also, limited financial and human resources mean that the reach of the communication activities may have been limited. Detailed information on different aspects of the intervention and its cost is being compiled in a separate paper focusing on the process evaluation and cost of this study. The intervention was broadly similar to the United Kingdom's (UK) salt reduction strategy. The UK successfully demonstrated a 15% reduction in the average population salt intake during a 7-year period [16] with parallel reductions in people suffering from strokes, heart attacks, and heart failures during the same time period [16]. Multiple other countries have also effectively reduced population salt intake through similar multi-faceted interventions [24]. While this implementation science study in Fiji was unable to demonstrate a reduction in salt intake after 20 months, evidence from the UK and other countries suggests that the intervention strategies are worthwhile and should continue [24]. Adherence to agreements to reduce salt in foods by the food industry requires effective industry engagement and transparent monitoring [25,26]. Further sustained efforts will be required in Fiji, to ensure that the voluntary sodium targets that were set and accepted by the industry are adhered to in the next few years. Challenges such as costs for re-formulation and lack of control on imported products of similar categories have been highlighted as reasons for slow progress by food industries in Fiji, yet multiple other countries have overcome such challenges, demonstrating feasibility [26].

In a parallel study in Samoa, population salt intake was 7.09 g (SE 0.09) [27] which is lower than Fiji yet still higher than WHO recommendations for salt intake. Whilst there has yet to be a reduction in salt intake in Samoa [28], the Samoan Ministry of Health has integrated the regional salt targets [7] into its draft food regulations as part of a comprehensive salt reduction strategy. This is in line with growing evidence from modelling which suggests that regulated targets are more cost-effective than voluntary targets [28]. Whilst regulatory approaches need to be supplemented with behavior change interventions [29], there is increasing evidence showing that education alone is not sufficient to reduce salt intake to the recommended levels [29], especially when the majority of salt is added to foods before it is sold [30]. Whilst implementing effective policy changes might pose challenges for low and middle-income countries (LMICs) due to limited expertise and resources, there is evidence that programs can be effective [31], and reductions in salt intake have been associated with substantial cost savings [28]. Cost saving has been estimated for reduction of salt intake of 15% in LMICs with 13.8 million deaths averted over 10 years at an initial cost of less than $0.40 per person per year [30] and salt reduction is therefore listed as a top priority for action to address the non-communicable diseases crises worldwide [32].

Iodine intake has been identified as an ongoing public health concern in some Pacific Islands including Vanuatu [33] and Samoa [34]. In particular, iodine deficiency during pregnancy and lactation can negatively affect fetal development and impact health. This study confirmed that the mean iodine concentration (207 μg/L) of non-pregnant women (*n*-131) between 25–45 years was in the WHO recommended range (200–299 μg/L) based on data collected in 2016 [35]. Iodine was recognized as a public health problem in Fiji in 1996 when mean concentrations of iodine amongst school children were found to be 26 μg/L with 45% prevalence of goiter amongst pregnant women and school children [10]. Universal salt iodization, including certification of iodized salt imports was mandated that year [10]. A subsequent survey in 2009 demonstrated that the iodine status amongst children and pregnant women was now sufficient with a median of 237 μg/L and 227 μg/L, respectively. Our study provides further evidence to support the fact that Fijian adults are no longer iodine insufficient. As salt is the vehicle for iodine fortification, it is important that efforts to reduce salt are aligned with continued efforts to maintain adequate iodine intakes [35]. This requires collaboration on monitoring changes in intake and adjusting the amount of iodine added to salt accordingly [35].

Study Strengths and Limitations

A number of strengths for the study can be noted. The study was designed to obtain a nationally representative sample of 24-h urines to assess population salt intake at baseline and after 20 months [36]. Whilst response rates were low, the comparison of the sample characteristics between the two surveys showed the samples were remarkably similar. Though 24-h urine collection can be onerous for participants and researchers, it is still regarded as a gold standard for assessing salt intake, as it accounts for around 95% of secreted sodium, although it still does not account for the possible 10% that can be lost through sweat, saliva, and gastrointestinal secretions [37]. Creatinine cutoff and total volume were used to ensure completeness of 24-h urine collections, in line with previous studies [16,38,39], so we are confident that the estimates of salt intake are fairly robust.

A weakness of the study is that the low response rates at baseline (28.2%) and at 20 months (22.5%), whilst comparable to other studies, resulted in the sample size likely being too small to measure changes in salt intake. The small sample sizes and sampling issues may have introduced biases, which may explain some of the observed findings and limit the generalizability of the findings to the Fijian population. As the study did not include a control group, it would also not have been possible to differentiate an intervention effect from secular trends. Lengthy policy change processes, which impacted intervention implementation, and the Cyclone, which delayed the planned 20-month monitoring and potentially impacted the results, were also major challenges. Restricting the intervention and monitoring to a smaller more defined geographic area—such as just the main island of Viti Levu, where the capital is based—might have been more achievable.

For future population-based implementation science studies measuring changes in salt intake, consideration should be given to having a longer, more intense intervention period and obtaining higher participant response rates for urine samples, to ensure adequate power to demonstrate an effect.

5. Conclusions

Whist measured salt intake was 11.7 g/day at baseline and 10.3 g/day after 20 months, it was not possible to draw firm conclusions about any possible changes due to the low response rates and high risk of sampling bias. However, this study provides credible nutrient intake data on sodium, potassium and iodine levels in Fiji through the assessment of urine samples. In order to achieve the global WHO target of reducing salt intake to less than 5 g p/d per person by 2025, existing policies and programs, which aim to change consumer behavior, reduce salt levels in foods and meals, and target schools and hospitals, need to be strengthened. Monitoring to assess population sodium and iodine levels should be built into future surveys such as the WHO STEPS survey of NCD risk factors and the National Nutrition Survey.

Acknowledgments: The authors wish to thank Fiji National University, C-POND, the Fijian Ministry of Health and Medical Services, the National Food and Nutrition Centre, Vanua Medical Laboratory, the World Health Organization, the members of the Food Taskforce Technical Advisory Group (FT-TAG) and all of the survey participants for their support and interest in the study. The Project is funded by the National Health and Medical Research Council of Australia under the Global Alliance for Chronic Disease (GACD) Hypertension Program (#1040178). K.T. is supported by a National Health and Medical Research Council of Australia postgraduate scholarship (#1115169) and VicHealth for work on salt reduction. M.M. is supported by a NHMRC Centre for Research Excellence in Obesity Policy and Food Systems (#1041020). J.W. is supported by a National Health and Medical Research Council/National Heart Foundation Career Development Fellowship (#1082924) on International strategies to reduce salt. J.W. has funding from WHO, VicHealth and the National Health and Medical Research Council of Australia for research on salt reduction. J.W. is further supported through an NHMRC CRE on food policy interventions to reduce salt (#1117300).

Author Contributions: J.W., W.S., M.M. and C.B. conceived the study. A.P., A.S., W.S. and J.S. implemented the project in Fiji. G.M. performed all urine iodine analysis. A.P., K.T., J.A.S., and K.R. did the data analysis. J.W. and A.P. interpreted the results. A.P. wrote the first draft of the manuscript. All other authors commented on various drafts and approved the final paper.

References

1.   He, F.J.; MacGregor, G.A. Salt, blood pressure and cardiovascular disease. *Curr. Opin. Cardiol.* **2007**, *22*, 298–305. [CrossRef] [PubMed]

2. World Health Organization. *Guideline: Sodium Intake for Adults and Children*; World Health Organization: Geneva, Switzerland, 2012.

3. Aburto, N.J.; Ziolkovska, A.; Hooper, L.; Elliott, P.; Cappuccio, F.P.; Meerpohl, J.J. Effect of lower sodium intake on health: Systematic review and meta-analyses. *Br. Med. J.* **2013**, *346*. [CrossRef] [PubMed]

4. Ministry of Health and Medical Services. *Annual Report 2015*; Ministry of Health and Medical Services: Suva, Fiji, 2016.

5. Ministry of Health and Medical Services. *Non-Communicable Diseases Strategic Plan 2015–2019; Fiji Health Sector Support Programme*; Ministry of Health and Medical Services: Suva, Fiji, 2014.

6. Snowdon, W.; Raj, A.; Reeve, E.; Guerrero, R.L.; Fesaitu, J.; Cateine, K.; Guignet, C. Processed foods available in the Pacific Islands. *Glob. Health* **2013**, *9*. [CrossRef] [PubMed]

7. Downs, S.M.; Christoforou, A.; Snowdon, W.; Dunford, E.; Hoejskov, P.; Legetic, B.; Campbell, N.; Webster, J. Setting targets for salt levels in foods: A five-step approach for low-and middle-income countries. *Food Policy* **2015**, *55*, 101–108. [CrossRef]

8. McLean, R.; Williams, S.; Mann, J. Monitoring population sodium intake using spot urine samples: Validation in a New Zealand population. *J. Hum. Hypertens.* **2014**, *28*, 657–662. [CrossRef] [PubMed]

9. National Food and Nutrition Centre. *Salt, Fat and Sugar Food Sources in the Fijian Diet*; National Food and Nutrition Centre: Suva, Fiji, 2009.

10. Khan, A. Elimination of Iodine Deficiency in Fiji. *IDD Newslett.* **2009**, *21*, 12–13.

11. Fiji Bureau of Statistics. *Census 2007, Population Size, Growth, Structure and Distribution*; Statistical News No. 45; Fiji Bureau of Statistics: Suva, Fiji, 2008.

12. Webster, J.; Snowdon, W.; Moodie, M.; Viali, S.; Schultz, J.; Bell, C.; Land, M.-A.; Downs, S.; Christoforou, A.; Dunford, E.; et al. Cost-effectiveness of reducing salt intake in the Pacific Islands: Protocol for a before and after intervention study. *BMC Public Health* **2014**, *14*. [CrossRef] [PubMed]

13. Trieu, K.; Neal, B.; Hawkes, C.; Dunford, E.; Campbell, N.; Rodriguez-Fernandez, R.; Legetic, B.; McLaren, L.; Barberio, A.; Webster, J. Salt Reduction Initiatives around the World—A Systematic Review of Progress towards the Global Target. *PLoS ONE* **2015**, *10*, e0130247. [CrossRef] [PubMed]

14. Christoforou, A.; Snowdon, W.; Laesango, N.; Vatucawaqa, S.; Lamar, D.; Alam, L.; Lippwe, K.; Havea, I.L.; Tairea, K.; Hoejskov, P.; et al. Progress on salt reduction in the Pacific Islands: From strategies to action. *Heart Lung Circ.* **2015**, *24*, 503–509. [CrossRef] [PubMed]

15. World Health Organization. *WHO STEPS Surveillance Manual: The WHO STEPwise Approach to Chronic Disease Risk Factor Surveillance*; World Health Organization: Geneva, Switzerland, 2005.

16. Land, M.-A.; Wu, J.H.; Selwyn, A.; Crino, M.; Woodward, M.; Chalmers, J.; Webster, J.; Nowson, C.; Jeffery, P.; Smith, W.; et al. Effects of a community-based salt reduction program in a regional Australian population. *BMC Public Health* **2016**, *16*. [CrossRef] [PubMed]

17. Woodruff, R. A simpe method for approximating the variance of a complicated estimate. *J. Am. Stat. Assoc.* **1971**, *66*, 411–414. [CrossRef]

18. Trevena, H.; Neal, B.; Dunford, E.; Haskelberg, H.; Wu, J.H. A comparison of the sodium content of supermarket private-label and branded foods in Australia. *Nutrients* **2015**, *7*, 7027–7041. [CrossRef] [PubMed]

19. Powles, J.; Fahimi, S.; Micha, R.; Khatibzadeh, S.; Shi, P.; Ezzati, M.; Engell, R.E.; Lim, S.S.; Danaei, G.; Mozaffarian, D. Global, regional and national sodium intakes in 1990 and 2010: A systematic analysis of 24 h urinary sodium excretion and dietary surveys worldwide. *BMJ Open* **2013**, *3*, e003733. [CrossRef] [PubMed]

20. Sacks, F.M.; Svetkey, L.P.; Vollmer, W.M.; Appel, L.J.; Bray, G.A.; Harsha, D.; Obarzanek, E.; Conlin, P.R.; Miller, E.R., III; Simons-Morton, D.G.; et al. Effects on blood pressure of reduced dietary sodium and the Dietary Approaches to Stop Hypertension (DASH) diet. *N. Engl. J. Med.* **2001**, *344*, 3–10. [CrossRef] [PubMed]

21. Adler, A.J.; Taylor, F.; Martin, N.; Gottlieb, S.; Taylor, R.S.; Ebrahim, S. Reduced dietary salt for the prevention of cardiovascular disease. *Cochrane Database Syst. Rev.* **2014**, *12*. [CrossRef]

22. Strazzullo, P.; D'Elia, L.; Kandala, N.-B.; Cappuccio, F.P. Salt intake, stroke, and cardiovascular disease: Meta-analysis of prospective studies. *Br. Med. J.* **2009**, *339*. [CrossRef] [PubMed]

23. Jones-Burton, C.; Mishra, S.I.; Fink, J.C.; Brown, J.; Gossa, W.; Bakris, G.L.; Weir, M.R. An in-depth review of the evidence linking dietary salt intake and progression of chronic kidney disease. *Am. J. Nephrol.* **2006**, *26*, 268–275. [CrossRef] [PubMed]

24. Barberio, A.M.; Sumar, N.; Trieu, K.; Lorenzetti, D.L.; Tarasuk, V.; Webster, J.; Campbell, N.R.C.; McLaren, L. Population-level interventions in government jurisdictions for dietary sodium reduction: A Cochrane Review. *Int. J. Epidemiol.* **2017**, *46*. [CrossRef] [PubMed]

25. Charlton, K.; Webster, J.; Kowal, P. To legislate or not to legislate? A comparison of the UK and South African approaches to the development and implementation of salt reduction programs. *Nutrients* **2014**, *6*, 3672–3695. [CrossRef] [PubMed]

26. Webster, J.; Trieu, K.; Dunford, E.; Hawkes, C. Target Salt 2025: A Global Overview of National Programs to Encourage the Food Industry to Reduce Salt in Foods. *Nutrients* **2014**, *6*, 3274–3287. [CrossRef] [PubMed]

27. Webster, J.; Su'a, S.A.F.; Ieremia, M.; Bompoint, S.; Johnson, C.; Faeamani, G.; Vaiaso, M.; Snowdon, W.; Land, M.A.; Trieu, K.; et al. Salt Intakes, Knowledge, and Behavior in Samoa: Monitoring Salt-Consumption Patterns through the World Health Organization's Surveillance of Noncommunicable Disease Risk Factors (STEPS). *J. Clin. Hypertens.* **2016**, *18*, 884–891. [CrossRef] [PubMed]

28. Hope, S.F.; Webster, J.; Trieu, K.; Pillay, A.; Ieremia, M.; Bell, C.; Snowdon, W.; Neal, B.; Moodie, M. A systematic review of economic evaluations of population-based sodium reduction interventions. *PLoS ONE* **2017**, *12*, e0173600. [CrossRef] [PubMed]

29. Trieu, K.; McMahon, E.; Santos, J.A.; Bauman, A.; Jolly, K.-A.; Bolam, B.; Webster, J. Review of behaviour change interventions to reduce population salt intake. *Int. J. Behav. Nutr. Phys. Act.* **2017**, *14*. [CrossRef] [PubMed]

30. Cappuccio, F.P.; Capewell, S.; Lincoln, P.; McPherson, K. Policy options to reduce population salt intake. *Br. Med. J.* **2011**, *343*. [CrossRef] [PubMed]

31. Do, H.T.; Santos, J.A.; Trieu, K.; Petersen, K.; Le, M.B.; Lai, D.T.; Bauman, A.; Webster, J. Effectiveness of a Communication for Behavioral Impact (COMBI) Intervention to Reduce Salt Intake in a Vietnamese Province Based on Estimations from Spot Urine Samples. *J. Clin. Hypertens. (Greenwich)* **2016**, *18*, 1135–1142. [CrossRef] [PubMed]

32. Beaglehole, R.; Bonita, R.; Horton, R.; Adams, C.; Alleyne, G.; Asaria, P.; Baugh, V.; Bekedam, H.; Billo, N.; Casswell, S.; et al. Priority actions for the non-communicable disease crisis. *Lancet* **2011**, *377*, 1438–1447. [CrossRef]

33. Li, M.; McKelleher, N.; Moses, T.; Mark, J.; Byth, K.; Ma, G.; Eastman, C.J. Iodine nutritional status of children on the island of Tanna, Republic of Vanuatu. *Public Health Nutr.* **2009**, *12*, 1512–1518. [CrossRef] [PubMed]

34. Land, M.-A.; Webster, J.L.; Ma, G.; Li, M.; Su, S.A.F.; Ieremia, M.; Viali, S.; Faeamani, G.; Bell, A.C.; Quested, C.; et al. Salt intake and iodine status of women in Samoa. *Asia Pac. J. Clin. Nutr.* **2016**, *25*, 142–149. [PubMed]

35. World Health Organization. *Salt Reduction and Iodine Fortification Strategies in Public Health*; Report of a Joint Technical Meeting Convened by the World Health Organization and the George Institute for Global Health in Collaboration with the International Council for the Control of Iodine Deficiency Disorders Global Network; Sydney, Australia, 26–27 March 2013; World Health Organization: Geneva, Switzerland, 2014.

36. McLean, R. Measuring Population Sodium Intake: A Review of Methods. *Nutrients* **2014**, *6*, 4651–4662. [CrossRef] [PubMed]

37. Ji, C.; Sykes, L.; Paul, C.; Dary, O.; Legetic, B.; Campbell, N.R.; Cappuccio, F.P.; Sub-Group for Research and Surveillance of the PAHO-WHO Regional Expert Group for Cardiovascular Disease Prevention through Population-wide Dietary Salt Reduction. Systematic review of studies comparing 24-hour and spot urine collections for estimating population salt intake. *Rev. Panam. Salud Pública* **2012**, *32*, 307–315. [PubMed]

38. Staessen, J.; Bulpitt, C.; Fagard, R.; Joossens, J.V.; Lijnen, P.; Amery, A. Four urinary cations and blood pressure a population study in two belgian towns. *Am. J. Epidemiol.* **1983**, *117*, 676–687. [CrossRef] [PubMed]

39. Charlton, K.E.; Steyn, K.; Levitt, N.S.; Zulu, J.V.; Jonathan, D.; Veldman, F.J.; Nel, J.H. Diet and blood pressure in South Africa: Intake of foods containing sodium, potassium, calcium, and magnesium in three ethnic groups. *Nutrition* **2005**, *21*, 39–50. [CrossRef] [PubMed]

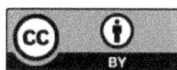

nutrients

MDPI

Article

The Sodium and Potassium Content of the Most Commonly Available Street Foods in Tajikistan and Kyrgyzstan in the Context of the FEEDCities Project

Inês Lança de Morais [1,2,*], Nuno Lunet [3,4], Gabriela Albuquerque [3], Marcello Gelormini [2], Susana Casal [3,5,6], Albertino Damasceno [7], Olívia Pinho [6,8], Pedro Moreira [3,8,9], Jo Jewell [2], João Breda [2] and Patrícia Padrão [3,8]

[1] Institute of Tropical Medicine and International Health, Charité-Universitätsmedizin Berlin, Campus Virchow-Klinikum, Augustenburger Platz 1, 13353 Berlin, Germany
[2] Division of Noncommunicable Diseases and Life-Course, World Health Organization (WHO) Regional Office for Europe, UN-City, Marmorvej 51, DK-2100 Copenhagen Ø, Denmark; marcello.gelormini@gmail.com (M.G.); jewellj@who.int (J.J.); rodriguesdasilvabred@who.int (J.B.)
[3] EPIUnit—Instituto de Saúde Pública, Universidade do Porto, Rua das Taipas nº 135, 4050-600 Porto, Portugal; nlunet@med.up.pt (N.L.); gabriela.albuquerque@ispup.up.pt (G.A.); sucasal@ff.up.pt (S.C.); pedromoreira@fcna.up.pt (P.M.); patriciapadrao@fcna.up.pt (P.P.)
[4] Departamento de Ciências da Saúde Pública e Forenses e Educação Médica, Faculdade de Medicina da Universidade do Porto, Alameda Prof. Hernâni Monteiro, 4200-319 Porto, Portugal
[5] Faculdade de Farmácia, Universidade do Porto, Rua Jorge de Viterbo Ferreira 228, 4050-313 Porto, Portugal
[6] REQUIMTE, Laboratório de Bromatologia e Hidrologia, Universidade do Porto, Rua Jorge de Viterbo Ferreira 228, 4050-313 Porto, Portugal; oliviapinho@fcna.up.pt
[7] Faculdade de Medicina da Universidade Eduardo Mondlane, Avenida Salvador Allende nº 702, 257 Maputo, Moçambique; tino_7117@hotmail.com
[8] Faculdade de Ciências da Nutrição e Alimentação da Universidade do Porto, Rua Dr. Roberto Frias, 4200-465 Porto, Portugal
[9] Centro de Investigação em Atividade Física, Saúde e Lazer, Universidade do Porto, Rua Dr. Plácido da Costa, 4200-450 Porto, Portugal
* Correspondence: ines.lanca-de-morais@charite.de; Tel.: +351-91-773-5562

Received: 27 November 2017; Accepted: 11 January 2018; Published: 16 January 2018

Abstract: This cross-sectional study is aimed at assessing sodium (Na) and potassium (K) content and the molar Na:K ratios of the most commonly available ready-to-eat street foods in Tajikistan and Kyrgyzstan. Four different samples of each of these foods were collected and 62 food categories were evaluated through bromatological analysis. Flame photometry was used to quantify sodium and potassium concentrations. The results show that home-made foods can be important sources of sodium. In particular, main dishes and sandwiches, respectively, contain more than 1400 and nearly 1000 mg Na in an average serving and provide approximately 70% and 50% of the maximum daily recommended values. Wide ranges of sodium content were found between individual samples of the same home-made food collected from different vending sites from both countries. In industrial foods, sodium contents ranged from 1 to 1511 mg/serving in Tajikistan, and from 19 to 658 mg/serving in Kyrgyzstan. Most Na:K ratios exceeded the recommended level of 1.0 and the highest ratios were found in home-made snacks (21.2) from Tajikistan and industrial beverages (16.4) from Kyrgyzstan. These findings not only improve data on the nutritional composition of foods in these countries, but may also serve as baseline information for future policies and interventions.

Keywords: sodium; potassium; sodium–potassium ratio; ready-to-eat food; street food; Tajikistan; Kyrgyzstan; low- and middle-income countries

Nutrients **2018**, *10*, 98

1. Introduction

Non-communicable diseases (NCDs) are the leading cause of death globally, accounting for 70% of the total estimated deaths in 2015 [1]. In the World Health Organization (WHO) European Region, NCDs alone are responsible for 89% of total deaths [1]. Approximately 80% of these deaths occur in low- and middle-income countries (LMICs) [2] and the situation is of particular concern in Newly Independent States (NIS) such as Tajikistan and Kyrgyzstan, where 57% and 47%, respectively, of all NCD-related deaths occur prematurely [3].

This epidemiological transition observed in LMICs (including the NIS) [4], has been accompanied by a nutrition transition with conspicuous changes in the supply, availability, and consumption of foods [5–8]. Dietary patterns are rapidly shifting towards a greater consumption of animal-source foods, refined grains, and processed foods, frequently high in saturated fat, *trans* fatty acids, free sugars, and/or salt [7,9], as well as lower consumption of fruits and vegetables [7,10]. Specifically, diets high in sodium (Na) and low in potassium (K) have long been identified as important drivers for NCD-related disability and mortality [11].

Sodium intake is closely associated with blood pressure (BP) [12,13] and high BP itself is an important risk factor for NCDs, particularly cardiovascular diseases (CVDs). [11]. The relationship between sodium intake and CVD morbidity and mortality is suggested to vary according to different sodium intake levels, following a J-shaped curve: low intakes (less than 2 g/day) show an inverse association with CVD outcomes; excessive intakes, particularly those above 4 g/day of sodium, show a direct impact; and intermediate intakes do not appear to have measurable effects [14]. The WHO recommends a maximum daily intake of 2 g of sodium per day [15].

Additionally, low potassium intake has been associated with increased risk of high BP and stroke, while an intake of 90 mmol/day ($\approx$3510 mg) is potentially protective against these conditions [16–18]. The role of potassium in diminishing the effect of high sodium intake in BP has also been established [19]. Furthermore, sodium-to-potassium (Na:K) ratios were shown to be key predictors of BP and CVD outcomes [20–23] and ratios close to 1.0 are considered beneficial for health [24]. As such, the WHO recommends that countries implement salt reduction strategies and promote increased consumption of fruit and vegetables, among other policies, to improve diets in the region [25].

New urban living patterns are marked by less time for home food preparation and increased consumption of food prepared away from home, notably street food [26,27]. Street food provides an accessible and affordable source of nutrition for many people living in LMICs. Nevertheless, little is known about the nutritional contribution of these foods to the diet, despite the high amounts of sodium that might be expected in many food products sold by street vendors [28].

This study is set in the context of the WHO project FEEDCities, which is a multi-country project in Central Asia, the Caucasus, and south-eastern Europe that aims to fill the gap of lack of information available on the nutritional composition of the available ready-to-eat street food in the WHO European Region [29,30]. The main objectives of this project are to characterize street food environments in urban contexts, to document the types of foods most commonly available on the streets, and to assess their nutritional composition. This paper will exclusively focus on the latter objective, in particular, on the analysis of sodium and potassium content of street foods (including beverages) sold in urban areas of Tajikistan and Kyrgyzstan. We aim to describe the variability across different types of foods and similar food products acquired in different vending places to illustrate the potential for improvement of street food availability and use.

2. Materials and Methods

The present study is a cross-sectional evaluation of the sodium and potassium content and the Na:K ratio of the most commonly available street foods collected from the streets of Dushanbe and Bishkek, the capital cities of Tajikistan and Kyrgyzstan, respectively. After approval (reference number CE16058) from the Ethics Committee of the Institute of Public Health of the University of Porto (ISPUP) and local authorities, the study was carried out between April and May 2016 in Dushanbe, and between June and July 2016 in Bishkek.

The study adopted the definition of street food proposed by the Food and Agricultural Organization (FAO) and the WHO of "ready-to-eat foods and beverages prepared and/or sold by vendors or hawkers especially in the streets and other similar places" [31]. This includes prepared or cooked foods to be consumed immediately or later on (e.g., at work), without any further preparation needed.

Through a first exploratory visit to the cities, it was observed that the street food vending was typically occurring in and around bazaars and public markets (hereinafter "markets"). A comprehensive list of these venues, including a total of 36 markets in Dushanbe and 19 in Bishkek, was provided by the local authorities. From each city, 10 markets were randomly selected, including small to large-sized markets, among those selling only food or food and other goods. In Dushanbe, the final list ensured a representation of all four districts of the city proportional to the corresponding number of markets. In Bishkek, the final list represented three out of the four districts.

The study area was defined by selecting a 500-m-diameter buffer for each selected market, with the centroid in the geographic midpoint of the market, which covered the market and its surroundings. Preliminary data on the street food on offer was collected from vending sites operating within this study area. Eligible vending sites comprised those selling ready-to-eat food from any venue, including both fixed and mobile vending units, selling directly on the street. Street hawkers were also covered. Vending sites selling exclusively fresh or dry fruits in natura were not eligible. In Tajikistan, all eligible vending sites within the study area were assessed, whereas in Kyrgyzstan, taking into account that the selected markets in Bishkek had a larger number of eligible vending sites, of every two vending sites, the second was systematically evaluated.

In the first phase of the study, 10 trained field researchers gathered preliminary data on the availability of the ready-to-eat food, mostly by direct observation. Data was collected through mobile phones. The existing android-based tool 'KoBoCollect' [32], by 'KoBoToolbox', was used to administer an electronic questionnaire, containing both closed- and open-ended questions that helped researchers record the characteristics of the food products sold. Operating in pairs, the researchers canvassed each selected market and all publicly accessible streets in their surroundings within predefined study areas. For the eligible vending places identified, the researchers registered the corresponding position through Global Positioning System (GPS) coordinates, and described the type of foods being sold as well specific serving sizes, and took photographs of the portions typically served. Data collection took place during weekdays and weekends to ensure the evaluation of the food on offer was representative.

Foods available were grouped into two broad types according to their elaboration and degree of processing [33]: (1) home-made food, defined as foods and beverages cooked and/or prepared at home or on the street; and (2) industrial foods, comprising foods and beverages that are industrially produced using industrial techniques.

The most commonly available street foods, both homemade (20 in Bishkek and 25 in Dushanbe) and industrial (10 in each country) were then selected for bromatological analysis by ranking the number of occurrences of each food registered during preliminary data collection on food offer. The larger number of home-made foods to be sampled is explained by the fact that the nutritional composition of these foods is often not known, as opposed to industrial foods. Fruits in natura, water, coffee, tea, and soft and alcoholic drinks were excluded from the sample collection as their nutritional values have been well studied and are not expected to vary significantly in terms of sodium and potassium contents.

2.1. Food Sample Collection

The most common home-made and industrial foods identified were split in equal sets of five in each country. For 10 consecutive days, including weekdays and weekends, two sets for home-made foods and two sets for industrial foods were collected in each of the 10 study areas of Dushanbe and

Bishkek, until four samples of each of the most common foods in each country were collected from four different vending sites. However, for some foods (from Tajikistan), it was only possible to collect three samples. A total of 254 food samples was collected.

The collection started in the study areas with the least number of vending sites registered during data collection. In each market and its surroundings, 10 GPS coordinates—corresponding to the location of the 10 previously assessed vending sites—were randomly selected for purchasing the corresponding sets for the day. In each market and for each day, only one sample of homemade and/or one sample of industrial food was obtained from the same vending site. In the case it was not possible to buy foods in the selected coordinates, a systematic selection procedure (north, clockwise) was followed until reaching vending sites where the selected foods were available.

Samples were purchased as part of regular transactions, and therefore no consent was required. For each item, the amount of food bought corresponded to the usual serving size, according to the typical consumption pattern observed.

All samples were weighed and prepared for analysis; liquids were homogenized and solid foods were triturated with a food grinder. Four portions of each sample were individually packed in small containers and weighed before being stored in freezer at –18 °C until analysis.

2.2. Bromatological Analysis

For analysis of the nutritional composition of the foods collected, samples were defrosted and each container weight was compared with the one registered before being frozen, with no significant variations detected. Each container was carefully homogenized for reincorporation of any condensate/leach and immediately analyzed.

Sodium and potassium were evaluated by flame photometry, on duplicate 2-g portions of each sample according to a previously validated method [34]. Sample extracts were diluted to fit the linear range of the photometric response, using both standard and sample controls through the determinations. The caloric values of samples were estimated after proximate analysis of food components (moisture, protein, total fat and ash) performed in accordance with standard methods, as recommended by the FAO, and using the general Atwater values [35]. All the analytical results are the average of at least two determinations, expressed with respect to 100 g of fresh food.

2.3. Data Analysis

Figure 1 shows a flow chart displaying the data analysis process. From the 254 samples collected, samples of industrial chocolate from both countries, as well as home-made ice-creams from Tajikistan, were omitted from the detailed analysis due to their low-sodium content. Therefore, 242 samples were taken into account, corresponding to the 62 most common foods from both countries.

These 62 foods were further assigned to eight broader groups that were created based on the groups of the WHO nutrient profile model [36] and new ones were extended when necessary: (1) beverages; (2) bread; (3) buns; (4) cakes and cookies; (5) main dishes; (6) sandwiches; (7) savoury pastries and (8) snacks. Based on these groups, a total of 10 (Tajikistan) and 12 (Kyrgyzstan) sets of a variable number of samples were created, each set referring to broader groups of home-made or industrial foods.

Average serving sizes per food, in grams, were calculated as the mean of the individual doses of each of the samples collected for the respective foods. For the food group analysis, the average of serving sizes of the respective food items included in the group was calculated.

Per-serving sodium and potassium levels were expressed in milligrams (mg)/serving. To calculate individual molar Na:K ratios, contents of sodium and potassium (mg/serving) of each sample were converted in millimoles (mmol) using the conversion 23 mg sodium = 1 mmol sodium and 39 mg potassium = 1 mmol potassium.

The average contents of sodium and potassium as well as the molar Na:K ratio of the foods was obtained from the mean of the individual samples collected for the corresponding food [37]. For food group analysis, the averages of sodium, potassium and molar Na:K ratios of the respective foods included in the groups were calculated and the contribution of the sodium and potassium contents of each group to these nutrients' recommended daily intake was computed.

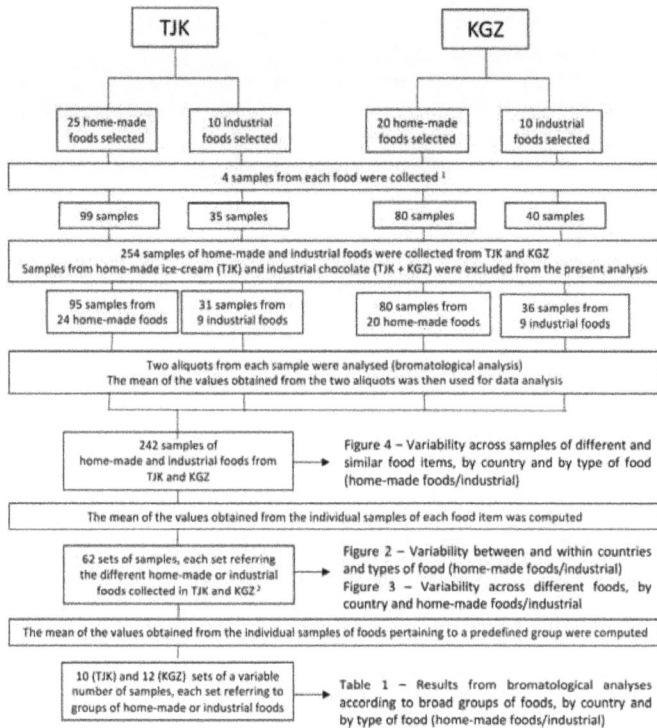

Figure 1. Flow chart of the data analysis process. TJK: Tajikistan; KGZ: Kyrgyzstan. [1] Except for home-made sweet pastries and industrial bread, chips, biscuit rolls, dry bread crumbs and wafers, all from Tajikistan, for which only three samples were collected. [2] The 62 sets of samples correspond to a total of 46 different foods.

Sodium and potassium contents of individual samples and foods were further calculated as mg/2000 kilocalories (kcal), taking into account the average daily energy intake in adults.

Statistical analysis was conducted with Stata. Descriptive statistics were used to present results from the nutritional composition of foods. Three box plots were produced to describe the distribution of sodium, potassium, and Na:K ratio/serving, by type of food (home-made vs. industrial) and by country. Mean values of foods were used to describe data of home-made and industrial foods. Scatter plots were obtained with the average sodium and potassium contents, per food, in mg/2000 kcal, and compared with the WHO's recommended limits [15,18].

A detailed analysis of sodium and potassium contents (mg/2000 kcal) of each food sample was also presented through scatter plots displayed by food groups.

The mean values were obtained from the individual samples of foods for presenting the results according to the predefined groups of foods.

The nonparametric Mann–Whitney U test was used for comparisons between home-made and industrial foods and between countries.

3. Results

Figure 2a–c, respectively, show the distribution of the average sodium and potassium contents and the molar Na:K ratios of the 62 most common home-made and industrial foods of Tajikistan and Kyrgyzstan. There were no significant differences between countries with respect to sodium (home-made, p-value = 0.211; industrial, p-value = 0.691), potassium (home-made, p-value = 0.158; industrial, p-value = 0.691) or Na:K ratios (home-made, p-value = 0.585; industrial, p-value = 0.965).

Overall, Figure 2a shows that home-made foods in both countries have higher levels of sodium when compared to industrial foods (Tajikistan, p-value = 0.032; Kyrgyzstan, p-value = 0.002), as well as greater variability in the average levels of sodium per serving. In Kyrgyzstan, nearly 75% of home-made foods had a content exceeding 500 mg Na/serving, while some of them reached almost 2000 mg Na/serving. In Tajikistan, the median sodium content per serving in home-made foods was 560 mg Na (335–751) although some foods reached 2500 mg of sodium per serving. Regarding sodium content in industrial foods, 75% of foods did not reach 500 mg Na/serving in both countries. However, in Tajikistan, this content ranged from 1 to 1511 mg/serving, while in Kyrgyzstan, sodium content of industrial food was in the range of 19 to 658 mg/serving, with larger dispersion of sodium contents above the median.

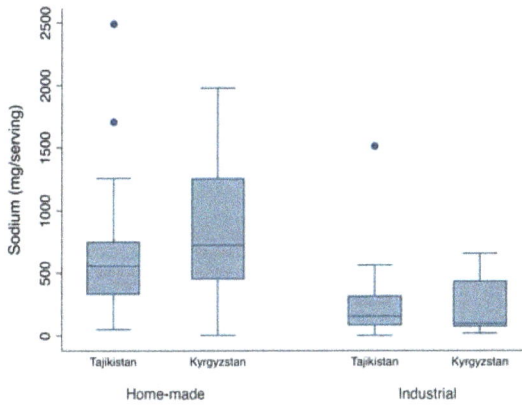

(a)

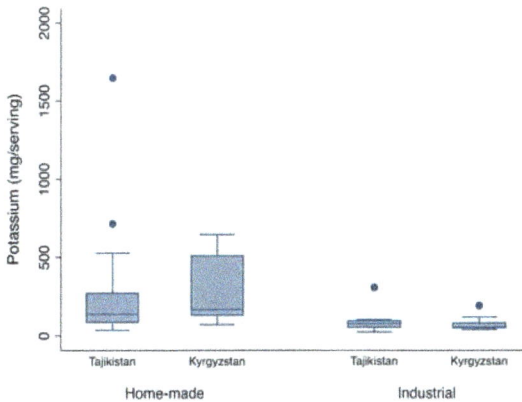

(b)

Figure 2. *Cont.*

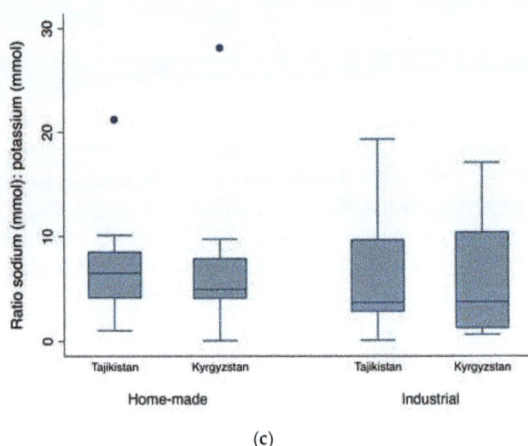

(c)

Figure 2. Per-serving average of (**a**) sodium; (**b**) potassium content; and (**c**) molar sodium:potassium ratio of the most commonly available ready-to-eat home-made and industrial foods in Tajikistan and Kyrgyzstan. Outliers are indicated by dots (•).

Figure 2b shows that potassium contents were also higher in home-made foods of both countries (Tajikistan, *p*-value = 0.019; Kyrgyzstan, *p*-value < 0.001), in comparison to industrial foods. The potassium content of home-made foods ranged between 35 and 1646 mg/serving in Tajikistan and between 78 and 634 mg/serving in Kyrgyzstan. The variability in potassium was much lower in industrial foods and per-serving medians were 75 mg (51–93)/serving, in Tajikistan, and 52 mg (47–79)/serving in Kyrgyzstan.

With respect to molar Na:K ratios, Figure 2c suggests that, on average, industrial foods present higher variability than home-made foods, though differences were not statistically significant (Tajikistan, *p*-value = 0.571; Kyrgyzstan, *p*-value = 0.354). In industrial foods, ratios ranged from 0.1 to 19.3 in Tajikistan, and from 0.7 to 17.1 in Kyrgyzstan. In Tajikistan, the ratios of home-made foods ranged from 1.1 to 10.1 and in Kyrgyzstan from 1.6 to 9.9, reaching up to 21.2 and 28.1, respectively.

Figure 3 displays the distribution of average sodium and potassium contents, adjusted to a 2000 kcal diet, in relation to WHO recommended limits for these nutrients [15,18].

In Figure 3a it is possible to identify two well-defined groups of foods (bottom left), where foods from both countries fell short of potassium recommendations and exceeded (Figure 3b) or complied (Figure 3c) with sodium recommended limits. Home-made fried potatoes (Tajikistan), presented the highest average of potassium content—almost twice the minimum daily recommendation. Carrot salad, corn and the industrial drink *chalap* (all from Kyrgyzstan) followed, with average potassium contents between 6000 and 4000 mg K/2000 kcal. The dried milk-based home-made snack *kurut* (Kyrgyzstan) and soups (Tajikistan) presented potassium contents, per 2000 kcal, slightly below the minimum potassium threshold. At the same time, these six foods exceeded maximum daily sodium recommended limits; yet *chalap* had over 20 times more the upper recommended limit for sodium, surpassed only by home-made *kurut* (also from Kyrgyzstan). This was the uppermost average sodium content value of all the foods collected from both countries (47,117 mg Na/2000 kcal). *Kurut* collected in Tajikistan also presented high sodium content, exceeding upper recommended limits by more than nine times. *Maksym*, a Kyrgyz drink usually sold together with *chalap*, and sunflower seeds (Tajikistan) were also high in sodium, with contents close to 20,000 mg Na/2000 kcal. In Kyrgyzstan, industrial chips, had an average sodium content below upper recommended limits and potassium content close to the threshold of 3510 mg K/2000 kcal (Figure 3a), while in Tajikistan chips had four times more sodium and potassium levels below 2000 mg K/2000 kcal (Figure 3b).

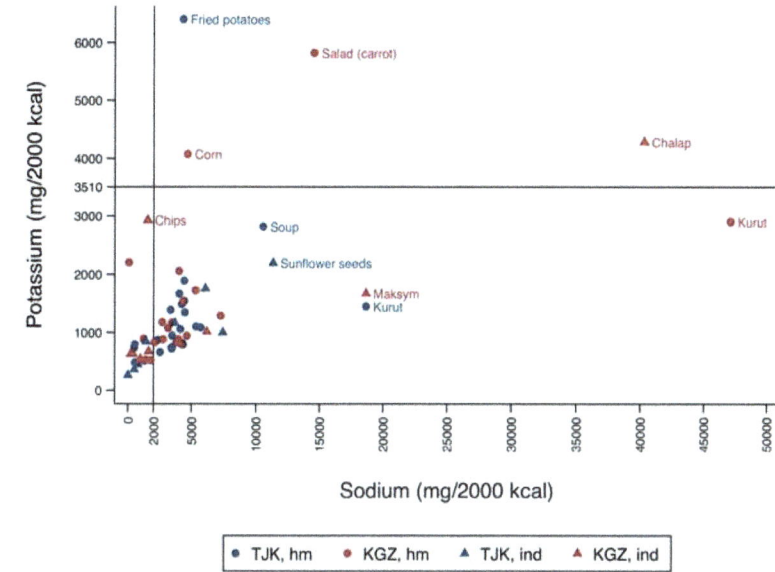

(a)

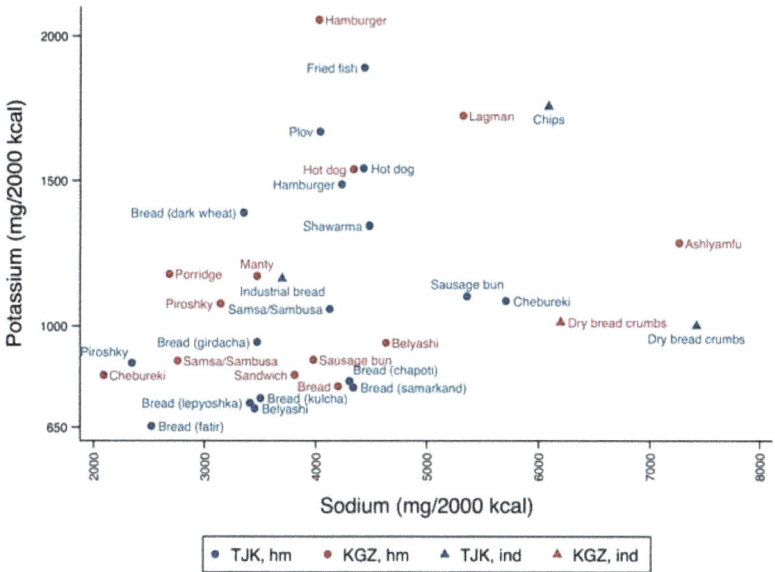

(b)

Figure 3. *Cont.*

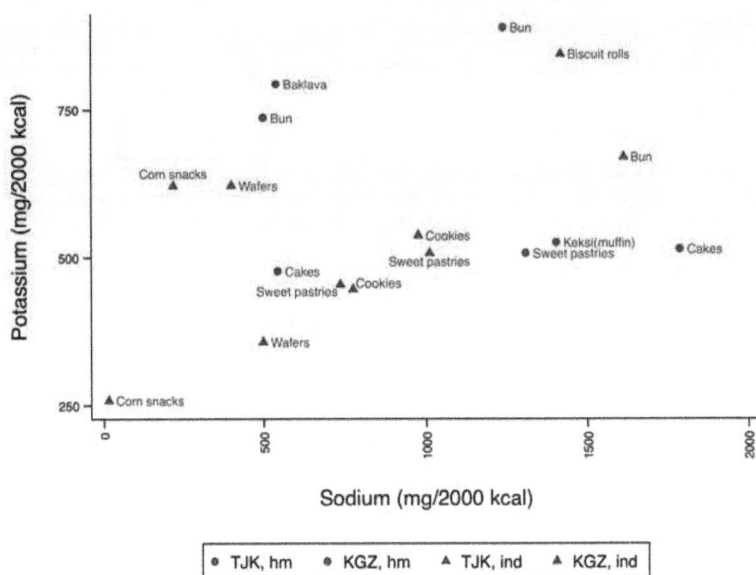

(c)

Figure 3. Distribution of average of sodium (Na) and potassium (K) contents (mg/2000 kcal) of the most commonly available home-made (hm) and industrial (ind) foods in Tajikistan (TJK) and Kyrgyzstan (KGZ) relative to the World Health Organization (WHO) sodium and potassium recommendations (less than 2000 and at least 3510 mg/day, respectively); 2000 kcal was assumed as the average energy requirement for adults. (**a**) A general view of these nutrients' content in all foods collected from both countries, and zoomed-in views of foods that tended to have contents that either (**b**) exceeded sodium upper recommended limits up to 8000 mg Na/2000 kcal and were below minimum potassium recommendations down to 650 mg K/2000 kcal; or (**c**) were below sodium upper recommended limits and below 1000 mg K/2000 kcal.

Figure 3b discloses 34 foods that exceeded maximum sodium recommended limits, presenting contents above 2000 and up to 8000 mg Na/2000 kcal. Four of these 34 foods are industrial foods, of which the dry bread crumbs collected in both countries stand out due to their high sodium contents—ranging from 6198 to 7422 mg Na/2000 kcal. Home-made traditional dishes also exceeded the upper recommended limits for sodium—around 4000 mg Na/2000 kcal (*plov*, in Tajikistan) and over 7000 mg Na/2000 kcal (*ashlyamfu*, in Kyrgyzstan). Regarding breads, all types (home-made and industrial) were in the range of 2500 to 5000 mg Na/2000 kcal; and presented potassium contents below or close to 1000 mg K/2000 kcal, with the exception of home-made dark wheat bread (Tajikistan), with 1389 mg K/2000 kcal. Home-made savoury pastries, such as *chebureki, piroshky, samsa/sambusa,* sausage rolls and *belyashi*, are also displayed in this group: sodium content varied between 2000 and 6000 mg Na/2000 kcal and most had potassium levels between 650 and 1000 mg K/2000 kcal. Hot dogs in both countries presented similar levels of sodium (more than 4000 mg Na/2000 kcal) and potassium (more than 1500 mg K/2000 kcal).

Figure 3c shows 17 foods with sodium contents below the upper recommended limits and the lowest potassium contents from all foods collected. Sweet foods predominate and more than half of these foods are industrial, including corn snacks, cookies, and sweet pastries. Home-made sweet pastries, buns, and cakes are also included in this figure. Notably, two sweet foods (e.g., cakes and buns) showed a sodium content per 2000 kcal above 1500 mg.

Table 1 shows the sodium and potassium contents per serving and molar ratios of the most common ready-to-eat predefined food groups, as well as their contributions to the daily recommended limits of these nutrients. In both countries, the main dishes were the principal home-made food source of sodium, contributing almost three-quarters of the maximum sodium recommended limits, followed by home-made sandwiches with a contribution of nearly half of the value. In Tajikistan, home-made breads and industrial snacks had a sodium content representing 31% of the maximum recommended limits each, while in Kyrgyzstan, home-made snacks, bread, and savoury pastries provided 43%, 36% and 33%, respectively, of sodium values with respect to the limits for daily intake. Beverages were shown to be the major sodium source of industrial foods collected in Kyrgyzstan. Main dishes and sandwiches were also the most important sources of potassium in both countries, although their contribution towards the minimum threshold ranged between 9.6% and 22.4%. Home-made snacks presented the highest mean molar Na:K ratio in Tajikistan (21.2), while in Kyrgyzstan industrial beverages had the uppermost molar Na:K ratio (16.4). Home-made buns (Tajikistan) and home-made beverages (Kyrgyzstan) showed the lowest molar ratios from all food groups—1 and 0.1, respectively.

Table 1. Sodium (Na) and potassium (K) content and molar Na:K ratio in different groups of the most commonly available street foods in Tajikistan and Kyrgyzstan.

		Mean Serving Size (g) *	Na				K				Molar Na:K Ratio		
			Mean (Min–Max) * mg/Serving			% Recom. [1]	Mean (Min–Max) * mg/Serving			% Recom. [2]	Mean (Min–Max) *		
Tajikistan													
Industrial foods	N *												
Bread	3	50.0	240	234	243	12.0	75	56	87	2.1	5.6	4.6	7.4
Cakes and cookies	14	59.1	103	30	238	5.2	66	21	133	1.9	3.1	0.7	7.2
Snacks	14	38.6	621	0	2218	31.0	129	17	447	3.7	10.2	0.0	42.6
Home-made foods	N *												
Bread	27	122.4	620	325	839	31.0	152	95	279	4.3	7.3	3.5	11.5
Bun	4	60.0	50	0	97	2.5	68	51	94	1.9	1.0	0.0	2.1
Cakes and cookies	11	88.2	112	45	275	5.6	105	31	169	3.0	2.4	0.6	4.9
Main dishes	16	361.4	1485	109	3724	74.2	788	55	1922	22.4	5.5	0.9	17.6
Sandwiches	12	222.4	962	442	1588	48.1	336	128	632	9.6	6.0	2.1	21.1
Snacks	4	18.0	559	50	1325	28.0	44	24	80	1.3	21.2	3.3	46.4
Savoury pastries	20	75.1	364	158	619	18.2	85	37	123	2.4	7.4	3.7	11.7
Kyrgyzstan													
Industrial foods	N *												
Beverages	8	200.0	579	432	986	29.0	67	42	115	1.9	16.4	8.8	29.4
Bun	4	45.5	127	5	381	6.3	47	37	65	1.3	3.8	0.2	10.0
Cakes and cookies	12	50.3	76	4	139	3.8	65	17	144	1.9	2.9	0.2	7.5
Snacks	12	31.6	183	9	528	9.2	104	25	244	3.0	4.0	0.2	12.3
Home-made foods	N *												
Beverages	4	200.0	4	0	15	0.2	82	13	122	2.3	0.1	0.0	0.2
Bread	4	120.0	720	521	867	36.0	135	117	149	3.9	9.0	7.5	10.6
Bun	4	66.2	132	115	157	6.6	91	63	116	2.6	2.6	1.8	3.5
Cakes and cookies	8	122.4	347	124	590	17.3	113	33	180	3.2	5.5	3.9	10.1
Main dishes	20	402.7	1409	241	2639	70.5	438	98	856	12.5	5.7	2.5	11.9
Sandwiches	12	222.1	1078	443	1858	53.9	423	107	1187	12.1	5.5	2.4	9.1
Snacks	8	150.5	861	66	1848	43.0	321	52	645	9.1	14.9	0.2	32.5
Savoury pastries	20	136.1	661	141	1424	33.0	178	90	407	5.1	6.3	2.7	12.2

[1] World Health Organization (WHO) recommends sodium intake of less than 2000 mg/day [15]. [2] World Health Organization (WHO) recommends potassium intake of at least 3510 mg/day [18]. * Mean, minimum and maximum values take into account sodium or potassium contents (in mg/serving) or molar Na:K ratios of individual samples included in each food group. *N* values correspond to the number of individual samples included in each food group.

Figure 4a–f presents the food groups with the highest average sodium content, disaggregated into all their constituent foods samples and distributed according to individual sodium and potassium contents (in mg/2000 kcal).

In the group of home-made savoury pastries (Figure 4a), the individual samples presented a great variability in their sodium contents, even between the four samples of the same food collected from different vending sites. Most samples had contents above the maximum sodium recommended limits, with some samples reaching up to 5000 mg Na/2000 kcal (Kyrgyzstan) and 7000 mg Na/2000 kcal (Tajikistan).

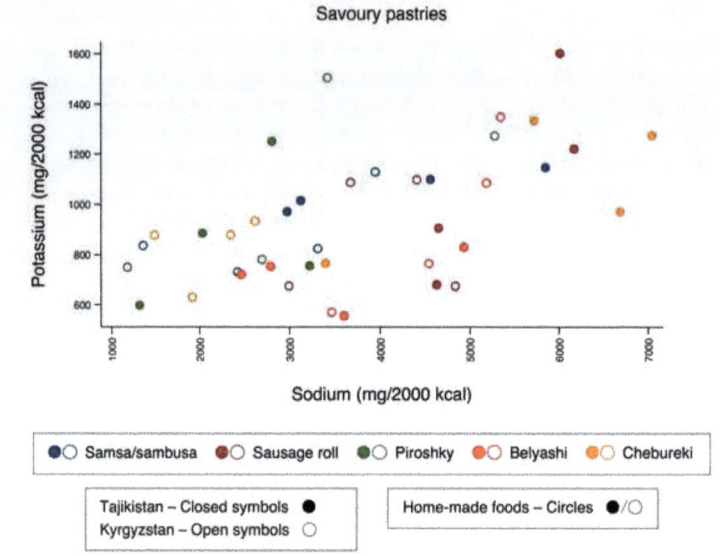

(a)

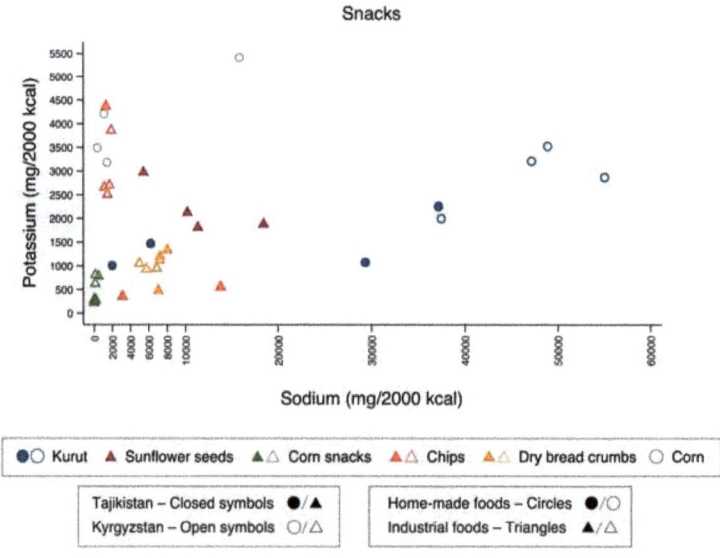

(b)

Figure 4. *Cont.*

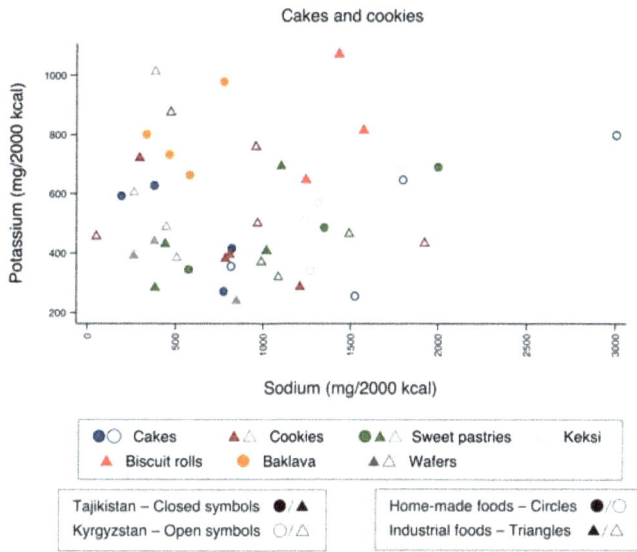

(c)

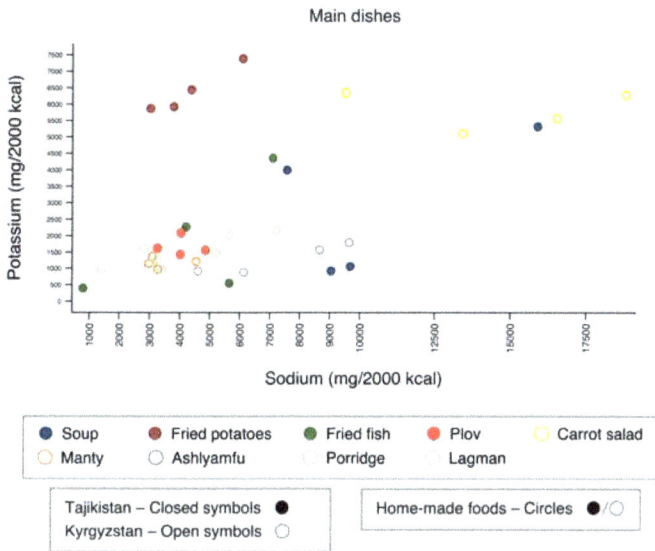

(d)

Figure 4. *Cont.*

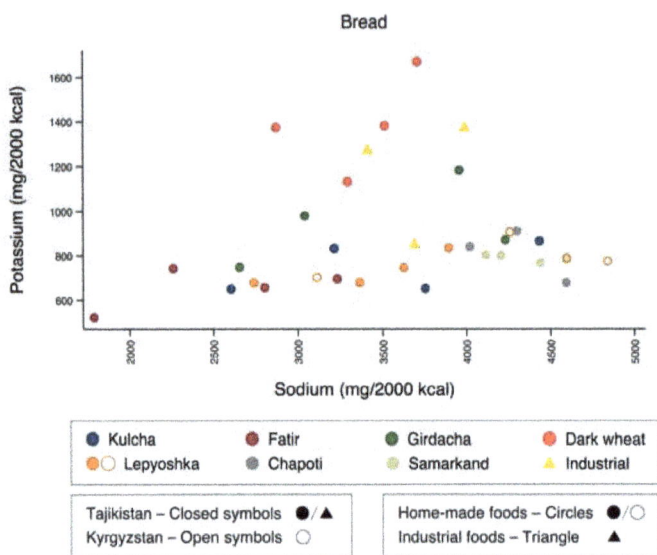

(e)

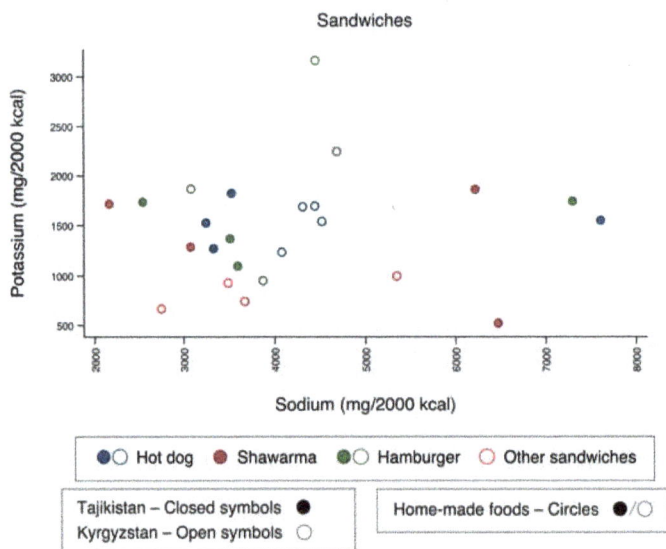

(f)

Figure 4. Distribution of individual sodium and potassium contents (mg/2000 kcal) of each of the samples collected for the most commonly available home-made and industrial foods assigned to six of the eight different predefined groups: (**a**) savoury pastries; (**b**) snacks; (**c**) cakes and cookies; (**d**) main dishes; (**e**) bread and (**f**) sandwiches. Closed symbols represent Tajikistan and open symbols represent Kyrgyzstan; circles indicate home-made foods and triangles indicate industrial foods.

Regarding snacks (Figure 4b), most samples of home-made *kurut* had extreme sodium contents—between 30,000 and 60,000 mg Na/2000 kcal. In Tajikistan, the majority of chips collected had values above maximum sodium recommended limits, reaching more than 10,000 mg Na/2000 kcal, while in Kyrgyzstan, all chip samples had borderline values with respect to the limits of sodium. In Kyrgyzstan, three out of four samples of corn on the cob had potassium values above 3510 mg K/2000 kcal and sodium content below upper recommended limits, although one of the samples contained almost 20,000 mg Na/2000 kcal.

Within cakes and cookies (Figure 4c), the majority of samples had sodium content below recommendations in both countries, although home-made sweet pastries (Tajikistan) and industrial cookies (Kyrgyzstan) were borderline in terms of the sodium threshold. Exceptionally, one sample of home-made cake (Kyrgyzstan) had a content of 3000 mg Na/2000 kcal.

In the main home-made dishes group (Figure 4d), overall the four samples of each dish were grouped in similar ranges of sodium contents. In samples of carrot salad (Kyrgyzstan) extreme values of between 10,000 mg Na/2000 kcal and more than 17,500 mg Na/2000 kcal were found. In Tajikistan, soups presented the highest sodium contents—between 7000 and more than 15,000 mg Na/2000 kcal; half of them had potassium contents above the minimum potassium recommended limits. Samples of fried potatoes (Tajikistan) had contents ranging between 2000 and around 6000 mg Na/2000 kcal and presented the highest potassium contents, with one of the samples containing approximately 7500 mg K/2000 kcal. Only two samples—porridge (Kyrgyzstan) and fried fish (Tajikistan)—had sodium contents below the upper recommended limits.

Regarding the group of breads (Figure 4e), all samples but one, collected for both countries, had sodium contents above the upper recommended limit, with some of them reaching almost 5000 mg Na/2000 kcal. Most potassium contents varied between 600 and 1000 mg K/2000 kcal. Industrial bread and home-made dark wheat bread samples (both from Tajikistan) presented higher potassium contents in comparison to other bread samples.

Within the samples of home-made sandwiches (Figure 4f), all presented sodium above 2000 mg Na/2000 kcal, with a great dispersion in the contents of this nutrient within the same types of sandwich from the same country. Most had potassium contents between 500 and 2000 mg K/2000 kcal, except two samples of hamburger (Kyrgyzstan) that presented higher levels of potassium.

4. Discussion

The results of this study show that street food in Dushanbe and Bishkek can be an important source of dietary sodium and may have a low potassium content and high Na:K ratio, though a large variability is observed across different types of foods or among samples of the same food items obtained from different vendors. As street foods have been shown to be important sources of dietary intake for many people living in LMICs [28], this study is timely and relevant for Tajikistan and Kyrgyzstan since these countries are exploring new ways of preventing NCDs and, in particular, are exploring how to strengthen the promotion of healthy diets [38,39].

In both countries, home-made foods, notably the main traditional dishes, are the leading sources of sodium among street foods, with one serving of these foods contributing, on average, to more than 70% of the maximum daily sodium recommended limits [15]. Other important sources of sodium are home-made sandwiches, snacks, bread, and savoury pastries, in line with previous evidence [40,41].

While in some countries industrial foods are the most important source of dietary sodium [42]; in others, sodium is mainly obtained from the preparation and cooking of foods, which can contribute up to 70–76% of the sodium intake [41,42]. In the case of countries from Central Asia, the high sodium content of traditional foods is suggested to be influenced by the "Silk Road" pattern, in which the tradition of using salt for food preservation strongly remains in the food culture [43]. Additionally, some traditional foods, such as *ashlyamfu* or carrot salads from Kyrgyzstan, contained soy sauce in their recipes, which can also add to the sodium content of the foods [40,41].

Even though home-made foods can be major sources of sodium, main dishes are also significant sources of potassium. For example, despite being sodium-rich, Kyrgyz carrot salad and some Tajik soup samples, including potato and vegetables (sources of potassium [44]), also presented important levels of this nutrient.

Industrial foods were shown to be key sources of sodium as well. The increasing availability of these foods, in the urban contexts of Dushanbe and Bishkek, reflects the nutrition transition that is ongoing in these countries [6,9]. In particular, commonly available industrial beverages from Kyrgyzstan, or industrial snacks from Tajikistan, were shown to largely contribute to the maximum daily sodium recommended limits.

Most food groups presented mean molar Na:K ratios well above the optimal ratio of 1 suggested by the WHO in order to prevent NCDs [19]. This also reaffirms the need for sodium reduction among these foods. The offer of healthy foods, low in sodium and high in potassium, should be encouraged in these settings [28].

In fact, promoting healthy diets should be a priority for Tajikistan and Kyrgyzstan. The prevalence of hypertension in these countries is increasing [45,46] and latest estimates indicate that Central Asia is the region with the highest sodium intake in the world, with a mean of 5.51g/day—almost three times the WHO maximum recommended limit [15]. Unhealthy food environments and diets contributing to a further increase in these sodium intake levels are of major concern [14].

Salt reduction strategies are considered best-buy interventions, as they are effective, feasible, and affordable to implement [2]. Reducing sodium intakes has shown to be beneficial in high-sodium environments, leading to a decrease in BP [47] and directly reducing CVD risk, resulting in long-term impacts on public health [14,42,48].

Different salt reduction strategies have been implemented worldwide, at population or individual levels, including food reformulation, front of pack labelling, regulatory schemes to limit sodium levels in foods, taxation of high-sodium foods, community interventions, and consumer education [49]. Multi-component approaches have been shown to have the most powerful benefits [50]. Combining interventions to engage individuals and relevant stakeholders in health behavior change and population interventions to create healthy food environments could be the best approach in contexts where high sodium contents come from both discretionary salt added while preparing/cooking home-made foods and industrial foods [51].

For home-made foods, one option would be focusing on salt reduction strategies in public education and consumer awareness, as previously done in countries like China and Japan, where, similarly, sodium intake comes typically from salt added during preparation of foods [49]. Particularly, in Tajikistan and Kyrgyzstan, strategies could involve education of street food vendors to both encourage the cooking of healthy local foods and limit the use of discretionary salt or sodium-rich sauces and condiments.

From our findings, the wide ranges of sodium content found with respect to individual samples of some foods show that there is room to cook, prepare, and/or produce foods from all food groups with less added salt [52]. Gradual and small reductions of sodium content in foods have been shown not to affect consumer taste preference, acceptability, and purchase intent [53–56]. In some cases, it was observed substantial differences even among different samples of the same food, brand and country (e.g., chips from Tajikistan), which reinforces the opportunity to efficiently produce products towards the lower end of the range of sodium content.

In addition, work could be done on increasing consumer education with respect to diet, health, and awareness of the harmful effects of high sodium and low potassium intakes [49,57].

Regarding the sodium content in industrial foods, an option would be that of setting sodium content targets (voluntary or mandatory) for encouraging reformulation. While some countries have set voluntary targets for specific foods, other countries have adopted more comprehensive legislative approaches to set a maximum sodium content of their foods (e.g., South Africa and Argentina) [49]. Setting up maximum limits for food groups that have shown to be major sources of sodium, such as industrial beverages (*maksym* and *chalap*), would be a priority for Kyrgyzstan. Tajikistan could prioritize industrial snacks, such as chips and dry bread crumbs. This approach would require mapping as well as engagement of local food suppliers and further efforts to monitor compliance with regulations or voluntary guidance.

Another approach could be working closely with the industry to improve information available on packaging of industrial foods, as well as educating consumers on label reading. This would entail setting rules for the provision of quantitative ingredient lists, nutrition declarations, and front-of-pack labelling, in order to provide consumers with the necessary information regarding the sodium contents of foods in order to make a decision [49,58]. If companies are required to provide compositional information, it might also serve as a further incentive for them to reduce the sodium in their food.

In addition to sodium-reduction approaches, the overall composition of diets is also of particular importance for determining the impact on CVD outcomes in high-sodium environments [14]. Population-level approaches to concurrently lower sodium and increase potassium intakes may subsequently produce a joint effect in the reduction of BP and CVD risk [17,19,21].

However, the simultaneous compliance with sodium and potassium daily recommendations may be a challenge which needs to be supported by the promotion of healthy and affordable eating patterns [59]. Diets, such as the Mediterranean and the Dietary Approaches to Stop Hypertension (DASH) diets—rich in fruits, vegetables, legumes, nuts, whole-grains, seafood and vegetable oils, with moderate consumption of dairy products and less red meat, processed foods, and added fats and sugars—have shown to be associated with lower BP and to improve cardiometabolic health and other chronic diseases [60–64]. With adjustments to locally available foods and taking into account cultural preferences, the dietary recommendations of these diets could be translated to the context of Tajikistan and Kyrgyzstan to help promote healthy and accessible diets, without increasing dietary costs in these settings [7].

For example, fruits and vegetables, which are low in sodium and high in potassium, were observed to be widely available in the markets of Dushanbe and Bishkek, despite the fact that their daily consumption continues to decline in these countries [10]. Their adequate consumption is associated with a lower risk of mortality, notably from CVDs, and could be promoted as a key component of a healthy diet in these countries [65].

Likewise, nuts and legumes, also linked to better cardiometabolic outcomes [66], were frequently found in all markets visited during the study and could also be promoted, rather than certain sources of animal protein such as red meat and, especially, processed meat [7].

Furthermore, dietary guidance could also be focused on sodium–potassium ratios [59]. Advice could be given based on the food groups with the highest Na:K ratios, which could include recommendations to moderate the consumption of industrial snacks and beverages as well as home-made snacks, which may greatly contribute to high sodium intakes. Boiled corn in the cob, commonly found in all markets, may be a healthy alternative snack due to its high potassium content, especially when no salt is added before consumption. The variability of sodium content in corn may be most dependent upon the quantity of salt commonly added by the vendor before selling or upon customer request. One particular sample may have been exceptionally salted in excess (i.e., purposely, to increase the flavor or added twice, by mistake), which reinforces the need for education strategies targeting the use of discretionary salt and consumer awareness about the risks of its excess consumption. In addition, seasonality may condition fruits and vegetables' availability and is an important element to take into account for dietary guidance.

To our knowledge this is the first study that provides data on the nutritional composition of ready-to-eat street foods in Central Asia. The study was carefully designed to provide an accurate and representative assessment of the nutritional content of these foods from Dushanbe and Bishkek. The number of different samples collected for each food, from different vending sites, gives us important insights into the ranges of sodium and potassium content, which may be helpful when planning interventions. However, the availability of street foods may not necessarily reflect the usual dietary intake of the urban population in both countries, although it is expected that the contribution of street food to total food consumption is high in these settings [28]. Results of this study also cannot be generalized to other settings (e.g., rural areas), where the availability and the nutritional composition of foods may differ. Other important sodium-rich and potassium-poor food sources sold in settings distinct from markets and their surroundings may have been missed.

In this sense, the study provides useful information on the quantity of sodium and potassium in commonly available foods and may be used as a starting point to promote dietary changes to help the population in Tajikistan and Kyrgyzstan to achieve recommendations for the intake of these nutrients. Nevertheless, it does not replace data on dietary intake nor does it provide information on the overall quality of diets in these countries.

Monitoring the impact of interventions on intake levels is crucial when implementing successful national strategies related to these nutrients [67]. Available methods include 24-h urine collection, spot urine collection and dietary surveys. Using 24-h urine collection is considered the gold standard method for establishing sodium baseline intake, for both individuals and populations [67]. Potassium baseline intake may also be accurately measured through 24-h urine excretion and 24-h dietary recall methods [68]. However, using 24-h urine collection method for monitoring and evaluation can pose a high burden for surveillance in LMICs, as it requires full capacity and financial and political support [69]. A less expensive, practical, and accurate monitoring approach, at an individual level, may include assessing repeated casual urine Na/K ratios, which may help to understand the features of high, intermediate and low Na/K ratio individuals [68]. Urinary Na/K ratios have shown to be a more precise index for tracking the contribution of changes in sodium and potassium intakes not only to BP but also to CVD risk, when compared to measuring the levels of these nutrients separately [70]. However, none of these methods substitute the identification and monitoring of changes in the nutritional composition of food sources.

Likewise, it is essential to assess baseline sodium and potassium contents in other important sources of these nutrients and to systematically monitor the impact of interventions on the nutritional composition of foods. Further evaluation may focus on food categories that present the highest average sodium contents and Na:K ratios, and for which specific targets should be set beforehand [71]. Alternatively, for industrial prepacked foods, analyzing both food labelling and sales data, may help identifying further sources and tracking the ones contributing the most to sodium exposure as a result of their high sodium content and high consumption by the population [72]. Nevertheless, this would require the main food retailers to be engaged in the reformulation process and willing to share data and accurate updates to the nutrient declarations of their products. In both countries, additional efforts aiming at commonly imported products are also needed.

5. Conclusions

In summary, promoting the nutritional quality of street foods should be a priority to be integrated into wider work on nutrition and food security in Tajikistan and Kyrgyzstan. The large variability observed in this study across different types of foods and similar products acquired in different vending places translates the possible patterns of consumption of street food, as well as shows the large potential for improvement of the street food environment by promoting the healthiest foods available. The creation of healthier food and drink environments and the regular monitoring of specific targets set for key food sources will contribute towards the delivery of national action plans on NCDs and the achievement of the WHO's voluntary global targets of a 30% reduction in mean population sodium intake and a 25% reduction in risk of CVDs by 2025 [73].

Acknowledgments: The project is funded by the World Health Organization Europe (WHO registration 2015/591370-0) and, in particular, work on FEEDCities project is funded by a voluntary contribution of the Ministry of Health of the Russian Federation. The authors would like to thank the staff from WHO Country Offices in Tajikistan and Kyrgyzstan as well as local authorities. The authors would also like to thank Andreia Lemos and Eulália Mendes for carrying out laboratory analysis.

Author Contributions: M.G., J.B., P.P. and N.L. conceived and designed the study. P.P., N.L., M.G. and J.J. coordinated all phases of study implementation. I.M. was responsible for data and food sample collection. S.C. was responsible for the nutritional analyses. P.P., N.L., G.A. and I.M. analyzed the results. I.M., N.L. and P.P. drafted the manuscript. All authors critically revised the manuscript for relevant intellectual content and approved the final version for submission.

Conflicts of Interest: João Breda and Jo Jewell are staff members of the World Health Organization Regional Office for Europe. The authors are responsible for the views expressed in this publication and they do not necessarily represent the decisions or stated policy of the WHO. The authors declare no conflict of interest.

References

1. World Health Organization. Global Health Estimates 2015: Cause-Specific Mortality. Available online: http://www.who.int/healthinfo/global_burden_disease/estimates/en/index1.html (accessed on 20 May 2017).

2. World Health Organization. *Global Status Report on Noncommunicable Diseases 2010;* World Health Organization: Geneva, Switzerland, 2011.

3. World Health Organization. Global Health Observatory (GHO) Data. Premature NCD Deaths. Available online: http://www.who.int/gho/mortality_burden_disease/causes_death/region/en/ (accessed on 20 May 2017).

4. Gaziano, T.A.; Bitton, A.; Anand, S.; Abrahams-Gessel, S.; Murphy, A. Growing epidemic of coronary heart disease in low- and middle-income countries. *Curr. Probl. Cardiol.* **2010**, *35*, 72–115. [CrossRef] [PubMed]

5. Popkin, B.M.; Gordon-Larsen, P. The nutrition transition: Worldwide obesity dynamics and their determinants. *Int. J. Obes. Relat. Metab. Disord.* **2004**, *28*, S2–S9. [CrossRef] [PubMed]

6. Popkin, B.M. Nutrition transition and the global diabetes epidemic. *Curr. Diab. Rep.* **2015**, *15*, 64. [CrossRef] [PubMed]

7. Anand, S.S.; Hawkes, C.; de Souza, R.J.; Mente, A.; Dehghan, M.; Nugent, R.; Zulyniak, M.A.; Weis, T.; Bernstein, A.M.; Krauss, R.M.; et al. Food consumption and its impact on cardiovascular disease: Importance of solutions focused on the globalized food system: A report from the workshop convened by the world heart federation. *J. Am. Coll. Cardiol.* **2015**, *66*, 1590–1614. [CrossRef] [PubMed]

8. Food and Agriculture Organization of the United Nations. *Europe and Central Asia: Regional Overview of Food Insecurity 2016. The Food Insecurity Transition;* Food and Agriculture Organization of the United Nations: Budapest, Hungary, 2017.

9. Popkin, B.M. Global nutrition dynamics: The world is shifting rapidly toward a diet linked with noncommunicable diseases. *Am. J. Clin. Nutr.* **2006**, *84*, 289–298. [PubMed]

10. Abe, S.K.; Stickley, A.; Roberts, B.; Richardson, E.; Abbott, P.; Rotman, D.; McKee, M. Changing patterns of fruit and vegetable intake in countries of the former soviet union. *Public Health Nutr.* **2013**, *16*, 1924–1932. [CrossRef] [PubMed]

11. Lim, S.S.; Vos, T.; Flaxman, A.D.; Danaei, G.; Shibuya, K.; Adair-Rohani, H.; Amann, M.; Anderson, H.R.; Andrews, K.G.; Aryee, M.; et al. A comparative risk assessment of burden of disease and injury attributable to 67 risk factors and risk factor clusters in 21 regions, 1990–2010: A systematic analysis for the global burden of disease study 2010. *Lancet* **2012**, *380*, 2224–2260. [CrossRef]

12. Mohan, S.; Campbell, N.R. Salt and high blood pressure. *Clin. Sci.* **2009**, *117*, 1–11. [CrossRef] [PubMed]

13. He, F.J.; MacGregor, G.A. A comprehensive review on salt and health and current experience of worldwide salt reduction programmes. *J. Hum. Hypertens.* **2009**, *23*, 363–384. [CrossRef] [PubMed]

14. Cohen, H.W.; Alderman, M.H. Sodium, blood pressure, and cardiovascular disease. *Curr. Opin. Cardiol.* **2007**, *22*, 306–310. [CrossRef] [PubMed]

15. World Health Organization. *Guideline: Sodium Intake for Adults and Children;* World Health Organization: Geneva, Switzerland, 2012.

16. Vinceti, M.; Filippini, T.; Crippa, A.; de Sesmaisons, A.; Wise, L.A.; Orsini, N. Meta-analysis of potassium intake and the risk of stroke. *J. Am. Heart Assoc.* **2016**, *5*. [CrossRef] [PubMed]

17. Aburto, N.J.; Hanson, S.; Gutierrez, H.; Hooper, L.; Elliott, P.; Cappuccio, F.P. Effect of increased potassium intake on cardiovascular risk factors and disease: Systematic review and meta-analyses. *BMJ* **2013**, *346*, f1378. [CrossRef] [PubMed]

18. World Health Organization. *Guideline: Potassium Intake for Adults and Children*; World Health Organization: Geneva, Switzerland, 2012.
19. Rodrigues, S.L.; Baldo, M.P.; Machado, R.C.; Forechi, L.; Molina Mdel, C.; Mill, J.G. High potassium intake blunts the effect of elevated sodium intake on blood pressure levels. *J. Am. Soc. Hypertens.* **2014**, *8*, 232–238. [CrossRef] [PubMed]
20. Zhang, Z.; Cogswell, M.E.; Gillespie, C.; Fang, J.; Loustalot, F.; Dai, S.; Carriquiry, A.L.; Kukina, E.V.; Hong, Y.; Merritt, R.; et al. Association between usual sodium and potassium intake and blood pressure and hypertension among us adults: Nhanes 2005–2010. *PLoS ONE* **2013**, *8*, e75289.
21. Cook, N.R.; Obarzanek, E.; Cutler, J.A.; Buring, J.E.; Rexrode, K.M.; Kumanyika, S.K.; Appel, L.J.; Whelton, P.K. Trials of Hypertension Prevention Collaborative Research, G. Joint effects of sodium and potassium intake on subsequent cardiovascular disease: The trials of hypertension prevention follow-up study. *Arch. Intern. Med.* **2009**, *169*, 32–40. [CrossRef] [PubMed]
22. Judd, S.E.; Aaron, K.J.; Letter, A.J.; Muntner, P.; Jenny, N.S.; Campbell, R.C.; Kabagambe, E.K.; Levitan, E.B.; Levine, D.A.; Shikany, J.M.; et al. High sodium:potassium intake ratio increases the risk for all-cause mortality: The reasons for geographic and racial differences in stroke (regards) study. *J. Nutr. Sci.* **2013**, *2*, e13. [CrossRef] [PubMed]
23. Okayama, A.; Okuda, N.; Miura, K.; Okamura, T.; Hayakawa, T.; Akasaka, H.; Ohnishi, H.; Saitoh, S.; Arai, Y.; Kiyohara, Y.E. Dietary sodium-to-potassium ratio as a risk factor for stroke, cardiovascular disease and all-cause mortality in japan: The nippon data80 cohort study. *BMJ Open* **2016**, *6*, e011632. [CrossRef] [PubMed]
24. World Health Organization. *Diet, Nutrition and the Prevention of Chronic Disease: Report of a Joint WHO/FAO Expert Consultation*; World Health Organization: Geneva, Switzerland, 2003.
25. World Health Organization. *European Food and Nutrition Action Plan 2015–2020*; WHO Regional Office for Europe: Copenhagen, Denmark, 2015.
26. Mendez, M.; Popkin, B.M. Globalization, urbanization and nutritional change in the developing world. *Electron. J. Agric. Dev. Econ.* **2004**, *1*, 220–241.
27. Langellier, B.A. Consumption and expenditure on food prepared away from home among mexican adults in 2006. *Salud Pública de México* **2015**, *57*, 4–13. [CrossRef] [PubMed]
28. Steyn, N.P.; McHiza, Z.; Hill, J.; Davids, Y.D.; Venter, I.; Hinrichsen, E.; Opperman, M.; Rumbelow, J.; Jacobs, P. Nutritional contribution of street foods to the diet of people in developing countries: A systematic review. *Public Health Nutr.* **2014**, *17*, 1363–1374. [CrossRef] [PubMed]
29. World Health Organization. *Feedcities Project: The Food Environment Description in Cities in Eastern Europe and Central Asia—Tajikistan*; WHO Regional Office for Europe: Copenhagen, Denmark, 2017.
30. World Health Organization. *Feedcities Project: The Food Environment Description in Cities in Eastern Europe and Central Asia—Kyrgyzstan*; WHO Regional Office for Europe: Copenhagen, Denmark, 2017.
31. Food and Agriculture Organization of the United Nations. *Selling Street and Snack Foods*; Food and Agriculture Organization of the United Nations: Rome, Italy, 2011.
32. KoBoToolbox. KoBoCollect (Version 1.4.3) [Mobile Application Software]. 2014. Available online: https://play.google.com/store/apps/details?id=org.koboc.collect.android (accessed on 3 April 2016).
33. Moubarac, J.; Parra, D.C.; Cannon, G.; Monteiro, C.A. Food classification systems based on food processing: Significance and implications for policies and actions: A systematic literature review and assessment. *Curr. Obes. Rep.* **2014**, *3*, 256–272. [CrossRef] [PubMed]
34. Vieira, E.; Soares, M.E.; Ferreira, I.; Pinho, O. Validation of a fast sample preparation procedure for quantification of sodium in bread by flame photometry. *Food Anal. Methods* **2012**, *5*, 430–434. [CrossRef]
35. Food and Agriculture Organization of the United Nations. Proximate Analyses. Available online: http://www.fao.org/docrep/field/003/ab479e/ab479e03.htm (accessed on 12 June 2017).
36. World Health Organization. *Nutrient Profile Model*; WHO Regional Office for Europe: Copenhagen, Denmark, 2015.
37. Krebs-Smith, S.M.; Kott, P.S.; Guenther, P.M. Mean proportion and population proportion: Two answers to the same question? *J. Am. Diet. Assoc.* **1989**, *89*, 671–676. [PubMed]
38. World Health Organization. *Better Non-Communicable Disease Outcomes: Challenges and Opportunities for Health Systems. Kyrgyzstan Country Assessment*; WHO Regional Office for Europe: Copenhagen, Denmark, 2014.

39. World Health Organization. *Better Non-Communicable Disease Outcomes: Challenges and Opportunities for Health Systems. Tajikistan Country Assessment*; WHO Regional Office for Europe: Copenhagen, Denmark, 2015.

40. World Health Organization. *Mapping Salt Reduction Initiatives in the WHO European Region*; WHO Regional Office for Europe: Copenhagen, Denmark, 2013.

41. Anderson, C.A.; Appel, L.J.; Okuda, N.; Brown, I.J.; Chan, Q.; Zhao, L.; Ueshima, H.; Kesteloot, H.; Miura, K.; Curb, J.D.; et al. Dietary sources of sodium in China, Japan, the United Kingdom, and the United States, women and men aged 40 to 59 years: The intermap study. *J. Am. Diet. Assoc.* **2010**, *110*, 736–745. [CrossRef] [PubMed]

42. He, F.J.; Campbell, N.R.; MacGregor, G.A. Reducing salt intake to prevent hypertension and cardiovascular disease. *Rev. Panam. Salud Publica* **2012**, *32*, 293–300. [CrossRef] [PubMed]

43. Powles, J.; Fahimi, S.; Micha, R.; Khatibzadeh, S.; Shi, P.; Ezzati, M.; Engell, R.E.; Lim, S.S.; Danaei, G.; Mozaffarian, D.; et al. Global, regional and national sodium intakes in 1990 and 2010: A systematic analysis of 24 h urinary sodium excretion and dietary surveys worldwide. *BMJ Open* **2013**, *3*, e003733. [CrossRef] [PubMed]

44. Weaver, C.M. Potassium and health. *Adv. Nutr.* **2013**, *4*, 368S–377S. [CrossRef] [PubMed]

45. World Health Organization. Global Health Observatory Data Repository. Raised Blood Pressure (sbp $\geq$ 140 or dbp $\geq$ 90), Age-Standardized (%), Estimates by Country. Available online: http://apps.who.int/gho/data/node.main.A875STANDARD?lang=en (accessed on 20 May 2017).

46. Batyraliev, T.A.; Makhmutkhodzhaev, S.A.; Kydyralieva, R.B.; Altymysheva, A.T.; Dzhakipova, R.S.; Zhorupbekova, K.S.; Ryskulova, S.T.; Knyazeva, V.G.; Kaliev, M.T.; Dzhumagulova, A.S. Prevalence of risk factors of non-communicable disease in Kyrgyzstan: Assessment using WHO STEPS approach. *Kardiologiia* **2016**, *11*, 86–90. [CrossRef]

47. Aburto, N.J.; Ziolkovska, A.; Hooper, L.; Elliott, P.; Cappuccio, F.P.; Meerpohl, J.J. Effect of lower sodium intake on health: Systematic review and meta-analyses. *BMJ* **2013**, *346*, f1326. [CrossRef] [PubMed]

48. He, F.J.; MacGregor, G.A. Effect of modest salt reduction on blood pressure: A meta-analysis of randomized trials. Implications for public health. *J. Hum. Hypertens.* **2002**, *16*, 761–770. [CrossRef] [PubMed]

49. Trieu, K.; Neal, B.; Hawkes, C.; Dunford, E.; Campbell, N.; Rodriguez-Fernandez, R.; Legetic, B.; McLaren, L.; Barberio, A.; Webster, J. Salt reduction initiatives around the world—A systematic review of progress towards the global target. *PLoS ONE* **2015**, *10*, e0130247. [CrossRef] [PubMed]

50. Hyseni, L.; Elliot-Green, A.; Lloyd-Williams, F.; Kypridemos, C.; O'Flaherty, M.; McGill, R.; Orton, L.; Bromley, H.; Cappuccio, F.P.; Capewell, S. Systematic review of dietary salt reduction policies: Evidence for an effectiveness hierarchy? *PLoS ONE* **2017**, *12*, e0177535. [CrossRef] [PubMed]

51. Campbell, N.R.; Johnson, J.A.; Campbell, T.S. Sodium consumption: An individual's choice? *Int. J. Hypertens.* **2012**, *2012*, 860954. [CrossRef] [PubMed]

52. Webster, J.L.; Dunford, E.K.; Neal, B.C. A systematic survey of the sodium contents of processed foods. *Am. J. Clin. Nutr.* **2010**, *91*, 413–420. [CrossRef] [PubMed]

53. La Croix, K.W.; Fiala, S.C.; Colonna, A.E.; Durham, C.A.; Morrissey, M.T.; Drum, D.K.; Kohn, M.A. Consumer detection and acceptability of reduced-sodium bread. *Public Health Nutr.* **2015**, *18*, 1412–1418. [CrossRef] [PubMed]

54. Girgis, S.; Neal, B.; Prescott, J.; Prendergast, J.; Dumbrell, S.; Turner, C.; Woodward, M. A one-quarter reduction in the salt content of bread can be made without detection. *Eur. J. Clin. Nutr.* **2003**, *57*, 616–620. [CrossRef] [PubMed]

55. Hendriksen, M.A.; Verkaik-Kloosterman, J.; Noort, M.W.; van Raaij, J.M. Nutritional impact of sodium reduction strategies on sodium intake from processed foods. *Eur. J. Clin. Nutr.* **2015**, *69*, 805–810. [CrossRef] [PubMed]

56. Goncalves, C.; Monteiro, S.; Padrao, P.; Rocha, A.; Abreu, S.; Pinho, O.; Moreira, P. Salt reduction in vegetable soup does not affect saltiness intensity and liking in the elderly and children. *Food Nutr. Res.* **2014**, *58*. [CrossRef] [PubMed]

57. Van de Vijver, S.; Oti, S.; Addo, J.; de Graft-Aikins, A.; Agyemang, C. Review of community-based interventions for prevention of cardiovascular diseases in low- and middle-income countries. *Ethn. Health* **2012**, *17*, 651–676. [CrossRef] [PubMed]

58. Kloss, L.; Meyer, J.D.; Graeve, L.; Vetter, W. Sodium intake and its reduction by food reformulation in the European Union—A review. *NFS J.* **2015**, *1*, 9–19. [CrossRef]

59. Drewnowski, A.; Rehm, C.D.; Maillot, M.; Mendoza, A.; Monsivais, P. The feasibility of meeting the WHO guidelines for sodium and potassium: A cross-national comparison study. *BMJ Open* **2015**, *5*, e006625. [CrossRef] [PubMed]

60. Estruch, R.; Ros, E.; Salas-Salvado, J.; Covas, M.I.; Corella, D.; Aros, F.; Gomez-Gracia, E.; Ruiz-Gutierrez, V.; Fiol, M.; Lapetra, J.; et al. Primary prevention of cardiovascular disease with a mediterranean diet. *N. Engl. J. Med.* **2013**, *368*, 1279–1290. [CrossRef] [PubMed]

61. Panagiotakos, D.B.; Pitsavos, C.; Arvaniti, F.; Stefanadis, C. Adherence to the mediterranean food pattern predicts the prevalence of hypertension, hypercholesterolemia, diabetes and obesity, among healthy adults; the accuracy of the meddietscore. *Prev. Med.* **2007**, *44*, 335–340. [CrossRef] [PubMed]

62. Sacks, F.M.; Svetkey, L.P.; Vollmer, W.M.; Appel, L.J.; Bray, G.A.; Harsha, D.; Obarzanek, E.; Conlin, P.R.; Miller, E.R.; Simons-Morton, D.G.; et al. Effects on blood pressure of reduced dietary sodium and the dietary approaches to stop hypertension (DASH) diet. Dash-sodium collaborative research group. *N. Engl. J. Med.* **2001**, *344*, 3–10. [CrossRef] [PubMed]

63. Struijk, E.A.; May, A.M.; Wezenbeek, N.L.; Fransen, H.P.; Soedamah-Muthu, S.S.; Geelen, A.; Boer, J.M.; van der Schouw, Y.T.; Bueno-de-Mesquita, H.B.; Beulens, J.W. Adherence to dietary guidelines and cardiovascular disease risk in the epic-nl cohort. *Int. J. Cardiol.* **2014**, *176*, 354–359. [CrossRef] [PubMed]

64. Reedy, J.; Krebs-Smith, S.M.; Miller, P.E.; Liese, A.D.; Kahle, L.L.; Park, Y.; Subar, A.F. Higher diet quality is associated with decreased risk of all-cause, cardiovascular disease, and cancer mortality among older adults. *J. Nutr.* **2014**, *144*, 881–889. [CrossRef] [PubMed]

65. Wang, X.; Ouyang, Y.; Liu, J.; Zhu, M.; Zhao, G.; Bao, W.; Hu, F.B. Fruit and vegetable consumption and mortality from all causes, cardiovascular disease, and cancer: Systematic review and dose-response meta-analysis of prospective cohort studies. *BMJ* **2014**, *349*, g4490. [CrossRef] [PubMed]

66. Afshin, A.; Micha, R.; Khatibzadeh, S.; Mozaffarian, D. Consumption of nuts and legumes and risk of incident ischemic heart disease, stroke, and diabetes: A systematic review and meta-analysis. *Am. J. Clin. Nutr.* **2014**, *100*, 278–288. [CrossRef] [PubMed]

67. World Health Organization. *Strategies to Monitor and Evaluate Population Sodium Consumptions and Sources of Sodium in the Diet: Report of a Joint Technical Meeting Convened by Who and the Government of Canada, October 2010*; World Health Organization: Geneva, Switzerland, 2011.

68. Iwahori, T.; Miura, K.; Ueshima, H. Time to consider use of the sodium-to-potassium ratio for practical sodium reduction and potassium increase. *Nutrients* **2017**, *9*. [CrossRef] [PubMed]

69. Hawkes, C.; Webster, J. National approaches to monitoring population salt intake: A trade-off between accuracy and practicality? *PLoS ONE* **2012**, *7*, e46727. [CrossRef] [PubMed]

70. Yatabe, M.S.; Iwahori, T.; Watanabe, A.; Takano, K.; Sanada, H.; Watanabe, T.; Ichihara, A.; Felder, R.A.; Miura, K.; Ueshima, H.; et al. Urinary sodium-to-potassium ratio tracks the changes in salt intake during an experimental feeding study using standardized low-salt and high-salt meals among healthy japanese volunteers. *Nutrients* **2017**, *9*. [CrossRef] [PubMed]

71. Zganiacz, F.; Wills, R.B.H.; Mukhopadhyay, S.P.; Arcot, J.; Greenfield, H. Changes in the sodium content of australian processed foods between 1980 and 2013 using analytical data. *Nutrients* **2017**, *9*. [CrossRef] [PubMed]

72. Pravst, I.; Lavrisa, Z.; Kusar, A.; Miklavec, K.; Zmitek, K. Changes in average sodium content of prepacked foods in Slovenia during 2011–2015. *Nutrients* **2017**, *9*. [CrossRef] [PubMed]

73. World Health Organization. *Global Action Plan for the Prevention and Control of Noncommunicable Diseases 2013–2020*; World Health Organization: Geneva, Switzerland, 2013.

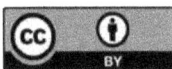

nutrients

MDPI

Article

Process Evaluation and Costing of a Multifaceted Population-Wide Intervention to Reduce Salt Consumption in Fiji

Jacqui Webster [1,2,*], Arti Pillay [3], Arleen Suku [3], Paayal Gohil [1], Joseph Alvin Santos [1,2], Jimaima Schultz [4], Jillian Wate [3], Kathy Trieu [1,2], Silvia Hope [5], Wendy Snowdon [6], Marj Moodie [5,6], Stephen Jan [1] and Colin Bell [6]

[1] The George Institute for Global Health, University of New South Wales, Sydney, NSW 2052, Australia; paayalgohil2@hotmail.com (P.G.); jsantos@georgeinstitute.org.au (J.A.S.); ktrieu@georgeinstitute.org.au (K.T.); sjan@georgeinstitute.org.au (S.J.)

[2] School of Public Health, the University of Sydney, Sydney, NSW 2006, Australia

[3] Pacific Research Centre for the Prevention of Obesity and Noncommunicable Diseases (C-POND), Fiji National University, Nasinu, Fiji; arti.pillay@fnu.ac.fj (A.P.); arleen.sukhu@fnu.ac.fj (A.S.); jillian.wate@fnu.ac.fj (J.Wa.)

[4] Independent Nutrition Consultant, Suva, Fiji; jimaima63@gmail.com

[5] Deakin Health Economics, Centre for Population Health Research, Faculty of Health, Deakin University, Burwood, VIC 3125, Australia; hope.silvia@gmail.com (S.H.); marj.moodie@deakin.edu.au (M.M.)

[6] Global Obesity Centre, Deakin University, Geelong, VIC 3216, Australia; wendy.snowdon@deakin.edu.au (W.S.); colin.bell@deakin.edu.au (C.B.)

* Correspondence: jwebster@georgeinstitute.org.au; Tel.: +61-280524520

Received: 20 December 2017; Accepted: 24 January 2018; Published: 30 January 2018

Abstract: This paper reports the process evaluation and costing of a national salt reduction intervention in Fiji. The population-wide intervention included engaging food industry to reduce salt in foods, strategic health communication and a hospital program. The evaluation showed a 1.4 g/day drop in salt intake from the 11.7 g/day at baseline; however, this was not statistically significant. To better understand intervention implementation, we collated data to assess intervention fidelity, reach, context and costs. Government and management changes affected intervention implementation, meaning fidelity was relatively low. There was no active mechanism for ensuring food companies adhered to the voluntary salt reduction targets. Communication activities had wide reach but most activities were one-off, meaning the overall dose was low and impact on behavior limited. Intervention costs were moderate (FJD $277,410 or $0.31 per person) but the strategy relied on multi-sector action which was not fully operationalised. The cyclone also delayed monitoring and likely impacted the results. However, 73% of people surveyed had heard about the campaign and salt reduction policies have been mainstreamed into government programs. Longer-term monitoring of salt intake is planned through future surveys and lessons from this process evaluation will be used to inform future strategies in the Pacific Islands and globally.

Keywords: evaluation; salt reduction; advocacy; public health policy; capacity building; costs; behavior change; food; nutrition; hypertension prevention

1. Introduction

Recent analysis from the Global Burden of Disease study revealed that 3.7 million deaths per year could be attributed to consuming too much salt and that globally salt intakes are around 10 g/person/day, which is twice the World Health Organization (WHO) recommended maximum amount of 5 g/day [1]. Whilst an increasing number of countries are developing national salt reduction strategies [2], most are in the early stages of implementation and only a handful have demonstrated an impact to date [3]. Furthermore, the majority of experience to date comes from high income countries, so there is an urgent need to build the evidence about how to effectively implement programs in low and lower middle income countries [4]. The Fiji Sodium Impact Assessment Project (FSIA), funded by the National Health and Medical Research Council (NHMRC) as part of the Global Alliance for Chronic Diseases hypertension research program [5], evaluated the impact of multifaceted interventions to reduce population salt intake in Fiji and Samoa.

The intervention strategies were based on the WHO's three pillars for creating an enabling environment for salt reduction [6], which is grounded in the theory that behavior change influencers span beyond education and information to include environmental and policy change [7]. The logic model for salt reduction programs (Figure 1) was informed by previous assessments of salt activities in the Pacific Islands [8]; baseline monitoring of salt intake, consumer knowledge attitudes and behaviors (KAB) related to salt and focus groups to understand stakeholder positions and barriers and opportunities for action in Fiji. The main causal assumption was that, given most salt consumed is already in processed foods and meals [9], reduction of salt levels in processed foods and meals would result in reduced salt intake.

The resulting multifaceted intervention in Fiji targeted the whole national population, and had three strands: encouragement of the food industry to reduce sources of salt in the diet (through engagement of manufacturers and food service operators); strategic health communication (through targeted advocacy and a health educator training program); and a hospital program (education and reduction of salt in meals). The intervention was planned and implemented through collaboration between the Pacific Research Centre for the Prevention of Obesity and Noncommunicable Diseases (C-POND), the Fiji National Food and Nutrition Centre (NFNC) and the Wellness Unit in the Fiji Ministry of Health and Medical Services (MOHMS). It was overseen by a Food Taskforce Technical Advisory Group (FT-TAG) consisting of government, research and consumer organizations.

The impact of the population-wide intervention program was assessed through cross-sectional surveys of salt consumption patterns in a national sample at baseline and after 20 months [10]. The results of the impact evaluation were recently published in Nutrients [11]. The evaluation showed a 1.4 g/day drop in salt intake from a baseline of 11.7 g/day, however, this was not statistically significant. Lack of significant effect could have been due to the low response rates and small sample sizes obtained in the survey. However, limited intervention dose and duration is also a possible explanation. The outcome evaluation showed some improvements in consumer knowledge, as well as attitudes and behaviors regarding salt, but it was difficult to draw firm conclusions in view of the low response rates.

In order to get a better understanding of whether the lack of the effect on salt intake was due to the fact that the intervention didn't work or whether it was because the intervention was not implemented effectively or over a long enough timescale, we conducted a comprehensive process evaluation. The results of this process evaluation will be used to inform future program implementation both in the Pacific Islands and globally.

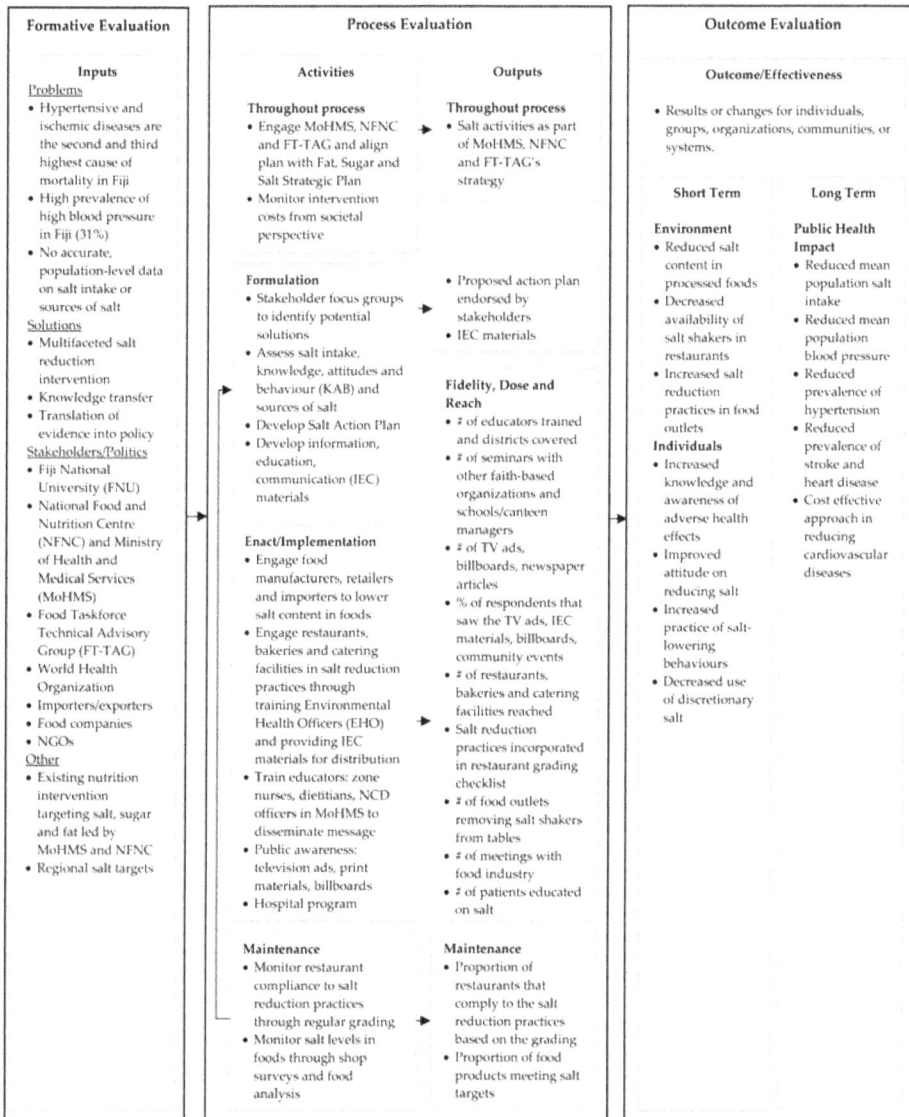

Figure 1. Centre for Training and Research translation logic model for Fiji Sodium Intervention Assessment Project (FSIA).

2. Materials and Methods

2.1. Research Questions

The process evaluation approach was informed by the Medical Research Council (MRC) framework and guidance for process evaluations of complex interventions [12] supplemented by a review of process evaluations of similar nutrition related interventions [13–18]. The first step was defining and understanding the causal assumptions underlying the intervention through the development of a logic model (Figure 1) and a detailed implementation plan during the project planning stages. We integrated the costing into the process evaluation as part of the routine monitoring.

The main questions for the process evaluation and costing were:

(1) Were the program interventions delivered with high fidelity, dose and reach?
(2) How did context affect implementation?
(3) What was the cost of different elements of the interventions?
(4) What lessons can inform continuation and/or replication of salt reduction strategies in other countries?

2.2. Data Collection

Data were collected through qualitative and quantitative measures integrated into the different stages of project implementation follows:

(1) Understanding the extent to which the intervention was actually implemented as planned (in line with the logic model and detailed implementation plan) through implementer self-report and collection of routine monitoring data supplemented through semi-structured interviews with key stakeholders (relevant government departments, consumer and health groups and food industry organizations that had been involved in the project).
(2) Understanding mechanisms of impact including whether specific groups were impacted differently through sub-analysis of the outcome data and routine monitoring data as well as semi-structured interviews with implementers and participants.

The semi-structured interviews were undertaken by the lead investigator who had a good understanding of the interventions without having been directly involved in program implementation. Interviews lasted approximately 40 min and were recorded. Additional questions were incorporated into the consumer, knowledge, attitudes and behavior survey at 20 months, as part of the intervention monitoring, to assess the extent to which people had been exposed to the campaign.

2.3. Intervention Costing

A societal perspective was adopted for the costing, meaning that costs to participants, government and all sectors of the economy involved in the delivery of the intervention were included. The costing was done using pathway analysis to specify resources associated with the intervention strategies. Resource use and cost data were collected by the FSIA project team and the NFNC project officer in Fiji and analysed by the health economist team based at Deakin University, Australia.

The costs included:

(i) program-level expenses associated with the delivery and management of activities including transportation, accommodation, catering, venue hire, and administration;
(ii) costs associated with dissemination of information through radio, TV and newspaper;
(iii) costs associated with consultation with industry including group and one-to-one meetings and production of materials
(iv) human resource costs based on the hours involved for all individuals participating in any interventions and the relevant hourly wage rate.

The following costs were excluded from the analyses:

(i) research costs associated with intervention evaluation rather than implementation. The interventions were assumed to be operating in a 'steady state'; therefore costs involved in set-up, research and development prior to the intervention were not included.

2.4. Data Analysis

Routine process monitoring data including activity logs, quarterly FSIA reports and annual reports were collated and tabulated according to the different intervention activities. The stakeholder interviews were transcribed verbatim. Each transcribed interview was individually imported to NVivo and the interviews were coded based on relevant themes in order to answer the process evaluation questions.

Ethical Approval for this work was granted by the Human Research Ethics Council at the University of Sydney, Australia (15359), Deakin University, Australia (2013-020) and the Fiji National Research Ethics and Review Committee, Suva, Fiji (FNRERC 201307).

3. Results

3.1. Data Sources

Routine monitoring data was collated from the costing spreadsheets, two FSIA annual reports, quarterly reports and reports on specific initiatives such as Salt Awareness Week 2014 and 2015.

Table 1 provides an overview of the activities based on routine monitoring data with specific costs for interventions detailed in Section 3.4. Fifteen stakeholder interviews were conducted, with respondents comprising: three NFNC staff members, three Ministry of Health staff, three food industry stakeholders, three C-POND members, one WHO officer, one media representative, one hospital dietitian and one politician.

3.2. Overall Findings

Most people interviewed had been closely involved in the project and had a good understanding of what it was trying to achieve. The most consistent feedback from interviewees was that FSIA had been challenging to implement given time and resources. Reach was limited with routine monitoring data showing that most of the communication (except TV and radio) and industry meetings did not extend beyond Suva (population = 300,000 compared to 800,000 total population) and the hospital program was also only in the main hospital in Suva. Participants noted that, while there was strong awareness of the project, the strategic approach, in terms of both health communication and food industry engagement, could have been more clearly defined and communicated.

> *"I think they really need to do that planning, the strategic planning to come out clear that okay this is a new program that has come in. This is what we need to achieve in the first year, second year, and third year. So these are the activities that we would expect."*

Government workers and project staff said that the relatively short timescale (four years for baseline monitoring, interventions and post-intervention monitoring) meant that interventions were immature and had yet to take effect and that it needed to be continued.

> *"So the time from planning to educating the educators and then getting them to get to the communities, being able to do something, getting information or us trying to go through the communities, the time frame was really short."*

> *"I don't think we can expect to have achieved much given the timescale of the intervention. But, we now know how to do it and can continue."*

Table 1. Summary of salt reduction intervention activities in Fij from routine monitoring data.

Target Group and Objective	Summary of Intervention Activity	Numbers	Distribution
Consumers and stakeholders To raise awareness of dangers of too much salt, recommended level of salt consumption, and hidden salt levels of food	• C-POND communication and advocacy materials (pamphlet, posters, booklets, DVD) • IEC materials distributed through nurses and dietitians and the NFNC and Wellness Centre • Information also available on NFNC and MoHMS websites • TV adverts, regular print media coverage and C-POND newsletter • Salt awareness week (SAW) events	• 681 Pamphlets • 731 Sets of 3 posters • 200 Salt facts booklets • 32 Salt The Hidden Danger Digital Video Disk (DVDs) • 2 TV adverts distributed free to air • Media coverage on salt 4–5 times per year • 2 SAW events 1 Motorway Billboard	- Materials distributed annually at national events such as Salt Week, Health Day, Nutrition Month, Hibiscus Festival, Noncommunicable disease (NCD) Month and World Food Day (mainly in Central Division) - Regular coverage through TV, radio and print media and information available on MoHMS website (available throughout the regions)
Health educators To provide training and resources so people already working in the community can integrate salt reduction into their programs	• Training of educators (nurses, dietitians, red cross workers etc) on salt reduction • Other government Ministries, faith based organizations and nutrition educators were consulted • PEN Model Training included a module on salt reduction • Presentation to Heads of Schools and Canteen Managers • Attempts to facilitate training and dissemination of materials through Ministry of Women, Ministry of Youth and Ministry of Education	• 75 educators trained, August–September 2014 • Meetings held with 9 organizations but only one group—Muslim Markaz Women's Group went on to deliver training (41 participants) • Pen training 7 groups October–December 2015 • 100 participants in schools and canteen manager training, August 2014	- Dieticians and nurses trained covered all 21 districts - Additional one-off trainings took place in Central Unit and Western Unit - Training for MoHMS Food Unit workers who cover all districts - Muslim Women's Groups in all districts - School Canteen managers in all districts

Table 1. *Cont.*

Target Group and Objective	Summary of Intervention Activity	Numbers	Distribution
Food business operators To encourage and support manufacturers and retailers to produce and sell lower salt Foods	• Promotion of voluntary targets for salt levels in foods agreed between government and food industry • Food industry consultation meetings held by C-POND • Nutrition consultant/WHO worker hired to support industry negotiations • FT-TAG group set up and met monthly to advise on progress and to develop salt, fat and sugar reduction strategy • Category specific Food and Beverage Health action groups established • One to one meetings with Food companies ($n = 9$): restaurants and takeaways ($n = 3$) and retailers ($n = 3$)	• Targets agreed September 2012 • Cross cutting industry consultation meetings held in September 2013 and July 2014 • C-POND held 15 meetings with industry organizations in 2014 • 6 Category specific groups established • No records of meetings with these groups.	- All industry meetings in Vitu Levi where companies operate.
Restaurants and catering facilities To raise awareness of the importance of reducing salt and provide incentives for taking action to reduce salt for restaurant and catering staff	• Posters distributed to the Environmental Health Officers for distribution in restaurants/catering institutes. • Taking salt shakers off the table integrated into MoHMS restaurant grading scheme	• 100 posters distributed, November 2014–2015 • No data on number of restaurants graded	- No record on numbers of restaurants graded
Hospitals To educate hospital staff and dieticians about the importance of reducing salt in diet so that they might introduce salt reduction initiatives into hospitals	• Salt reduced in hospital meals (from 4.8 g/head per day (2014) to 3.7 g/head/day) • Salt shakers have been removed from the staff dining room • Food Service staff trained on preparation of low salt meals • Education of patients and relatives through hospital dietitians	• 1 hospital in Suva, 2015 • No numbers available on staff trained • 50 patients educated	- Suva only

Notes: C-POND—Pacific Research Centre for the Prevention of Obesity and Noncommunicable Diseases; IEC—Information, Education and Communication; PEN—Package of Essential NCD interventions; MoHMS—Ministry of Health and Medical Service; NFNC—National Food and Nutrition Centre; WHO—World Health Organization; FT-TAG: Food Taskforce Technical Advisory Group.

Despite these challenges, some interviewees thought FSIA had helped to build research capacity and added value to existing efforts to improve the food supply.

"There were already some interventions but the FSIA project really added value in terms of research which strengthened the case for further action. It also led to celebration of national salt week and stronger focus on salt through salt, fat and sugar strategy."

"The project has helped us in relation to our NCD work and working with industry, but also in relation to research."

Whilst the results of the outcome evaluation were unknown at that stage, most interviewees, including those from government, research and industry, felt that the intervention strategies should be continued through integration into government programs. In fact, the recommendations from the project have already been used to inform the new Fiji Nutrition and Food Security Policy and Framework 2018–2022 and there are plans to repeat the monitoring of salt intake through the next WHO STEPwise approach to surveillance of noncommunicable disease risk factors (STEPS) survey (scheduled for 2018).

"This is a great project. We now know what the nations' salt intake is and we have structures and strategies in place to reduce it. It would be a shame now if it didn't continue. The work needs to be incorporated into the Wellness Centre and the FT-TAG group needs to be mandated to oversee ongoing implementation."

3.2.1. Project Governance

Project governance was seen as both a strength and a weakness of the project. Most people felt that it was appropriate that the research project was led by the research organization, C-POND and overseen by a multi-stakeholder advisory group. Also, there was strong recognition of the achievements and resilience of the C-POND team in effectively completing the project, particularly in view of the relatively short timescale and Cyclone Winston which affected post-intervention monitoring. Involvement of government was seen as a key strength of the project.

"Certainly for Fiji I think the willingness of the Ministry of Health to be a full partner in this and to be involved throughout, I think has been absolutely key. Running this sort of intervention research project just from academia would be a huge problem and just be a mistake."

However clearer allocation of the roles of different agencies might also have supported more effective implementation of the industry strategy and led to greater reach for the communication of the health messages.

"Task forces were set up, meetings were held, targets were agreed, IEC [Information, Education, Communication] materials were produced. But how far did the materials actually reach, who was responsible for making sure the industry even knew about let al.one adhered to the targets?"

"Would have been useful to have regular dissemination about the project—some sort of stakeholder newsletter, to keep people up to date and remind them of commitments, feedback on progress etc."

3.2.2. Engaging the Food Industry to Reduce Salt in Foods and Meals

Food Business Operators

Based on the fact that most salt is in processed foods and meals a priority strategy was the get food businesses to reduce salt in foods and meals. However, interviewees indicated the strategy to engage companies was unclear. Whilst the voluntary targets for salt levels in foods had been agreed with industry in 2012, no mechanism was put in place to ensure compliance. The FT-TAG group was never formally established (so there was no clear Ministerial mandate). Also, the remit of the FT-TAG expanded to include fat and sugar reduction strategies so the focus on salt was less strong. At the same time, responsibility for the industry engagement work passed from C-POND to a WHO sponsored worker based at the NFNC during the intervention period. Many industry contact people changed, meaning some of the momentum was lost, which was a further barrier to effective engagement.

> "If they could just properly share with us the contacts ... what are the commitments the food industry have mentioned to them. And for me to just follow up from there so there's a continuity and a link between the two."

Previous effective salt reduction interventions with industry have relied on strong government leadership. However, stakeholders interviewed highlighted the political changes (elections leading to new Ministers), industry lobbing and lack of food technological expertise as additional challenges.

> "It's the way our system is at the moment ... Facing a big challenge. Particularly when you're fighting against people like Coke and Nestle. Marketing is a big ... "

> "I really need somebody who can actually talk across to the food industry."

One food manufacturer interviewed said that most food companies were now fully aware of the importance of reducing salt in food products. Another company reported reformulating products in line with the voluntary targets that had been agreed prior to the project commencement. Most of the people interviewed reported that there appeared to be greater availability of "reduced salt" or "low salt" options in stores. However, one person indicated that companies were unclear about whether they should to act now or wait for government regulation. Several other stakeholders said that companies were not convinced about the health benefits of reformulating their foods, that they were not aware of any involvement of the Department of Trade and Industry and would not prioritize salt reduction in the absence of government regulation.

> "They were very honest in saying that until and unless it's mandatory, we don't see the priority to do this"

> "The other big thing is voluntary. I have a feeling you need to regulate. But how to do it is the challenge ... "

Restaurant and Catering Facilities

The restaurant and catering sectors were engaged through the Environmental Health Officers (EHOs) (employed by the MoHMS) who were given two training session on salt reduction and provided with posters for distribution in restaurants/catering institutes. Taking salt shakers off the table was also integrated into MoHMS's restaurant grading scheme which was communicated and enforced through EHOs. This was identified as a positive outcome of the project.

> "And one of the divisional environmental health officers from the northern division had advised us that they had removed salt from all their tables, as a rule in the northern division. So those were some outcomes of the intervention education that we had."

> "And there has been some visible changes. Most of the main restaurants we go to, they don't give salt ... It's no longer on the table, you have to ask."

However, there was no follow-up activity to assess the extent to which the posters were distributed. The stakeholder interviews revealed that the Food Enforcement Unit in the MoHMS did not consider that it had a role in monitoring voluntary targets, and said the team would be unable to take on additional work without the provision of additional resources. Therefore no records were collected on how many restaurants had included salt reduction activities as part of the restaurant grading scheme.

3.2.3. Health Communication: Targeted Advocacy and Training of Educators

Targeted Advocacy

The routine monitoring data (Table 1) showed that various communication materials (pamphlets, posters, booklets and DVDs) were produced and distributed fairly widely through events and educator training sessions. Faith-based organizations, The Ministry of Women, Children and Poverty Alleviation and Ministry of iTaukei affairs, are usually considered effective channels for disseminating information to communities in Fiji. However, neither the faith-based groups nor these two ministries were interested in engaging (citing other priorities) which limited the project reach. Instead, information was mainly disseminated through routine health promotion work of the NFNC and MoHMS and annually at national events. Two TV adverts were screened and there was media coverage on TV/radio to coincide with national events which means the messages were disseminated to regions beyond Suva. Based on the KAB survey post-intervention ($n = 272$), 73% of respondents reported that they had heard about the campaign from one or more sources. The most common source of exposure to the salt reduction campaign was through TV (32%), followed by health workers (27%), radio (26%), IEC materials (20%), community events (8%) and billboards (4%).

Those interviewed reported a much greater recognition of the importance of reducing salt in the diet amongst the general public as well as key government and health organizations However, some people expressed doubt about the reach of the campaign and reported the need to sustain efforts to so that this new knowledge could be translated to behavior change.

> *"My concern is what percentage of the community we've reached regarding this information. Particularly the rural . . . "*

> *"But people are being now more aware. I don't know how much of it gets it into behavior change, but they do know and I have started talking about it in terms of groups when they're getting along."*

Training of Educators

Information was also disseminated through a training program for health educators covering Fiji's 21 health districts. Seventy-five educators—zone nurses, dietitians, NCD project officers and health workers participated in workshops that covered the adverse effects of salt, using of salt substitutes for cooking and flavoring food, identification of reduced sodium products in similar categories of products by reading nutrient information panels and creation of demand for reduced salt products and meals. Twenty-seven per cent of the people who completed the KAB survey at the 20 month time point, said they were aware of the campaign through health workers. Interviewees thought the training sessions were informative but several people noted that there was no clear strategy or guidance for how the increased knowledge of the participants should then be disseminated at the community level.

> *"FSIA (The project) should have worked more strategically with NFNC to get to the schools and through the Head of the NHS dietitians to get the messages to the community via the dietitians. And there needed to be a strategy—not just one-off communications."*

3.2.4. Salt Reduction in Hospitals

The Colonial War Memorial Hospital (CWMH), the main hospital in Fiji, located in Suva, made a commitment to reducing salt for staff and patients. Whilst some of this work to reduce the salt in patient meals was initiated prior to the FSIA project, activities reported during the project included training food service staff in the preparation of low salt meals, reducing salt in staff meals and taking salt shakers off the table and patient trays. The amount of salt available per person (hospital staff) per day from meals was reduced from 4.8 g in the second quarter of 2014 to 3.7 g in the same quarter of 2015. Dietary training covering the why and how of reducing salt was also provided for around 50 patients and relatives in the Special Outpatients Department.

Unfortunately, due to limited time and resources, these activities were not replicated in hospitals in the other geographic divisions of the country although there were plans to replicate in other Divisions and extend to workplace catering guidelines thereafter. Materials were distributed widely to the sub-divisional hospitals but it is not clear to what extent they were used.

> *"Because we have the lovely bags with the posters. . . . when I go through the sub-divisional hospitals, I don't see them in the outpatients clinics where they sit around and wait . . . Hypertension and diabetes clinics . . . So I guess the extra step we should've taken was to ensure that we just go around again and make sure they have it up."*

3.3. Sub-Analysis of Outcome Data

One of the recurring themes from the stakeholder interviews was the fact that Cyclone Winston had devastated much of the country during the 20 month follow-up monitoring which may have impacted the results. Sub-analysis of the main outcome data showed no differential impact of the intervention by age or ethnicity. However, there was a large and statistically significant reduction in salt intake of females in the Central division, compared to the other divisions. There was also a large and significant difference in salt intake between people in areas affected by the cyclone and those in areas not affected by the cyclone, with the cyclone areas consuming much more salt. Examination of reported exposure to the communication campaign (Table 2) showed that 73% of those surveyed had been exposed to the campaign by one or more sources—the most common source was TV, followed by health workers, radio and then posters/information materials. Exposure was fairly similar between the Central division and other divisions, for both males and females.

Table 2. Percentage of respondents who heard about the campaign by sex and division.

		Any Source	Radio	TV	Bill Boards	Posters, Information Materials	Community Event	Health Worker	Others
Total Sample	Overall	72.7	25.9	32.0	3.5	20.4	8.1	26.5	1.6
	Male	67.3	23.4	27.0	3.5	13.7	8.9	20.6	0.8
	Female	78.3	28.4	37.1	3.5	27.3	7.2	32.6	2.3
Central Division	Overall	69.1	18.1	30.0	3.2	14.9	5.3	21.1	1.0
	Male	62.5	16.7	29.7	2.1	8.2	9.8	15.2	2.1
	Female	75.3	19.4	30.2	4.3	21.2	1.1	26.6	0.0
Other Division	Overall	75.3	31.2	33.3	3.7	24.1	9.9	30.3	1.9
	Male	70.4	27.6	25.3	4.3	17.1	8.3	24.0	0.0
	Female	80.6	35.2	42.1	2.9	31.9	11.8	37.1	4.0

3.4. Intervention Costs

The overall cost of implementing the sodium reduction interventions in the specified time period was FJD $277,410. This equates to $0.31 per person based on the 2013 population of Fiji (881,065). Approximately half (49.5%) of the costs were related to human resources. Of the balance, the largest component was for printing of promotional materials (39.2%), with the largest expense being the purchase of TV adverts (33.9%) whilst meeting expenses (catering) accounted for 9.6% and travel expenses (1.7%) (Table 3).

Table 3. Intervention costs.

(a) Breakdown of Total Costs by Resource Type (FJD)			
Type of Cost	Total Cost	% Consumable Costs	% Total Costs
Personnel	$138,506 *		49.93%
Promotional materials	$106,685	76.80%	38.46%
Meeting expenses (catering)	$16,001	11.52%	5.77%
Travel	$16,219	11.68%	5.85%
Total costs	$277,410	100.00%	100.00%
(b) Breakdown of Total Costs by Activity Type (FJD)			
Activity Type	Cost		% Total Costs
Consultation (meetings, focus groups)	$49,757		17.94%
Salt Awareness weeks	$9801		3.53%
Training	$8030		2.89%
TV adverts	$94,226		33.97%
Activities across all above	$115,596		41.67%
	$277,410		100.00%

* Participant time was costed as the average wage in Fiji. For persons involved in a professional capacity, an average hourly rate (based on 45-h week) was calculated based on average annual salaries according to different salary levels within each profession. It was assumed that the FSIA Research Fellow and Research assistant spent 50% of their time over the 20 months intervention period on intervention delivery activities.

4. Discussion

This is the first comprehensive process evaluation of a population-wide intervention to reduce salt. It demonstrated that the fidelity, dose and reach of FSIA was relatively low, partly due to the fact that the intervention was vulnerable to contextual issues such as poorly defined organizational roles, political changes, and natural disasters (Cyclone Winston). It also highlighted a timeframe that was insufficient for delivering the intervention with full fidelity. On the other hand, the process evaluation highlighted added value of the project in providing a robust estimate of how much salt people in Fiji are eating and the importance of reducing salt, strengthening research capacity and establishing mechanisms for engaging with the food industry to improve the food supply. The project also influenced government policy, with salt reduction activities now integrated into the work of the NFNC and MoHMS and plans to repeat monitoring of salt intake as part of the next WHO STEPS survey of NCD risk factors planned for 2018.

The likely impact of Cyclone Winston on the project was further highlighted through the process evaluation. Analysis of intervention exposure (Table 2) showed no differential exposure by division, thus challenging the theory that the significant effect in females in the Central division might be explained by the intervention dose being stronger there. The alternative explanation is that this was the only area where the monitoring took place before the cyclone hit in February 2016, and that the cyclone, which delayed the monitoring and affected diets due to the provision of rations, might have negated any potential impact of the intervention. Whilst the small sample sizes, meaning that the main outcome analysis was likely underpowered, make it impossible to draw firm conclusions, it is highly plausible that the cyclone had some sort of impact on the results.

Routine monitoring data showed the distribution of resources was fairly even, meaning the reach of the communications was wide. However, there was no data to show the extent to which resources were used and participant feedback suggested dissemination strategies were unclear. Likewise, whilst 73% of the population were exposed to the campaign, only a third (33%) and just over a quarter were exposed to TV or radio respectively and it is not clear how many times. The CDC recommends that 75–85% of the target audience need to be exposed each quarter of the year and that a campaign should run at least three to six months to achieve awareness of the issue, six to 12 months to influence attitudes, and 12 to 18 months to influence behavior [19]. A recent comprehensive review of salt reduction communication campaigns also suggested that behavior change programs on salt are more likely to be effective if grounded in a theoretical framework [20]. Future communication strategies need to identify and target specific salt related behaviors to change and develop clear strategies for broader dissemination of behavior change communications over an extended time frame to increase the likelihood of effectiveness [21].

Complex interventions to reduce salt include policy changes which require adequate time and strong governance to implement. The importance of establishing robust and transparent mechanisms for engaging and monitoring industry in relation to salt targets has been highlighted by previous research [22]. Whilst the agreement on voluntary targets to reduce salt intake was established in Fiji, strategies to ensure these targets were adhered to, were not effectively implemented during the timescale of the research project. Considering the large contribution of processed foods to salt in the diet, this is likely one of the main reasons for the lack of intervention impact and emphasises the importance of strengthening policy implementation, potentially through the use of legislation, and ensuring adequate time for interventions to take effect as part of future salt reduction efforts.

Lack of effective governance mechanism to implement and monitor nutrition polices in Low and Middle Income Countries (LMICs) has been identified as an ongoing challenge in previous research [23–25]. The salt reduction research project was led by C-POND, a regional research organization working on NCDs. It was intended that the intervention be implemented primarily through the MoHMS and the NFNC. However, the roles of the NFNC and MOHMS in implementing the program were never clearly defined and much of the salt reduction intervention effort was left to C-POND, which had limited financial resources (the total cost of the intervention was FJD227.410 including personnel time).

The process evaluation has identified a range of lessons that will be useful in informing future salt reduction interventions, both in the Pacific Islands and globally. Firstly, four years is not long enough to develop, implement and evaluate a project. Whilst this project did not show what time frame is required to impact on dietary sodium levels at a population level, other countries have demonstrated an impact after five years [26]. Secondly, adequate resources need to be provided to implement and monitor program impact. The cost of this intervention was moderate resulting in a relatively low intervention dose. Likewise, greater resources for monitoring could have helped to increase sample size, increasing the power of the study to detect change. Thirdly, strong multisectoral governance mechanisms need to be established for implementation and monitoring of policies. Strong government leadership is preferable, particularly to ensure that the food industry adheres to agreements to reduce salt in processed foods and meals. Health ministries often have established mechanisms for communicating to communities and undertaking health surveillance that salt reduction interventions need to harness. Ministries of trade and industry and education should also be involved in planning and implementation. Fourthly, there needs to be a clear strategic approach to communication activities to change behavior with adequate replication. Also, whilst policy initiatives are usually best implemented at a national level, limited resources and the challenges of reaching all areas means communication campaigns might be better piloted in certain regions before being rolled out nationally. Lastly, communication with key stakeholders to ensure that everyone is clear about the objectives and approach at different stages throughout the project is important. Maintaining an up-to-date stakeholder database can help facilitate this. Training to support project implementation, including food industry engagement, needs to be repeated regularly, particularly when new project staff are engaged.

Many of these lessons are relevant to other implementation science projects and some have been highlighted in previous process evaluations of food-related interventions in the region. [16–18]. Common to all these interventions is that they were being implemented in the "real world" working through government institutions where it is harder to control processes as part of a research project. On the other hand, increased research capacity and mainstreaming of programs into government policies and practices increases the likelihood of programs being sustained and longer-term benefits being realized.

Strengths and Weaknesses

Strengths of this process evaluation include the mapping of causal assumptions at the start of the intervention, transparency of the process and the openness and willingness of stakeholders, including government and industry organizations, to discuss challenges related to the project. A weakness was the fact that the main outcome study was underpowered which made it difficult to draw firm conclusions on many of the issues. The limited number of interviews, particularly with representatives from industry, may have biased the views obtained. Also, the multiple players involved in the intervention meant that routine monitoring data was not collected effectively by all parties so it was not always possible to quantify the extent of the activities, making it difficult to determine dose and reach as well as to assess the cost of some activities. The costing data is fairly comprehensive and indicates a low-cost intervention, but does not capture the pre- and post-intervention monitoring, which is a challenging and expensive element of all salt reduction interventions [27].

Whilst an extensive sub-analysis of the main outcome data was undertaken, only some of the issues are reported here and the low response rates means that the sub-analysis was also likely underpowered.

5. Conclusions

This process evaluation demonstrates the impact of the project in terms of policy outputs and increased research capacity in Fiji and has identified lessons to inform ongoing salt reduction efforts in the Pacific Islands and globally.

Acknowledgments: The authors wish to thank the people who give their time freely to participate in the process evaluation as well as to assist with the interventions and monitoring. In addition we would like to thank Fiji National University, C-POND, the Fijian Ministry of Health and Medical Services, the National Food and Nutrition Centre, Vanua Medical Laboratory, the World Health Organization, and the members of the Food Taskforce Technical Advisory Group (FT-TAG) for their support throughout the project. The project was funded by the National Health and Medical Research Council of Australia under the Global Alliance for Chronic Disease (GACD) Hypertension Program (#1040178). J.We. is supported by a National Health and Medical Research Council/National Heart Foundation Career Development Fellowship (#1082924) on International strategies to reduce salt. J.We. has funding from WHO, VicHealth and the National Health and Medical Research Council of Australia for research on salt reduction. J.We. and M.M. are supported through an NHMRC CRE on food policy interventions to reduce salt (#1117300). K.T. is supported by a National Health and Medical Research Council of Australia postgraduate scholarship (#1115169) and VicHealth for work on salt reduction. M.M. and C.B. are researchers within a NHMRC Centre for Research Excellence in Obesity Policy and Food Systems (#1041020).

Author Contributions: J.We., W.S., M.M., C.B. and K.T. conceived the study. A.P., A.S., W.S. and J.S. implemented the project in Fiji. J.We. conducted the process evaluation interviews. P.G. completed the data analysis of qualitative information. J.S. did the sub-analysis of the main outcome data. J.We. and A.P. interpreted the results. J.We. wrote the first draft of the manuscript. All other authors commented on various drafts and approved the final paper.

Conflicts of Interest: J.We. is Director of the World Health Organization Collaborating Centre on Population Salt Reduction with a remit to support countries to implement and evaluate salt reduction programs in line with the WHO target for all countries to reduce population salt intake by 30% by 2025. All other authors declare that they have no conflicts of interest related to this study. The founding sponsors had no role in the design of the study; in the collection, analyses, or interpretation of data; in the writing of the manuscript, and in the decision to publish the results.

Abbreviations

C-POND	Pacific Research Centre for the Prevention of Obesity and Noncommunicable Diseases
EHO	Environmental Health Officer
FNU	Fiji National University
FSIA	Fiji Sodium Impact Assessment Project
FT-TAG	Food Taskforce Technical Advisory Group
GACD	Global Alliance for Chronic Diseases
IEC	Information, Education and Communication
KAB	Knowledge, attitudes and behaviors

LMIC	Low and Middle Income Countries
MoHMS	Fiji Ministry of Health and Medical Services
MRC	Medical Research Council
NCD	Noncommunicable diseases
NFNC	National Food and Nutrition Centre
NHMRC	National Health and Medical Research Council of Australia
NNS	National Nutrition Survey
PEN	Package of Essential NCD interventions
SAW	Salt Awareness Week
STEPS	WHO STEPwise approach to surveillance of noncommunicable disease risk factors
WHO	World Health Organization

References

1. World Health Organization. *Guideline: Sodium Intake for Adults and Children*; World Health Organization: Geneva, Switzerland, 2012.
2. Trieu, K.; Neal, B.; Hawkes, C.; Dunford, E.; Campbell, N.; Rodriguez-Fernandez, R.; Legetic, B.; McLaren, L.; Barberio, A.; Webster, J. Salt Reduction Initiatives around the World—A Systematic Review of Progress towards the Global Target. *PLoS ONE* **2015**, *10*, e0130247. [CrossRef] [PubMed]
3. Barberio, A.M.; Sumar, N.; Trieu, K.; Lorenzetti, D.L.; Tarasuk, V.; Webster, J.; Campbell, N.R.; McLaren, L. Population-level interventions in government jurisdictions for dietary sodium reduction: A Cochrane Review. *Int. J. Epidemiol.* **2017**, *46*, 1551. [CrossRef] [PubMed]
4. Trieu, K.; McLean, R.; Johnson, C.; Santos, J.A.; Raj, T.S.; Campbell, N.R.; Webster, J. The Science of Salt: A Regularly Updated Systematic Review of the Implementation of Salt Reduction Interventions (November 2015 to February 2016). *J. Clin. Hypertens.* **2016**, *18*, 1194–1204. [CrossRef] [PubMed]
5. GACD Hypertension Research Programme, Writing Group; Peiris, D.; Thompson, S.R.; Beratarrechea, A.; Cardenas, M.K.; Diez-Canseco, F.; Goudge, J.; Gyamfi, J.; Kamano, J.H.; Irazola, V.; et al. Behavior change strategies for reducing blood pressure-related disease burden: Findings from a global implementation research programme. *Implement. Sci.* **2015**, *10*, 158. [CrossRef] [PubMed]
6. World Health Organization. *Creating an Enabling Environment for Population Salt Reduction Strategies: Report of a Joint Technical Meeting held by WHO and the Food Standards Agency, United Kingdom, July 2010*; World Health Organization: Geneva, Switzerland, 2010.
7. Michie, S.; van Stralen, M.M.; West, R. The behaviour change wheel: A new method for characterising and designing behaviour change interventions. *Implement. Sci.* **2011**, *6*, 42. [CrossRef] [PubMed]
8. Christoforou, A.; Snowdon, W.; Laesango, N.; Vatucawaqa, S.; Lamar, D.; Alam, L.; Lippwe, K.; Havea, I.L.; Tairea, K.; Hoejskov, P.; et al. Progress on salt reduction in the Pacific Islands: From strategies to action. *Heart Lung Circ.* **2015**, *24*, 503–509. [CrossRef] [PubMed]
9. Webster, J.; Trieu, K.; Dunford, E.; Hawkes, C. Target salt 2025: A global overview of national programs to encourage the food industry to reduce salt in foods. *Nutrients* **2014**, *6*, 3274–3287. [CrossRef] [PubMed]
10. Webster, J.; Snowdon, W.; Moodie, M.; Viali, S.; Schultz, J.; Bell, C.; Land, M.A.; Downs, S.; Christoforou, A.; Dunford, E.; et al. Cost-effectiveness of reducing salt intake in the Pacific Islands: Protocol for a before and after intervention study. *BMC Public Health* **2014**, *14*, 107. [CrossRef] [PubMed]
11. Pillay, A.; Trieu, K.; Santos, J.A.; Sukhu, A.; Schultz, J.; Wate, J.; Bell, C.; Moodie, M.; Snowdon, W.; Ma, G.; et al. Assessment of a Salt Reduction Intervention on Adult Population Salt Intake in Fiji. *Nutrients* **2017**, *9*, 1350. [CrossRef] [PubMed]
12. Moore, G.F.; Audrey, S.; Barker, M.; Bond, L.; Bonell, C.; Hardeman, W.; Moore, L.; O'Cathain, A.; Tinati, T.; Wight, D.; et al. Process evaluation of complex interventions: Medical Research Council guidance. *BMJ* **2015**, *350*, h1258. [CrossRef] [PubMed]
13. May, C.R.; Mair, F.S.; Dowrick, C.F.; Finch, T.L. Process evaluation for complex interventions in primary care: Understanding trials using the normalization process model. *BMC Fam. Pract.* **2007**, *8*, 42. [CrossRef] [PubMed]

14. Rosecrans, A.M.; Gittelsohn, J.; Ho, L.S.; Harris, S.B.; Naqshbandi, M.; Sharma, S. Process evaluation of a multi-institutional community-based program for diabetes prevention among First Nations. *Health Educ. Res.* **2008**, *23*, 272–286. [CrossRef] [PubMed]

15. Baranowski, T. Environmental Influences and What Have We Learned from Dietary Behavior Change with Children? *Nutr. Today* **2002**, *37*, 171–172. [CrossRef] [PubMed]

16. Fotu, K.F.; Moodie, M.M.; Mavoa, H.M.; Pomana, S.; Schultz, J.T.; Swinburn, B.A. Process evaluation of a community-based adolescent obesity prevention project in Tonga. *BMC Public Health* **2011**, *11*, 284. [CrossRef] [PubMed]

17. Mathews, L.B.; Moodie, M.M.; Simmons, A.M.; Swinburn, B.A. The process evaluation of It's Your Move!, an Australian adolescent community-based obesity prevention project. *BMC Public Health* **2010**, *10*, 448. [CrossRef] [PubMed]

18. Waqa, G.; Moodie, M.; Schultz, J.; Swinburn, B. Process evaluation of a community-based intervention program: Healthy Youth Healthy Communities, an adolescent obesity prevention project in Fiji. *Glob. Health Promot.* **2013**, *20*, 23–34. [CrossRef] [PubMed]

19. Centers for Disease Control and Prevention. *Best Practices for Comprehensive Tobacco Control Programs—2014*; National Center for Chronic Disease Prevention and Health Promotion Office on Smoking and Health U.S. Department of Health and Human Services, Ed.; Centers for Disease Control and Prevention: Atlanta, GA, USA, 2014.

20. Trieu, K.; McMahon, E.; Santos, J.A.; Bauman, A.; Jolly, K.-A.; Bolam, B.; Webster, J. Review of behavior change interventions to reduce population salt intake. *Int. J. Behav. Nutr. Phys. Act.* **2017**, *14*, 17. [CrossRef] [PubMed]

21. Do, H.T.; Santos, J.A.; Trieu, K.; Petersen, K.; Le, M.B.; Lai, D.T.; Bauman, A.; Webster, J. Effectiveness of a Communication for Behavioral Impact (COMBI) Intervention to Reduce Salt Intake in a Vietnamese Province Based on Estimations From Spot Urine Samples. *J. Clin. Hypertens.* **2016**, *18*, 1135–1142. [CrossRef] [PubMed]

22. Downs, S.M.; Christoforou, A.; Snowdon, W.; Dunford, E.; Hoejskov, P.; Legetic, B.; Campbell, N.; Webster, J. Setting targets for salt levels in foods: A five-step approach for low-and middle-income countries. *Food Policy* **2015**, *55*, 101–108. [CrossRef]

23. Sunguya, B.F.; Ong, K.I.; Dhakal, S.; Mlunde, L.B.; Shibanuma, A.; Yasuoka, J.; Jimba, M. Strong nutrition governance is a key to addressing nutrition transition in low and middle-income countries: Review of countries' nutrition policies. *Nutr. J.* **2014**, *13*, 65. [CrossRef] [PubMed]

24. Wolfenden, L.; Wiggers, J. Strengthening the rigour of population-wide, community-based obesity prevention evaluations. *Public Health Nutr.* **2014**, *17*, 407–421. [CrossRef] [PubMed]

25. Wolfenden, L.; Wyse, R.; Nichols, M.; Allender, S.; Millar, L.; McElduff, P. A systematic review and meta-analysis of whole of community interventions to prevent excessive population weight gain. *Prev. Med.* **2014**, *62*, 193–200. [CrossRef] [PubMed]

26. McLaren, L.; Sumar, N.; Barberio, A.M.; Trieu, K.; Lorenzetti, D.L.; Tarasuk, V.; Webster, J.; Campbell, N.R. Population-level interventions in government jurisdictions for dietary sodium reduction. *Cochrane Database Syst. Rev.* **2016**, *9*, Cd010166. [CrossRef] [PubMed]

27. Webster, J.; Su'a, S.A.F.; Ieremia, M.; Bompoint, S.; Johnson, C.; Faeamani, G.; Vaiaso, M.; Snowdon, W.; Land, M.A.; Trieu, K. Salt Intakes, Knowledge, and Behavior in Samoa: Monitoring Salt-Consumption Patterns through the World Health Organization's Surveillance of Noncommunicable Disease Risk Factors (STEPS). *J. Clin. Hypertens.* **2016**, *18*, 884–891. [CrossRef] [PubMed]

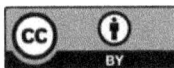

MDPI

St. Alban-Anlage 66

4052 Basel

Switzerland

Tel. +41 61 683 77 34

Fax +41 61 302 89 18

www.mdpi.com

Nutrients Editorial Office

E-mail: nutrients@mdpi.com

www.mdpi.com/journal/nutrients